THE EQUITY FUNDING PAPERS

**WILEY/HAMILTON Series on
Accounting and Information Systems**

Consulting Editor   John W. Buckley

THE EQUITY FUNDING PAPERS

The Anatomy of a Fraud

Lee J. Seidler
Frederick Andrews
Marc J. Epstein

John Wiley & Sons
Santa Barbara   New York   Chichester   Brisbane   Toronto
A Wiley/Hamilton Publication

Library of Congress Cataloging in Publication Data.

Main entry under title:

The Equity Funding papers.

  (Wiley/Hamilton series on accounting and information systems)
  "A Wiley/Hamilton publication."
  1. Equity Funding Corporation of America.
2. Securities fraud—United States. I. Seidler, Lee J. II. Andrews, Frederick. III. Epstein, Marc J.

HV6698.Z9E654	364.1'63	77-9921
ISBN 0-471-02275-X		

Printed in the United States of America

10 9 8 7 6 5 4 3 2 1

Design and Production by Graphics Two, Los Angeles

ABOUT THE AUTHORS

Lee J. Seidler is Professor of Accounting at New York University Graduate School of Business Administration. He is a Consulting Financial Analyst to the investment firm of Baer, Stearns & Company and was selected by *Institutional Investor* as the outstanding accounting financial analyst in 1976. He is Deputy Chairman of the AICPA Commission on Auditors' Responsibilities.

Fred Andrews is Deputy Financial Editor at the *New York Times*. Prior to joining *The Times* he was, for eight years, a staff reporter with *The Wall Street Journal* where he edited the weekly page one column "Tax Report" and wrote about accounting, auditing, taxes, and security law. His *Wall Street Journal* article in May 1973 was the first to raise questions about Equity Funding's auditors, two of whom were later convicted of securities fraud.

Marc J. Epstein is Associate Professor at California State University, Los Angeles where he teaches both graduate and undergraduate courses in accounting. The author of numerous books and articles he has also been active in research and consultant work to both business and government.

THE EQUITY FUNDING FRAUD: WHAT HAPPENED?

On January 1, 1973, the shares of Equity Funding Corporation of America were trading on the New York Stock Exchange, in moderate volume, at about $37. Three months later, on March 28, trading in Equity Funding shares was stopped by the SEC, after a week of fevered activity had reduced their price to $14.

On January 1, 1973, Equity Funding was one of the darlings of Wall Street, a company that had managed to produce continued high earnings growth for a decade. By early April, it was, instead, a gigantic fraud. The machinery of the American financial and justice systems roared into action; hordes of accountants and lawyers descended on the plush Los Angeles offices of the company. When the investigations were completed, it became clear that the fraud was unique in American financial history. Despite its spectacular "record," Equity Funding had not actually earned a penny of profit—it had lost money. And the fraud was not a sophisticated, computer operation run by a small cabal, as was first suspected. Instead, a large number of employees had systematically developed and maintained a completely false picture of sustained growth and prosperity, which pervaded the company's operations. Using the inflated values of the shares of the company, they were able to acquire a small empire of other companies, with real assets. As one method of extending the fraud outlived its usefulness, the conspirators turned to another. From falsifying their "funding programs," they moved to producing and selling false insurance policies to other insurance companies. Eventually, they even began to "kill" the fake insured bodies, to collect real proceeds.

Even more unbelievable, with dozens of people intimately acquainted with the details of the fraud, with audited financial statements, the secret was kept—for a decade. Only when Equity Funding fired the "wrong employee," Ron Secrist, did the story begin to unfold. The stock price plunged. Huge blocks changed hands at the last minute, resulting in an endless series of lawsuits as buyers and sellers tried to conclude or renege on transactions. Eventually, twenty-two people pled guilty, and the auditors were convicted of fraud. In January 1977, the lawyers were able to fashion an enormous settlement of much of the litigation.

The key question remained: How did they do it? How could a false shell be built and sold to the public for so long? How could it remain undetected? How could it have been detected? These are the questions this book tries to answer.

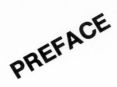

Why and How This Book Was Assembled

There is no shortage of articles and books about the Equity Funding fraud. Why add yet another volume to the pile?

The answer is both simple and complex. The editors—a financial reporter and two accounting professors—felt that the existing available materials, voluminous though they are, do not provide the answers to a deceptively simple series of questions: What really happened? What were the mechanics of the fraud? Why didn't the auditors blow the whistle? Why didn't sophisticated creditors and investors find the fraud? Where were the legions of state and federal regulators who are supposed to protect the investing public and holders of insurance policies? Can it happen again?

The conventional responses—that Stanley Goldblum and his cohorts were too clever, or that the auditors "sold out"—were just not good enough. The fraud continued for over a decade; perhaps 100 people knew about it. The three editors had studied the available materials extensively, as a reporter and as researchers. The more study, the less clear the conclusion.

What then can one teach to business students, or explain to the executives who read the financial press?

When we decided that we had no neat answers to these questions, the need for this volume became clear. Equity Funding is too complex, has too many implications, for simple, direct analysis. Each interested person must first learn the facts and then try to decide for himself.

This book contains the facts. It contains the statements of the company itself, financial results as well as the public utterances of the officers. It has the best descriptions yet developed of the mechanics of the fraud, as written by the people forced to pick up the pieces, and as testified to at the trial of those who actually perpetrated the fraud. True, we have indulged in a bit of speculative analysis, but only for the purpose of pointing the reader in the general direction of the answers.

The rest is up to the reader.

What This Book Does and Does Not Contain

It was difficult to decide what to include in this volume. The guideline we established was to provide original materials that were not readily available.

The trustee's report, the financial information, and the transcript of the auditors' trial form the core of this volume. The trustee's report, as discussed in the introductory essay, is the basic source of factual information about the fraud and its operation. The proxy statements, prospectuses, financial statements, interim reports, and the supplementary insurance schedules are the raw materials for those who wish to determine for themselves whether outside financial analysts, creditors, and investors should have been able to scent the fraud.

The trial transcript included here is only a small part of the total, distilled after review and consultation with prosecution and defense attorneys, but these portions provide the best insight yet available into the behavior and motivation of the Wolfson, Weiner auditors.

The text of the trustee's report is complete; the financial statements that make up about half the report are not included. The original report includes reproductions of Equity Funding financial statements from published annual reports. However, the exhibits in the text of the trustee's report were developed from statements that can be found only in prospectuses, listing applications, etc. To aid in the examination and possible further development of the trustee's calculations, relevant financial materials have been substituted.

Thanks to the dedication of the Securities and Exchange Commission to the concept of full disclosure—and Equity Funding's financial complexity—many of the numerous prospectuses run to well over 100 pages. They are a gold mine of information about the structure and operations of the company. Since we were unable to include all of them in full, we have excerpted the parts we believe will be most useful. Some potentially important prospectuses that have not been reproduced are noted. They can usually be found in stock brokerage libraries.

We have not included Forms 10-K or annual reports (except for a few text portions). A prospectus contains more information than either of these documents, and EFCA issued enough prospectuses to provide continuity of financial information. On the other hand, we have reproduced some quarterly reports because they have information not found in the prospectuses.

The testimony about Peat, Marwick's mini-audit of Equity Funding Life became available as depositions were taken in the civil litigation. The Peat, Marwick staff would certainly have disclosed the fraud if they had found it. Their testimony and notes provide unique insight into the problems—some mechanical, but most psychological—faced by conscientious auditors working in the middle of a fraud. The nagging harrassment by Equity Funding will make future auditors more suspicious of uncooperative clients. The memoranda of the staff auditors first considering, then rejecting the possibility of a fraud, show better than any text or AICPA pronouncement how hard it is for an honest man to perceive the face of massive dishonesty. The PMM testimony became the fourth major part of this book.

The Hudes and Grosman articles on auditing, after the fraud was discovered, while less dramatic, seemed to provide a good contrast to the Peat, Marwick episode. In addition, they allow the reader to evaluate the claim of the defense in the auditor's trial that only an audit such as Grosman's would have discovered the fraud. The AICPA's report provides the finale to the auditing story.

After these larger parts, it became a matter of selecting the *most* interesting items from a mass of materials. We could not resist Stanley Goldblum's last presentation to the New York Society of Security Analysts, or the notice to the employees of Equity Funding assuring them that all was well. The two Goldblum speeches give the flavor of the message he presented to Wall Street over the years.

Equity Funding was the subject of many brokerage firm research reports, most of which were optimistic and none of which found or even seemed to suspect the fraud. We have selected one as representative of many, neither more nor less perceptive than the other reports generated by Wall Street. In fairness, we have omitted the names of the one lucky analyst and firm selected. The report demonstrates an aspect of Wall Street's view of Equity Funding: a view that may explain one reason why no securities analyst discovered the fraud. Equity Funding was considered by many a glamorous "financial services" organization rather than a more mundane insurance company. As such, it was often followed by analysts less familiar with the complex, often tedious details of insurance company statement analysis.

Several business publications gave coverage to the Equity Funding story as it unfolded. *The Wall Street Journal,* in particular, has provided continuing reporting in considerable depth. Some of the stories were written by one of the editors. We have not duplicated these materials, because much of their content is found in other sources already reproduced here. In addition, the newspaper stories are easily available in most libraries. We have, however, included the sequence of *Wall Street Journal* articles just before and after the revelation of the fraud. With the share price and volume figures, they provide a vivid picture of the frenetic activities of that short period when the myth of Equity Funding fell apart.

Lee J. Seidler

Fred Andrews

Marc Epstein

1977

CONTENTS

THE EQUITY FUNDING PAPERS

INTRODUCTION

The Equity Funding Fraud: The Cast, the Times, and the Place

Few white-collar crimes have seized the nation's attention more dramatically than Equity Funding. None has been more disquieting. An established, nationally known insurance and securities company was abruptly exposed as a beehive of fraud, the seat of an enormous swindle that had gone undetected for years. Behind a facade of confident prosperity, Equity Funding had been forging documents, falsifying accounts, and manufacturing phony insurance business on an assembly-line scale. And, most puzzling and disturbing, this wholesale swindle was not simply the work of a tiny cadre of out-and-out conmen. From the first, fragmentary reports, it appeared that the swindle was helped along, or winked at, by dozens, perhaps scores, of ordinary office workers who apparently took to the fraud as a lark, a gigantic black prank.

The revelations of early April 1973 startled a public whose faith in American institutions and in itself was already eaten away by a long and dismaying war and whose capacity for disbelief was once again being assaulted by the opening barrages of the Watergate disclosures. But Equity Funding had less in common with Watergate than with another wrenching episode that had grown into a national trauma. Equity Funding hit the headlines like a white-collar Mylai. It was a tough serving of headlines to get down. American GIs, your sons and ours, the appealing dogfaces we recall from World War II, do not rape, brutalize, and murder women and children. Nor do ordinary Americans, middle-class people, the folks who work for insurance companies, fall willingly, even gleefully, into a blatant swindle. Scores of people privy to an enormous fraud? Why didn't anybody *tell?*

Why didn't anybody tell? Though, of course, Ron Secrist, for reasons of his own (he was fired), eventually did tell, that question remains one of the riddles of Equity Funding. Perhaps in a strict sense it is unanswerable, an invitation to prove a negative; but it is as important today as it was then to try to understand what happened. Nothing to date has refuted the broad outlines of the original revelations about Equity Funding. Some hasty explanations have proved half-baked or worse (most notably, the notion that it was all done by computers), and other impressions have been tempered. It appears, for instance, in cold light that probably fifty to seventy-five Equity Funding employees, rather than hundreds, knew or suspected something was wrong; that most were passive observers or reluctant participants, not avowed accomplices; that the fraud was not common knowledge in the corridors at Equity Funding or routine lunchtime chatter; that, in fact, some people most intimately concerned with the company's affairs (for example, Rodney Loeb, its house counsel) seem never to have caught on to the fiction they worked within.

These corrections notwithstanding, fifty to seventy-five employees remain a large number, certainly large enough to shake prevailing assumptions of everyday honesty. And if some questions, such as the breadth and blatantness of complicity by employees, appear less alarming with time, new and equally troubling issues have come into sharp focus. The more that is learned about Equity Funding's principal outside auditors, for instance, the worse their part in the debacle looks. As glaring contradictions in Equity Funding's published data become more apparent, it is difficult to understand the lack of suspicion by qualified outsiders.

*   *   *

This collection of papers began with the recognition of a gem, the 239-page *Report of the Trustee of Equity Funding Corporation of America*,[1] filed in federal court in Los Angeles on November 1, 1974, by Robert M. Loeffler, trustee. Though filed in compliance with a routine provision of the Bankruptcy Act, the trustee's report was anything but routine. The trustee took to heart his mandate to report "any facts ascertained by him pertaining to fraud, misconduct, mismanagement and irregularities and to any causes of action available to the estate." The resulting report is a unique document, a superior piece of work, probably without equal in financial annals. It is, and will remain, the starting point for anyone seriously concerned with Equity Funding. In its details, Loeffler's report is much richer than anything else in print, and the interpretation it advances, though debatable, must be reckoned with. Indeed, until the trustee's report came along, there was no coherent account of how the Equity Funding fraud happened. Ray Dirks' book, *The Great Wall Street Scandal*,[2] tells much more about how the fraud finally came unglued than about how it managed to hold together all those years. *The Impossible Dream*,[3] by Soble and Dallos, lacks detail and documentation.

Small wonder that the trustee's report is the mother lode, the point of departure. The trustee in bankruptcy was able to command access and draw on resources that no news reporter or scholarly researcher could hope to attain. Not only did the trustee have the run of Equity Funding's files, but he also obtained the workpapers of Equity Funding's main auditors, the Wolfson, Weiner firm, later merged into Seidman & Seidman. He had the cooperation of federal and state authorities. And the trustee was in an enviable position to elicit the assistance of key participants in the fraud who presumably thought it never too late to join the right side.

The bankruptcy trustee also had at his disposal some of the most skillful legal and auditing talent available. The trustee's report is an important byproduct of tens of thousands of hours of investigation by the lawyers and accountants the trustee retained to help carry out the seemingly impossible task of keeping Equity Funding alive and nursing it through bankruptcy reorganization.

The report's accounting and auditing foundations are the work of Touche Ross & Co., the international accounting firm, which almost overnight assembled the equivalent of a fully staffed metropolitan office for the Equity Funding job.[4] At one point Touche Ross had seventy accountants working on Equity Funding, and the firm's total fees for the enormous undertaking exceeded two million dollars. Norman Grosman, who headed the Touche Ross team, was the government's principal expert witness in convicting three of Equity Funding's outside auditors (Julian Weiner, Solomon Block, and Marvin Lichtig) for securities fraud.[5] The Weiner, Block, and Lichtig convictions are under appeal.

As legal counsel, the trustee hired the Los Angeles firm of O'Melveny & Myers, probably the preeminent law firm in Southern California. In short order, O'Melveny had a score of lawyers up to their ears in Equity Funding. The O'Melveny people were split into groups to handle the trustee's various legal chores, and it fell to a "fraud task force" (composed of Richard C. Warmer, Richard J. Stone, Robert C. Vanderet, and Sally A. Treweek) to draft the trustee's report. According to Loeffler, that group's first draft, prepared over the summer of 1974, pretty much stood up. The trustee himself began working over the draft that August, and the final report was filed on November 1 (after Stanley Goldblum had pleaded guilty, but before the auditors' trial). Loeffler authorized a printing of 2,000 copies, which disappeared almost overnight.

Though the creation of a committe, the trustee's report bears distinctly the imprint of Robert Loeffler, the trustee. In particular, the concluding section ("A Final Postscript") strikes the reader as set down by an individual hand, quite different in tone from the impersonal, all-purpose legal prose of the preceding sections. Loeffler has confirmed that these concluding reflections were largely his work alone.

Robert M. Loeffler, the trustee, is not an imposing figure. A short, soft-spoken man of bland appearance and with an air of reserve, Loeffler betrays no notable sparkle. Nevertheless, by persistence and skill, he accomplished what many others never believed possible. In the morning-after, when the fraud revelations had shattered Equity Funding, he held the torn company together and kept it limping along. In the three years that followed, Leoffler pieced and pulled together a plan of reorganization that salvaged the company's untainted operations and enabled it to emerge alive (if shrunken) from Chapter 10 bankruptcy proceedings as Orion Capital Corp.

An Oklahoma native, Loeffler majored in accounting at the University of Oklahoma and went on to Harvard Law School, where he was law review and graduated with honors. After law school, he joined the Wall Street firm of Donovan, Leisure, Newton & Irving and practiced securities law for two decades. When the Equity Funding scandal broke, Loeffler was drafted as trustee from a comfortable job as senior vice-president and general counsel of Investors Diversified Services Inc., the huge, Minneapolis-based mutual-fund complex.

"I said to myself, 'What do you need this grief for?'" the trustee later told William E. Blundell of *The Wall Street Journal,* "and as soon as that crossed my mind, I said, 'Hold on, Loeffler. If you're in that much of a rut at fifty, you *need* this job.'"

*   *   *

The trustee's report is a fascinating document. It unravels complexity within complexity, first laying out what Equity Funding's business purported to be, no simple task, and then showing how that web was corrupted into a tangle of fraud. And while the explanation imposes a coherent order on the sequence of events, the concrete detail hits/with an impact that no summary can convey. (The spectacle of Jim Banks et al. being caught at the death-benefit scheme, only to be put to work at the selfsame larceny for the company's account, speaks volumes about a corporation cancerous with fraud.)

As a caveat for the unwary reader, however, one must note that the trustee's report is not the work of a detached and impartial scholar poking through the long-cold embers. The report must be read partly as a legal brief, laying out the trustee's case against the accounting firms. The trustee, one recalls, has the duty of reporting not only any findings pertaining to fraud, etc., but also "any causes of action available to the estate"—in short, any likely target he can sue.

In a financial mess, the outside audit firms involved typically present an inviting target, if for no other reason than that when the dust settles, the auditors are usually among the few survivors with any money. In legal parlance, they have "deep pockets," eminently deep pockets.

In this case, of course, the auditors' financial resources are hardly the only reason for proceeding against them. The trustee's report nevertheless tends to blur the distinction between the Wolfson, Weiner firm, Equity Funding's long-time auditor, and Haskins & Sells, the international accounting firm that audited the life-insurance subsidiary. For all its criticism, the report seems too easy on Wolfson, Weiner (particularly in the light of testimony at the subsequent trial of the Wolfson, Weiner auditors) and too harsh on Haskins & Sells (which may have made mistakes, but has yet to be accused of anything criminal or shown to be grossly negligent). This blurring appears to reflect, on the one hand, the trustee's concern not to completely prejudge the criminal charges against the accused Wolfson, Weiner auditors and, on the other, the fact that Haskins & Sells is as prosperous a source of compensatory damages as Wolfson, Weiner and its successor firm, Seidman & Seidman, indeed decidedly more prosperous.

One also gets the impression that the trustee, like most of us, enjoys telling a good story. His account of the foreign phase of the fraud, that comedy of errors, is so good that only a spoilsport could object to its running on at much greater length than its importance merits. Admittedly, the hapless misadventures abroad do support Loeffler's contention that Goldblum and crew, far from being evil geniuses, were a bunch of clowns.

That is precisely the point. It's questionable that Goldblum and his confederates were as manifestly incompetent as the trustee's report suggests. For years, Goldblum and his key lieutenants managed to deal successfully with much of the financial community, deceiving, among others, nationally prominent lawyers, auditors, investment bankers, commercial bankers, financial analysts, the New York Stock Exchange, the National Association of Securities Dealers, and the Securities and Exchange Commission, and various other regulators. They also worked at close quarters with Equity Funding officers whose honesty and competence the trustee has accepted (such as Rodney Loeb, general counsel; Lawrence Williams, his assistant and a former SEC enforcer; and Herbert Glaser, in charge of real estate). And no one caught on.

True, this is a matter of shading. Undoubtedly, Goldblum and his crew were shallow, petty, second- and third-rate people whose performance never matched their posture. Nevertheless there is danger in deprecating the skill required to keep things going. It involved considerably more than "a degree of inventiveness in extricating themselves from near hopeless situations."

The foreign affairs were something of a sideshow that should not upstage the action in the center ring, the funding phase and the reinsurance phase. At a minimum, there were numerous episodes touching on these phases where one would have appreciated the kind of blow-by-blow attention the report gives the foreign capers. As one intriguing example, exactly what happened when Pennsylvania Life, in the trustee's bland phrasing, "became aware of the 'special class' nature of the business ceded to it and negotiated an additional $40 million of face value"? Or to take another example, was there much more to the merger of Seidman & Seidman and Wolfson, Weiner than the trustee's simple statement that the two firms combined practices? The trial testimony suggests that the merger was midwived by Goldblum, who until he hit upon that solution seemed to think that he was faced with the unhappy choice of either giving up Wolfson, Weiner, his tame auditor, or forgoing a highly desirable listing on the New York Stock Exchange.[6]

The trustee's report explains too well or, rather, too confidently. A model of clarity and thoroughness in tracing cash flows or matching debits with credits, the report turns curiously flat and unsatisfying when it deals with human beings. The trustee's matter-of-fact approach does not leave much place for uncertainty. One does not get the impression that Loeffler is a man who savors ambiguity, or is much in touch with the darker side of the human psyche.

Incredibly, the report never explicitly grapples with the question that in the public eye has become synonymous with Equity Funding, with what we have called the Mylai theme: *Why didn't anybody tell?* The trustee's explanation of how the fraud survived so long all but ignores that question.

> If the EFCA fraud was truly as haphazard and disconnected as it has been portrayed in this report, then it is legitimate to ask how it persisted for a decade without detection. . . . Foremost, of course, were the lies, audacity and luck of the ringleaders. Of almost equal importance was the surprising ability of the originators of the fraud to recruit new participants over the years. Closely related was the moral blindness of those participants, including several who helped execute the scheme and then left the Company, but remained silent.[7]

These references to "moral blindness" and the "surprising ability" to recruit new people are apparently the closest Loeffler comes to taking account of the fact that dozens of Equity Funding people helped the fraud, knew about it, glimpsed it, or strongly suspected it. "Moral blindness" has a nice ring to it, but the notion doesn't shed much light on the many different degrees of complicity or acquiescence. It is almost astonishing that Loeffler isn't more perturbed by the large number of employees with some knowledge of the fraud. That is especially so inasmuch as the trustee later invokes "the presumption of good faith and honest dealing which customarily prevails in American business practice" to explain why persons outside the company were only remotely likely to have suspected the fraud. At a minimum, fifty persons either helped the swindle along, or knew something of it and stood silent. What does *that* mean for Loeffler's presumption?

One possible explanation is that Loeffler apparently believes that the number of employees involved has been grossly exaggerated. As previously noted, that may well be true. It doesn't offer much solace, however, when twenty-two men were convicted of taking part in the swindle (all but three pleaded guilty), and four others were acknowledged coconspirators. That is a big number of any scale. And, perhaps more troubling, what of the people who discovered the fraud, or were told about it, and though largely or wholly unimplicated, either stood silent or left quietly, having made a separate peace? No certain means exist to pinpoint how many people belong in this category, but from Ray Dirks' account, Bill Blundell's findings, and our own interviews, two dozen is a conservative estimate. Indeed, Dirks identifies a dozen such persons in his book and, concerning the likely total, speculates that 100 "seems like a reasonable guess."[8]

(As an intriguing aside, it's remarkable that no *woman* is anywhere identified as having been aware of the fraud, much less as having assisted it. This seems surprising when one considers not only that women fill the ranks of clerical help, but also that secretaries who serve the executive suite are continually at their boss's elbow and seem to know whatever there is to know about corporate goings-on. It strains the imagination—not to mention one's respect for the corporate grapevine—to believe that nothing at Equity Funding ever struck these typically perceptive women as out-of-line.)

The reasons different people at Equity Funding did what they did are endlessly fascinating. Like survivors of some harrowing natural disaster, each of the Equity Funding crew has his own tale to tell. For a perceptive treatment of this human dimension, see Bill Blundell's narrative essay, "Equity Funding: 'I Did It for the Jollies.'"[9] Though indeed some participants *did* do it for the jollies, Blundell's essay also makes it clear that motives were diverse and human and often understandable. "Moral blindness" (or the ringleaders' luck) doesn't begin to do them justice.

Even among the avowed participants, motives varied greatly. The trustee's report goes into the financial benefits, the fat salaries, the stock options, the plush surroundings, that the inner-circle people—Goldblum, Fred Levin, Sam Lowell, Jim Smith, Michael Sultan, Art Lewis, to name the main ones—enjoyed. But the lesser participants, the spear-carriers, weren't getting rich. To them, Equity Funding was at most a job. Financially, the fraud game couldn't have been worth the candle.

It is also true that Equity Funding's executive cadre was young and callow. The trustee's report notes the participants' "curious flippancy" and observes that some of them "appeared to have looked upon the fraud as a game." Undoubtedly, there's a lesson in that. Older, more experienced businessmen, individuals whom life had knocked down a time or two, would likely have seen with greater clarity that the bubble had to burst. Nevertheless, it seems improbable that things were all that casual, even allowing for the nonchalance of youth. It stands to reason that, at least for some, the flippancy was a kind of gallows humor masking an inner agony over their suicidal course. Consider Bill Symonds, a middle-level manager who later pleaded guilty to securities fraud. One participant who watched Symonds at close hand recalled, "It preyed on his mind, like a death wish. He wanted the whole thing to collapse, it bothered him so much."[10] Given the pressure of keeping the scheme going, given the burning anxiety that must have mounted, it is a wonder that some participant did not go off the deep end and blow the scandal wide open (suicide in despair is a classic way for wrongdoing to be brought to light).

The question of silence and complicity deserves careful, discriminating analysis. Apparently few people outside Goldblum's inner circle realized the staggering magnitude of the fraud. Equity Funding is another instance of the blind men and the elephant. Many who tumbled to the scheme were drawn into the gigantic fraud by going willingly along with lesser cheating. "Like wow!" a computer programmer recalled later.[11] "I was kind of wondering what to do about it. I was told that this was a short-lived financing to acquire Bankers and Northern." Once initiated, he resisted in a half-hearted but understandable way. Under continual pressure from Art Lewis and others, the programmer always tried to keep his distance by delivering less than they demanded, as though he could preserve his purity by stopping short of full commitment. Inevitably, it wasn't long before he became deeply involved. When the bubble burst, he was at work on a computer program to take over the intricate task of "killing off" selected policyholders of the phony policies reinsured. He developed a certain pride in this work. The problem, he explained, was to kill off as many of the fictitious policyholders as possible without producing a pattern of "deaths" that would arouse the reinsurers' suspicions.)

The programmer's tale can be repeated again and again. In those early years, the Wolfson, Weiner auditors seemed willing to buy Goldblum's dubious cover story of the give-up commissions that supposedly had to be concealed in the accounts. Similarly, Bill Blundell quotes the reaction of Gary Beckerman, a young advertising specialist convicted of fraud, to the "special class" insurance (the policies given away to employees and then ceded to reinsurers): "I asked myself, 'Is it honorable?' No. 'Who's hurt?' The reinsurers. 'Is the reinsurer a big boy?' You bet."[12]

A little larceny is a dangerous thing. If incomplete knowledge of what was going on permitted active participants to rationalize their conduct, it isn't surprising that people who merely stumbled over something fishy hesitated to blow the whistle. To be sure, some had no inclination to do so. In his book, Ray Dirks describes an occasion when Pat Hopper, an Equity Funding executive who suspected fraud, was puzzling over why the company's reported sales far exceeded five times the total of any one of its five sales regions. One region's sales were $65 million. " 'If you're trying to multiply that by five, forget it,' the sales chief said (to Hopper). He added: 'I don't really care so long as the earnings go up and the stock price goes up.' "[13]

In other instances, however, employees searched their souls before determining to remain silent. One employee, a native of another country, talked out the situation at home and made a conscious decision not to do anything. The employee and spouse had already decided to leave the United States for their home country. "We weren't going to be here," the employee related later.[14] "We decided it was none of our business."

For a morality play in shades of gray, it is hard to improve upon the John Templeton vignette in the trustee's report:

> According to Templeton, throughout the 1968 audit he complained . . . about the problems he was having with the fund loans receivable. . . . He told his boss that there was a large discrepancy between the general ledger balance and the underlying detail, but got little sympathy. By the close of the audit, Templeton had reached the conclusion that the 1968 financial statements were not good enough to release to the public. He informed no one of his decision until, in the presence of a roomful of EFCA officials and attorneys, he refused to sign a Form S-1 containing the financials for filing with the SEC. Templeton recalls that when asked to explain his conduct, he said he was unable to describe what was wrong. So he was ushered out of the room, and [his boss] signed the Form S-1 in his place.
>
> About a week after Templeton refused to sign the form S-1 he was summoned to Goldblum's office. Templeton told Goldblum he thought there

was fraud at the Company. Goldblum responded . . . by asking Templeton if he was going to settle down and work. Templeton recalls that he exclaimed "No, effective now!" and walked out of the office. Later in the day, he was called back. This time Goldblum offered the Controller a substantial sum to stay and help fix EFCA's problems. After thinking it over, Templeton asked for a larger sum in immediate cash, plus stock options and additional money to exercise them. Goldblum agreed. After talking with his wife, however, Templeton had a change of heart and decided to quit. He wrote a note of resignation, left it on Goldblum's desk late at night and never went back to EFCA.[15]

It isn't very useful to dismiss Templeton's confusion as "moral blindness." In his predicament, many of us would have done no better, possibly worse. Isolated in a lonely and uncertain stand against one's superiors, first balking, then yielding, then stiffening again, a great many people would doubtless be content to close the chapter by saying good riddance. If, in hindsight, one can say that Goldblum all but acknowledged the fraud by offering to buy Templeton off, at the moment such overtures are advanced, their meaning is usually ambiguous. Note the sly subtlety, the invitation to rationalization, in Goldblum's request that Templeton stay on "and help fix EFCA's problems." Balm for the conscience. Bribes don't come with labels; they aren't subject to truth-in-packaging. It takes moral courage, a willingness to step up to the plate, to stamp a bribe for what it is.

Clearly, these episodes have pragmatic as well as moral lessons. Consider again Loeffler's presumption "of good faith and honest dealing which customarily prevails in American business practice." That presumption does exist, probably necessarily so (it is hard to conceive of a thriving economy founded on distrust and the expectation of dishonesty at every turn), and the Equity Funding scandal doesn't rebut it, at least not as a general proposition. (In fact, the swindle provides a vivid illustration of the strength of that presumption: The Peat, Marwick accountants, sent in to check policies ceded to a reinsurance company, could not bring themselves to believe the manifest signs of fraud. They deliberated over the possibility of fraud, only to explain it away.)[16]

The failure of any Equity Funding employee to report anything about the fraud has ominous implications for independent auditors. Traditional audit doctrine assumes that, as a practical matter, management fraud will be contained within a small circle, or fall of its own weight. As one experienced auditor, perplexed by what he read of Equity Funding, asked, "Why didn't somebody come up to the auditor in the john and tip him off? That's what I don't understand." (Certainly the later conviction of three Wolfson, Weiner auditors for fraud helps explain why, but those defendants were by no means the only outside auditors on Equity's premises.) Obviously, Equity Funding *wasn't* contained within a small circle. If auditors assume a broader conspiracy *must* topple of its own weight, their confidence is unwarranted.

The implications are enormous. Corporate internal control systems and audits both depend on an assumption that one individual's work can be used as a check on that of another. Obviously, such checks will fail if the individuals are colluding, passively or actively. If Equity Funding is anything more than the accident of the century, some fundamental concepts will have to be reexamined. Indeed, reexamination may be too mild a term; if massive collusion can exist with any frequency, control systems and audits, as now conceived, just won't work.

The failure of Equity Funding's directors to exercise control over its choice of auditors was glaring, and its results were tragic. "It really has been a shattering experience for me," lamented Robert Bowie, an internationally known Harvard University professor who said he accepted a place on Equity Funding's board mainly as a favor to a friend. "I was really relying on their auditing reports . . . to make sure I was abreast of what was going on. I was really rather appalled that these accountants apparently had not been making the kinds of tests to bring this out."[17]

From its inception as a public company until its spectacular demise, Equity Funding relied for auditors on the Wolfson, Weiner firm, principally on Julian Weiner, the firm's dominant partner, and Solomon Block, manager of the Equity audit. Both Weiner and Block were later convicted of securities fraud, but their poor reputations long antedated their indictments and were well known at Equity Funding, where Block in particular was held in low regard. The Wolfson, Weiner firm's deficiencies were so obvious that in 1970, when it sought a merger partner, at least two nationally known accounting firms turned it down because of misgivings over its work. Then, when Wolfson, Weiner secured agreement by a larger national firm (Seidman & Seidman) to take it over, the merger was effected in questionable circumstances and left the Equity Funding audit in Weiner's and Block's hands—as Stanley Goldblum had insisted. And as we shall see, there are allegations that Seidman & Seidman itself swallowed misgivings about Weiner and knew that Block, a former Seidman employee, was a poor auditor. (See p. 363 for the SEC's views on the acquisition.)

Julie Weiner, fifty years old when he was indicted, was known in California financial circles as a "creative" accountant, a specialist in intricate tax-shelter schemes and in taking new companies public. On occasion, Weiner boasted at cocktail parties that he and the late Mike Riordan had thought up Equity Funding's basic gimmick, the notion of selling mutual-fund shares and having investors borrow against the shares to buy life insurance. Several disgruntled clients had sued Weiner for one thing or another. (One episode involved International Recreation & Sports, Inc., a company created from a reactivated shell corporation. Weiner, who was a director and treasurer of International Recreation, was accused of concocting a tax scheme in which clients were to pay $10,000 for counseling in how to set up their own corporations, whose stock International Recreation would later acquire in an exchange of shares. A disgruntled client charged that the scheme was a sham to sell stock in International Recreation while permitting investors to deduct their $10,000 payment as investment-advisory fees. Weiner denied any wrongdoing, and the suit was settled.)[18]

In separate interviews[19] (all after Equity Funding had come to light, but before any public questioning of the auditors' part), several of Weiner's business associates described him in strikingly similar terms. A Century City lawyer who had worked on registration statements with Weiner said he had "a very facile mind, but extremely poor judgment. In a tight spot, he panics." Another securities lawyer considered

Weiner "a very, very brilliant guy . . . a very weak guy. He can be the tool to help you build up a company or help you destroy it."

If Weiner's reputation was dubious, Solomon Block, forty-five years old when indicted, was considered crude and dull-witted. "He whines. He's an excuse-maker," Rodney Loeb, the general counsel, said (in April 1973). Block apparently lacked any semblance of an "audit presence," anything in his bearing or conduct to suggest independence. Ordinary employees at Equity Funding who knew him vaguely considered him a fellow employee. Indeed, Block's name appeared in the Equity Funding telephone directory without any special designation, and his office door on the premises didn't indicate it was the outside auditor's office.

During the four years Block managed the Equity Funding audit, he wasn't even a CPA. In 1961, when Block first sat for the CPA examination, he flunked all four parts: law, theory, practice, and audit. He didn't attempt the exam again until 1969, when he passed law and audit (with a bare minimum of 75), but failed theory and practice. He finally passed those two in November 1972. Ironically, Block wasn't issued his CPA certificate until the following April, after the scandal had burst wide open. At the same meeting, the California State Board of Accountancy instructed its staff to investigate what role, if any, accountants had played in the fraud.

To be sure, it isn't unusual for candidates to flunk the CPA exams, but it isn't common (or commendable) for eight years to elapse before a second try. Nor is there a rule that an audit manager must have a CPA certificate, although many firms have such a requirement. It's highly unusual, however—and questionable on its face—for an accountant without a certificate to manage the audit of a company as large and prominent as Equity Funding. And it's unheard of, for an accounting firm to relegate to an audit manager (CPA or not) the partner's responsibility for signing the firm's opinion letter, as was the practice at Wolfson, Weiner.

Nor was that the worst about Block. In a breach, or near breach, of independence, Block's son was on Equity Funding's payroll (though nothing has come to light to indicate that the younger Block didn't do an honest job). Still worse, Sol Block testified before the SEC that on several occasions he had borrowed $300 or $350 from Marvin Lichtig, the former Wolfson, Weiner auditor who had become Equity Funding's treasurer (and was later convicted of fraud alongside Weiner and Block). According to the complaint in the shareholders' lawsuit against Equity Funding and its auditors, Block was an inveterate gambler who became financially dependent on the company. When Block took personal bankruptcy after the scandal broke, among the creditors' claims was $2,000 owed Equity Funding.

Even if (to accept Loeffler's contention) Equity Funding's directors couldn't have known about the fraud, how could they have missed all this? Wolfson, Weiner was known in business circles as wheeler-dealers, too clever by half, even shady. The man in charge of the audit was manifestly uninspiring, ill-trained, and unqualified. How could the directors have missed the odor?

One might ask that same question of the corporate officers—Rodney Loeb, for example—who weren't implicated and who, after the fact, brim over with denunciations of Wolfson, Weiner. Their complaints are a sword that cuts both ways. If the Wolfson, Weiner crew were so bad, and known to be so bad, why did those officers acquiesce in keeping them?

Wolfson, Weiner was a small firm, tiny by today's standards, and Equity Funding was by far its largest and most important client. At the auditors' trial, the prosecution put Equity Funding's audit fees at $300,000, compared with $75,000 and $40,000 for Wolfson, Weiner's next two largest accounts. A Seidman & Seidman witness testified that Wolfson, Weiner drew 20 percent of its revenues from Equity Funding. He put the annual fees at $200,000, though there were hopes, he said, that with Wolfson, Weiner's merger into a larger firm, the total might grow to $500,000 because the larger entity could take on more work. Weiner testified that by 1971, revenues had grown to $1.5 million, of which $250,000 was from Equity Funding. (He also claimed the account required so much overtime it wasn't profitable.)

It's hard to argue that small firms should be barred from auditing publicly held companies of national importance. Certainly the gargantuan international accounting firms with their strings of far-flung offices have botched their share of audits. It is sometimes argued that sheer size promotes independence by an audit firm because no single client then provides more than a tiny fraction of its fee revenues. Though that argument certainly can be pushed too far (one would not wish to be the Arthur Andersen & Co. partner who loses its International Telephone & Telegraph Corporation account), it does have merit, other things being equal. A small firm (or an office of a large one that bases partners' pay on each office's profits) may more easily slip past that tipping point where a prominent client becomes simply too important, the auditor's mindset of independence—his sense of apartness—is eroded, and auditor and client become too close. In particular, this seems a danger when auditor and client have worked together since time immemorial, as did Wolfson, Weiner with Equity Funding.

The continual tension between independence and bread-and-butter is obvious, but that conflict is put into especially sharp focus when an accounting firm goes on the auction block, as did Wolfson, Weiner. Not only was Wolfson, Weiner actively shopping for a merger partner (it broached the possibility with at least four other accounting firms roughly the size and prominence of Seidman & Seidman), but it was also asking an unusually stiff price, twice the firm's annual billings. Wolfson, Weiner's most notable asset, probably the only thing it had that another firm might covet, was the Equity Funding account. The merger talks, with one firm or another, apparently went on for well over a year. One might ask how much independence an audit firm seeking to sell itself might be expected to show toward its principal selling point.

The circumstances under which Wolfson, Weiner was merged into Seidman & Seidman, while the Equity Funding audit remained in the same hands, might well have troubled a board of directors concerned with the integrity of its audit. It appears that Stanley Goldblum shoved Wolfson, Weiner into merger (which isn't to say Wolfson, Weiner resisted), and it is clear that Goldblum clung to Weiner and Block for dear life. Surprisingly, the trustee's report doesn't mention this flagrant breach of independence.

Though in retrospect it seems highly unlikely that Goldblum ever would have given up the compliant Wolfson, Weiner firm, at the time there was at least the possibility of their being forced out. Early in 1970, Goldblum dispatched emissaries to scout the possibility of Equity Funding's being admitted to listing on the New York Stock Exchange. The emissaries got the distinct impression that one of three conditions was that the company retain a better-known audit firm. Though the exchange denies it ever dreamed of imposing such a requirement (as well it might deny it, unless it wants protests from every small or medium-sized accounting firm in the country), and no mention of the point appears in minutes of formal negotiations, both Rodney Loeb and Sam Lowell have said they understood a change of auditors to be a prerequisite for listing. (At the auditors' trial, Lowell did testify that the requirement could have come from the underwriters. Of course, underwriting houses, which have to sell the issues, are usually eager to have a nationally known audit firm's imprimatur on a prospectus.)

Loeb recalled that he reported the condition to Goldblum and found him most unreceptive. "He said he had a great deal of loyalty to Julie Weiner,' Loeb remembered[20] "In the early days, Weiner had been very helpful [Goldblum said]. He said he felt a tremendous loyalty toward Julie Weiner. I admired the trait." Discussions with the stock exchange nevertheless proceeded, and in mid-1970, according to Loeb, Goldblum himself met with exchange officials, and the matter of a better-known audit firm again came up. By Loeb's recollection, Goldblum reiterated his extreme reluctance to change auditors, but added an element that came as a surprise to Loeb: Goldblum said he had reason to believe Wolfson, Weiner intended to merge with a larger firm. According to Loeb, those assurances satisifed the exchange.

How much trouble Wolfson, Weiner had recruiting a merger partner isn't known. Two firms, Alexander Grant & Co. and another that wishes to remain anonymous, have said they rejected Wolfson, Weiner's overtures; and at his trial, Weiner mentioned two other firms, Wolf & Co. and Laventhol & Horwath, that he allegedly negotiated with. Be that as it may, once Wolfson, Weiner and Seidman & Seidman were ready to tie the knot, Goldblum expressed worries about Weiner and Block. Sam Lowell testified about one meeting:

> Julie . . . assured us that he had been assured by them (Siedman & Seidman) that he would continue to be on the audit and that we would continue having Sol on the audit. And he says, "There might be changes in the lower level staff."
>
> And as I recall, Phil Wolfson reaffirmed this, that this was the case.[21]

Lowell's testimony goes on to suggest that Equity Funding and Seidman & Seidman had agreed on a *quid pro quo.*

> Stanley brought up the topic of our wanting Julie and Sol to continue on the audit and not wanting any change of personnel. And I continued on in the same vein. . . . And that if Seidman & Seidman was going to put somebody else on the account, then we would just have to think about going to a Big Eight firm, but we would much rather be with Seidman & Seidman if we knew we were going to have the same quality of work [!!] that we had with Wolfson, Weiner.
>
> Then the discussion immediately turned to which audits Seidman & Seidman was going to get.
>
> They wanted the insurance company and the savings and loan, and so forth. And I left the meeting, it was my impression that we had an agreement.

The charge that Seidman & Seidman cut a deal to get more business is an extremely serious accusation. It has been denied under oath by Robert L. Spencer, partner in charge of Seidman's Los Angeles office and the man who negotiated the Wolfson, Weiner merger, and it is not included in the SEC's allegations against Seidman. In testimony at the auditors' trial, Spencer denied ever discussing Weiner and Block with Goldblum or Lowell, much less agreeing to keep them on the audit. But Seidman & Seidman did take over as auditor for Equity Funding Life Insurance Co. and for Liberty Savings & Loan, another subsidiary. And in the audit for 1972, the first where Seidman & Seidman was in charge, Weiner and Block stayed on the job.

Entirely apart from the accusation, Seidman & Seidman was derelict on other grounds. Though Equity Funding's financial statements for 1971 were certified by Seidman & Seidman (in the 10-K and prospectuses, Seidman signed indicating they were successors to Wolfson, Weiner; in the annual report, the plain Seidman & Seidman signature appeared), by its own admission, Seidman merely reviewed Wolfson, Weiner's work. (It appears that Wolfson, Weiner and Seidman & Seidman reached agreement in early January of 1972 and signed the formal papers around February 18, retroactive to February 1; Equity Funding's 1971 results came out the first week in March.) Though Seidman & Seidman has cited the cursoriness of its review as evidence that the firm shouldn't be held accountable for the 1971 audit, other auditors say Seidman was asking for trouble. As another firm's managing partner explained, it is always touchy when a larger firm is moving in to assume charge of its smaller merger partner's accounts, "and jobs spanning the merger date are particularly crucial," he warned. It's too easy for something to fall between the chairs. As a further caveat, he added, "One thing you learn very quickly to do is rotate the personnel."

At best, Seidman & Seidman blundered into trouble by linking up with a sorry outfit whose people it didn't know and whose work, according to the SEC, it hardly checked. Somehow it missed the bad odor that was well known in business circles and apparent to others whom Wolfson, Weiner approached. That is the best face one can put on Seidman & Seidman's actions. The stockholders' class-action lawsuit against Seidman & Seidman has charged that things were worse than that, however—that Seidman swallowed its own reservations in forging ahead with the merger. In pre-trial maneuvering, the class-action plaintiffs filed papers showing that Sol Block had once worked for Seidman & Seidman, where his personnel record described his performance as "poor" and characterized Block as "light category only at this time," rather than senior material.

That same filing included excerpts from a deposition given in 1974 by L. William Seidman, the firm's managing partner when it acquired Wolfson, Weiner and more recently a senior economic adviser to President Ford. In the deposition, Seidman described a March 1972 meeting of the firm's "policy group," at which Julie Weiner and Phillip Wolfson, its newly admitted partners, were discussed. "The discussion was to the effect that after listening to the two of them talk, we better be very careful about the work they did," Seidman related. In particular, he said, concern was expressed that "Mr. Weiner tended to have an attitude that implied he didn't have sufficient concern for the public." (The observation is consistent with Weiner's testimony that in January 1972, William Seidman had told him "my talent would be better served if I concentrated on bringing in business"—which can be read as a desire to keep Weiner away from audit work.)

According to the plaintiffs' filing, that March policy group meeting went on to stress the need for more thorough review of prospective merger partners and closer supervision of their post-merger work. But the filing also quoted a January 13, 1972, memo attributed to Robert Spencer in which he purportedly urged the firm to approve the Wolfson, Weiner acquisition without the usual review "because of our stringent timing problem, " a reference that isn't explained. The plaintiffs also cite documents that they contend show Seidman & Seidman rushing into the merger because its earnings were lagging and it needed money. William Seidman has called that allegation "absurd."

As we have noted, Robert Loeffler is a mild-mannered man, the soul of reasonableness, and the last person one would expect to assume an extreme stance on anything. Yet to grasp the full weight of the burden seemingly put on an independent auditor's shoulders, one need only consider the trustee's concluding throughts in "A Final Postscript." In Loeffler's view, not only should Equity Funding's outside auditors have detected the swindle, but they also were the *only* outsiders with half a chance to do so. The crowd of other outsiders—investment analysts, bankers, underwriters, reinsurers, state regulators—"probably could only have discovered the fraud at EFCA by blind luck." Loeffler concedes that in hindsight Equity Funding's financial statements do contain discrepancies, but "only someone examining the statements thoroughly, regularly and with a critcal eye would have found them. And only someone with an exceedingly skeptical bent of mind would have then inferred massive fraud."[22]

So the fraud went on so long because the auditors did not do their job. And why didn't they do their job? Because they were crooked or stupid? "There is strong evidence," the report concludes, that the Wolfson, Weiner people "were aware of or suspected the fraud and cooperated in its concealment. Such a conclusion seems irresistible to the trustee if only because Wolfson, Weiner's performance was so manifestly incompetent for so many years as to be inexplicable on any other basis."[23] For a document blessed by lawyers, that is pretty strong language.

No doubt, bolstered by the conclusions of the AICPA committee (see p. 338), the trustee is technically correct; if the Wolfson, Weiner auditors had simply done their job, they would have detected and disclosed the fraud in its earliest stages. The massive, unsupported journal entries creating nonexistent commission income should have caught the attention of even the most inept auditor.

That answer might do for a small, privately held manufacturing company in upstate New York, but not for a huge, publicly held insurance conglomerate. The United States has created a web of corporate regulation probably unmatched in complexity anywhere in the world. Equity Funding had auditors, but it also had a board of directors with supposedly competent outsiders. Its numerous debt and stock issues each resulted in a voluminous, highly detailed prospectus, duly filed with and reviewed by the United States Securities and Exchange Commission. Its securities were traded first on the American Stock Exchange, later on the New York Stock Exchange, both of which have staffs eyeing the trading and filings of listed companies.

Equity Funding's shares and debt issues were offered to the public repeatedly by established underwriting firms who—in principle at least—exercise considerable professional diligence in investigating the companies whose shares they bring to the public. Nelson Loud, a senior partner of the leading underwriter, sat on the board of directors of Equity Funding, where he had a continuing, inside view of the operation and the perpetrators.

Equity Funding shares were analyzed by many security analysts, none of whom noted the discrepancies pointed out by the trustee and easily seen in the quarterly reports reproduced here.

Equity Funding's tax returns were examined by the United States Internal Revenue Service. Indeed, the trial testimony suggests that the steps taken by the IRS to verify the falsified revenues of the company should have presented the fraud in full flower to the IRS. Did an IRS agent ignore the fraud and merely collect his 48 percent in taxes?

Nor were the hapless Wolfson, Weiner auditors the only ones to inspect the books. As noted above, the EFCA December 31, 1971, financial statements, included in the prospectus of September 11, 1972, were signed by Seidman & Seidman, and Haskins & Sells, a Big Eight accounting firm of undoubted competence, audited Equity Funding Life Insurance Company. As chronicled later in this volume, another Big Eight firm had a crack, albeit under thoroughly inhospitable conditions, at Equity Funding Life.

Equity Funding was (in theory) mainly an insurance operation. The insurance regulators of some of the largest states—including New York, California, and Illinois—examined the company. (One must note, in justice to these regulators, that actual policyholders of real Equity Funding policies suffered no losses from the fraud.)

Insurance companies use actuaries. The financial statements of Equity Funding Life in the prospectuses included the certificates of an outside actuarial firm certifying to the adequacy of its reserves.

Thus Equity Funding was crawling with regulators and quasi-regulators, none of whom seemed to question the staggering good fortune of a company that could virtually double sales every year, year after year.

Not quite in the category of regulators, but nevertheless under obligations to their own shareholders, were some of the entities with whom Equity Funding did business. One obviously thinks of some of the creditors. A consortium of large banks, including Citibank, Wells Fargo, and the ill-fated Franklin National Bank, gave EFCA a line of credit of over $100 million, only nine months before the fraud broke.

Bank credit analysts, however expert, are not in the insurance business. Insurance companies are. Five experienced insurance companies reinsured about $1.2 billion (face amount) of EFLIC policies for which they paid fees of about $12 million through the end of 1971 (1972 figures are not available).

If anyone in this entire spectrum of regulators, quasi-regulators, and very interested parties should have been able to spot EFLIC's inflated insurance operations, it would have been these insurance companies. Indeed, as materials on pages 70–116 chronicle, the largest of the reinsurance customers, Ranger National Life, apparently had suspicions when it rushed Peat, Marwick to start its special review. Yet no evidence has been unearthed to suggest that even the people in the same business perceived any more than the most innocent shareholder of Equity Funding.

In the same class as the reinsurers, in terms of knowledge and skills, if not responsibilities, were the former shareholders of some of the companies acquired by Goldblum and Co. For example, the shareholders of Bankers National Life received 1.6 million shares of EFCA stock in that merger. Fidelity Corporation, a Virginia-based insurance company owned 36.2 percent of Bankers (acquired through a 1970 merger with Bankers) and thus ended up with about 580,000 shares or 7.4 percent of EFCA outstanding stock, a significant block.[24] Insurance men who owned another insurance company also did not seem to have any inkling of the fraud.

Perhaps the reader will add others to the list, but the point is clear. Goldblum, Levin, et al. carried out their fraud for years while they were constantly observed, examined, audited, regulated, directed, controlled, and even owned by a veritable horde of people, every one of whom was capable of recognizing and understanding the fraud, and none of whom did.

Why not? We have no clear answer. Perhaps that is the great attraction of Equity Funding. It might just be that we live in an overregulated, overcontrolled society, where there are so many regulators, that everyone, including the regulators, assumes that someone else is checking. As Bob Krenske, the Peat, Marwick auditor who was kicked out of the EFLIC offices, noted in his memo titled "Possibility that EF (Equity Funding) is Ceding Fraudulent Policies":

> I do not feel that there is evidence of fraud. I base this on . . . examinations by H & S as EF's CPAs, also by state ins. examiners and independent actuaries which have not indicated any fraud.

This is not to argue that any single lapse caused the Equity Funding fraud. At this juncture, it serves no purpose to sift after the one supposedly critical element but for which the fraud would have been exposed much sooner. That would be a wrong-headed approach, which might be called the want-of-a-nail fallacy, and the trustee slips into it. Equity Funding happened. It cannot be explained away. The best one can do is try to comprehend what happened, in all its complexity.

Notes

[1]*Report of the Trustee of Equity Funding Corporation of America Pursuant to Section 167(3) of the Bankruptcy Act (11 U.S.C. §567(3)),* October 31, 1974, (Robert M. Loeffler, Trustee); cited hereafter as *Trustee's Report.*

[2]Raymond L. Dirks and Leonard Gross, *The Great Wall Street Scandal,* New York (McGraw-Hill Book Company), 1974.

[3]Ronald L. Soble and Robert E. Dallos, *The Impossible Dream: The Equity Funding Story,* New York (G. P. Putnam's Sons), 1974.

[4]For a view of the Touche Ross "fraud audit" in progress, see Albert Hudes, "Behind the Scenes at Equity Funding," and Norman C. Grosman, "How to Audit a Known Fraud," *Tempo* (Vol. 22, No. 1, 1976). Reproduced at p. 294.

[5]Grosman's testimony is excerpted at pp. 319–323 below.

[6]The trial testimony is excerpted at pp. 303–337 below.

[7]Trustee's Report, pp. 140-1.

[8]Dirks, pp. 69-71, 73, 137-138, 142-143, 186-187, 203-204, 239, and *passim.*

[9]William E. Blundell, "Equity Funding: 'I Did It For The Jollies'", Donald Moffitt, Editor, *Swindled! Classic Business Frauds of the Seventies,* Princeton, New Jersey (Dow Jones Books), 1976.

[10]In an interview with one of the editors.

[11]In an interview with one of the editors.

[12]Blundell, p. 64.

[13]Dirks, p. 63.

[14]In an interview with one of the editors.

[15]*Trustee's Report,* p. 36.

[16]See the selections on Peat, Marwick at pp. 71–116 below.

[17]In an interview with one of the editors.

[18]*Gurasich v. International Recreation & Sports, Inc.,* United States District Court, Central District of California, No. 70-1204-HP, *passim.*

[19]With one of the editors.

[20]In an interview with one of the editors.

[21]Lowell's testimony is excerpted at pp. 313–318 below.

[22]*Trustee's Report,* pp. 145-146.

[23]*Trustee's Report,* p. 141.

[24]The details of the Bankers merger with Fidelity may be found in the Bankers proxy statement dated April 27, 1970. An indication of Fidelity's and other holdings of EFCA is on p. 64 of the September 11, 1972, EFCA prospectus reproduced here.

EQUITY FUNDING SELLS ITSELF TO WALL STREET

Technically, it was a financial analyst who blew the whistle on Equity Funding. However, Ray Dirks' information came from a fired employee, not through security analysis. As a practical matter, after reviewing a number of reports on Equity Funding by brokerage house analysts, we found no indication that any of them found, or even suspected that something was amiss. It is possible, of course, that analysts working directly for investment institutions, who do not publish their reports, did find the fraud. Considering the speed and ferocity with which Ray Dirks was punished for the way he broke the fraud, financial analysts may well be leary of heroics in the future.

It must be admitted that a former student of one of the editors did submit a term paper setting forth some strong—and in retrospect accurate—suspicions of fraud at Equity Funding well over a year before public disclosure. With a notable lack of perception, the professor failed to follow up.

It is impossible to determine why financial analysts missed it. As the introduction to the financial materials demonstrates, a minimum of pencil pushing would have revealed some very suspicious, if not conclusive, figures. Indeed, there is no indication that any analyst even noticed the $50 million difference between the company's January and February 1971 press releases on its 1970 new insurance placements and the figure that later appeared in the 1970 annual report published in March 1971.

We can make a guess. Equity Funding was neither sold nor analyzed as an insurance company. It was that classic of the market of the 1960s, a "concept stock." It was, as Stanley Goldblum said in his 1968 speech, a "fully integrated financial service organization." In what appears to be his last published speech to analysts made only two months before the fraud broke, Goldblum was still calling EFCA "a life insurance marketing organization," which had "succeeded in identifying unfilled needs in the financial services area."

Analysts and the stock market seemed far more interested in the "concept" of Equity Funding. Note that Goldblum explains the gimmick in virtually the same terms in both speeches, although they were years and hundreds of speeches apart.

Insurance company financial analysis is tedious work. It must have been easier to contemplate the golden promise of exciting financial services products than to calculate persistence ratios. We found little indication that Equity Funding was subject to searching financial analysis, which is somewhat more common today than in the 1960s, and which might well have revealed the numerous examples of incompatible figures.

We have also included an analyst's report, typical of many written about the company. In fairness to the fact that this report is no more or less perceptive than many others, we have identified neither the analyst nor the firm.

A Progress Report to The New York Society of Security Analysts

By Stanley Goldblum, President Equity Funding Corporation of America

November 15, 1968

Gentlemen:

It is a pleasure to have this opportunity to talk to you about Equity Funding Corporation of America. If corporate performance is measured in terms of earnings and earnings growth; then our published record of past performance certainly speaks for itself.

Since 1962 Equity Funding's compound annual rate of growth of earnings per share has been 66%. Interestingly, 1967 showed an increase of 82% over 1966 and earnings for the first 9 months of 1968 increased by 100% over the same 1967 period.

We are pleased by that record, primarily because it was not an accident. It was achieved as a result of careful analysis, planning, and execution. However as pleased as we are with the past, we continually recognize the necessity to not only realize results in each particular year, but to concurrently plan for the continuation of similar results in future years.

I would like to tell you about the elements that we have already built into our business that we believe should make it possible for Equity Funding to continue its past earnings growth rate into the future.

In order to recognize the interrelationship of those growth-producing elements and their impact on the Company's future, I must touch briefly on the history and marketing concepts of our Company.

Equity Funding started operations as a corporate entity in 1960, and was primarily engaged in the sale of mutual fund shares and to a lesser degree of life insurance policies. Our sales organization consisted of approximately 150 representatives. We recognized then the market potential for a dynamic new financial program that would coordinate the benefits of mutual funds and life insurance ownership.

A number of organizations offered various such programs at the time, but with little commercial success. The Program that we intended to develop had to meet the tests of fulfilling the actual public need and of producing profit for the insuring company, distributing company and sales representatives. This was not a simple problem. The need to develop a program objectively was very apparent to us.

For example, the statistical fact that most men in their 40's live to 65, retirement age, made it apparent that as strong an emphasis as possible should be placed on directing the greatest amount of our clients' dollars to mutual fund purchases. On the other hand, the fact that not all men in their 40's live to retire, makes it obvious that the purchase of life insurance in sufficient amounts in each client's circumstances also was essential.

The problem of properly dividing the estate building funds was solved through the use of a credit function. An arrangement was developed whereby all of the client's available out-of-pocket dollars are invested in mutual fund shares, and through the extension of credit—using the shares as collateral security—monies are advanced to pay the premiums on a life insurance policy. The form of insurance utilized is ordinary life (also known as straight life or whole life). This form of insurance provides the greatest death benefit for the lowest net cost and thus is best suited to solve the problem of creating the estate for the dependents.

Through this arrangement—the purchase of mutual fund shares, the use of credit with the shares as security, and the purchase of an ordinary life insurance policy with the credit proceeds—the individual client can significantly lessen, or eliminate the problem of determining in what proportion his dollars should be divided between the purchase of mutual fund shares and life insurance. After an initial investment, these shares are usually purchased monthly, in sufficient amount to meet the collateral requirements of the credits advanced. An objective of the Program is thus to enable the participant to utilize the hoped-for appreciation of the fund shares—plus any dividends or capital gains distributions—to aid in offsetting the principal and accumulated interest on the loans and related charges and fees.

Here is how a typical Program might be proposed to a client:

The client takes out a life insurance policy. Under the Program, the annual premium must be at least $301. The Program also requires that his initial mutual fund investment be 2.3 times the amount of the annual insurance premium or at least $692.

The Company pays the initial insurance premium by loaning the client $301 upon the pledge of his fund shares. Thus, the client's initial out-of-pocket expense is $692—yet all of his $692, less the mutual fund sales charge, is working for him in equity investment. Moreover, he has the life insurance protection which he needs. He then continues a monthly investment of approximately $50.

What are the merits of such an arrangement for the client?

1. He has no out-of-pocket current premiums to pay.
2. He has all the money he puts into the Program invested in a diversified portfolio of American industry stocks and supervised by professional investment managers.
3. He has the cash value savings portion of his life insurance policy built up for him with borrowed capital.
4. He has coordinated both his living estate and death estate objectives in one "two estate" program in which both are maintained by his regular investment in the mutual fund.

Marketing of the Program met with immediate initial success, and our sales organization and profits grew very satisfactorily during 1960 and 1961. In 1962 the Program as briefly outlined above was deemed to be a security by the regulatory agencies and consequently required registration. As a result, the offering of our Program was interrupted until registration could be completed. This was accomplished in the fall of 1963, at which time Program sales were resumed. The Company had continued the separate sale of mutual funds and life insurance during the interim period while registration was pending.

Concurrently with the original development of the coordinated financial program as a principal marketing concept, we had initiated the first of a continuing series of annually updated 5-year plans for overall corporate development. Full implementation of all of the elements of the first 5-year corporate development plan was not accomplished until 1967, and 1968 actually represents the first full year of operation with all elements on stream.

I would like to outline for you the principal elements of the initial 5-year plan and indicate our status in regard to each. At the same time I will be able to indicate in general terms the contribution to future earnings that we have in mind for each element. Finally, I will outline our current status in terms of the newly-emerging areas of corporate activity. I might point out that we are continuously modifying our overall thrust as we interpret both the external environment in which the Company finds itself operating, and the environment we create for ourselves as a result of the impact of plans initiated in prior years.

First, the principal elements of our initial 5-year plan.

A. After the marketing impact of a coordinated mutual fund/life insurance program became apparent, we determined to expand the sales operation nationally. The 5-year objective was 2,000 sales representatives. We reached that objective early in 1968, and allowing for the 18-month interruption of Program sales this objective was on schedule. The importance of the sales organization on future earnings cannot be under-estimated. Since the sales force growth has been rapid, a large number of representatives are really only just now reaching the stage of career stablization and sophistication, so it is not unreasonable to expect them to produce increasing volume in the future.

At the present time the organization totals approximately 2300 representatives operating from 103 sales offices in 28 States and continues to grow in total size and in overall skill and quality.

In view of the Company's emphasis on expanding the direct-selling organization which consists of sales representatives paid entirely on a commission basis, it was necessary for us to devise an incentive program for sales representatives that would motivate them to develop their careers over a long period of time with the Company. This was accomplished through the use of an unusual production stock option plan keyed by its terms to each individual agent's commission production. The plan makes it possible for each representative of the Company to share in the growth that he helps to create and is based strictly on personal performance. One element of the plan requires that the agent remain with the Company over a 5-year period in order to realize the full benefit of his stock options. The plan has been extremely successful and has made it possible for us to meet our sales force objectives and to build stability into the sales organization.

B. Once a reliable distribution network had been established, we had planned for the vertical integration of our life insurance operations to include a wholly-owned life insurance company, and of our mutual fund operations to include the distribution of shares of a fund managed by the Company. The latter objective was accomplished in 1966 with the establishment of Equity Growth Fund of America. At the present time, the Fund's total assets are approximately $35,000,000.

This aspect of the plan was supplemented this year with the acquisition of the management company of Republic Technology Fund. Republic's total assets are approximately $30,000,000. At the present time, approximately 40% of our total mutual fund sales are directed to these two funds.

We consider that the impact on earnings in the future should be substantial with respect to management fees. By way of illustration, the total management fees received by the Company in 1967 equalled $39,000. The 1967 fees were as a result of our management of Equity Growth Fund of America. In 1968 management fees are being earned from the management of Equity Growth Fund, and as of September 12, 1968 from Republic Technology Fund, and are anticipated to total $180,000 for the year. However, in 1969, and based on our estimate of the assets that will be under management, it is anticipated that gross fees from the management of Equity Growth Fund, Republic Technology Fund, and Fund of America will exceed $1,000,000. This, of course, contemplates that the Investors Planning Corporation acquisition, which includes the management company for Fund of America, which I will discuss later, will have been completed.

C. Integration of a life insurance operation was completed late in 1967 with the acquisition of The Presidential Life Insurance Company of America. Essentially all of our life insurance sales, outside of New York, are now directed to Presidential. Presidential's total insurance in force at the end of 1967 was approximately $100,000,000. It is expected to be $300,000,000 at the end of 1968, and our budgeting is based on an in-force amounting to approximately $800,000,000 by year end 1969.

D. Since we define our market as the "thrift market," which consists of savings, insuring and investing, we implemented our entry into the savings aspect of the thrift market through the acquisition of Crown Savings & Loan Association in late 1967. Crown's total savings at the time were $32,600,000. As of today, they have been increased by approximately 25% to $40,700,000.

E. As part of our corporate planning in terms of marketing, we determined to, and in fact have, broadened the financed insurance program to include both A & H and general insurance in addition to life insurance, and to our knowledge we have the only IRS approved Keogh Plan in the country, utilizing the financed premium principle. In addition, this year we began the marketing of limited partnership units in the Equity Resources Limited Partnership 1968.

This product affords those of our clients whose investment objectives so require, an opportunity to participate in an oil and gas exploration program with favorable tax advantages. In addition, through the sophisticated use of leverage, we believe we have developed a substantially more valuable program than is presently marketed anywhere in this country, from the standpoint of tax advantages.

The program is also advantageous to the Company which earns the interest profit, a 5% management fee, and a 9% overriding royalty on future production. This kind of sophisticated marketing technique builds the potential for future profits for Equity Funding. This year's oil drilling program totals $2,500,000. Assuming the success of the program, we anticipate offering additional programs in the future.

F. One of the most essential elements of our corporate development plan was the expansion of the Company's capital base so that we could adequately provide the funds necessary to finance the programs and expansion. This was accomplished through earnings and supplemented through both debt and equity offerings. To implement the latter, it was determined to list the Company's stock on a national exchange and this was accomplished on November 30, 1966 when trading on the American Stock Exchange began. As of September 30, 1968 the capital base or stockholders' equity had reached $24,394,234.

Just to summarize to this point briefly, Equity Funding Corporation of America today is a fully-integrated financial service organization. Our sales team consists of approximately 2,300 representatives licensed to sell mutual funds and life insurance, operating out of 103 company-owned offices in 28 States. They are marketing sophisticated financial programs consisting principally of the insurance policies of our wholly integrated subsidiary, Presidential Life, and the shares of Equity Growth Fund of America and Republic Technology Fund, managed by our fully-integrated subsidiaries. In addition, they are selling coordinated A & H-mutual fund programs, casualty insurance-mutual fund programs, separate insurance policies, separate mutual fund investment plans, and oil partnerships in a program managed by our subsidiary, Equity Resources Corporation.

This vertical integration of our operation has enabled us to capture a greater percentage of the profit generated by each sale since we are in a position to receive the sales commission, distributor commission, insurance operating profits, management fees and financing profits. In addition, because of our philosophy of fully-integrated management, we are able to eliminate administrative duplication that could otherwise exist.

I believe you can begin to see that the sources of future earnings have been built solidly into the operation. We are often asked our estimate of those future earnings. Obviously, we cannot make specific comments or assurances in that regard. However, to the extent that the past is a prologue, you will be interested in just a few figures reflecting some elements of past performance.

Our life insurance sales from 1963 through 1967 were as follows:

$25 million, $70 million, $156 million, $226 million, $309 million. This year we are selling at the rate of $425 million.

Our mutual fund sales from 1963 through 1967 were as follows:

$3.6 million, $8.4 million, $19.7 million, $29.9 million, $36.2 million. This year we expect sales will total $65 million.

I might point out that in terms of the total insurance industry in 1963 we had .03% and in 1967 we had .23% and in terms of total mutual fund new sales our penetration increased from .15% to .78% during the same period. While we have been growing at a faster rate than either of these growing industries, there is still a great potential ahead of us in terms of the total market.

Our net after tax earnings per share adjusted for all splits and dividends including the recent 2 for 1 split for the years 1963 through 1967 were $.02, $.16, $.28, $.41, $.73 on an increasing number of shares.

Our total earnings after taxes from 1963 through 1967 have been $52,800, $389,468, $795,944, $1,177,355, $2,530,380.

Before I discuss some of our plans for the future, I would like to spend a few minutes on our recently announced acquisition of the assets of Investors Planning Corporation of America. Essentially, we are acquiring all of the assets of this mutual fund sales company, except for its non-U.S. based sales organization. In addition, we are acquiring 80% of Pension Life Insurance Company in New Jersey. The purchase price will be approximately $8.8 million plus the net worth of Investors Planning Corporation. The price will be paid in cash and notes as to 81% of the total price and in stock as to 19% of the contract amount for Investors Planning Corporation.

Just what are we acquiring? First, the sales organization consisting of approximately 1,800 representatives, which together with our present organization of representatives will bring our total to approximately 4,100. Second, we are acquiring the management company of Fund of America—approximately $108 million in assets—bringing our total of assets managed to approximately $170 million. Third, we are acquiring contractual plan trail commissions with respect to approximately $800 million in face amount of plans. Next, we are acquiring a fine field sales management group which has displayed great sales talent in the past in becoming one of the largest organizations of its type in the country. Finally, we are acquiring a real potential in terms of future life insurance and mutual fund sales. Assuming that we complete the acquisition no later than early spring of 1969, our budgeting is based on mutual fund cash sales next year for the over-all organization in the area of $225 to $250 million and insurance sales for 1969 approaching $600 million. In addition, once the administration of the company subsequent to the completion of the acquisition has been fully integrated, we expect substantial pro-rata reductions in unit operating costs. In other words, we will be able to leverage our existing administrative structure. We expect, however, that at least a full year will be required to realize the full benefit from this latter area.

Briefly as to some of our plans for Equity Funding in the future, we recently announced our intention to enter the European equity market. The flight from currency and the strong U.S. stock market are furthering the developing of this market. Plans are now being completed which include the initiation next year of operations in France, Germany, and Italy in conjunction with established companies in each of the respective countries. We see a fresh challenge to utilize our marketing techniques within a framework that is traditional to Europe. We are confident we can accomplish these goals.

In addition, plans for the Company's entrance into the investment counsel business are now being developed. We believe that the trend toward further institutionalization of the market will result in increased demand for sophisticated investment advice. Small banks, trust companies, pension and profit-sharing funds, as an example, have an increasing need for this kind of service. Their problem is primarily caused by the growing shortage and rising cost of good investment management people. We believe we can efficiently build this service as an extension of our existing investment team.

In conclusion, there is one final point that I believe is important. While our record of earnings and earnings growth has certainly been a good one, it has been accomplished in a somewhat different environment than we would have chosen. We pioneered the coordinated sale of mutual funds and life insurance. The idea passed through the stages of being ridiculed, and then violently opposed; until now it is accepted as being self-evident throughout the field of modern financial planning.

This can only be interpreted as a positive development. We

believe the market potential is still relatively untapped. For example, more than 50 million families do not own mutual funds. So with a now friendly environment, and a self-evident and accepted marketing idea, an expert management team, and a sales staff growing in both size and effectiveness and professionalization, we expect to maintain and strengthen our leadership position in the future, and we further expect that the future will bring even more impressive earnings results than the past.

Insertion to Report to New York Society of Security Analysts

by Stanley Goldblum, *President,* Equity Funding Corporation of America

November 15, 1968

On December 10, 1968, the Federal Reserve Board proposed an extension of Regulation G so that loans made under Progams initiated subsequent to the proposed effective date of the Regulation—January 31, 1969—would be subject to the margin requirements of that Regulation. If the revision is adopted, the Program would be modified so that the initial mutual fund investment will be 4 times the amount of the annual insurance premium and the subsequent total yearly investments will be 2.5 times the annual premium.

The Company has been advised that the margin requirements were not intended to apply to and would not affect any subsequent renewal loans made in connection with the completion of the originally-specified terms of Programs initiated prior to the effective date of the proposed Regulation.

MAY, 1970

EQUITY FUNDING CORPORATION OF AMERICA

SUMMARY AND CONCLUSION

The common stock of Equity Funding Corp. (19 - ASE) has been under severe pressure for several months, reflecting both general market weakness and apprehension that the mutual fund and funding businesses are in difficulty. It is a fair comment that the poor general stock market could have a dampening effect on future fund sales, but to date, the balance between new sales levels and existing program cancellations has not deteriorated markedly. Based on numerous management contacts* this year, we believe that EQF is making excellent earnings progress. Results for the first quarter were 48¢ a share, a 30% advance over year-earlier profits of 37¢ per share. We estimate earnings for 1970 at $2.30 per share fully diluted, up 22% from the $1.89 per share of 1969.

Longer term, the common stock of Equity Funding Corp. appears to be well situated to exploit a burgeoning market for life-equity funding programs, a growth sector in which the company pioneered and one in which others are now expected to join. The key variable is the ability to expand sales in an otherwise lack-luster economic financial period of indeterminate length.

EQF recognized the need for a better financial product; created a product to fill that need, the Equity Funding program; developed a marketing force to sell the product; and, then, integrated vertically all the profit centers created by the sale of the product. In these terms, we believe EQF's equity could recoup in time a multiple commensurate with its extraordinary record and bright prospects despite the generally desultory stock market. Meantime, the shares, held institutionally by several hedge funds and other heretofore aggressive performance-oriented accounts, could continue to be buffeted by inordinate degrees of forced liquidation.

*   *   *   *   *

The pertinent data concerning Equity Funding Corp. of America will enable the reader to evaluate better the company's present operations and future potential. The general field of activity in which the company operates can be described broadly as financial services. That description has been expanded to "multiple, integrated, individually programmed" financial services to describe more fully EQF's operating philosophy, and it is an important definition. Its services are considered "multiple" because the company offers a number of financial services to the public through its sales organization and continues to add new ones at all times. It is "integrated" be-cause, as a basic management philosophy, all operating entities involved in providing a particular financial service to the public should be wholly under one supervision and control and should be integrated for the client and in its presentation. EQF defines

---

*   Stanley Goldblum, President; Fred Levin, Executive Vice President; and Sam Lowell, Vice President at information meetings in each of the past several months.

-2-

itself as selling an "individually programmed" service, for it provides financial service to each client based on <u>his</u> unique circumstances and requirements. However, in order best to understand the company, because there are some difficulties in doing so, since the operation is somewhat complex, it is necessary to have a general familiarity with the primary financial product marketed, known as the Equity Funding Program. It was developed and perfected in response to the public need for a better solution to the basic financial problem each individual faces -- creating a retirement estate for himself while concurrently providing an immediate and continuing estate for his family in the event of his death. In the program, the retirement estate is achieved through the continuing purchase of mutual fund shares and the family estate is created through a policy of ordinary life insurance. It is really quite basic in its concept. These two financial vehicles, however, are integrated in one program as follows:

Having assisted a client in identifying and determining his retirement and family protection objectives and in determining, equally importantly, what funds he has available to achieve his objectives, an initial mutual fund investment is recommended and generally made. Concurrently, the client, through EQF's services, obtains sufficient life insurance in the form of an individual ordinary life insurance policy to fulfill his stated family needs. The mutual fund shares are pledged as security for a loan to pay the life insurance premiums. Each month thereafter additional pre-programmed, monthly purchases of mutual fund shares are made by the client. Each subsequent year the life insurance premiums are again paid by adding to the collateralized loan account and increasing it. This arrangement has the unique advantage of making it possible for all of the client's out-of-pocket available dollars to be invested in mutual fund shares and the borrowed dollars pay the life insurance premiums. This use of leverage provides the client the potential of creating a larger fund for his retirement. This program was developed in its present form in 1964.

There are obviously a number of other methods which the client might use to achieve these very same personal financial planning objectives. However, an objective comparison with five other methods indicates the clear-cut advantage of the Equity Funding program. *

The other five forms selected are: (1) a split-dollar level term type program; (2) a split-dollar ordinary life type program; (3) a straight savings and loan investment; (4) a retirement income at age 65; and (5) a 20-year endowment policy. The latter two are insurance policies.

In each of these assumptions a potential client makes an initial investment of $1200 and maintains his program on the basis of $100 per month. At the end of ten years, the funded program based on the results of the Keystone S4 Fund over the last ten years, will provide the client with a living result of approximately $38,400. This result is provided to the client after the repayment of the premium indebtedness and it

* An illustration of this comparison is attached on p. vii of the appendices.

- 3 -

also assumes an interest charge of 8 1/2% * per annum on the premiums being
borrowed. This compares with the other living results ranging from $33,000 down
to $11,000 for method #6. In the event that the client were to die after the 10-year
program, the death estate result, which is the investment results of the fund purchases,
plus the life insurance, less the amount of the indebtedness including the interest at
8 1/2%, would provide his family with a death estate of $58,000 comparing with the
other investment media available to him ranging down to $17,000. If the program were
to be carried for 20 years, the living results provide the client, if he had invested in a funding
program, with a living estate of approximately $162,500, comparing favorably to the others'
benefits downward to $26,000. This twentieth year assumption in connection with the funded
program again assumes the repayment of all indebtedness and again assumes interest at the
rate of $8\frac{1}{2}\%$. The death estate, the amount of benefits to be derived from the funded
program, is comparably advantageous to the client. Suffice it to say that with very
rare exceptions and at almost every age for clients for whom this program is suitable,
the potential advantages of EQF's plan are superior. The impact of the sale of an Equity
Funding program on both the corporate development and profitability of the company is
noteworthy here as well.

There are four basic profit sources available to the company as the result of
the sale of an Equity Funding program:

First is the life insurance sales commission that is available as a result of the
sale of the ordinary life insurance policy, for both first year and renewal commissions.

Secondly, there is the potential of the life insurance company statutory operating
profit available as a result of having underwritten this policy of life insurance.

Third, in connection with the sale of mutual fund shares in the program, there
is the broker-dealer sales commission, the distributor's commission and the management
fees available as the result of the cash flow from the sale of the mutual fund shares.

Fourth, there is the interest profit or spread between the interest cost and the
interest charged.

The company's chief financial service is the funded program. Its profitability for the
company is significant. The profit flow from $100 of assumed premium in the funded program
achieves the following results. The key assumptions that underlie the analysis presented
include a lapse ratio of 10% for the policies sold in the first year, and continuing at that rate for
the next two years, but at 5% per annum thereafter. Thus, at the end of a ten-year period,
approximately 55% of the original policies sold are still outstanding as funded cases. This is a
conservative projection and actual lapse ratios could be significantly lower. Also assumed is,
that 88% of the agent's commissions will vest after the first year. This is based upon the
vesting of commissions earned by agents in 1968, and paid in 1969. No consideration is given
in this analysis to increase or decrease in the market value of mutual fund shares. The client
is charged interest at $8\frac{1}{2}\%$ per annum and Equity Funding externally finances approximately 50%
of the premium at an average cost of 10%. There is a three month delay assumed in the

* Prime rate extant at date of this presentation and synopsis.

-4-

analysis between the time the client begins paying the interest and the time Equity
Funding finances the portion of the premium that is not carried for the company's
account.   The analysis includes all direct expenses of selling and processing the clients
order for all the years of the program.   It includes only historical profit centers.   Some
of the newer profit centers; e.g., brokerage commissions and earnings on cash flow
while the clients money is in company hands are not considered in this analysis.   The coinsurance rate assumed for EQF's Presidential Life Insurance Co. subsidiary is 90%.

        Chart "A", shows an analysis of the first year income based upon the assumption
that the annual premium paid by the client was $100.   The $100 premium generates pre-
tax income for EQF of approximately $102; and after-tax income of approximately $70,
over 92% of which comes from insurance earnings.   It is also interesting to note that,
without the downstream integration, the securities income in the first year would
be approximately a break-even situation, i.e., the securities income comes from
mutual fund distributor's fees. Brokerage commissions could add an additional $0.78
to after-tax earnings, with respect to the $100 assumed program, and the company
could earn an additional $0.03-$0.04 after taxes by having the use of the clients' payment
for his mutual fund purchase, again with respect to each assumed $100 of program
premium. (Page ii - appendices)

        Chart "B" presents the income over the life of the program.   It shows the ten
years of total after-tax income earned each year.   As the downstream profit centers
become more significant, securities, management fees and particularly interest become
a more significant part of the total income picture, while the insurance still remains
the primary factor, representing approximately 50% of total after-tax income during the
ten year period.   The total after-tax income of $314, is, of course, a function of the
assumed lapse ratio.   If there were no lapses, i.e., if 100% of the policies were to
remain on the books for the entire life of the program, this income after taxes would
be in excess of $450 for the initial $100 premium.   Similarly, projections of Brokerage
commissions and float would add about another $27 to total earnings. (P. iii)

        Chart "C" presents the earnings picture over the life of the program.   This $314
of after-tax earnings flows in the pattern indicated in this chart, approximately 22% in
the first year.   There is a dip in the second year, and then as the downstream profit
centers begin to contribute, income continues to grow, reaching the final peak of 12.1%
of total income in the tenth year of the program. (P. iv)

        These figures have been extrapolated as presented in Chart "D" which portrays
results if sales remain constant for the next ten years, that is every year $100
worth of premium were sold, and the clients continued to renew assuming the lapse ratio
given earlier. The first year earnings of approximately $70 grew at the rate of 27%,
with no sales increase, to $87.   Earnings continued to grow at a rate of approximately
20% until nearly the end of the period.   Over the ten year period cumulative earnings
would be 450% of the first year earnings. (P. v)

-5-

As an example of what happens when sales increase at a 10% compounded rate each year, Chart "E" (p. vi) reveals the first year sales were $100 of premium, the second year sales $110 of premium. The first year growth rate, compared to 27% as indicated by Chart "D", is now 35%, and the compound growth over the ten year life of the program, instead of representing 450% of the first year income, in the tenth year represents an excessive 733%. It is generally assumed that when mutual fund sales go down, Equity Funding Corporation's earnings will be affected. The charts however, indicate clearly that the major profit source to the company is really highly weighted in the direction of the insurance operation. As a matter of fact, during 1969 new mutual fund cash sales which were approximately $100 million, as compared to $64 million in 1968, were down from earlier projections. Mutual fund sales generally divide into two categories, those which are program mutual fund sales and those that are non-program mutual fund sales. Non-program mutual fund sales are purchases not related to the Equity Funding program. Non-program sales during 1969 were somewhat less than anticipated at the beginning of the year. However, the sales of mutual funds that were made in connection with the program met the expected levels. These sales have been continuously increasing, as the total number of mutual fund programs continues to increase month after month. This is most significant. The sale of the program, while somewhat related to the market, appears to be in reality more related to long term planning. In order to realize the full profit potential of the program sales, the company had to achieve two objectives: First, to recruit, train and organize a sales force to sell the product, and second, to form or acquire and then integrate the activity of the following corporate entities to capture the potential upstream profit centers as described earlier, which can each add to the profits available from every program sold: 1) an insurance agency to make the direct life insurance sale to the public. In that regard, the company has a number of life insurance agencies that are wholly owned subsidiaries operating in about 35 states throughout the country; 2) a life insurance company obviously in order to capture the life insurance statutory operating profits. Presidential Life Insurance Company is a wholly owned subsidiary, licensed in 45 states at this time; 3) a mutual fund management company. EQF's wholly owned subsidiary, EFC Management is the investment advisor to three mutual funds, Equity Growth Fund, Fund of America and Public Technology Fund, which are all operating in the program; 4) a mutual fund distribution company in the form of EFC Distribution Company; and 5) the finance operation.

Equity Funding has achieved those two objectives of the sales force and the companies. At the present time, the sales force consists of approximately 4,500 representatives. They are operating from 135 company-owned offices in 35 states. The sales organization is constantly being augmented (and pruned), trained and improved in quality and effectiveness. Presidential Life Insurance Company and the various insurance agencies are a corporate vehicle, then, for capturing the insurance sales and operating profits. Equity Funding Service Corporation is a subsidiary that handles the financing of the programs along with a more recently acquired company, Bishops Bank and Trust Company, which provides additional financing through utilization of foreign funds. Each of the acquisitions made or each of the companies formed and developed

- 6 -

has a coordinated objective, which is to capture upstream profits from the sale of the Equity Funding program.

There are several new profit centers recently put on stream. One of them is a subsidiary, North American Equity Corp., which is a member of the Pacific Coast Stock Exchange. Its primary objective will be to capture brokerage commissions to the extent feasible from the Mutual Fund portfolio transactions. The primary financial product market is the funding program. There are several additional financial products marketed of a more highly specialized nature. Essentially these have been developed to service the need on the part of many clients for investments that can provide income tax shelters in the fields of natural resources, oil, cattle and real estate. They generally take the form of limited partnership interests, purchased in partnerships formed by subsidiaries of the company which act as the general partners and managers of the enterprise. Here again is the management principle of filling a public need and capturing the upstream operating as well as selling profits that can be available from each sale of the product or the service. Last year, EQF acquired Au Kony Angus Corporation which is one of the leading Angus cattle breeding companies in the United States. The company is now making available through its sales organization limited partnership interests in an Angus breeding herd. Au Kony Managment Corporation is the general partner and manager of the programs. Equity Resources Corporation acts as the general partner and manager of a series of limited partnerships created by the sale of limited partnership interests through the company's sales force to the public. The monies are then invested in oil and gas exploration programs. To date, three such programs have been offered. Equity Funding Development Corporation is a real estate construction company, building various commercial and residential real estate projects in the southern California area. EFC Property Management, Incorporated will act as the general partner of a limited partnership offering limited partnership interests to the public. The partnership will then purchase buildings from the Equity Construction Company. In that same regard to assist in some of the operations that are connected with the financing, is another EQF arm, Crown Savings & Loan, a wholly-owned savings and loan association located in California.

In the course of developing each of the many operations which are potential profit centers in the sale of the Equity Funding programs and in the sale of the oil, cattle and real estate interests, management has developed substantial in-house expertise and capability in each of these specialized fields. Equity Funding takes advantage of this executive capability by investing surplus corporate funds in the very operations that are necessary to provide the respective service to its clients. Thus, some corporate funds are involved in real estate development, oil exploration, cattle breeding operations,and,to some extent,in stock market investments.

- 7 -

       Future prospects appear bright. The company's primary product, the Equity Funding program has proven acceptable. The potential number of prospects who are proper candidates for the program in terms of the profit potential of each program as explained earlier, is significant. At the present time, a total of approximately 25,000 programs are in force, but a potential many times that sum still exists. This is based on an analysis of the statistical profile of the typical present program holder and the number of individuals in the general population of similar financial circumstances. With such a vast potential and continuing opportunity to improve internal efficiency and profitability, Equity Funding Corporation of America's future appears exciting.

     *   *   *   *   *

Questions and Answers

Question: What are the capital requirements in Chart "D"?

Answer: $100 of first year premium renewed over the life of the program with the lapse ratio assumed required an average total premium per year of approximately $70. Therefore, the company needs $35 worth of financing per year on the average to carry the program plus interest.

Question: Does the company have programs to market that take into account the existing insurance that a client has?

Answer: All programs are designed to do that. It is not the objective of the program to recommend to a client that he terminate his present life insurance. When management analyzes his present circumstances and his future needs, and there is a gap, the salesman tries to fill the gap. Many clients analyze their present insurance policies and come to the personal decision that there is possibly a more advantageous method to employ the monies that are invested in cash values of life insurance policies. When they do arrive at that decision, EQF may have some recommendations as to where they might consider investing those monies, probably into mutual fund shares. However, this must be done in the context of an overall program. Life insurance companies are experiencing drains on their reserves, because people are utilizing their cash values. That is not only due to the possible activity of companies that are trying to convince people to do that. Today, with interest rates so high, people can borrow generally from their cash values at 5-5½%. It does not really take much financial acumen to figure out that they could borrow that money and do better with it. Thus, the drain that life insurance companies are experiencing is due to several factors. If the client has other stocks, EQF might suggest that he could be in a better position with some other medium.   It may offer other forms of insurance that he may want to rearrange. A total financial planning job for each client is attempted. Each sale is a two interview sale. The first interview is merely fact finding. No sale is made.

- 8 -

The information is sent back to the home office, and a recommendation is prepared for each of the clients. This is then sent back to the EQF representative who goes back on a second call at which time he presents the company's recommendation.

Question: During 1969 were any of the clients required to put up additional collateral and what was the lapse ratio?

Answer: Yes, some clients were asked for additional collateral. It was a very low percentage, about 2% of the cases, that required additional collateral. The lapse ratio was 9% on new cases. In general the lapse ratio has been below the industry average and a little better than that which had been assumed as the basis of the projections supplied earlier.

Question: Does the company assume a level interest rate during the life of the plan?

Answer: For the purposes of illustrating a plan to a client, a level interest rate is assumed; however, the interest varies from year to year. During the last five years, the interest rate has ranged from 5% to the present level of $8\frac{1}{2}$%. If interest rates come down, the company may wait a while and decrease its interest rates afterward, too. The interest rate charged is (at its option) in the range of 6% minimum to the prime plus $1\frac{1}{2}$% maximum. The client is not locked into any fixed charge of any kind; it is a completely voluntary arrangement. He enters into the program and at the end of each year, unless the company is told otherwise, the premium is automatically renewed for the following year at the rate of interest then in effect. This continues each year of the program. Generally speaking, the client makes an initial investment of perhaps $1,200 and then he invests an additional $100 a month. The $100 a month is an almost automatic investment because, in almost all the cases, the clients utilize EQF's automatic bank draft procedure. Each month, a pre-authorized investment is made in the mutual fund account. When the twelfth month or the anniversary of the policy occurs, an automatic increase in the loan balance is made, collateral shares are mechanically withdrawn from the custodian account, a new loan is made, and the client receives a statement. This occurs year after year, automatically. The interest rate charged is the rate in effect with the company at that time. The client can terminate at any time with no penalty.

- 9 -

Question: Can the client sell his mutual fund shares?

Answer: The client can liquidate all shares not required by EQF to be
                 held as loan collateral.

Question: What are the company's sales and earnings objectives for 1970?

Answer: The target for 1970 is about a 40% increase in mutual fund
                 sales and 70% increase in life insurance sales. New cash
                 mutual fund sales were $100 million in 1969; therefore, this
                 year management is expecting $140-$145 million. Life
                 insurance sales are expected to be in the neighborhood of
                 $650-$750 million in 1970, bringing to slightly in excess of
                 $1 billion the amount of business in force in Presidential
                 Life by the end of this year. In 1969, some 9,000 funded
                 programs were sold. The target for 1970, considered attainable,
                 is to double this sum. To date in the first quarter of 1970, the
                 results are close to expectations. Company earnings for 1969
                 were in the range of $10 million net after taxes, and the
                 objective is to maintain a 25% annual compound rate of growth
                 in earnings per share over the intermediate term.

Question: With respect to the sales force, what is the approximate turn-
                 over ratio that EQF is experiencing, what techniques is the
                 company employing to improve the quality of the manpower being
                 recruited, and the manpower already in house?

Answer: The turnover ratio being experienced is somewhere between
                 20%-30%, and that is perhaps midway between what the
                 securities industry and the insurance industry have been
                 experiencing. With respect to the improvement of manpower,
                 EQF's program for 1970 includes a selection technique designed
                 to add those men with greater potential than have been employed
                 in the past. For the first time the professional life insurance
                 agent is being pursued with good success. Only of late has he
                 begun to accept an Equity Funding concept and the Equity Funding
                 program. In addition a series of regionalized training programs
                 has been initiated both to qualify new National Association of
                 Security Dealers insurance examinations and then to commence
                 a three part formal training program within the first twelve months
                 that a man joins the company. This will qualify him to sell the
                 funded program and then qualify him to sell some of the more
                 sophisticated variations of the program. The company's 1970
                 plan has allocated a substantial percentage of the budget that the
                 marketing department has assumed upon itself towards this training
                 activity. Equity Funding will be training more in 1970 than it did
                 in the 1960's. It will be looking for more professional men to train

- 10 -

constantly in the sale of programs. With these training programs and with the personnel recruited to date plus those to be recruited, earnings per man should increase rather dramatically during 1970.

Question:

What are the compensation incentives?

Answer:

EQF is currently compensating its men at between 50%-70% on an incentive bonus arrangement contingent upon production. The commission structure is competitive. There have been no requests from either the men being sought or those currently within our organization for any increase in this commission structure. In addition to the recruiting and training programs developed for 1970, EQF also has a very active prospecting campaign to be activated sometime during the middle of the year.

Question:

Presumably EQF earns more from larger sales; what prevents the company from "over-selling" a customer?

Answer:

There is an economy of scale, but it is not dramatic. The program itself is a separate registered security. It is not a common stock or straight bond or a convertible bond or a debenture; rather it is an <u>investment contract</u> which is a security for statutory purposes. Consequently, every time a new sale is made, a client receives a program prospectus, he also gets a supplementary prospectus based on whether he is buying life, casualty or "A and H" insurance. In view of the fact that the company is selling a security and in view of the fact that in connection with the whole establishment of this security in earlier years, new regulations were adopted, which determined the methods by which the presentation and sale must be made, e. g., the suitability requirements. They are far more severe than the suitability requirements that one would have in the sale of a security like a mutual fund or a share of conventional common stock. There is a much greater responsibility on EQF's part to determine whether the program is suitable for the client. That is why the company has "a two interview sale": because it really cannot be determined suitably on one interview. A presentation is prepared showing the client all the charges that he will specifically have for the ten years of the program based on the assumptions. When a recommendation is made by the Program Analysis Department, in fact, if it turns out to be unsuitable at some future date, the company might have to buy it all back from him. Consequently, if anything there is probably a greater tendency to sell him a little less, than a little more.

- 11 -

Each year the program for the client is reviewed in light
of his current circumstances. Generally, people require
more as they mature in their professions.

Question:

What is the profile of a typical client?

Answer:

The industry results have been that a salesman generally
sells to people within three years of his age, hence, a 35
year old man would sell to a man between 32 and 38.
Professional men have been in business longer; therefore,
they would be expected to have slightly more assets, but if
they get to a certain age their need for insurance begins
to diminish. The client EQF is looking at is a man generally
between 30 and 50. He probably is a white collar worker,
earning about $12,000 to $15,000 a year, married with two
children, and carrying some life insurance.

Question:

Who is your major competition?

Answer:

There are about a dozen other companies that are known as
"funding companies". None of them has yet matured
sufficiently to be considered real competition, particularly
in view of the relatively untapped market that exists for
Equity Funding programs.

Question:

What is the status of the company's investment in overseas
oil exploration program?

Answer:

Progress has been encouraging but it must be conceded that
benefits of these programs will be relatively small for the
near term. In Equador EQF and Swift Company are members
of an eight company consortium. EQF has an interest in the
2.6 million acres held by this consortium for drilling rights
in the Gulf of Guayaquil.

- 12 -

EQUITY FUNDING CORPORATION OF AMERICA

Comparative Year-End Statistics

Income: (Millions)	1964	1965	1966	1967	1968	1969
Life Insurance Commissions	$1.9 (66%)	$3.5 (65%)	$4.7 (63%)	$6.9 (62%)	$10.5 (55%)	$15.2 (33%)
Mutual Fund Commissions	0.5 (17%)	1.1 (20%)	1.7 (23%)	2.1 (19%)	5.0 (26%)	19.9 (44%)
Natural Resources	n.a.	n.a.	n.a.	n.a.	0.1 (1%)	3.5 (8%)
Investment Management	n.a.	n.a.	n.a.	n.a.	1.4 (7%)	2.5 (6%)
Interest Income	0.5 (17%)	0.7 (13%)	0.9 (12%)	1.3 (12%)	1.8 (9%)	2.9 (6%)
Real Estate Income	n.a.	n.a.	n.a.	n.a.	---	1.0 (2%)
Other Income	---	0.1 (2%)	0.2 (2%)	0.9 (7%)	0.4 (2%)	0.5 (1%)
Totals	$2.9	$5.4	$7.5	$11.2	$19.2	$45.5
Net Income Per Share: (Ex-Capital Gains)	$0.16	$0.28	$0.41	$0.72	$1.35	$1.99
Net Income Per Share: Fully Diluted(Ex-Capital Gains)	$0.16	$0.28	$0.34	$0.56	$1.10	$1.90

-i-

FUNDED ACCOUNT ANALYSIS

The succeeding assumptions include historical information only
and give no consideration to new profit centers, e.g., reciprocal
brokerage and earnings on cash float.

Lapse ratio of 10% for the first three years, 5% thereafter, leaving approximately
54% of the original accounts sold outstanding at the end of the program. (In fact,
the assumed lapse ratio should be lower in view of actual experience.)

Eighty-eight per cent of agent's commissions vest after the first year, but based on
last year, this proportion may be higher.

No consideration is given to any potential increase in the market value of the mutual
fund shares.

Client is charged interest at 8 1/2% per annum. Equity Funding uses external sources to finance 50% of the total premium loans at an average cost of 10%
per annum.

There is a three month delay between the time the client begins paying interest and
the time Equity Funding finances the premium. (In fact, between 3 to 6 weeks lapse
on the actual cash outlay.)

Coinsurance rate of 90%.

Expenses include direct selling and back office processing costs.

-ii-

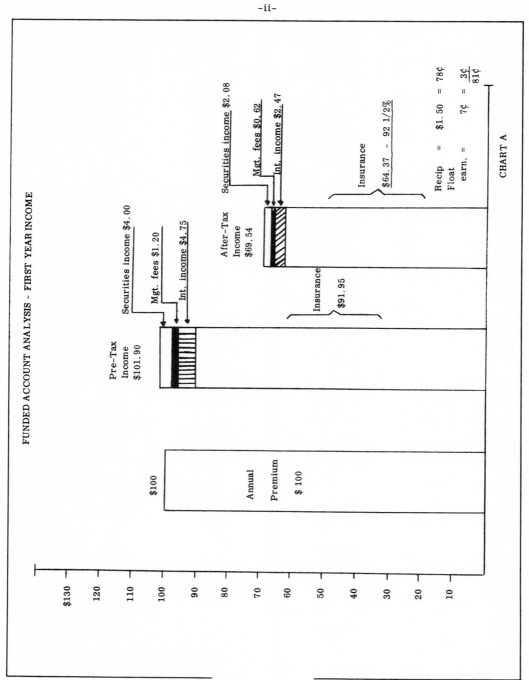

FUNDED ACCOUNT ANALYSIS - FIRST YEAR INCOME

$130
120
110
100
90
80
70
60
50
40
30
20
10

$100

Annual
Premium
$ 100

Pre-Tax
Income
$101.90

Securities income $4.00
Mgt. fees $1.20
Int. income $4.75

Insurance
$91.95

After-Tax
Income
$69.54

Securities income $2.08
Mgt. fees $0.62
Int. income $2.47

Insurance
$64.37 – 92 1/2%

Recip   = $1.50   =   78¢
Float
earn. =   7¢   =   3¢
                          81¢

CHART A

-iii-

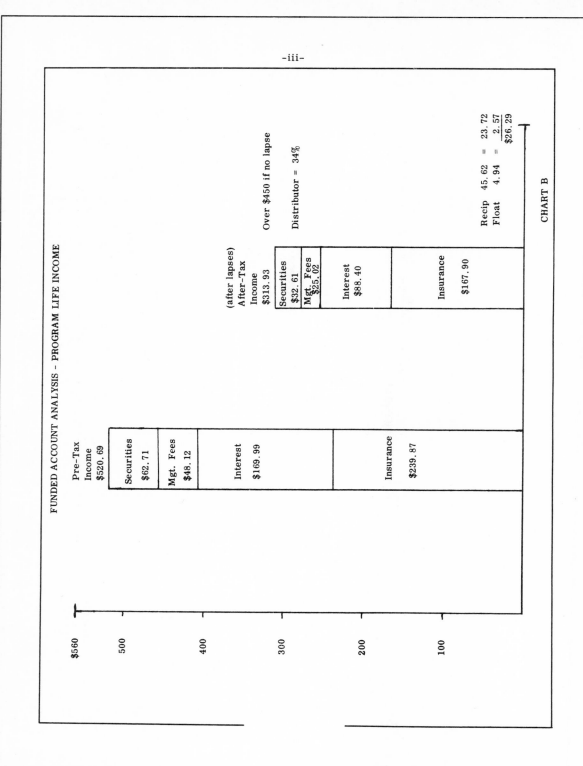

FUNDED ACCOUNT ANALYSIS - PROGRAM LIFE INCOME

CHART B

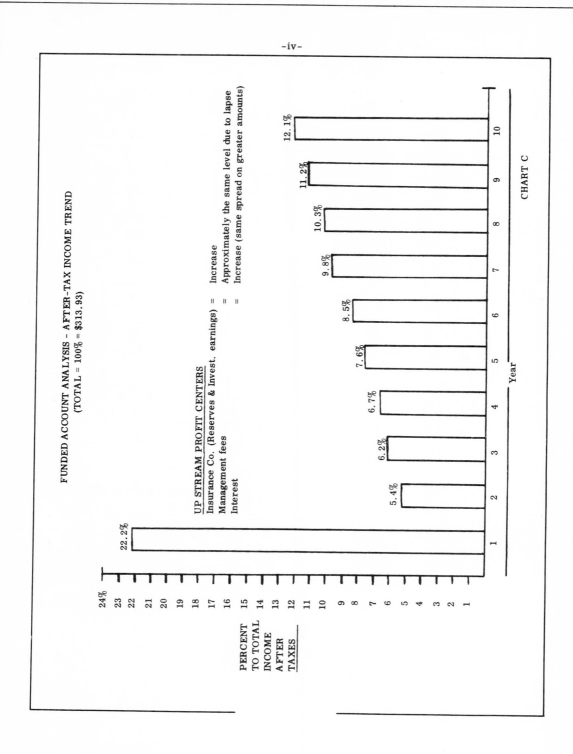

-iv-

FUNDED ACCOUNT ANALYSIS - AFTER-TAX INCOME TREND
(TOTAL = 100% = $313.93)

UP STREAM PROFIT CENTERS
Insurance Co. (Reserves & Invest. earnings) = Increase
Management fees = Approximately the same level due to lapse
Interest = Increase (same spread on greater amounts)

CHART C

-v-

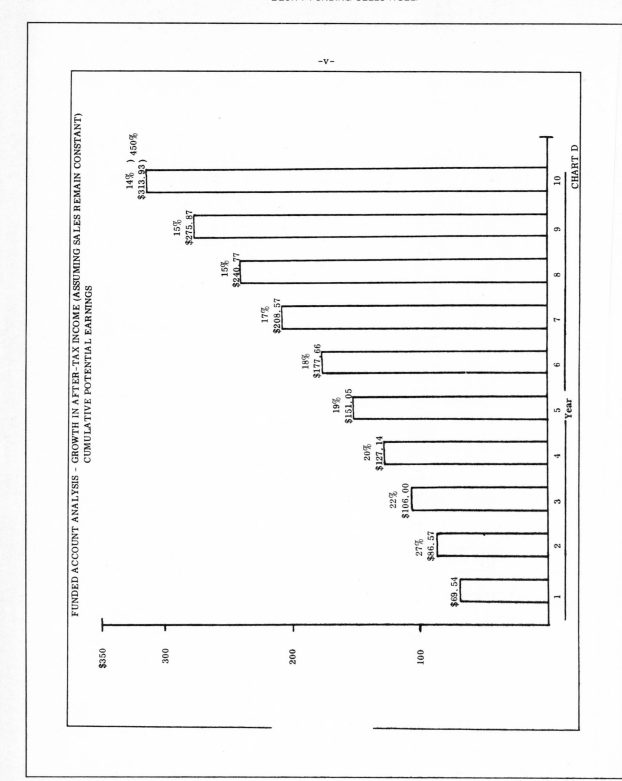

FUNDED ACCOUNT ANALYSIS - GROWTH IN AFTER-TAX INCOME (ASSUMING SALES REMAIN CONSTANT)
CUMULATIVE POTENTIAL EARNINGS

CHART D

-vi-

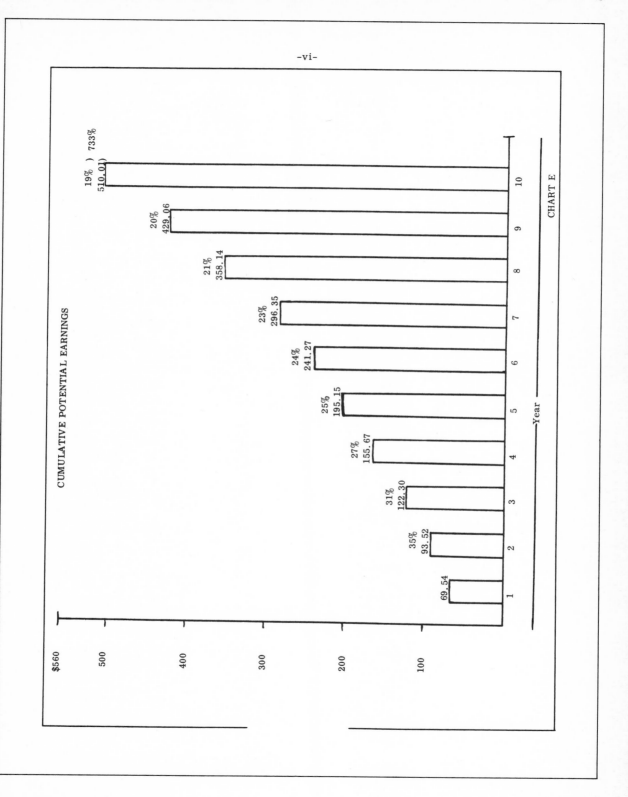

CUMULATIVE POTENTIAL EARNINGS

CHART E

-vii-

ILLUSTRATIONS COMPARING OTHER INVESTMENT PROGRAMS*

Age: 45   This Comparative Summary Assumes an Initial Outlay of $1,200 and a Monthly Outlay of $100 Thereafter.

(A) Type of Investment	(B) Annual Premium	(C) Face Amount	(D) 10th Yr. Living Results	(E) 10th Yr. Death Estate	(F) 20th Yr. Living Results	(G) 20th Yr. Death Estate
1. Funded Program	480	21,703	38,434	58,184	162,400	180,978
2. Split Dollar Level Term to 65	374	21,703	33,961	54,666	145,303	167,006
3. Split Dollar Whole Life	480	16,253	32,650	46,026	137,144	146,928
4. Savings & Loan	-	-	17,764	17,764	45,733	45,733
5. Retirement Income at 65	1,200	16,315	10,262 / 2,012(S&L) / 12,274	16,315 / 2,012(S&L) / 18,327	26,512 / 3,372 / 29,884	26,512 / 3,372 / 29,884
6. 20-Year Endowment	1,200	23,393	9,287 / 2,012(S&L) / 11,299	23,393 / 2,012(S&L) / 25,405	23,393 / 3,372 / 26,765	23,393 / 3,372 / 26,765

*See Pages viii and ix for assumptions and definitions used in this analysis

-viii-

The illustrations on the attached page are based on the assumptions and definitions listed below:

General: For all comparisons, we have selected investment programs offered by major companies with competitive benefits and premium rates. All equity investments are based on the net investment results of the Keystone S-4 Fund from January 1, 1949 to December 31, 1968. The savings and loan rates are assumed to be 5.25% per annum compounded annually. In no case was provision made for taxes on dividends, sales or exchanges.

Line 1:   The Funded Program.

Initial investment plus monthly investment after sales charges are accumulated for 20 years. The premiums for the insurance are borrowed at an interest rate of 8.5% per annum. The loan, including both principal and interest, is liquidated after each 10 year period by selling appropriate amounts of the mutual funds. The insurance premium is used to purchase a Double Whole Life to age 65 policy as well as disability income for the amount of monthly contribution. The Double Whole Life policy has level premiums, but the face amount reduces by 50% after age 65.

Line 2:   Split Dollar - Level Term to Age 65.

Enough Level Term to Age 65 was purchased to provide the same face amount as under the funded program. The excess of the amount paid under the funded program and the amount of insurance premium was invested in the Keystone S-4 Fund.

Line 3:   Split Dollar - Whole Life.

The same insurance premium as used in the funded program was used to purchase permanent life insurance. The excess of the money put into the funded program over this amount was invested in the Keystone S-4 Fund.

Line 4:   Savings and Loan.

The entire amount invested under the funded program was put into a savings and loan account.

Line 5:   Retirement Income at 65.

The Retirement Income Policy is a permanent insurance policy with premiums payable to age 65. It matures at age 65 for an amount sufficient to purchase a specified monthly retirement income. In this illustration, the entire annual contribution was assumed to be paid for the insurance policy. The initial $1,200 investment was put into a savings and loan and credited with 5 1/4% interest.

-ix-

Line 6:   20-Year Endowment.

In this example, the entire annual investment was used to purchase insurance with the excess being put in a savings and loan.

Col. B: Annual Premium.

This is the annual insurance premium payable under each of the types of investment shown in Column A.

Col. C: Face Amount.

This is the face amount of the insurance policy purchased under each of the programs in Column A.

Cols. D
  & F: Living Results.

The amounts shown in this column represent the cashout value at the end of either 10 or 20 years. They include the market value of investments, cash value of life insurance policy and amount of savings and loan accounts. In the case of the funded program, the amount of the loan is deducted from this value.

Cols. E
  & G: Death Estate.

The amounts shown in this column represent the amount payable to the beneficiary in the event of the client's death at the end of either 10 or 20 years. It includes the face amount of insurance, the market value of mutual fund investments and the value of the savings and loan account. In the case of the funded program, the amount of the loan is deducted from this value.

Equity Funding Corporation of America

Presentation by Stanley Goldblum, President, and Sam Lowell, and Fred Levin, Executive Vice Presidents, before the New York Society of Security Analysts January 22, 1973

Mr. Goldblum: Good afternoon, ladies and gentlemen. It's a pleasure to once again have this opportunity to talk to you about Equity Funding Corporation of America.

I'll lead off our presentation with an overview of our corporate structure and objectives. Then Sam Lowell, Executive Vice President of corporate operations and finance will talk to you about our finances, management and internal controls.

Fred Levin, Executive Vice President of insurance operations and marketing will conclude with a more detailed review of our insurance operations and our marketing organization.

Following that, all of us, including Yura Arkus-Duntov, Executive Vice President of investment management operations will be available for questions.

Equity Funding Corporation of America last appeared before the New York Society of Security Analysts in late 1968. Since that time the Company has grown, matured, and has made some important acquisitions. But, its primary thrust and long range objectives have not changed.

We are basically a life insurance marketing organization. In the last few years we have integrated vertically through the acquisition of life insurance companies. There were several objectives in making the more recent acquisitions, Banker's National and Northern Life. We wanted to capture the operating profits that flow from the insurance sales we generate; and to expand our operations geographically. The acquisitions have worked out very well for us in both respects.

We also desired to gain direct control over the creation of new financial products based on life insurance. Acquisition of life companies gave us the opportunity and the capacity to design new products and get them to market quickly.

As an organization, Equity Funding's great strength is marketing. We have succeeded in identifying unfilled needs in the financial services area, and have the technical capability to develop new products to satisfy those needs. Finally, we have the organization, manpower, and know how to effectively market those products.

Our primary product has been, and is, ordinary life insurance, marketed both separately and in equity-linked programs. These equity Funding Programs account for about forty-five per cent of our life insurance sales, which now have passed the two billion dollar mark annually.

Our total insurance in force at the end of 1972 was over $6.5 billion.

In the past year our individual insurance in force has been rising at an average rate of two per cent a month, approximately three times the average for all life insurance companies.

During 1971, only one stock life insurance company exceeded the $1.2 billion dollar gain of insurance in force which we achieved, independent of the effect of acquisitions.

In fact, including all of the mutual companies, there were only nine companies in the United States that had a greater net increase in insurance in force in our group. And none matched its rate of growth.

While acquisitions have augmented our expansion, it has been mainly growth plus the revitalization of the organizations we acquired that brought us to our present level of sales.

I mentioned that through our insurance acquisitions we have the control necessary for the development of new financial products, and an opportunity to broaden our geographic coverage.

With regards to the latter point, we have attempted to acquire strong regional life insurance companies and build on their base, rather than trying to carry a new name into every part of the United States.

The name, reputation, and marketing organization of an existing insurance company provides a good operating base for entering a new market. It's most likely that our objectives for expansion in the Southeast and Midwest would be implemented in that manner.

Our first insurance acquisition was Presidential Life, which we acquired in 1967 and renamed Equity Funding Life Insurance Company.

It is now the third largest company in California. In 1971 we acquired Banker's National Life Insurance Company of New Jersey, and their New York subsidiary, now known as Equity Funding Life Insurance Company of New York. Last year we acquired Northern Life in Seattle, Washington.

Our primary marketing method is the co-ordinated sale of life insurance and mutual funds in the Equity Funding Program.

For those of you not familiar with the concept, briefly, it brings the use of leverage and financial planning into the reach of approximately twenty-five million American families in the $10,000 to $25,000 income range.

There's nothing especially complicated about an Equity Funding Program. The investor buys mutual fund shares through our representative and borrows enough from us to pay the annual premium on life insurance purchased at the same time. As collateral he puts up his mutual fund shares. The total premium loan is due at the end of ten years. The investor can pay by liquidating some of his shares, or use the insurance policy cash value built up over the term of the program, or use other cash resources, or any combination of ways.

The benefit to him is that his full payments through the entire program are invested in equities, with no cash outlay for ten years for his insurance premiums.

The benefits to us are the opportunity to sell both life insurance and mutual fund shares, and to derive earnings from insurance operations and mutual fund management fees. Because, in effect, we lend the client his premium dollars each year for ten years, we have been a consumer of capital. Netting in other factors, our cash flow was negative by about $20 million in 1972. And it should be negative by about $12 million this year. We project break even cash flow in 1974, and about twelve million dollars on the positive side in 1975.

Subsequently, positive cash flow should continue to build. The big swing comes as the Equity Funding Programs mature. After ten years, for example, a client with a $1,000 annual insurance premium owes us ten thousand dollars, plus interest of about $4,000, or a total of about $14,000.

When he pays off the loans, we realize enough cash to fund fourteen new programs of comparable size. The number of programs maturing begins to rise in 1974, paralleling the rapid growth of program sales starting in 1964.

Our equity-linked insurance business also interfaces with our mutual fund activity. We manage three mutual funds with combined assets of approximately $210 million.

We sell about $100 million of fund shares per year, of which about $35 million is in shares of our own funds. As a matter of perspective, our total mutual fund activity accounts for just under ten per cent of our pre-tax earnings.

At the present time, we have approximately four thousand representatives operating from a hundred branch offices in thirty-eight states. In addition, our general agency system has nearly one thousand sales representatives, for a total of approximately five thousand sales personnel.

In addition to our life insurance, and equity-linked life insurance sales, in the past we marketed a series of proprietary tax shelter programs.

In both 1968 and 1969, when we were aiming our tax shelter products at the very high income bracket, we marketed limited partnership oil exploration programs. However in view of the limited profitability of this particular operation and the market saturation that began to develop, we discontinued this particular activity in 1969, and no further proprietary oil programs have since been offered. 1970, and '71, again aiming at the same high income market, we offered tax shelter limited partnerships in cattle breeding and feeding.

These programs were developed through a cattle breeding subsidiary, Ankony Angus Corporation, which we acquired in 1969.

However, our analysis of changes in the political and tax environment led us to decide, about a year ago, that no further proprietary programs would be offered in cattle. And in fact, in 1972 none were offered, and none are presently contemplated for the future.

In 1970, '71 and again in '72, we offered tax shelter investment programs in real estate. These programs, which consist of investments in apartment buildings constructed and managed by the company, prove to be a very desirable investment for a much broader market and for clients in a somewhat lower tax bracket.

This type of investment is particularly attractive for people who are seeking not only some measure of tax shelter, but a source of income as well. Our real estate programs have in fact fulfilled these objectives and we anticipate continuing offering this type of tax shelter investment in the future.

As a by-product of our real estate operations we have available the additional expertise in this area that is needed also by our life insurance companies for their real estate investments, and by our savings and loan subsidiary for its mortgage lending activities.

That should give you an overview of where Equity Funding has been, and where it is today. Where we plan to be tomorrow I believe is apparent as well. We plan to continue the expansion of our life insurance and sales activities, both geographically and by developing new insurance products designed to serve the changing needs of the public.

And in that context, I would like to mention one particular product with which I'm sure you're all familiar, variable life insurance, which we believe will be available in individual policy form in the very near future.

Briefly, variable life insurance, as the name implies, offers the insured a policy, which, for fixed premium, will provide a varying death benefit as well as a varying cash value dependent upon the investment experience of reserves that are invested essentially in equities. Stability is provided by including a guaranteed minimum death benefit so that the variations are only on the upside.

We are developing a marketing approach which will be based on the sale of variable life policies both separately and linked to mutual funds, with the possibility of deferring premium payments by utilizing the Equity Funding leverage principle.

In that regard, we are also studying a form of insurance that would guarantee a minimum mutual fund performance over the ten year life of such a program.

We belive that variable life will constitute about twenty per cent of a $200 billion annual life insurance market by 1980—perhaps some $40 to $45 billion of variable life a year. We believe that Equity Funding Corporation is eminently well-positioned to capture a substantial share of that market. Since we have been selling an equity-linked insurance product for the last twelve years, we already have a sales organization which is licensed and operating successfully in that kind of marketing environment.

In analyzing both the changes and the direction taken by the financial services industry over the last decade, we have learned that financial service products can become obsolete just as readily as other consumer products. And that research and development are therefore just as vital to the future success of financial service companies as they are in industrial manufacturing.

What Equity Funding Corporation has achieved to date is the product of a management team which was attracted to our company early in its development and continues on the job, applying the same talents which have brought the company to its present structure.

Mr. Samuel Lowell, our executive vice president for corporate operations and finance, will now discuss our financial picture and the internal control system so vital to producing continued growth.

Mr. Lowell: As Mr. Goldblum indicated, my segment of the presentation will cover first some of the financial statistics which, as you know, have made us the fastest growing company listed in the Fortune top fifty diversified financial services companies, and secondly, the financial controls we use to avoid surprises. And believe me, our management likes surprises even less than you gentlemen do.

Revenues have grown from $60.5 million in 1968 to $131 million in 1971. Through the nine months of 1972, total revenues stood at $104.9 million.

Revenues are increasingly at an extremely satisfactory rate. Being financially oriented, we all realize that, unless revenues grow, no company can continue to increase its profits.

An important point to note is that companies we have acquired such as Bankers, had large but relatively flat revenues under previous management. The size of those revenues tends to mask our growth when you look at pooled figures. In other words, while pooling increases our absolute figures, it tends to lower the apparent historical growth rate.

Insurance revenues account for over sixty per cent of total revenues and they continue to grow at a faster pace than total revenues.

Bankers represented $38 million of the total in 1968 and $45 million in 1971. Our growth, as you can see, has been basically internal.

It is customary in our business to use the past to predict the future. In looking at the past, we must be careful to segregate that which was run by Equity Funding and the kind of growth it produced, from the results of acquired companies before they were brought under our management.

Our earnings per share before extraordinary items, on a primary basis, have grown from $1.17 per share in 1968 to $2.45 per share in 1971. On a fully diluted basis, earnings per share were $1.04 in 1968, rising to $2.36 in 1971. For the nine months of 1972, primary earnings were $1.93 per share while fully diluted earnings were $1.73

Total earnings before extraordinary items have grown from $7.1 million in 1968 to $19.3 million in 1971. Again, for the nine months last year, we reported $15.5 million in earnings before extraordinary items.

Fully diluted earnings in 1972 appear to be somewhat less satisfactory than the growth indicated in primary earnings. The reason is that in December of 1971 we had a $38.5 million convertible debt issue, which works out to roughly a million shares, affecting fully diulted earnings but not primary earnings. As a result, the year-to-year comparisons were hurt in 1972. Looking ahead, in 1973 we are once again on a comparable basis, without this sort of distortion in the growth rates of fully diluted versus primary earnings.

Looking at the percentage composition of earnings, we find that an increasing share of our profits come from insurance. In 1970, sixty-five per cent of our total profits came from insurance operations and insurance sales. In 1971, it had grown to 72 per cent, and in the first nine months of 1972, to 77 per cent. Our profit plan for 1973 indicates that roughly 80 per cent of our profits will be coming from our insurance operations.

For the first nine months of 1972, securities income was only six per cent of total income compared to 10 per cent in 1970. Securities income includes sales commissions on mutual fund shares and limited partnership interest, and the earnings of our security brokerage subsidiary, which has seats on the regional exchanges. The significant drop from th 1970 figures reflects growth in the insurance end of the business, and also a drop in contractual plan sales. There was no such drop in straight mutual funds sales—and certainly not in funded program sales.

As a matter of fact, equity Funding's group of mutual funds has never had net redemptions. This is largely attributable to the funding program. I'll repeat it again. We have never had net redemptions in any month in our Equity Funding group of funds.

An important side issue of interest is that with the three years ended December 31, 1972, securities sales income has been less than 15 per cent of total income. Consequently, as of January 1, 1973, Equity Funding stock can now be legally purchased by mutual funds. I believe most fund managers are waiting to see the third year ratio in writing, so I think that we'll begin to see the positive effects of this after our next annual report or prospectus becomes available.

Savings and loan operations, which are shown separately because they are an unconsolidated subsidiary, have been accounting for about four per cent of net income. The last item which includes net interest income and management fees decreased from 17 per cent in 1971 to 13 per cent at the nine months of 1972. This drop obviously reflects more than just the tremendous growth of our insurance business. The main reason is the carrying cost on the Northern Life acquisition, completed in June, 1972. The interest costs were quite substantial as it was basically a cash acquisition, and this reduces our net interest figure.

Total assets, as of September 30, 1972, were in excess of $682 million. Stockholders equity was $136 million, and including subordinated debt of some $65 million, effective equity is approximately $200 million. Total debt outstanding, including notes on funded programs, was $148 million. Again, these results are as of September 30, 1972.

Even after taking into consideration roughly $33 million in intangibles (principally) excess costs over net assets of the companies previously acquired) our debt-equity ratio is about .88, not at all insignificant in a company that Mr. Goldblum described just a few moments ago as historically capital-intensive.

In an era of complex capitalizations, we have a relatively straightforward capital structure—common stock, a minor amount of preferred stock issued in connection with an acquisition, two convertible bond issues, and some warrants in connection with our debt issue in 1970.

There are, of course, stock options, a key factor in motivating and retaining our sales force. And these also have an effect on diluted earnings per share.

One last point on the balance sheet. There is a line that I object to—the caption "deferred policy acquisition recapture cost," which appears on the asset side of the balance sheet.

I object to this caption, because the word "deferred" seems to imply something intangible. Obviously, this is as real an asset as are General Motors plants. In fact, if General Motors had to sell their automobile plants, I don't know if there would be much of a market for them. If we had to sell off our book of insurance, there would be an almost instant market. In fact, historically, we've been able to prove that insurance has an instant market.

Let me now discuss our cash flow situation. As Mr. Goldblum indicated, our cash flow has been negative historically. We feel the turning point is 1974.

The last topic I want to discuss is financial and operating controls. As you know we're a marketing company. But no manager can be really effective unless he has an effective control system behind him. The best way I can think of to illustrate our financial controls is to talk about our budgeting process.

This process begins with a statement by senior management defining our corporate objectives and policies in very broad terms. This statement, in turn, is distributed to all operating heads throughout the company and becomes the basis for individual plans developed by each operating department. The plans are not only numerical (I know almost every company of any sophistication has a numerical budget) but we also use an extensive narrative budget. The first question we want our managers to ask is—"What business am I in and what business do I want to be in?"

We ask every executive to focus on that question, and not only write a detailed report every year, but revise his report quarterly. It becomes an intensive analysis of what he is doing, what his goals and objectives are—and why. The obvious purpose is to relate the year's goals to our long-range planning process at the executive level.

Each department head prepares a one-year budget and profit plan of our entire monitoring system. We don't burden all the operating heads with detailed plans beyond one year, although we do ask them to go into broad plans for their natural operating cycle.

From these plans, budgets are developed which are consistent with the goals indicated. Then the department plans are reviewed and consolidated at each level as they rise upward in the organization. The final step, of course, before approval by the board, is a summary by each of the seven executive vice-presidents of their particular operating plans for the year.

This book in turn is submitted for distribution to the board. When approved, these summaries are the end result of some three hundred control units used in the budgeting process.

It's really a very detailed analysis. A valuable side benefit of the budget is that it enables us to get computerized models of our operations. It's particularly important in reporting, not only for information, but also for control. We are able to extract sensitivity factors by analyzing the computer models of our operation. We function on a management-by-exception basis. One report sometimes comes to me blank, because the operations people only report problems of which I should be aware. Of course, it's a very good week when I receive a blank report.

After the master plan is made, we continually monitor it not only with the computerized mathematical models I mentioned, but also with a regular analysis on both a weekly and monthly basis.

Management meetings are held at all levels. The executive vice-presidents have a regularly scheduled executive planning committee meeting every two weeks, and a daily luncheon meeting to discuss specific problems, so we keep on top of what we're tracking.

We also commission special studies which we call "white papers." When a problem arises and we want more detailed information on it, we set up a project team and study it.

I trust that I've made the point that we not only have a powerful management but that computer techniques are widely used throughout the company. This leads me to comment on the trend of selling, general and administrative expense. Our SG&A expenses, in relation to total revenues, reflect substantial reduction from mid-1970. Of course, part of the reason is that the control system we've installed really became effective in late 1970 and early 1971.

The second reason has been the increasing effectiveness of our computer operations. The insurance business is a high transaction business, and therefore, very adaptable to computerization.

The rather large jump in SG & A in 1969 principally reflected the acquisition of Investors Planning Corporation, a large mutual fund sales organization in the East. This acquisition was completed prior to the establishment of a special department which now employs techniques, such as PERT networks, to facilitate the integration of acauired corporations.

Finally, let's examine Equity Funding's organization structure. The company is divided into two distinct parts—the operating management and control or administrative management. None of our operating executives has his own controller, legal counsel or administrative facilities man. All of these functions report to the other parts of the organization.

Because they don't control their own financial people, our executives cannot mask problems until it is too late for senior management to do anything about it. We know about it as soon as the executive knows about it and sometimes before.

Summarizing: Equity Funding has a corporate structure which is organized vertically by product area and horizontally by function. The systems is flexible, responsible and adaptable to our needs. I think it has been, second to marketing the key element in our past growth: and we believe it will continue to serve us well in the future. Thank you.

Mr. Levin: A few days ago, I received confirmation that during 1972 we sold over $2.1 billion of new business. Three quarters of that business was ordinary life.

I believe this is particularly significant, as it moves us into the top one per cent of the life insurance industry in terms of ordinary sales.

This accomplishment was made possible by two key aspects of our business—our marketing organization and our life insurance subsidiaries.

Let me review first some statistical operating information: Equity Funding Life in 1972 had ordinary life sales of approximately $1.4 billion, up from approximately $1.1 billion in 1971. Bankers National sold $127 million in 1971, and increased that to $157 million in 1972.

During 1972 Bankers also increased its proportion of ordinary life sales, and this is reflected in the rise in Bankers first year premium from $1.8 million in 1971 to slightly over $3 million in 1972.

Let's analyze life insurance in force by company: Insurance in force for Equity Funding Life rose to $3.3 billion, a $2.1 billion increase from 1971. I should point out that Equity Funding Life's business is 99 per cent ordinary. (The only exception is group term on our own employees.)

At Banker's approximately 55 per cent of the business in force is group insurance. At Northern, most of the $721 million of life insurance is ordinary life.

Total premium income. We estimate that for the year ended December 31, 1972, Equity Funding will have received $89 million in premium income from its four life insurance subsidiaries. There was an increase in permanent insurance premium from $37 million in 1971 to $45 million in 1972 and terminsurance premiums from $9.9 million to $17 million in 1972. There was virtually no group insurance added during the year. The group insurance business currently on the books will be continued mainly as an accommodation.

I think in analyzing what we've accomplished, we first have to begin with our marketing operation. At the end of 1972, we had about one hundred company-owned branch offices with approximately four thousand sales representatives, and one thousand agents operating out of two hundred and fifty general agencies throughout the country. These general agencies represent Bankers National, Equity Funding Life of New York and Northern Life.

For those of you who have been following our company over a period of time—at least with respect to the branch office organization and the number of its sales representatives—I think you will have observed a reduction from an all-time high of about 5,600, immediately after the acquisition of Investors Planning to which Sam Lowell referred.

Over the last three years we have implemented a control system requiring a certain minimum production on the part of representatives in order to remain with the branch operation.

In addition, these controls have been applied to the branch offices themselves. You may remember that at our high we had as many as 140 branch offices. Currently, we have about 100.

The key figure—the one constantly reviewed by management—relates to productivity per agent of our branch operations. Production from the branches over a period of two years, has doubled, and production per man has risen from $138,000 in 1969 to approximately $310,000 in 1972.

In addition to upgrading the selection of men and setting certain minimum criteria for the branches, we established a dual distribution system: branches and general agencies. We take stock at quarterly intervals to determine which branches, if any, should be converted to general agencies and which general agencies should be converted to branches.

We find that the more entreprenurial individual is better suited to remaining with the general agency operation, and that an individual who requires closer supervision and more company administrative support, functions better in the branch operation.

I think a classic example of this is what has just occurred in St. Louis and Phoenix. In St. Louis, we had a branch operation grossing about $7,500 a month in premiums, about half our objective for that branch.

We also had a general agency in St. Louis, so we transferred the agents and the accounts from the branch operation to the general agency. That strengthened the general agency by $90,000 a year in premiums and ten or twelve men.

On the other hand, we had a general agency in Phoenix that was writing about $120,000 in premiums a year. The general agent indicated that he wanted a little more company support and closer supervision. He was most amenable to converting his general agency to a branch office operation.

Throughout 1973, as we've done in 1972, we anticipate converting branches grossing under $15,000 a month to general agencies. Conversely, we are contacting general agencies writing in excess of $120,000 a year in premiums, and asking them if they would like to convert to a branch office operation.

I think the $1.4 billion of ordinary life insurance written by Equity Funding Life during 1972 graphically indicates the reason the company implemented in 1968 the co-insurance concept, as part of our long-term planning. During 1971, about 50 per cent of our business was reinsured and about 50 per cent retained.

In 1972, writing $20 million of new ordinary life premiums, approximately 60 per cent was retained and 40 per cent was reinsured. The company plans during 1973 to co-insure 20 to 25 per cent of the new premiums generated. Beginning in 1974, we expect to co-insure only that amount which exceeds our retention—perhaps five per cent of the total written.

One last comment with respect to co-insurance: The quality and persistence of the business we write has led to co-insurance allowances of 180 to 200 per cent of first year premiums, compared to an industry norm of 110 to 120 per cent.

Appropriate renewal allowances are also paid, varying between 10 and 15 per cent. In each of our 10 reinsurance treaties, there are recapture privileges or provisions. Some permit recapture beginning with the sixty policy year, others at the eighth or eleventh years.

We intend to recapture at the first opportunity the business that has been co-insured. A cash flow drain occurs at the time of recapture, as the re-insurer will pay the cash values over to the ceding company, while the ceding company must set up a full reserve. Because of this drain, we have set up an appropriate policy recapture reserve in our GAAP conversion. The cost of the recapture, therefore, is amortized throughout the period of the co-insurance agreement.

The key to both our marketing and operations at Equity Funding is the Equity Funding Program. While we don't have full figures for 1972, we do anticipate record sales. At September 30, 1972, over 48,000 programs were in force. About 11,500 programs were sold during the first nine months of the year, and approximately 4,300 on a base of 48,000 were terminated during the period.

Mr. Goldblum indicated that program sales account for about 45 per cent of all life insurance sales. I think it's fair to say that the Program is the company's principal prospecting and recruiting tool.

I would estimate that, in about 90 per cent of the prospecting done by our field organization, the Equity Funding Program is the chief door opener. It also gives our agents the confidence to prospect aggressively because they know that the Program has unusual appeal to the client.

In addition, we've been successful over the past 15 months in recruiting professional life insurance men because of the availability of the Equity Funding Program, both in its simplest form and as it applies to pensions and profit sharing plans and key-man insurance programs.

The financial services business, and ours more than most, generally requires a large investment in sales manpower. This investment can be productive or not—depending on five fundamentals: **marketing structure, compensation, recruitment, training** and **supervision.** From the very start of our company, a policy decision was made and successfully adhered to: maximize sales incentives and minimize sales overhead. In practice, this means that our entire marketing structure is based upon commissions and overrides, so that every man is rewarded according to his productivity. We are now looking into ways of trying field management compensation to profitability as well as productivity.

Our salesmen, with very few exceptions, get no long-term draws or advances. This is made possible by the nature of our product line and our training methods, which help get new men off to a fast start. They don't become dependent on financing arrangements, and the company avoids building up a large and risky book of agent debit balances.

Our training operations were greatly expanded during 1972, and week-long basic schools now operate on a nearly continuous basis on the East and West coasts. Later this year, we will be introducing both a management training program and an advanced course for experienced salesmen. Our training systems have proved remarkably effective, and our financial sales representatives generally are licensed and trained in both life insurance and equities. As a matter of sales policy, we don't attempt to train all of our men in every product or service we offer. In highly technical areas, such as tax shelter programs and qualified pension and profit sharing plans, most of our men are trained only to prospect and qualify their prospects. Technical counseling and closing the sale are the responsibility of specialists who work with the men on a split commission basis. Here again, we have been able to build an effective marketing force without large numbers of salaried staff people.

I have deliberately left for last what really should be first—recruiting—but I wanted to provide you with background on what we are recruiting into. Our recruiting efforts are now concentrated largely in the life insurance area, where we have been very successful in attracting qualified, experienced people. This has been facilitated by our compensation system, which pays our men a dual commission for selling our Equity Funding programs. Our full product line—including funding programs, tax shelters and qualified retirement plans—are made available to appropriately licensed members of both distribution systems.

To summarize: I would say that we're aggressive in our marketing posture within our own industry. I would say that we're conservative in our financial management to keep each operation economical and profit-oriented.

I would also say we are innovative in product development, and certainly we are very traditional in our conviction that by serving the public's real needs, we will continue to grow in accordance to the objectives we set for ourselves.

Thank you.

QUESTIONS AND ANSWERS

Chairman: Thank you very much, Fred, and Sam. Tradition calls for us to have questions now.

Question: In making projections on variable life, what kind of first year commission assumptions have you made?

Mr. Levin: We've made the assumption that the variable life policy will be available on a traditional commission structure basis, and that variable life will not be subject to the 1940 Act, but will be subject to the 1933 Act. The first year commission is assumed to be 50 per cent under those conditions.

Question: Would you review the investment performance in your own funds relative to the broader market indices?

Mr. Arkus-Duntov: The performance of Equity Growth Fund, which is the primary fund in our funded programs, has been quite satisfactory. The performance of the two other funds have been somewhat less than satisfactory.

Fund of America this year has come up in its performance. Equity Progress is still lacking. But I repeat again that the fund which is used for the Equity Funding Programs had a satisfactory performance over the last five years.

Question: When do you expect the prospectus to be available which would confirm that Equity Funding stock is now eligible for purchase by mutual funds?

Mr. Goldblum: Financial figures would be available by March. However, there's no doubt that the contribution to total earnings of our securities operation was around ten per cent.

In fact, based on the information that we have, we have completed three full years where securities income was less than fifteen per cent. . .

Question: Would you care to make some comment on the Ecuadorian situation and what implication that would have for long-range attitudes toward the oil business?

Mr. Arkus-Duntov: Let me begin by suggesting that the remark which I'm about to make relates to a highly sensitive area involving international and domestic affairs of another country. Accordingly, I would like to keep my remarks brief and would prefer not to expand the discussion beyond this remark.

As you are aware the government of Ecuador issued a decree at the end of November alleging improprieties in the original grant of a concession in the Gulf of Guayaquil to a consortium in which our subsidiary owns a 23.75 per cent interest.

The allegations of the improprieties were not directed against the consortium and came as a surprise to us. At the December meeting of the board of directors of our company the management decided a representative should go to Ecuador to investigate the matter in order to make a first-hand report to the board.

I was designated as that representative and spent most of the week of January 7 in Quito. During that time I had the opportunity to visit with many of the officials of the government, who were involved in and concerned with the hydrocarbon area. Our meetings were without any question cordial, and I believe they were quite frank.

Concurrent with those conversations I had further conversations with persons familiar with other facets of Ecuador's international relations.

On the basis of what we have learned, we are convinced now that it is in the best interest of Ecuador to negotiate a new arrangement with our group, for development of the discovered dry gas reserves. We believe that this fact is fully recognized by the government.

The government, by various public statements as well as private statements, has led us to believe that it will shortly embark on negotiations. These negotiations may take different forms. But the Ecuadorian government will embark upon them with a full appreciation of our investment, and the unique economic problems involved in the development of these reserves.

Chairman: Does that answer the question?

Question: Well, partially. My understanding as of perhaps six or eight months ago was that the Company had intended getting out of the oil business entirely. How does that stand now?

Mr. Goldblum: We have no plans to go any further in the oil business in any regard, whether or not things develop successfully or otherwise in Ecuador.

The policy decision was made. This is not a business for our Company to be in. We intend to implement that policy at the most appropriate time.

Question: The question has to do with the cost of the programs. Assuming a thousand dollars a year payment, what would be the cost of buying the fund? And secondly, the interest on the loan?

Mr. Levin: The sales cost in connection with the purchase of a mutual fund would be eight and three quarters per cent. A thousand dollars of fund shares collateralizes a $400 annual premium, and the interest rate on the $400 loan would currently be 7¾ per cent.

Question: What would be the start up costs involved in variable life insurance?

Mr. Levin: It's very difficult to indicate what the start up costs will be until the SEC announces their final conclusion. A great deal of research and development work has already been done in 1972. A separate account has been established. The policy forms have been prepared and filed, and investments simulation has been done with respect to a typical portfolio over the last ten years. Our real costs will be directly contingent on what the requirements are imposed by the SEC. Let's assume that only the 1933 Act is applicable. The costs would then include the preparation and filing of a prospectus, but the main cost will be in selling the product to our own distribution operation, that is, in training our own sales force. Until such time as we have a better handle on what the requirements will be, we couldn't even hazard a guess as to what that cost will be.

We can say that because our distribution operation is already oriented to the sale of an equity-linked life insurance product, our start up costs will perhaps be appreciably less than those of some others in the life insurance industry.

Chairman: This, then, completes the luncheon meeting for the Equity Funding Corporation. Thank you very much.

PRESS RELEASES AND A FEW SLIPS

Equity Funding issued a large number of press releases, most of them confined to routine announcements of quarterly earnings and acquisitions. Some, however, are of particular interest. (For those who wish to read other EFCA press releases, most stock brokerage libraries tend to keep fairly complete files.)

The January 6, 1971, release announces that sales of new policies during 1970 were "over $750 million" (face value), an obviously impressive figure compared to the "approximately $350 million" the prior year. The $750 million also appeared in a *Wall Street Journal* story on February 5, 1971.

However, a March 4, 1971, release notes that EFCA's representatives wrote "over $800 million" of new insurance in 1970. The $800 million appeared in the annual report. It might be argued that the January and February figures were only preliminary, but the company did not label them as such, nor was any explanation of the difference offered. In retrospect, the difference equal to 3½ weeks' sales was another possible indication of the last minute 1970 falsification of policies.

The supposed doubling of insurance in force was accomplished in a year when the industry total increased by less than 4 percent and when, according to its prospectuses,

Equity Funding's sales force increased by only 16 percent. The remarkable productivity of the EFCA sales force hit new levels in 1971, when sales continued to increase in the face of a supposed decrease in the sales force.*

Shareholders were not the only ones who failed to tumble to the EFCA fraud. As a June 29, 1972, release indicates, only nine months before the fraud broke, a group of banks, including First National City and Wells Fargo (as well as the ill-fated Franklin National Bank) was willing to increase EFCA's line of credit by $35 million to $105 million. Note that the first $70 million line was announced only a few months earlier on April 7, 1972.

Undoubtedly, the March 12, 1973, release is the most interesting. Here are the infamous 1972 results, which were never issued in an audited annual report. Note that there is no mention that the figures are unaudited.

*The prospectus dated November 6, 1969 gave the sales force as being "approximately 5000". The December 9, 1970 prospectus said 5800. In the December 7, 1971 prospectus the figure is back to 5000.

EQUITY FUNDING CORPORATION OF AMERICA

NEWS RELEASE

NR-4014
Further Information: Gary S. Beckerman
                       Advertising/Communications

1900 Ave. of the Stars
Los Angeles
California 90067
(213) 553-2100
Cable: Equifund

FOR IMMEDIATE RELEASE

EQUITY FUNDING LIFE CROSSES $1 BILLION MARK OF INDIVIDUAL LIFE
INSURANCE IN FORCE

LOS ANGELES - January 6, 1971 - Equity Funding Life Insurance
Company, a wholly-owned subsidiary of Equity Funding Corporation of
America, has crossed the $1 billion mark of individual life insur-
ance in force, according to Stanley Goldblum, president of the
parent organization.

Goldblum said EFCA's dually-licensed sales representatives
wrote over $750 million of new individual insurance during 1970,
and approximately $350 million the year before. The bulk of this
insurance, Goldblum pointed out, was written as part of the
"Equity Funding" Coordinated Mutual Fund/Insurance Program.

"The strong increase in life insurance production during the
last two years reflects the growing public acceptance of the 'Equity
Funding' Program," he said.

Organized in Illinois in 1959 as Presidential Life Insurance Co.,
the insurer was acquired by EFCA, an integrated financial services
company, in October, 1967, and was renamed Equity Funding Life last
August.

"Reaching the one billion dollar milestone in such a short
period of time is a tremendous tribute to our field force," Goldblum
continued. "Quite obviously, this kind of production can only be

Equity Funding Life Crosses $1 Billion Mark   NR-4014   Page 2

generated by a professional, thoroughly dedicated group of people."

        Equity Funding Corporation of America has 125 offices nation-
wide. Other wholly-owned subsidiaries include a mutual fund
management company which manages three domestic mutual funds,
a mutual fund distributing company, a savings and loan association,
a company holding a seat on three regional stock exchanges, and
companies operating investment programs in cattle breeding, real
estate and oil and gas.

                                   #

EQUITY FUNDING CORPORATION OF AMERICA

News Release

CONTACT: Gary S. Beckerman -- Director of Communications
           Christopher Godchaux -- Argosy Group   (213) 655-5533
           Victor Kramer -- Argosy Group (212) 753-6715

NR-4020

                                        FOR IMMEDIATE RELEASE

▶ EQUITY FUNDING REPORTS
   RECORD EARNINGS AND REVENUES FOR 1970

LOS ANGELES, March 4, 1971 - Equity Funding Corporation of America
today reported record earnings from operations of $2.21 per share
for the year ending Dec. 31, 1970 compared with $1.91 a share a
year ago.

     Stanley Goldblum, President and Chairman of the Board of the
Los Angeles based integrated financial services company, said
consolidated net income before extraordinary items was $12,694,434
in 1970, up from $10,093,530 in 1969.

     Gross revenues rose to a record $60,912,874 in 1970 compared
with $48,033,408 the year before.

     Net income for the fourth quarter ended December 31, 1970 was
$4,203,654 equal to 71 cents per share on gross revenues of $26,059,377.
In the fourth quarter of 1969, the company netted $3,416,019 or 62
cents a share on $15,573,511 of gross revenues.

     On December 31, 1970 the company had approximately 5,750,000
shares outstanding compared to 5,290,000 the previous year.

                                        (more)

1900 Ave. of the Stars. Los Angeles. California 90067 (213) 553-2100 Cable: Equifund

NR-4020
Equity Funding Reports
Record Earnings and Revenues for 1970

Page 2

Goldblum said the increase in earnings is largely attributable to the growth of Equity Funding's insurance operations. He noted that net earnings for the company's wholly-owned life insurance subsidiary, Equity Funding Life, increased to $5,094,646 in 1970, or more than double the $2,116,415 reported for 1969.

The company's insurance subsidiary recently announced the crossing of the $1 billion mark of life insurance in force. EFCA's dually licensed representatives wrote over $800 million of new individual insurance during 1970, and approximately $350 million the year before. The bulk of this insurance, Goldblum pointed out, was written as part of the "Equity Funding" coordinated mutual fund/insurance Program which the company pioneered in 1960.

On February 25, 1971 Equity Funding Corporation of America declared its annual cash dividend of 10 cents a share.

Equity Funding Corporation of America, listed on the New York Stock Exchange, operates 100 offices nationwide. Wholly-owned subsidiaries include a life insurance company, a mutual fund management company which manages three domestic mutual funds, a savings and loan association, a company holding a seat on three regional stock exchanges, and companies operating investment programs in cattle breeding, oil and gas and real estate.

(more)

NR-4020
Equity Funding Reports
Record Earnings and Revenues for 1970

Page 3

EQUITY FUNDING SUMMARY OF CONSOLIDATED OPERATIONS

	1970	1969 (a)
Twelve Months to December 31:		
Total income.....................	$60,912,874	$48,033,408
Net earnings after preferred dividend of $42,500 in 1970......	$12,694,434 (b)	$10,093,530 (b)
Per share (c).....................	$ 2.21 (b)	$ 1.91 (b)
Approximate number of shares outstanding.....................	5,750,000	5,290,000
Fourth Quarter to December 31:		
Total income.....................	$26,059,377	$15,573,511
Net earnings after preferred dividend of $42,500 in 1970......	$ 4,203,654 (b)	$ 3,416,019 (b)
Per share (c).....................	$ .71 (b)	$ .62 (b)

(a) Restated to reflect an acquisition on a pooling of interest
     basis, 2% stock dividend in April 1970, and a change in reporting
     of income from its life insurance subsidiary from statutory to
     generally accepted accounting principles, which amounted to a
     decrease in ordinary earnings of $332,461 and a decrease in
     extraordinary income of $70,000 for 1969.

(b) Excludes extraordinary loss of $1,021,309 in the quarter and
     $1,021,309 in the twelve months of 1970, compared with an extra-
     ordinary loss of $3,790 and extraordinary income of $636,006,
     respectively, in the like 1969 periods.

(c) On a fully diluted basis, per share earnings were 70 cents in
     the quarter and $2.14 in the twelve months of 1970 compared with
     61 cents and $1.83, respectively, in the like 1969 periods.

#####

EQUITY FUNDING CORPORATION OF AMERICA

News Release

CONTACT:

Gary Beckerman, EFCA Director of Communications -- (213) 553-2100
Christopher Godchaux, The Argosy Group -- (213) 655-5533
Victor Kramer, The Argosy Group -- (212) 753-6715

<u>FOR IMMEDIATE RELEASE</u>

    EQUITY FUNDING EXPANDS
<u>CREDIT ARRANGEMENT TO $105 MILLION</u>

LOS ANGELES, June 29, 1972 -- Equity Funding Corporation of America
(NYSE) said today it has expanded a recently negotiated $70 million
credit arrangement with a group of institutional lenders to $105
million.

The previous $40 million unsecured revolving term loan portion
of the arrangement, which went into effect April 5, 1972, has been
supplanted by a new $75 million secured revolving credit term loan
arranged by a group of banks headed by First National City Bank of
New York.

A previously established $30 million line of credit arrangement
to finance <u>Equity Funding</u> Insurance Premium Funding Programs remains
unchanged.

Approximately $35 million of the new $75 million revolving
credit term loan will be used in connection with Equity Funding's
acquisition of Northern Life Insurance Co. of Seattle. The remainder
will be available as needed for general corporate purposes.

.....more

1900 Ave. of the Stars, Los Angeles, California 90067 (213) 553-2100 Cable: Equifund

2)

Participating with First National City in the new $75 million revolving credit term loan are Wells Fargo Bank (San Francisco), Franklin National Bank (New York) and the National Bank of North America (New York).

#####

EQUITY FUNDING CORPORATION OF AMERICA

News Release

CONTACT: Victor M. Kramer, EFCA Director of Marketing Services (213) 553-2100
           Dean Erickson, Booke & Co. (213) 657-6460
           Robert Frost, Booke & Co. (212) 593-8600

                        FOR IMMEDIATE RELEASE

▶   EQUITY FUNDING REPORTS RECORD EARNINGS
    AND REVENUES FOR 1972

LOS ANGELES, March 12, 1973 --Equity Funding Corporation of America
(NYSE/PCSE), a life insurance-based financial services company,
today reported record earnings from operations of $2.81 per share
for the year ending December 31, 1972, up from $2.45 per share in
1971.

    Stanley Goldblum, president and chairman of the board, said
consolidated net income rose to $22,617,000 in 1972, a 17% increase
over 1971 earnings of $19,332,000.

    The company reported no extraordinary gains or losses in 1972.
In 1971 it had reported an extraordinary loss of $1,140,000 or
$.14 per share.

    Earnings per share are based on approximately 8,036,000 shares
in 1972 and 7,883,000 shares in 1971.

    Consolidated gross revenues increased to a record $152,601,000
in 1972, up 17% from $130,951,000 the year before.

    Net income from operations for the fourth quarter ended December 31,
1972, was $7,132,000 or $.88 per share on gross revenues of $47,696,000.
In the comparable period in 1971, the company earned $6,149,000 or
$.79 per share on revenues of $44,616,000.

1900 Ave. of the Stars, Los Angeles, California 90067 (213) 553-2100 Cable: Equifund   more...

- 2 -

Mr. Goldblum said that the company's 1972 figures include Northern
Life Insurance Company since its acquisition on June 29, 1972.
Northern Life contributed $10,667,000 to 1972 gross revenues and
$437,000 to net earnings, after deducting amortization of goodwill
and interest expenses related to the acquisition.

Life insurance sales in 1972 amounted to a record total of $2.5
billion, Mr. Goldblum said, compared with $2.0 billion in 1971.
The company's 1972 sales consisted of $1.6 billion in individual
policies and $872 million under group plans. As of December 31,
1972, Equity Funding's life insurance company subsidiaries had
$6.5 billion of life insurance in force, compared to $4.6 billion
at the end of the previous year. Individual insurance accounted
for $4.8 billion of the 1972 total in force and $3.1 billion of
1971's insurance in force. The 1972 figures include Northern
Life's insurance in force of $602 million and sales of $40 million
in the six months since acquisition.

On March 8, Equity Funding's board of directors declared a
fourth consecutive annual cash dividend of 10 cents per share.
The dividend is payable on May 7, 1973, to stockholders of record
on April 6, 1973.

more...

- 3 -

EQUITY FUNDING SUMMARY OF CONSOLIDATED OPERATIONS

	1972(b)	1971
Twelve Months to December 31:		
Total Income (a)	$152,601,000	$130,951,000
══
Net earnings from operations		
-before extraordinary items	$ 22,617,000	$ 19,332,000
-extraordinary items (loss)	-	(1,140,000)
-after extraordinary items	$ 22,617,000	$ 18,192,000
══
Per share from operations(c)		
-before extraordinary items	$2.81	$2.45
-extraordinary items (loss)	-	(.14)
-net earnings after extra-		
ordinary items	$2.81	$2.31
══
Average number of common &		
common equivalent shares		
outstanding	8,036,000	7,883,000
══
Fourth Quarter to December 31:		
Total Income (a)	$ 47,696,000	$ 44,616,000
══
Net earnings from operations(c)		
-before extraordinary items	$ 7,132,000	$ 6,149,000
-extraordinary items (loss)	-	(1,140,000)
-after extraordinary items	$ 7,132,000	$ 5,009,000
══
Per share from operations		
-before extraordinary items	$.88	$.79
-extraordinary items (loss)	-	(.14)
-net earnings after extra-		
ordinary items	$.88	$.65
══

more...

- 4 -

(a) Includes the consolidation of all subsidiaries other than
    Liberty Savings & Loan Association.

(b) Includes the operating results of Northern Life Insurance
    Company, acquired on June 29, 1972. Northern Life's contri-
    bution to 1972 gross revenues was $10,667,000 from date of
    acquisition, and $4,806,000 for the three months ended
    December 31, 1972.

    Primary 1972 net earnings of Northern Life, after deducting
    amortization of goodwill and interest expenses related to
    the acquisition, were $437,000. Both primary and fully di-
    luted earnings of Northern Life were $.05 per share from the
    date of acquisition and $.03 per share for the three months
    ended December 31, 1972.

(c) On a fully diluted basis, per share earnings from operations
    were $2.51 in the twelve months of 1972 and $.78 in the quart-
    er, compared with $2.36 and $.74 respectively in the like 1971
    periods. Fully diluted earnings after extraordinary items
    were $2.51 in 1972 and $2.23 in 1971.

- 30 -

ANOTHER AUDITOR LOOKS AT EQUITY FUNDING AND ALMOST FINDS THE FRAUD

Not everyone who dealt with Equity Funding was totally lacking in suspicion. In early 1970, Ranger National Life Insurance Co., one of the largest reinsurers of Equity Funding's (fake) life insurance policies asked its auditors, Peat, Marwick, Mitchell & Co., to check Equity Funding Life to see that the policies it held were not "written on fence posts." Thus started another strange episode in the Equity Funding saga.

Realistically, the Peat, Marwick auditors had little chance of satisfying their colorful charge. Ranger asked them only to look at the support for a few policies, not to do a complete audit. Haskins & Sells, a Big Eight accounting firm with no connections to the inept Wolfson, Weiner crew, performed full, annual audits of EFLIC and apparently found nothing. Nevertheless, PMM came pretty close. So close that Equity Funding officers mounted a not very gentle campaign to get them thrown out—and succeeded.

The Equity Funding civil litigation resulted in depositions being taken from the Peat, Marwick auditors who worked on this engagement. The following pages are taken directly from the transcript of the deposition, including many of the exhibits from the PMM workpapers. The interaction between the Equity Funding personnel, the PMM auditors, and their client, Ranger, may be familiar to some practicing CPAs, but this may be the first time such interchanges have been published. It is interesting to conjecture the reaction of the Peat, Marwick partner to the final item. Here, notice that Seidman & Seidman had been engaged to replace Peat, Marwick.

NOON & PRATT

UNITED STATES DISTRICT COURT

CENTRAL DISTRICT OF CALIFORNIA

IN RE EQUITY FUNDING

CORPORATION OF AMERICA

SECURITIES LITIGATION

M.D.L. Docket
No. ___142___.

VOLUME I

Deposition of WILLIAM C. SUTTLE, taken

on behalf of Certain Plaintiffs, at

515 South Flower, 47th Floor,

Los Angeles, California, commencing at

9:40 A.M., Wednesday, December 17, 1975,

pursuant to Notice of Deposition and Pre-

Trial Discovery Order.

Reported by:

WENDY MORRIS, C.S.R. #2585
Notary Public

NOON & PRATT
Certified Shorthand Reporters
1930 WILSHIRE BLVD., SUITE 400
LOS ANGELES, CALIF. 90057
PHONE: 484-9770

NOON & PRATT

APPEARANCES OF COUNSEL:

    FOR CERTAIN PLAINTIFFS:

        SACHNOFF, SCHRAGER, JONES & WEAVER
        By: LOWELL SACHNOFF, ESQ.
                -and-
                NATHAN DARDICK, ESQ.,
        1 IBM Plaza,
        Chicago, Illinois 60611.

    FOR DEFENDANT HASKINS & SELLS:

        LOEB & LOEB
        By: ALFRED I. ROTHMAN, ESQ.
                -and-
                LESLEY A. ANDRUS, ATTORNEY-AT-LAW,
        One Wilshire Building,
        Wilshire at Grand Avenue,
        Los Angeles, California 90017.

    FOR DEFENDANT P. J. WOLFSON:

        FISCHMANN & WALLERSTEIN
        By: ROBERT WALKER, ESQ.
        1880 Century Park East,
        Los Angeles, California 90067.

    FOR DEFENDANT MILLIMAN & ROBERTSON, INC.:

        HAHN & HAHN
        By: RICHARD HALL, ESQ.,
        301 East Colorado Boulevard,
        Pasadena, California 91101.

    FOR DEFENDANT SEIDMAN & SEIDMAN:

        MITCHELL, SILBERBERG & KNUPP
        By: THOMAS P. LAMBERT, ESQ.,
        1880 Century Park East,
        Los Angeles, California 90067.

APPEARANCES OF COUNSEL: (cont'd.)

    FOR DEFENDANT MARVIN LICHTIG:

        RICHARD A. DeSANTIS, ESQ.
        By: PAUL SALERNO, ESQ.,
        1901 Avenue of the Stars,
        Los Angeles, California 90067.

    FOR DEFENDANT RANGER NATIONAL LIFE INSURANCE COMPANY:

        OVERTON, LYMAN & PRINCE
        By: SAMUEL E. ERICSSON, ESQ.,
        550 South Flower Street,
        Los Angeles, California 90017.

    FOR DEFENDANT PEAT, MARWICK, MITCHELL & CO.:

        GIBSON, DUNN & CRUTCHER
        By: IRWIN WOODLAND, ESQ.
                -and-
            JOHN LUCAS, ESQ.,
        515 South Flower Street,
        Los Angeles, California 90071.

NOON & PRATT

VOLUME I

I N D E X

THE WITNESS: EXAMINATION

    WILLIAM C. SUTTLE

        By: Mr. Sachnoff (a.m. session)   4

                    (p.m. session)   68

INDEX OF EXHIBITS *

DEPOSITION EXHIBIT NO.	DESCRIPTION	IDENT.
221-001	Memorandum in reference to a discussion Mr. Suttle had with Bill Vann, consisting of one page	8
221-002	2-page handwritten series of notations by Mr. Suttle, dated March 19, 1970	11
221-003	Short handwritten notation, entitled "Ranger - re: Presidential", dated March 24, 1970, by Mr. Suttle	17
221-004	Handwritten memorandum dated March 24, 1970, entitled "Ranger Insurance - Vann, Vitek and Smith", by Mr. Suttle	18
221-005	Communication from Mr. J. R. Brown to Mr. Ed Jones dated April 3, 1970, re: Ranger National Life Insurance Company	25
221-006	Memorandum dated April 13, 1970 from Mr. Brown to Mr. Jones, re: Ranger	27
221-007	Handwritten memorandum by Mr. Balint, dated May 1, 1970, entitled "Ranger Insurance - Ed Jones called"	29

  *Editors note: Most of the exhibits are reproduced at the appropriate point in the testimony or are repeated in the testimony.

Volume I - Suttle

DEPOSITION EXHIBIT NO.	DESCRIPTION	IDENT.
221-008	Handwritten note in Mr. Suttle's handwriting dated May 11, 1970, entitled "Ranger Insurance"	31
221-009	Handwritten memorandum, dated May 19, 1970, entitled "Ranger National Life"	31
221-010	Handwritten memorandum dated May 19, 1970, entitled "Ranger National Life Insurance"	32
221-011	2-page document with 2-page rider, dated June 16, 1970, addressed to Board of Directors, Ranger National National Life Insurance Company	37
221-012	3-page document which is a report on the letterhead of Peat, Marwick, Mitchell and addressed to the Directors of Ranger with 3-page rider, dated November 9, 1970	37
221-013	Report to Ranger on Peat, Marwick stationery, dated July 23, 1971	37
221-014	1-page document dated July 20, 1970 on letterhead of Equity Funding Corporation, an inter-office communication from Lloyd Edens to Jim Smith, Subject, "Peat, Marwick, Mitchell"	44
221-015	Letter dated August 7, 1970 from James Smith to Charles Rathbun	47
221-016	Memorandum on letterhead of Ranger Pan American Insurance Companies with handwritten "Confidential" on top of memo, to Mr. Vann from Mr. Vitek, dated August 31, 1970	48-49

iii

Volume I - Suttle

DEPOSITION EXHIBIT NO.	DESCRIPTION	IDENT.
221-017	Letter from Mr. Vann to Mr. Rathbun, dated January 29, 1971	56
221-018	Letter from Mr. Vann to Mr. Suttle, dated February 9, 1971	61
221-019	Memorandum on Peat, Marwick stationery from Mr. Suttle to Dale Dodge, dated February 12, 1971, consisting of two pages	63
221-020	1-page document in Mr. Suttle's handwriting dated February 19, 1971, entitled "Ranger National Life"	73
221-021	2-page document in Mr. Suttle's handwriting dated March 12, 1971, entitled "Ranger - Equity Life Deal"	74
221-022	Letter from Mr. Suttle to Mr. Vann, dated March 22, 1971	80
221-023	Letter dated March 2, 1971 from Fred Levin to Charles Rathbun	81-82
221-024	Short handwritten note in Mr. Suttle's handwriting dated April 23, 1971, headed "ACCO, Vann called"	83
221-025	Handwritten note by Mr. Suttle, dated December 15, 1971, indicating "Call Vann"	87
221-026	2-page document with initials RNL-EF, entitled "Meeting on progress of job", dated 12-15-71	91
221-027	2-page document with same heading, dated 12-16-71	91
221-028	2-page document with same heading, initialed FK, dated 12-28-71	91
221-028	(Re-marked copy of the above) which is a clearer copy	109

NOON & PRATT

1   <u>Volume I</u> - Suttle   *iv*

2

3   DEPOSITION

4   <u>EXHIBIT NO.</u>   <u>DESCRIPTION</u>   <u>IDENT.</u>

EXHIBIT NO.	DESCRIPTION	IDENT.
221-029	4-page document with initial FK, dated January 17, 1972	91
221-030	Document with initials FK, to Mr. John Brown, dated January 17, 1972	91
221-031	Inter-Office Memorandum from Mr. M. F. Wilson to T. L. Holton, dated September 29, 1971	103
221-032	Document entitled "Ranger - Equity Funding", dated January 28, 1972	129
221-033	7-page document entitled "The Board of Directors Ranger National Life Insurance Company", undated	135
221-034	1-page letter dated November 20, 1972 to Mr. Vann from Mr. Davis	138

<u>UNANSWERED QUESTIONS</u>

PAGE	LINE
93	2
93	14
97	9
112	14
112	22

WILLIAM C. SUTTLE,
having been duly sworn, testified as follows:

Examination

By Mr. Sachnoff:

Q. Mr. Suttle, would you state your name, please.

A. William Suttle.

*   *   *

Q. By whom are you now employed?

A. Peat, Marwick, Mitchell & Co.

*   *   *

Q. Mr. Suttle, what is your present position at Peat, Marwick, Mitchell?

A. I am a partner.

Q. How long have you been a partner?

A. Since 1959.

Q. Do you have any official position, other than being a partner, at Peat, Marwick, Mitchell?

A. I am the partner in charge of the Professional Practice Audit Department in Houston.

Q. How long have you held that position?

A. About ten years, I guess.

Mr. Sachnoff: I am going to mark for identification a one-page document and we will mark this as Exhibit 221-001.
(The document referred to was marked by the notary public as Deposition Exhibit No. 221-001 for identification, Witness Suttle.)

Mr. Sachnoff:

Q. Mr. Suttle, would you state for the record what this document is?

A. It is a memorandum I made of a discussion with Bill Vann.

Q. When you name someone, if you can identify them it would be very helpful to all of us in the room.

A. As to who Mr. Vann is?

Q. Yes.

A. He was the Vice-President and Controller of Anderson, Clayton & Co.

Mr. Rothman: Is there a date on that document?

Mr. Woodland: Let me try to identify the document on the record.
 Exhibit 221-001 is a handwritten memorandum in the handwriting of Mr. Suttle dated 3-16-70.

Mr. Rothman: Thank you, Mr. Woodland. That is exactly what I wanted.

Mr. Sachnoff:

Q. Will you explain the circumstances surrounding your writing of this handwritten memorandum?

A. As I recall, this had to do with the accounting by Anderson, Clayton in their consolidated financial statement of reinsurance business with Presidential Life Insurance Company, converting that to which we considered GAAP accounting at that time.

Q. In this document you indicate that it is not clear who it is who was to do these things but the words appear, "Want to move as fast as can."
 Who is "Want to move as fast as can" in connection with this special audit?

A. This is somewhat confusing and it is hard to recall. It appears that this memo may have also covered the fact that Anderson, Clayton wanted a special report on the reinsurance contract and wanted us to move as fast as we could to make that special report. I believe this covers two different things.

Q. Who at Anderson, Clayton made this request to you?

A. Mr. Vann.

Q. Did he indicate to you the reason why he wanted this special report?

A. At this date I do not know. The first time this came up, this subject came up, I did not know and I am not sure that he did and their special report, I am assuming at this point, was the work on the contract and not the other item which had to do with the generally accepted accounting principles.

Mr. Woodland: Perhaps for the sake of the others, I can just read this memorandum. As I said before, it is a handwritten memorandum and it says:
 "Anderson, Clayton & Co.—3-16-70, Ranger Insurance, Bill Vann.
 "Presidential Life reinsurance earnings look high.
 "12/31/69—Have actuary review reserve method using—also re: GAAP—Partner look at principles involved in accord with GAAP. Need accountant familiar with accounting and insurance business—Dunn.
 "Resolve before June 30.
 "Want as part of audit far as management concerned.
 "Special report wanted. Get in touch with Joe Vitek.
 "Want to move as fast as can."
 ". . . as fast as can" is underlined.
 "Van thinks concern with timing differences. Vitek thinks only conservative."
 Then there is an asterisk which says,
 "Done at Vann's request as part of year-end audit to be sure."

*   *   *

Mr. Sachnoff:

Q. Would you look at the document that has been marked as Exhibit 221-002, Mr. Suttle.

A. Yes.

Q. Would you tell me whether that is your handwriting?

A. Yes, sir, it is.

Mr. Sachnoff: The second page of this exhibit is very short and I am going to read this.

"Anderson, Clayton & Co.—Ranger 3-19-70. B. Vann called me to look at Presidential and GAAP in normal course of audit—alarm over.

"Want audit by PMM & Co. to determine policies valid, et cetera, on business buying—that is good business on people and not on fence posts.

"To have Los Angeles do and have Charles Smith work along with us.

"Three thousand policies a month—their man picked up only twenty-nine as test.

"Want regular audit on that business to satisfy ACCO that valid policies, et cetera—that we usually do in an audit.

"Start as soon as can."

Page 1 of that exhibit is a Xerox of a 5 x 8 piece of paper which says:

"Called B. Dunn *(Ed. Note–PMM Chicago insurance partner)* re Presidential Insurance. Do more test work than usual—really internal test audit work—special report—thinks L.A. can handle—shouldn't be big problem. We not concerned with underwriting or evaluation."

Mr. Suttle's initials are at the bottom.

Q. Mr. Suttle, what do you mean when you wrote that Ranger wanted an audit by Peat, Marwick to determine whether the policies were valid?

A. This memo is notes I made during the telephone conference and it is kind of my shorthand-type thing. This, basically, was recording what Vann had told me that he wanted.

Q. So Mr. Vann wanted you, as part of your assignment to determine whether these policies that were being ceded by Presidential to Ranger were valid?

A. That was his request at that time.

A. And then you go on and say, "That is good business on people and not on fence posts."

A. Yes, sir.

Q. Whose words were "fence posts"?

A. Those were his words.

Q. What did he mean by "fence posts"?

A. I have found out since that that is a common term in the insurance industry, fence posting, which normally applies to agents who are creating policies for sales promotion to get bonuses or this type of thing. That generally was the term that was used, as I understood it.

Q. Do you mean by creating policies that don't exist or—

A. Yes, or reporting that they have sold some life insurance that they have not sold. It has been submitted but it may not actually be issued.

*   *   *

Q. Would you describe for the record how you set up the special audit program in response to Mr. Vann's request to do this special audit of the Presidential Insurance policies?

*   *   *

A. It evolved over a period of some time. As I recall, my Auditor Manager, I believe he was the manager at the time, John Brown, Jr. worked with Mr. Vitek and Mr. Smith to determine what tests they wanted and what they thought should be needed. It was a combination of those things and then I reviewed this program and Mr. Vann reviewed the program. They added some things and we added some things and they took some things out and we took some things out and what have you and it was sort of a joint effort.

I might say that we worked with them on all of our audits very closely with their internal auditors. It was a joint program.

*   *   *

Mr. Sachnoff:

Q. I am looking at Exhibit 221-010.

This is your report, is it not, of a telephone conversation with Charlie Rathbun?

A. He is the President of Ranger National Life Insurance Company.

Q. And in your telephone conversation with Mr. Rathbun he told you he was in Los Angeles and had talked to Mr. Jones. He also indicated to you that—I am going to read the second paragraph. It says:

"Two of Presidential's men were swamped and referred to others. Gave us impression we were getting the runaround."

Can you tell me what Mr. Rathbun meant by that or what else he said about getting a runaround?

A. I think this gets back to this delay we had in getting files and he had called and was explaining what the delay was; that the men that were supposedly helping us were swamped with work and had sent us to some other people because they could not help us at the time. We got the impression that we were getting a runaround.

I think that is what he was telling me.

Q. Was there any discussion in this conversation about bogus insurance policies or fence posts or whether the policies were valid that were being examined?

A. No, sir.

Q. Was there any talk about fraud in this conversation?

A. No, sir.

Q. Was it Mr. Rathbun who said that he talked to Fred Levin?

You have a reference to Fred Levin in the third paragraph.

A. Yes, "CR talked to him."

That is Charles Rathbun.

Q. What did he say about that conversation to you?

A. From what he says here, he said that he requested cooperation from Mr. Levin; that he didn't get the impression that Mr. Levin was unhappy with our people. He said that if we had any more problems because they were not cooperating to call him and he would call Mr. Levin.

     *   *   *

Q. Is it safe to say that Exhibit 221-009, which is Mr. Brown's memorandum, involves the same subject matter, that is the lack of cooperation?

A. Yes.

Q. Did you talk to Mr. Brown on that day?

A. I would assume that I did. He and I were in pretty close touch on this thing. If he got a call on this thing, he would tell me and vice versa.

Mr. Woodland: Could we ask the witness to read Exhibit 221-009, please.

     *   *   *

The Witness: . . . it says:

"Wednesday—requested extend tests—Gresi"—I presume he meant the President of Equity—"says no. Called and explained situation and Edens said OK. Ranger has worn out their welcome—one week should be enough.

"Pulled off the job.

"Edens of Presidential says no more work until August.

"Rathburn (ACCO) man called Vogt and Jones—said he would try and improve cooperation—no feedback from Rathbun.

"Jones will call Edens again and send me memo re status.

"125 files reviewed. 125 files more now were requested."

I guess that is "required" instead of "requested." I am not sure.

Mr. Woodland: Tell me who Vogt was and who Edens was.

The Witness: Vogt was a partner in our Los Angeles office that I was working with at that time. Mangum had turned this over to Mr. Vogt.

I do not know Mr. Edens but, apparently, he was with Equity Funding Life Insurance Company.

Mr. Sachnoff:

Q. Mr. Suttle, what did "pulled off the job" mean?

A. I think it meant that we ran out of work because we didn't get these additional files and our Los Angeles people left the job because there wasn't any work to do. They had done their tests on the files that they had.

Q. He didn't say that you were kicked off of the job, did he?

A. This says, "Ranger has worn out their welcome."

I don't know what that meant.

It says, "Edens says no more work until August."

I presume what he means is that he was not going to pull any more files at that time. I do not know.

Q. When did you expect to have this report done?

A. I don't recall the date. I assume it was as soon as possible. We probably were working toward some deadline but I don't recall what it was.

Q. Was the work on the report taking longer than you expected?

A. Yes, because of this delay which we just talked about.

     *   *   *

Mr. Sachnoff: I am going to mark now for identification several exhibits, all of which have to do with the Peat, Marwick reports to Ranger.

The first one, which will be Exhibit 221-011, is a document on the letterhead of Peat, Marwick, Mitchell & Co., a two-page document with a two-page rider, dated June 16, 1970 and addressed to the Board of Directors Ranger National Life Insurance Company (Ed. Note: Not reproduced here)

W. P.

Cont. 115-1C037-11

PEAT, MARWICK, MITCHELL & CO.

CERTIFIED PUBLIC ACCOUNTANTS

700 CHAMBER OF COMMERCE BUILDING

HOUSTON, TEXAS 77002

The Board of Directors
Ranger National Life Insurance Company:

We have performed a review of certain of the accounting records of
Equity Funding Life Insurance Company of America (formerly Presidential Life
Insurance Company of America) for the nine months ended September 30, 1970,
for the purpose of determining: (a) that the terms of the reinsurance agreement between Ranger National Life Insurance Company (Ranger) and Equity Funding
Life Insurance Company of America (Equity Funding) are being adhered to; (b)
that the policies reinsured under such agreement are in force; (c) that the
information submitted to Ranger by Equity Funding on the quarterly reinsurance
bordereaux is in agreement with the individual policy contracts; and (d) that
the net quarterly settlements between Ranger and Equity Funding are substantially
correct. Our review included such tests of the accounting records and such
other auditing procedures as we considered necessary in the circumstances, in the
following general manner.

1. We reviewed the operating procedures of Equity Funding regarding
   policy underwriting, policy accounting, and reinsurance reporting
   to Ranger.

2. We made tests to determine that only approved policy plans and
   riders were included in the reinsurance bordereaux and that the
   approved individual life reinsurance dollar limit was being
   followed.

3. We selected policies from the reinsurance bordereaux and compared
   the reinsurance bordereaux information to the information contained
   in the individual policy files. We reviewed the selected policy
   files for underwriting approval, premium calculation, and policyholder signature.

4. We selected policies from the Equity Funding's transaction bordereaux,
   traced the transaction bordereaux information to the reinsurance
   bordereaux, and compared the selected reinsurance bordereaux information
   to the information contained in the individual policy files. We reviewed
   the selected policy files for underwriting approval, premium calculation,
   and policyholder signature.

5. We verified the calculation of the net reimbursement of Ranger to Equity
   Funding.

2

Our policy test work is summarized as to items below:

Items tested without exception	320
Items tested with exception, but cleared satisfactorily	24
Items tested with exception, but not cleared satisfactorily	39
Files not located for our review	32
Total items tested	415

A listing of all exceptions not cleared has been made available to Equity Funding.

The following were noted as exceptions during the test work performed by us:

1. Reinstatements of policies lapsed in 1970 were not included as part of the first two quarterly renewal settlements in 1970. Reinstatements should be added to renewed ceded premiums in the quarter reinstatement is effective.

2. During examination of quarterly settlements of renewed business it was noted that for policies lapsed or cancelled, when of a mode other than annual, and where a full annual premium had not been paid, the 180% commission paid by Ranger is not refunded for the portion of the annualized premium not paid by the insured. Similarly, on policies which were cancelled from inception or designated as "not taken out", adjustments of first year commissions and allowances have not been made. Since the basis for issuance of the policies was never met, the commission paid by Ranger should be refunded. Equity Funding management is of the opinion any settlement of this nature should take place on the next anniversary date of the policy.

3. Testing of lapsed policies revealed several policies with original issue dates prior to June 30, 1969 with less than ninety percent (90%) of the face amount of the policy ceded to Ranger. The Reinsurance Agreement as amended by Addendums 1 through 4 states that 90% of the insurance written will be ceded. No amendment to the agreement or correspondence has been noted that allows a cession of less than 90% of qualified business written.

4. Commissions on temporary substandard life premiums are on the policy reinsurance bordereaux and require manual adjustment of the commission percentage applicable thereto (10% on first year premium) prior to remittance to Equity Funding.

5. Testing of the policy reinsurance bordereaux disclosed two plans of coverage which were included that are not authorized by the Reinsurance Agreement: policy form R-4, payer waiver rider, and plan code 735, disability rider.

3

6. Tracing of policies from the transaction detail (a premium bordereaux of new business) to the reinsurance premium bordereaux disclosed five policies out of 100 tested that qualified for the 90% cession to Ranger but did not appear on the Reinsurance Bordereaux.

7. Tracing of reinsured policies from the reinsurance bordereaux to the policy files disclosed keypunching errors or errors in transcription. Policy date, sex of the insured and premium mode errors were note. This occurred on ten policies out of 200 policies tested.

8. Equity Funding personnel were unable to locate thirty-two policy files or 12% of the sample of two hundred-seventy policy files requested for test purposes. In addition, the company was unable to locate thirteen of the sixteen files which were not located during our previous audit work in May 1970. These exceptions indicate a deficiency in policy file physical control and because they are of a material number when compared to our testwork sampling, we consider this a material exception.

9. A substantial number of exceptions which were disclosed during our previous audit work in May, 1970 have not been cleared. Lists of the May, 1970 uncleared exceptions and the current exceptions have been provided to Ranger management.

Except for the items discussed above, no other matters came to our attention which would indicate that (a) the terms of the reinsurance agreement between Ranger and Equity Funding are not being adhered to; (b) the policies reinsured under such agreement are not in force; (c) the information submitted to Ranger by Equity Funding on the quarterly reinsurance bordereaux is not in agreement with the individual policy contracts, and (d) the net quarterly settlements between Ranger and Equity Funding are not substantially correct.

Peat, Marwick, Mitchell & Co.

November 9, 1970

RANGER NATIONAL LIFE INSURANCE COMPANY
PRESIDENTIAL WORK UNCLEARED EXCEPTIONS

Policy files which were not located by Presidential personnel:

6903658
6904613
6903273
6903545
6909459
6908668
6910789
6911099
6904333
6904686
6905188
6902184
6911078

List of Ranger reinsurance bordereaux to policy files:

6850676	Premium and in force differences
6905416	Premium difference
6907001	Acceptance authorization not in file
6904174	Acceptance authorization not in file
6905836	Wife's age difference
6908824	Plan code difference
6903658	In force difference on Presidential in force list file unlocated
6904986	In force key punch error on Presidential in force list
6908403	Plan code error on Presidential in force list
6904248	Plan code error on Pres. in force list, agrees to policy file
6905616	Wife's age difference
6905077	In force difference
6905530	Plan code for rider not on approved list
6905720	Unable to check substandard rate table
6903572	Premium difference
7000127	Unauthorized plan code, policy file code agrees to premium amt.

List of Presidential policy register to Ranger reinsurance bordereaux:

6900365	Not on reinsurance bordereaux - should be
6903868	Not on reinsurance bordereaux - should be
6905297	Not on reinsurance bordereaux - should be
6904184	Premium and in force differences
6908455	Plan code difference - reinsurance bordereaux correct, prem. diff.
6906435	In force difference
6903923	Premium difference
6906096	Wife's age difference
6908446	Policy date difference
6909756	In force difference

RANGER NATIONAL LIFE INSURANCE COMPANY
EQUITY FUNDING EXCEPTIONS
NOVEMBER 9, 1970

Policy files which were not located by Equity Funding personnel:

Selected from Ranger Reinsurance Bordereaux	Selected from Equity Funding Transaction Detail
7000465	7001114
7000801	7002859
7002859	7004806
7006617	7005268
7006857	7008002
7008039	6804464
7010293	
7038640	
7005983	

Coverage over $100,000	Lapsed Policies
7036651	6815975
7038862	6902470
7039041	6903163
7046860	6903998
7048200	6906023
7001107	6902752
7006483	
7007180	
7008610	
7020920	
7033880	

Trace from reinsurance bordereaux to policy valuation register:

7000924	Not on policy valuation register
7000581	In force difference
7000821	Not on policy valuation register
7003047	Plan code difference

Test of policy file data - selected from Ranger reinsurance bordereaux:

6908329	Rider 805 recorded for ½ unit
7004307	Policy date and sex difference
7005143	Policy date difference
7005373	Policy date difference
7005597	Policy date difference
7007348	Mode difference
7007540	Mode difference
7014470	Premium error
7006370	Policy date and age difference

RANGER NATIONAL LIFE INSURANCE COMPANY
EQUITY FUNDING EXCEPTIONS
NOVEMBER 9, 1970
2

Test of policy file data - selected from Equity Funding premium bordereaux:

6910720	Policy should appear on Ranger reinsurance bordereaux
6902700	Policy should appear on Ranger reinsurance bordereaux
7000762	Issue date difference
7003218	Plan code and in force difference
7018391	Policy should appear on Ranger reinsurance bordereaux
6804464	Policy should appear on Ranger reinsurance bordereaux
7003977	Policy should appear on Ranger reinsurance bordereaux
7024130	Sex difference on rider
7036651	Policy fee charge error
7043110	Age and sex difference

Test of over $100,000 coverage:

7024540	Improperly on Ranger reinsurance bordereaux
7007670	Policy not taken out - refund due

Test of lapsed policies:

6900274	Cession at less than 90%
6900351	Cession at less than 90%
6900294	Cession at less than 90%
6901974	Cession at less than 90%
6905649	Policy never lapsed
6900352	Cession at less than 90%, reinstated
6900420	Cession at less than 90%
6900837	Lapsed, but not credited in proper quarter
6903777	Lapsed in error
6905093	Policy not taken out, refund due
6904699	Canceled after quarterly premium earned, refund due
6903711	Reinstated in same quarter lapsed
6905287	Policy not taken out, refund due
6904042	Policy not taken out, refund due

Exhibit 221-012 is a three-page report on the letterhead of Peat, Marwick, Mitchell and addressed to the Directors of Ranger with a three-page rider, dated November 1970.

Exhibit 221-013 is also a report to Ranger on Peat, Marwick stationery and dated July 23, 1971.

Mr. Sachnoff:

Q. Mr. Suttle, I am referring to Exhibit 221-011, the first report dated June 16, 1970.

A. Yes, sir.

Q. Have you ever seen that document before?

A. Yes, sir.

Q. Who prepared that document?

A. There would have been a number of people involved in the preparation of it. It was issued by the Houston office.

Q. Could you tell me who was involved in preparing this report?

A. As I recall, a draft of a report on this work was originally prepared by the Los Angeles office and furnished to us with the work papers. John Brown and I would have worked on the report making revisions. I don't recall whether anyone else worked on it or not.

* * *

Mr. Sachnoff: I am going to mark as Exhibit 221-014 a one-page document dated July 20, 1970. It is on the letterhead of Equity Funding Corporation, an inter-office communication from Lloyd Edens to Jim Smith, subject "Peat, Marwick, Mitchell."

Mr. Sachnoff:

Q. Have you ever seen this document before?

A. Yes, sir.

Q. Are those your handwritten notes on the bottom of the page?

A. Yes, sir.

Q. I would like you to explain for the record what you mean by your first handwritten notation, "Untrue but."

* * *

Mr. Woodland: It is irrelevant for this purpose but go on.

Mr. Sachnoff:

Q. What did you mean by, "Untrue but"?

A. What did I mean by "Untrue but"?
That is not "but", those are my initials WCS.

Q. I am sorry about that.
You have "Untrue," and then you say, "I doubt this," and does that last one read, "Refused to help us"?

A. Yes.

Q. How do you know that?

A. This is what I was told by our Los Angeles people.

Q. Which Los Angeles person?

A. I don't know whether it came from Vogt, his first name was Hub, or Mr. Jones. It could have been the memos in the working papers that we got.

Q. You have a bracket after your three handwritten notes and then you have the cryptic notation, "This fellow is on the defense. W. C. Suttle."

* * *

Can you explain the time difference between the date of the memorandum, July 20, 1970 and the day you wrote this note?

A. This thing was not sent to Peat, Marwick, Mitchell. This was an internal Equity Funding memorandum; it was not meant for us.

* * *

Mr. Sachnoff: I am going to mark for identification now the second document that came in that package that Mr. Woodland referred to before. This will be Exhibit 221-015 a letter dated August 7, 1970 from James Smith to Charles Rathbun.

* * *

Q. On page 3 of the report (*Ed. Note: Exhibit 221-012*) Item 8 indicates that Equity Funding personnel were unable to locate 32 policy files or 12 percent of the sample of 270 policy files requested for test purposes. In addition, the company was unable to locate 13 of the 16 files which were not located during the previous audit work in May, 1970.
Can you explain why you considered the inability to locate 32 files out of 270 to be material whereas you didn't conclude that 16 out of 259 in the prior report was not material?

A. You go through a lot of things in reaching conclusions and I don't recall what my thinking was at that point, but I would assume the fact that we were still at that point unable to locate quite a few files from our previous audit work, I would assume that that, on top of this would have caused us to take exception. If you will recall, one of the purposes of this work was physical control policies. At this point we were going to have problems with that feature of it.
They would tell us, "The files are being worked on here or there and we cannot put our fingers on them."

* * *

Equity Funding Corporation   JUL 2? 1970

ER-OFFICE COMMUNICATION   Please use a separate letter for each subject

Jim Smith   Office Home Office   Dept. 6th Floor

Lloyd Edens   Office Home Office   Dept. Funding

Peat, Marwick & Mitchell   Date July 20, 1970

Basically the auditors representing Ranger National Life approached the problem of auditing the records of Presidential Life with a marked lack of planning. They began by making a selection of policy files from the Ranger National listing without first determining or discussing what their ultimate goals were to be. Had they scheduled the operation, they could have made their selections in their office and sent them to us with instructions in advance of their arrival. This would have allowed us time to gather the files rather than have the auditors wait for them.

Their attitude was more one of "snooping" than of auditing and therefore lacked much of the professionalism associated with outside auditors. On several occasions when told that a particular person would supply certain files or listings, the auditors would take it upon themselves to search file cabinets, vacant offices, etc. Many times this resulted in their obtaining an incorrect listing. When finished, the items were almost never returned properly.

In the future, I would suggest that the principals meet to discuss the plans for the audit beforehand. This would allow both parties time to schedule the various steps as well as eliminate the confusion associated with our first audit.

LDE/css

5141 0

OE 5141 0

_SIDENTIAL LIFE INSURANCE COMPANY OF AMERICA

August 7, 1970

RECEIVED

AUG 13 1970

C. R. RATHBUN

1900 Ave. of the Stars
Los Angeles
California 90067
(213) 553-2200

Mr. Charles R. Rathbun
President
Ranger National Life Insurance Co.
P. O. Box 2807
Houston, Texas 77001.

Dear Charlie:

The attached memorandum describes the difficulties which we incurred
with Peat, Marwick and Mitchell during their recent audit. I hope,
in the future, we will have more warning of an impending audit and
that we will have the opportunity to discuss the basic plan of attack
in advance. This will save all parties concerned much wasted
effort and expense.

Best regards,

James C. Smith
Executive Vice President

JS:cb

Attachment

DEPOSITION   EXHIB.
NO. 221-015 FOR IDENT.
WENDY MORRIS, NOTARY PUBLIC
WIT. Suttle
12-7-75

Q. I would like you, on the basis of your own recollection, to tell me if you can recall how it was that you were directed to prepare the second report.

A. I would normally get a call from Mr. Vann, "I would like for you to go out and do another examination."

Q. During the course of a telephone conversation with Mr. Vann directing you to go out and do another audit, was there any discussion of fictitious or bogus policies?

A. No, sir.

Q. Was there any more talk about fence posts?

A. Not that I can recall.

Q. Was there any reason why in connection with the November 9th report you looked at 415 policies as opposed to a smaller number, 259, in the June report?

A. Well, by this time, the nine months, the number of policies reinsured had grown substantially.

* * *

Q. What kind of feedback or contact did you have from the client concerning this report?

A. Sometime thereafter I recall talking to Mr. Vann that they wanted Equity Funding to locate the missing files and for us to go back and look at them, inspect them.

* * *

Q. Do you think it was Mr. Vann who called you and told you to see if you could locate the missing policies?

A. He would not have called and asked us to see if we could locate the missing policies.

He called and told me that they were going to have Equity Funding locate the missing policies and get them together and they were to go back and inspect them, as I recall. We had several discussions about that and my instructions, normally, for any work like that would come from Mr. Vann.

Q. Who did you have discussions with concerning that question, that is Equity Funding finding the missing policies?

A. It seems to me that I had some discussions with Mr. Vann and Bert Baker, Jr., the Administrative Vice-President of Anderson, Clayton & Co. It is possible that Mr. Rathbun would have been in on part of the discussion or Joe Vitek, John Brown in our office.

Q. Mr. Suttle, in the course of these conversations—by "these conversations," I mean the ones that you referred to in your immediately preceding answer relating to instructions to Equity Funding to locate the missing files—was there any discussion of bogus or fictitious policies?

A. Not that I recall.

Mr. Sachnoff: I would like to mark as the next exhibit, Exhibit 221-017, a letter from Mr. Vann to Mr. Rathbun dated January 29, 1971.

(The document referred to was marked by the notary public as Deposition Exhibit No. 221-017 for identification, Witness Suttle.)

Mr. Sachnoff: The second paragraph of that letter says:

"Peat, Marwick, Mitchell & Co. will be requested to confirm directly with the policyholders on the 13 files missing in May and selectively on the 32 policy files missing during the last examination."

Do you know if that was ever done, that is did Peat, Marwick & Mitchell ever request direct confirmation from policyholders?

A. Not to my knowledge.

Q. Why not?

A. Well, this was an initial decision by Anderson, Clayton people of what they wanted to do on the missing files. There were a number of discussions after that between them and Equity Funding and between them and us as to what would be done in—This whole thing got involved. One day they would decide that they would do this and then they would decide that they would do something else and then Equity Funding would decide, "No, you are not going to do this."

Q. Who was involved in these discussions?

I am talking about these discussions in which you said that Equity Funding people said, and I am quoting you now, "No, we are not going to do this."

What Equity Funding people?

A. I did not talk to them and I am giving you this third hand.

Q. I understand.

A. As I recall, Mr. Levin, for one, was concerned about these policyholders getting confirmations. They wouldn't know who Peat, Marwick was, to start with; that was the explanation that came back.

Q. That that would be upsetting to them or something; is that what you are saying; that that would be upsetting to them if they got a letter—

A. That is what he felt.

Q. Did you ever talk to Mr. Levin at all at this time?

A. No, sir.

Anderson Clayton
P. O. Box 2538   Houston, Texas 77001   (713) 224-6641

January 29, 1971

Mr. C. R. Rathbun
Ranger/Pan American Insurance
Houston, Texas

Dear Charlie:

      This will confirm the conclusions we reached in our discussion today concerning the audit of the Equity Funding business. It was agreed that —

1. Equity Funding would be requested to locate the 32 policy files that could not be located during the last examination, as well as the 13 files which were not located during the audit work in May, 1970.

2. Peat, Marwick, Mitchell & Co. will be requested to confirm directly with the policy holders on the 13 files missing in May and selectively on the 32 policy files missing during the last examination.

3. Peat Marwick should extend its test of policy files beyond the last sample to assure that the 12% missing files is not representative.

      The extent to which this test is expanded will depend to a large extent on the results of the above Steps 1 and 2.

      It is my understanding that you will contact Mr. Stanley Goldblum to inform him of our concern and of the steps we would like to take to clear this matter. As soon as you have cleared this matter with him, we would like to get PMM&Co. moving.

      In order to save PMM&Co.'s time, I should think the Equity Funding people would locate all the missing files for their examination.

      If this does not adequately explain the conclusions we reached, please let me know.

                      Yours very truly,

                      W. W. Vann

shb
cc: Mr. T. J. Barlow
    Mr. Burke Baker, Jr.
    Mr. Joe Vitek
    Mr. W. C. Suttle, Peat, Marwick, Mitchell & Co.

Q. Who was in charge of the project in Los Angeles at that time, in January of 1971?

A. Dale Dodge.

Q. Dale Dodge was a partner in the Los Angeles office?

A. Yes.

Q. Did you ever talk to Mr. Dodge about the possibility of Peat, Marwick making a direct confirmation with policyholders in connection with missing files?

A. I am sure we had a discussion on this.

Q. Why didn't you do that?

A. This was not a normal audit procedure at that time, to confirm policies with policyholders.
   To my knowledge, it is still not a policy or a generally accepted auditing standard, to confirm policies with policyholders.

Q. Why do you suppose that Mr. Vann, he was your client, would suggest an undertaking that was not a standard auditing procedure?

A. Well, Mr. Vann was an auditor and he understood auditing.

Q. I know that.

A. This was an extension of auditing procedures. You have got some missing files and you are thinking of extending auditing procedures and one thing that comes to mind is, "Well, why don't we confirm with policyholders."

Q. Mr. Suttle, if that is a logical thought or step, to satisfy yourself, why wasn't this procedure undertaken; who rejected it?

*   *   *

A. It was a mutual agreement, as I recall, that the client and Peat, Marwick agreed that confirmation with the agents of record would be sufficient because you would have so many agents scattered around the United States that these policies came in from—At this point, Anderson, Clayton was interested in following these up. This was their instigation of this work because they were concerned about these missing files. This was not instigated by us.

Q. I understand that.

A. So they had to decide what they wanted to do. Mr. Rathbun was concerned that we were going to get—when I say, "we," they and the auditor—were going to get Equity Funding so upset if they kept coming in that they were going to cancel the Reinsurance Agreement which they felt was a good investment, I gather, so in talking to them they agreed that confirmation with the agents would be satisfactory and that took place sometime later.

*   *   *

Mr. Sachnoff: I am going to mark for identification as Exhibit 221-018 a letter from Mr. Vann to Mr. Suttle, himself, the first letter to Mr. Suttle, dated February 9, 1971.

*   *   *

Q. The statement, "We all agree that a certain number of policyholders should be contacted directly to confirm the existence of the policies," didn't you take that as a direction from your client to, in fact, make direct contact with the policyholders to verify their authenticity?

A. This was a followup of this discussion that they had had internally; that we were going to confirm policies. This got changed. They did not discuss this with Equity Funding. In the "We are all agreeing," the "we" did not include Equity Funding.
   This is one of the documents that I was talking about a minute ago in the continuing subsequent discussions of this thing.

*   *   *

Mr. Sachnoff:

Q. Mr. Woodland has characterized your previous testimony by saying that it was not your opinion as of February 12, 1971 that Peat, Marwick ought to confirm directly with policyholders.

A. That is correct. It was not my opinion; it was not my instigation or Peat, Marwick's that they do any of this additional work. I was passing on to them (Ed. Note: in the interoffice memo to the PMM Los Angeles office identified as Exhibit 221-019) what I thought was the intent of this letter of Mr. Vann's to Mr. Rathbun, of what the company was going to do at that point. I was telling Dodge, "They may want you to do this work and I will notify you when it will be done".

Q. I am going to ask you again if you can be more specific as to why this work wasn't done, why the direct contact was not done?

A. Well, I think I answered that earlier. As I understand it, it was primarily because Equity Funding objected, so then we had more discussions and the client had to decide whether they wanted to insist on it and possibly lose their contract or whether there were some other alternative procedures.

Q. On Page 2 of the exhibit, that is Exhibit 221-019, the third full paragraph reads as follows:
   "The President of Anderson, Clayton & Co. looks upon Equity as a stranger and is quite concerned over the large amount of money Ranger is spending under the Reinsurance

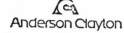

Anderson Clayton

P. O. Box 2538   Houston, Texas 77001   (713) 224-6641

February 9, 1971

Rec'd 2/10/71

Mr. W. C. Suttle, Partner
Peat, Marwick, Mitchell & Co.
700 Chamber of Commerce Bldg.
Houston, Texas 77002

Dear Bill:

Charlie Rathbun has contacted Mr. Fred Levin, President of Equity Funding Life Insurance Company in Los Angeles, regarding the exceptions which arose during your last examination.

Equity Funding has been requested to locate the missing files and get in contact with Charlie so that your people can return to examine them. We all agree that a certain number of the policy holders should be contacted directly to confirm the existence of the policies. I think the number will be dependent upon what your examination of the files indicates. We leave this to your discretion.

As soon as Equity Funding notifies us that the files are ready for examination, we shall immediately contact you.

Yours very truly,

W. W. Vann
Vice President - Controller

shb

cc: Mr. T. J. Barlow
    Mr. C. R. Rathbun

DEPOSITION   EXH:3.
NO. 221-018 FOR IDENT.
WENDY MORRIS, NOTARY PUBLIC
WIT: Suttle
12-17-75

PEAT, MARWICK, MITCHELL & CO.   *Corres.*

PRINTED IN U.S.A.

TO MR.	Dale Dodge	**DATE** February 12, 1971
OFFICE	Los Angeles	**STENO** BP
		ENC.
FROM MR.	Wm. C. Suttle	**CONTRACT NO.**
OFFICE	Houston	**CLIENT CLASS.**
CC:		

YOUR LETTER DATED:

SUBJECT   Ranger/Presidential (Equity Funding) Life Insurance Special Reviews

PRIVATE AND PERSONAL - To be opened by only Mr. Dodge

As a result of the material number of missing policy files encountered during the subject reviews, additional work must be performed in order for us to satisfy ourselves regarding the propriety of such files and to determine additional audit procedures for future reviews. Upon notification from Houston you should arrange for the following two steps to be performed:

1. Examine each of the previously missing files for proper contents and apparent validity.
    > Equity Funding has agreed to locate all missing files and have them together for your examination. Tentatively, Mr. Levin proposes to have them in his office on February 23, 1971, but you will be notified by us later as to the specific date and time.

2. Confirm positively with a selected number of the policyholders represented by the previously missing folders.
    > While the number to be confirmed will depend upon the findings during step 1, I suggest you confirm (1) all the policies for which files were missing in our first examination and still not located in our second examination and (2) fifty percent of the policies representing files missing in the second examination.

I also want to reemphasize a few matters for your consideration:

1. We were requested to do these audits by the President of Anderson, Clayton & Co., the parent company of Ranger National Life Insurance Co., the reinsuror.

2. Anderson, Clayton & Co. is a large, important client and it is most imperative we render good service.

3. The client has been most critical of the two examinations made to date and in each instance has received criticisms of the Los Angeles staff from Equity Funding Life Insurance Company President, Mr. Fred Levin, and other officers.

4. Please refrain from making any comments to Mr. Levin or other personnel of Equity regarding any findings or results of our examination, good or bad.

M C-18

PEAT, MARWICK, MITCHELL & CO.

PRINTED IN U.S.A.

TO	MR.	Dale Dodge	DATE	February 12, 1971
	OFFICE	Los Angeles	STENO	BP
FROM	MR.	Wm. C. Suttle	ENC.	
	OFFICE	Houston	CONTRACT NO.	
	CC:		CLIENT CLASS.	

SUBJECT   Ranger/Presidential (Equity Funding) Life Insurance Special Reviews   YOUR LETTER DATED:

-2-

I am sure Mr. Levin and his people are on the defensive because of their poor procedures, dissatisfaction with the audit request, etc., and looking for any excuse to be critical of us.

I have no way of refuting such statements with our client here and I was informed Mr. Levin was extremely unhappy to learn so many files were missing without him being informed and we not demand inspection of them plus confirmation. Consequently, any discussion with Equity people should be limited to what is absolutely necessary to do the requested audit work; this should prevent Mr. Levin from misconstruing any of our remarks or exaggerating events that transpire. It might even help for you to have two people present each time there is a conversation with the Equity people. It is not going to solve anything for two parties to cast aspersions on each other without support.

The President of Anderson, Clayton & Co. looks upon Equity as a stranger and is quite concerned over the large amount of money Ranger is spending under the reinsurance agreement. In his words, he wants to make certain he is not insuring "fence posts."

All of this is extremely confidential and for your personal information. If at any time you have any questions or problems or feel you have learned anything of interest to our client it is imperative you call me or John Brown, Jr. (audit manager) immediately.

I most certainly do not want to get in a position of having to do the audit work in Los Angeles with Houston office personnel which has been suggested once or twice by our client.

I do not intend this letter to be a personal criticism of you or your people, but thought it would be helpful to let you know how the client feels about the work.

Agreement. In his words, he wants to make certain he is not insuring 'fence posts'." Who was the president at that time of Anderson, Clayton?

A. Jim Barlow.

Q. Did you talk to him around the time that you wrote this memo to Mr. Dodge?

A. I don't know whether that came from Mr. Barlow or Mr. Vann, but somewhere in there I have the impression—This is when I learned that this original concept of the fenceposts came from Mr. Barlow. . . .

*   *   *

Mr. Sachnoff:

Q. Directing your attention to Exhibit 221-020, would you describe this memorandum? (Ed. Note: not reproduced)

A. I presume that Equity Funding had gotten a mess of documents together and I was calling Dodge to tell him that they were supposed to be available on February 22nd for us to inspect them. I would assume that because of the date, February 1971.

Q. How did you know that Levin would have the records on February 22nd?

A. This would have been conveyed to me from Anderson, Clayton or Bill Vann called and told me. That is why I put this, here. This is a phone message from Bill Vann.

Q. When you called Dodge, why did you tell him not to leave any of the records in Mr. Levin's office?

A. Because, as I recall, with this problem we had had back and forth, personnel problems, I could imagine Mr. Levin getting the records there and saying, "I am ready for you," and Dodge shows up a week later and Levin is screaming, "Every time I get ready for you you don't show up or something like that.

That is the only thing I can think of. It was part of this continual harassment saying, "Your people want to do this and that."

I don't recall any other reason. It was this conflict type of thing.

Q. In the last paragraph you reemphasized that decision to do additional work.

What did you mean by "additional work"?

A. I mentioned to you earlier that examining the missing files was instigated by Anderson, Clayton. They did not want Equity Funding to know this; they wanted Peat, Marwick to come out and say, "We have now decided we want to do some more work on the missing files."

That is why I said that this was the client's request. I guess because of every relationship

in this contract, trying to keep their relationship with Equity Funding, they wanted this to be Peat, Marwick's request and they asked me to write a letter to this effect, that this was our suggestion.

Mr. Sachnoff: I am going to mark for identification as our next exhibit, which is 221-021, a two-page handwritten document in Mr. Suttle's handwriting dated March 12, 1971 and entitled "Ranger—Equity Life deal."

*   *   *

Q. You were concerned, weren't you, about the possibility that Equity Funding Life was creating policies at that time?

A. No, sir.

Q. Why did you say, ". . . no chance to recreate"? What did you mean by that?

A. This gets back to Anderson, Clayton wanting us to go out and look at the missing files. In addition, if I recall the letter that Mr. Vann wrote Mr. Rathbun, he wanted us to look at some new files at that time, in addition to these. In an audit procedure when you are having this type of problem, you normally would not give these people, I don't think, in advance the files you want to look at if you have some concern about it, so we were talking about going in and we had discussions with Anderson, Clayton about this, about going in and asking for the files the morning you get them, which is what caused all of the problems the first time we went out there.

Q. From here on in, I am going to refer to Presidential and EFCA Funding as EFLIC. That is the shorthand acronym.

I am asking you whether you were concerned if they were creating files?

A. I was not concerned if they were; I was concerned with an audit procedure as an extension of work because we had missing files. We had no concern at that time that there was any fraud. The exceptions were not unusual; there were explanations for things that we run into all of the time on any insurance examination, but if you are going back to do some specific work because of some prior exceptions, you have a different thought. If you go to look at these additional files, because the client is concerned about missing files, then an audit procedure would be not to tell them in advance the files you want to see, if there is a possibility that they might be creating files.

We had no feelings that they were doing this.

Exhibit No. 221-021
Notes of William Suttle
3-12-71
(typed from original)

Ranger - Equity Life deal   3-12-71

Called Dale Dodge:

He is to confer Levin & decide procedures we should do & can
or cannot do -- probably monday. Then we'll write letter to ACCO
& await their decision.*

We will not reissue report.

To satisfy ourselves we must do new test & write new report
so files can all be located at visit & no chance to create (ed. note:
    the previous word is "create", although in the testimony it
    is referred to as "recreate")

I told Dale "Monkey on our back" & we must be judge of audit
procedures to satisfy us. If we decide have to confirm w/policy holders
and this costs company the contract, client will accept, per Bill
Vann (on 3-9-71) (ed. note: At this point in the memo, there is a
note in the left margin which reads, "Company changed mind later,
WCS, 4-9-73") *Minimum -- we are to confirm w/agents (or have H&S
do) and inspect funding records also to confirm (ed. note: portion
unintelligble)

I subsequently talked to Vann and he will set up meeting for me
to talk with Barlow, Vann and Rathbun. I called Dodge & told him to
hold up until after my meeting (at request of Vann).

Q. When did you first become concerned, if at all, that EFLIC was creating files?

A. I don't think I can answer that question; I don't think that I could say that I was ever concerned that they were creating files. Anything along that line would have been in the nature of an extension of audit procedures.

I don't know whether that is clear or not.

Q. Did you ever tell any of your associates at Peat, Marwick at any time during 1971 that you were concerned about fraud, fictitious policies at EFLICO

A. Not in the manner you are talking about, no.

Q. In what manner, then?

A. Well, it goes on into the next examination.

Q. Maybe we should wait until we get into the next examination. I am just trying to pin down when you were first concerned about the creation of files.

A. Any auditor would assume this many missing files—When you go back the second time because you could not find them the first time, then there is always the possibility that the files did not exist. We had no reason to believe that; these people were moving offices back in there, changing their IBM system and having registration statements. There were a lot of reasons why they were so busy and we were a nuisance to them coming in there and we had explanations for those things.

Q. In the next paragraph you told Dale, Dale Dodge, that there was "a monkey on our back."

A. I think I mentioned this, indirectly, earlier when I was talking about the phase of deciding the confirmations, that at one time Anderson, Clayton decided that if they lost the contract they were going to go ahead and confirm the policies.

Q. If what?

A. At one time—You have to remember that this was a whole series of events and at this point, apparently, they had decided that if we told them that they should confirm with the policyholders and that we felt that there was no alternative to satisfy them on the missing files, that they would do so, even if it cost them this contract. That was, at that point in time, the thinking.

*   *   *

Q. What is the meaning of the note in the margin, Mr. Suttle?

It says, "Company changed mind

later—and then there is what looks like a date of 4-9-73.

*   *   *

A. 4-9-73 would have been after all of this business came out in March of 1973 and I was reviewing the papers. I don't know if it was in connection with getting ready to send them to my New York office or what. I apparently made that note there on that date. It just got changed later.

Q. What does "Company changed mind later" mean?

A. About confirming with it.

Q. With the policyholders?

A. With the holders and losing the contract, if it came to that.

Editors Note: Testimony then continued with discussions of the letter to Rathbun from Fred Levin (Exhibit 221-023) in which Levin continues to resist confirmation with policyholders. The handwritten marginal notes on the letter are by Suttle and read:
Met with Vann and B. Baker. Recommended: 1. check all files that were missing to Funding files; 2. confirm above with agents; 3. confirm all five still missing files with policyholders; 4. inspect and completely account for 25 additional files—confirm any missing with policyholders in person, if necessary. They agreed to submit to Barlow.
This letter and subsequent discussions led to the writing of the letter from PMM to Vann on March 22, 1971, which is Exhibit 22, 1971. Suttle described the letter as follows:

The Witness: This letter was written at the request of Mr. Vann for him to take to Equity Funding and it said that Peat, Marwick says that they have got to do all of these things.

(Editors Note: The discussion then turned to the report issued by Peat, Marwick on July 23, 1971, labeled Exhibit 221-013.)

*   *   *

Q. Is there any reason why you did not include in this report any mention of what you have called the continuing problems at EPLIC, locating files, cooperation?

You have characterized it in several ways.

Is there any reason why you did not mention that in this report?

A. They were more aware of that than we could have ever spelled out in our letter, than all of the discussions and conversations and meetings and what have you.

Could I make a brief statement about this special report?

EQUITY FUNDING LIFE INSURANCE COMPANY

← CORRESPONDENCE FILE

RECEIVED
MAR 3 1971
C. R. RATHBUN

1900 Avenue of the S
Los Angeles
California 90067
(213) 553-2200

March 2, 1971

3/16/71 met with
Vann + B. Baker Recommended:
① Check all files that were
missing to funding files
② Confirm about which
③ Confirm all still missing
files with policyholders
④ Inspect + completely
account for 2 additional
files

Mr. Charles R. Rathbun
President
Ranger National Life Insurance Company
Post Office Box 2807
Houston, Texas 77001

Dear Charlie:

This letter will document the telephone conversation we had today
with respect to recent activities by your public accounting firm.
As I indicated on the telephone, Peat, Marwick & Mitchell have
asked for permission to send confirmations to policyholders of
Equity Funding Life verifying the information contained in the
actual policy files. When I spoke to you last you indicated that
Peat Marwick was withholding certification because of the fact
that 44 policy files could not be located. I stated to you at this
time that we indeed had the policy files, but that they were in
the process of being worked on by other departments within the
insurance company. When you asked me to accommodate Peat
Marwick, once again I instructed our staff to collect the 44 files
for purpose of examination. Peat Marwick then came and requested
the ability to verify coverage by transmitting confirmations to policyholders.

We are reluctant to assent to this request because of our desire not
to disturb the policyholder, nor to disturb the agent of record.
Recognizing your public accountant's desire to verify coverage, I
would like to suggest the use of any or all of the following alternative procedures:

1.   Increase the size of the sample of policy
      files to be examined.

2.   Verify coverage by sending confirmation
      letters to the agents of record.

Mr. Charles R. Rathbun
March 2, 1971
Page Two

3. Examine our agents' commission files to
    verify the payment of commissions on the
    policies being examined.

✓ 4. Examine the funding files to verify that an
    annual premium has in fact been paid.

5. Examine the general ledger to verify the
    sampled policy forms.

6. Examine the cash receipt journals.

7. Examine the retention computer runs
    to verify that the retained portion
    has been included in our insurance
    in force.

While I am not an accountant, nor am I familiar with audit procedures,
I think that the procedures suggested above could replace direct communications by an unrelated public accounting firm with our insurance
clients.

Please advise which of the alternatives listed above are satisfactory
so that the appropriate information necessary could be made available without any further delay.

Thank you for your cooperation in this matter.

Sincerely,

EQUITY FUNDING LIFE INSURANCE COMPANY

Fred Levin
President

FL:ml

March 22, 1971

Mr. W. W. Vann, Vice President
Anderson, Clayton & Co.
P. O. Box 2538
Houston, Texas 77001

Dear Mr. Vann:

The purpose of this letter is to summarize the current status of our
test examination in November 1970 of insurance policies issued by Equity
Funding Life Insurance Company, which are reinsured by Ranger National
Life Insurance Company.

Because a number (44) of files, which were deemed material in relation to
the size of our test sample, were not made available for inspection at
the time of our initial field work, we were unable to complete the
examination to our satisfaction.

You informed us the Equity people had agreed to locate the files so we
could inspect them and clear up our exceptions. We returned to Equity's
office in February and inspected 39 of the 44 files--5 were still not
located. Primarily because of the time lapse from the time of our field
work until the time of our inspection of the previously unlocated files
(some three months or so), we requested that we be permitted to extend
our procedures to include confirmation with the policyholders for the 44
policies.

The Equity people were reluctant to disturb their policyholders and you
have asked us to consider alternative procedures. Consequently, I am
setting forth below the minimum procedures we think are necessary at this
point. I say minimum as application of these procedures could produce
some questionable matters that might require additional procedures.
Extension of audit procedures is a normal thing in any audit. We presently
have no reason to believe that we would have to extend the procedures
beyond those set forth below and the procedures we are recommending are

DEPOSITION   EXHIB.
NO. 221-022 FOR IDENT.
WENDY MORRIS, NOTARY PUBLIC
WIT Suttle
12-17-75

Mr. W. W. Vann, Vice President
March 22, 1971
2

required because of unlocated files; they are not intended to imply we
are suspicious of any procedures or transactions that we have examined
to date. We consider these as routine procedures that we think are
minimum requirements under generally accepted auditing standards.

1. For the 44 files previously unlocated-
   A. Examine the funding files and
   B. Confirm the policies with the agents.

2. For any of the 44 files still unlocated-
   Confirm with the policyholders. It is my understanding
   there are still 5 unlocated files.

3. Select 25 policies not previously selected for test, apply
   all audit procedures used in our previous examination
   including examination of funding files and if there are
   any unlocated files, confirm them with the policyholders.
   It is anticipated we will obtain positive confirmation
   replies on all confirmations sent to policyholders. If
   necessary to obtain the replies, we will consider the
   advisability of making personal contact with the policyholders.

                     Very truly yours,

                     PEAT, MARWICK, MITCHELL & CO.

                     Wm. C. Suttle, Partner

WCS:bh

W.P.   Cont. 115-10039-10

Peat, Marwick, Mitchell & Co.
CERTIFIED PUBLIC ACCOUNTANTS
4300 ONE SHELL PLAZA
HOUSTON, TEXAS 77002

                                                          8
                                                1 wp; 1 index
                                                     2 - Brown
                                       December 9, 1971

The Board of Directors
Ranger National Life Insurance Company:

On November 9, 1970 we reported on our review of certain of the
accounting records of Equity Funding Life Insurance Company of America for the
nine months ended September 30, 1970. In our report, we indicated that the
number of unlocated files was a material exception. Subsequent to that date,
we have performed additional audit procedures to determine the propriety of
forty-four (44) policy files reported as unlocated during previous testwork
and to otherwise satisfy ourselves to the extent necessary to clear this
exception. Our review included such tests of the accounting records and such
other auditing procedures as we considered necessary in the circumstances, in
the following general manner:

1. We examined forty-two (42) policy files listed as being unlocated
   during our previous review. Policy files for policies 6904333
   and 6903273 were still not located. In addition, twenty-five
   (25) reinsured policies were tested that had not previously been
   selected. Twelve (12) policies were selected at random from the
   reinsurance bordereaux and thirteen (13) policies were selected
   from the Equity Funding premium bordereaux.

2. We subjected the sixty-seven (67) policies mentioned above to
   the same testwork described in our letter dated November 9,
   1970 and, in addition, agreed policy file data to funding file
   data where applicable.

3. We requested direct confirmation from the agents or branch
   managers as to correct policy information on sixty-six (66)
   files. It was determined from our testwork that policies
   6902470, 6902184 and 6911078 were never accepted by the prospective insured and, therefore, confirmation was not requested.
   Sixty-four (64) confirmation replies were received and exceptions
   were adequately cleared.

The following were noted as exceptions during the current testwork
performed by us:

Test of policy file data - selected from Ranger reinsurance bordereaux:

   7001402 - Payor Waiver of Premium Rider (R-4) improperly
             included in reinsurance bordereaux.

2

Test of over $100,000 coverage:

    6904613 – Reinsured premium per bordereaux was less than
                actual cession per policy file because of a
                programming error.

Test of lapsed policies:

    6906023 – Policy never lapsed.

    6903998 – Policy never lapsed.

Examination of policy files unlocated during test of 1969 cessions:

    6903273 – Policy number coded wrong on reinsurance bordereaux
                and premium bordereaux-should have been 6903773.

Each of the above exceptions were of the same nature as those indicated
in our report dated November 9, 1970.

Based on the results of the test procedures outlined above, we do not
believe the unlocated files and other exceptions are material in the accounting
for the transactions related to the reinsurance agreement between Ranger
National Life Insurance Company and Equity Funding Life Insurance Company of
America.

Peat, Marwick, Mitchell & Co.

July 23, 1971

Q. Sure. Go ahead.

A. In most special reports, normally there is some specific thing a client wants you to do and you get with the client on what he wants you to do and you agree to do it or you don't agree to do it and, usually, you go out and do the work and then you give him the exceptions. He asks you to do certain things and you find the exceptions and give them to him. Normally in a situation of that type it is up to him to evaluate the exceptions and decide whether they are material and how serious they are. That is what these reports were. We were telling them what we found. This personality-type thing, I don't think we would normally put that in a report of this type. If I were going to do that, it would be a separate letter.

Q. Did you write that report, Mr. Suttle?

A. I signed it.

Q. Is it fair to say that you probably signed it fairly close to date that appears in the stamp on the top, December 9, 1971?

A. Somewhere around that date, I would assume

Mr. Sachnoff: I am going to mark as Exhibit 221-025 for identification a handwritten note in Mr. Suttle's handwriting dated December 15, 1971. It says at the top, "Ranger Equity."

This is very short and I am going to read it into the record.

"Call Vann. If don't get files today may have to pull off (this per call from J. Brown via Krenzke).

"I called Vann and relayed above.

"In our conversation yesterday Tom Collerain told Mr. Vann of problems Gene Howard and Krenzke are having in securing files. W. C. Suttle."

Q. What did that phone call relate to?

A. The next examination. They had started the next examination that they had asked us to make.

Q. Who called whom; did you call Vann or did he call you?

A. This is, "Call Vann," so I called Mr. Vann to report what I had just gotten from Mr. Brown.

Q. What did Mr. Brown tell you that prompted this call to Mr. Vann?

A. He had gotten a call from Mr. Krenzke who was in Equity Funding's offices and was told that they were having problems getting files and that they were about to run out of work if they did not get the files and would have to pull off of the job.

Q. Did Mr. Brown tell you that he got this information from Mr. Krenzke?

A. Yes.

Q. So that this memorandum related to the next series of examinations?

A. That is right, the final work we did. That was the beginning of that work.

*   *   *

This was the first mention of Gene Howard and Krenzke.

Do you want me to identify them?

Q. Yes, if you would, please.

A. Gene Howard was the internal auditor with Ranger National Life Insurance Company and Fred Krenzke was an audit senior with PMM & Co., Peat, Marwick, Mitchell & Co. Tom Collerain, we have not mentioned him either, he was an officer of Ranger National Life Insurance Company.

*   *   *

Mr. Sachnoff:

Q. I am now going to direct your attention to Exhibit 221-027. . . .

*   *   *

At that time, that is December 16, 1971, did you have any indication that Fred Levin had requested that the Peat, Marwick audit team be pulled off? A. Yes, either on that day or the next day. Would have been notified by Mr. Krenzke on that fact.

*   *   *

Q. What did you tell Mr. Krenzke when you talked to him on the phone about this event?

A. I don't recall whether I talked to Mr. Krenzke or Mr. Brown but, somewhere in there I am sure we told him that there wasn't anything he could do but come on back to Houston.

Q. Did he, in fact, come back to Houston?

A. Yes, he did.

Q. When was that?

A. Well, I assume that he left pretty quickly. Mr. Levin asked him to leave.

*   *   *

Q. Do you recall having any discussion with Mr. Brown in the one or two-day period after December 16th when you became aware of that fact that your audit team had been directed off of the premises by Mr. Levin?

A. I am sure we had a number of conferences.

Q. Do you remember what you said to Mr. Brown and what he said to you?

A. That is a difficult question.

Q. Do you remember whether you discussed

Exhibit No. 221-027
Memorandum of F. Krenske
PMM audit staff, Los Angeles
(retyped from handwritten
original)

12-16-71

Request by Levin that PMM-RNL Audit Team Pull Off

At 6:00 pm on Thurs., 12/16/71, Mr. Fred Levin, President of
EFLIC, called me (Fred Krenzke) & Gene Howard into his office.

Mr. Levin asked that Gene & I leave as soon as possible. He
was very positive in his request and without saying it he left no
doubt that He intended for us to go.

The reason he stated for the request was that he wanted to
free Art Lewis & Lloyd Edens from having to work with us. He said
they wore exhausted physically & mentally. (Howard & I concur with
this.) He noted that they would have to go to New Jersey next week
& needed time to prepare. He referred to us and our audit as "straws,
straws on camels backs." He noted he had already removed some other
straws (no further identification given.)

We noted that we were trying to work around them & had some of
their underlings assigned to us. We asked if we could continue the
audit to conclusion under these circumstances. He said no.

He suggested that we leave a list of things we need to finish
& that ----------unintelligible----------these items for a couple
of days between Christmas & New Years.

We agreed that we would do this (he quite really left us no choice.)
As we left his office hes parting remark was how soon would we be out.

It is my feeling that Levin is only looking out for his men & does not intend any malice toward RNL or PMM. Lewis & Edens are extremely overworked. I feel Levin is acting in their best interests although it means sacrificing the efficiency of the RNL-PMM audit.

Read and conur - Gene Howard
                    12-16-71
                    6:45 PM

with him at all anything to do with fraud at Equity Funding?

A. I can't say. We were discussing other procedures and the fact that we were not able to complete that work and, I think, it ties into some subsequent discussions of what they had proposed to do about this.

Q. What were those discussions, sir?

A. The company, Equity Funding, was proposing to fly some records to Houston, some microfilm, whatever we needed to complete the work and I objected to that.

Q. Why did you object to that suggestion?

A. As an auditor I don't think I can make an audit on microfilm.

Q. You think it is better to go on site and examine original files?

A. That is right.

*   *   *

Q. Let me go back to Exhibit 221-028 which we have marked for identification. This exhibit is entitled "Memo on Possibility That EF is Ceding Fraudulent Policies." This is dated December 28, 1971.

     Have you ever seen this document before?

A. Yes, sir.

Q. Can you tell me when you first saw it?

A. To the best of my knowledge, it was in April 1973.

Q. What was the occasion for your seeing that document in April of 1973?

A. When this business came out in the paper, in the news about the fraud, I took these papers out to review them in connection with sending them to our legal counsel, I guess.

*   *   *

Q. Do you recognize the handwriting in the margins?

A. Yes.

Q. Whose handwriting is that, sir?

A. That is John Brown's.

*   *   *

Q. Did you ever tell Mr. Brown that you were concerned that Equity Funding might have been ceding fictitious policies to Ranger?

A. There would have been some discussions to that effect but I don't know whether I would have said that I was concerned. It gets around to audit procedures and the scope of an audit.

Q. Did you ever tell Mr. Brown that the problems of the matters that Mr. Krenzke discussed in Paragraph 1 of Exhibit 221-028 are, "the kind of treatment we would have received if there was fraud"?

A. Yes.

Q. When did those discussions take place?

A. I don't know. I guess, according to this memo, it must have been prior to December 28.

Q. Do you remember how much prior?

A. It would have to have been, I presume, between the time Mr. Krenzke came back to Houston and the 28th, whenever that was.

     I direct your attention to Page 2. Up at the top of the page there is a statement by Mr. Krenzke, which I am going to read, the introductory paragraph, and then I am going to read subparagraph C and ask you a question.

     "I have discussed my feeling with Mr. Brown that I do not feel that there is evidence of Fraud. I base this on: C, examinations by H & S as EF's CPA's, also by State Insurance Examiners and independent actuaries which have not indicated any fraud."

     Do you recall ever having any discussions with Mr. Brown, during the period that you earlier testified that you had talked off and on to him about these things, about whether he or any other Peat, Marwick employee contacted Haskins & Sells about EFLIC?

A. No, I don't recall.

*   *   *

Q. Mr. Suttle, during the period from the 16th of December through year-end of 1971 did you ever discuss with anyone at Ranger, your client, concerns that you earlier talked to Mr. Brown about, the ones that you testified about?

     I am specifically referring now to—

A. During that period?

Q. Yes.

A. I don't recall.

Q. You don't recall?

A. No, I don't know whether I did or not.

Q. You testified earlier that you did tell Mr. Brown that—I am quoting again—"this is exactly the kind of treatment we would have received if there was fraud."

     I asked you whether you talked to Mr. Brown about that and you said, "Yes."

     You are now testifying that you did not have any conversations concerning that subject with anyone at Ranger, with your client, or you don't recall whether you did; is that right?

*   *   *

Q. In your opinion should an account auditor that has concerns about the possibility of fraud occurring in connection with a special examination, such as the one involved with

Ranger - Equity Funding,
Memo on Possibility that
EF is Ceding Fraudulent Policies
9-30-71

W. P. No.	4-9
ACCOUNTANT	FL
DATE	12-28/71

This memo is prepared to set down the present status of the examination as I understand it.

① As conveyed to me by John Brown, Mr. Bill Suttle, engagement partner, is concerned about the possibility that Equity Funding may be ceding fictitious policies to RNL. He founds his concern in the slowness of with which Gene Howard I received files while at EF & the request by Fred Levin, Pres. of EF, that we leave in the midst of the examination. His position that ~~that~~ this is exactly the kind of treatment we would have received if this was fraud.

② I have discussed my feeling with Brown ~~that I~~ do not feel that there is evidence of ~~collusion~~ fraud. I base this on.

   ⓐ No serious exceptions noted in file examination
   ⓑ First hand knowledge of EF growing problems which would seem to explain the delays in obtaining files (this includes microfilm conversion bottlenecks & EF management's general

RNL-EF		W. P. No.	H-9-
		ACCOUNTANT	R
9-30-71		DATE	1 2/LE/

attitude that they didn't have time
for us.)
© Examinations by H+S as EF's CPA's,
also by state ins. examiners &
independent actuaries which have
not indicated any ~~possibility of~~
fraud.

Mr. Suttle has indicated we
may need to examine funding
files in California.
        I have pointed out to VB
that I do not think this
is necessary + that it seems
such an examination would ~~not~~
yield no better evidence than
we now have. If EF is
manufacturing policy files they
could just as easily manufacture
funding files. However, I also
recognize that Mr. Suttle
draws from much greater experience
than me + can see problems I
might miss. I have requested
that should Mr. Suttle deem
this work necessary that he
advise me of his reasons so
I can recognize what I have
overlooked + can convey these
reasons to RNL

EFLIC—Ranger, communicate those concerns to his client immediately?

Mr. Woodland: You can answer it now. *(Ed. note: Woodland's remark relates to a long legal wrangle that preceded this question.)*

The Witness: Yes.

Mr. Sachnoff:

Q. Mr. Suttle, at any time after December 16, 1971 did you communicate to any representative of Ranger your concerns about the possibility of fraud at EFLIC?

A. I would have to say that I don't recall, to start with, that I said that I had concerns about fraud.

Q. Mr. Suttle, your testimony earlier was that you had discussions with Mr. Brown in which you expressed your concerns about "the possibility of fraud at EFLIC."

I think the record will show that if we read the answers back.

A. Well, it didn't come out as me being concerned with fraud. If you let me amplify this, I will tell you what I am talking about.

Q. By all means, sir.

A. We had had an examination that aborted; we had been sent back to Houston and they wanted to send microfilm back for us to look at. Somewhere in here during discussions with the client, the client already knew of this because Mr. Howard was the representative for the client there, purposely from Ranger, with Mr. Krenzke. He reviewed all of these memos with Mr. Krenzke. The client knew everything that we know.

Mr. Howard was there as an internal auditor. I was concerned and that was discussed with the client, I was concerned in trying to do an audit looking at microfilm. I wanted to go back to California to do certain things. I felt we had reached a point where the scope of my examination was being limited and they, of course, were arguing, "No, we have got to do all of this and get this done. We want the support and we will have these people fly in whatever you need."

In one of these discussions I said, "No, we don't have any evidence there was any fraud but, in hindsight, if something is wrong, people will look back and say that these were signs of fraud."

What I was getting at was audit procedures that I needed to do to issue a report on this work.

Q. Let me direct your attention to Exhibit—

A. These memos did not reflect what I said to Mr. Brown in the way it was said in these discussions.

Q. I think your answer is clear.

Exhibit 221-027 on the second page contains a notation and it says:

"Read and concur—Gene Howard 12-16-71 6:45 p.m."

I would like to now direct your attention to the next exhibit, Exhibit 221-028, which is also a memorandum by Mr. Krenzke. . . . *(Ed. Note: not reproduced here)*

*　　　*　　　*

Would you look at Item 1B, please. It says:

"Pending: Policies have not been compared to cash receipts or in force listings. Both documents have been requested but are yet to be received.

Will you explain what is meant by the first sentence, "Policies have not been compared to cash receipts or in force listings"?

A. As I recall, that was part of the test work. The in force listing is a listing of policies in force that Equity Funding would have which they use in computing reserves on policies. We had not tested those yet to that listing to see that the records showed that these policies were in force because they had not furnished, apparently, the microfilm of the in force listings. I presume it would have been microfilm. The same way with cash receipts; we had not compared them back to see that there had been premiums received on these policies as part of the test work.

Q. Why is that; why didn't you do that?

A. We had not been furnished those records.

Q. But would those two procedures have normally been included in your special report as part of tests that you would do, that is comparing?

A. Yes, this was in the program and it was subsequently done when they flew back the microfilm, these records to Houston. Apparently Brown must have asked certain questions, "What do we need to finish this work," and "What is left pending," and this was one of the things that had not been done yet because we had not received those records. We didn't get all of this work completed while in California.

Q. We are not talking about work on the next report now.

A. This is the same job. They weren't through when Mr. Levin asked them to leave back in December. This is still part of that work.

Q. Why is it that you were trying to do work on this matter after your representatives were kicked off the premises of EFLIC on December 16, 1970?

A. Because Ranger was trying to get us to go ahead and complete this audit by using microfilm in Houston and their man, Gene Howard, did a lot of this subsequent checking and they wanted to go ahead and do that and have us issue a report. That is what I was objecting to. "You can go ahead and do the work to see if you find exceptions or whatever you want to do, but I am not going to give you an audit report because of the scope of my examination. You have limited my scope."

Q. But then, Mr. Suttle, why didn't you tell your associate to stop all of this work if you were not going to render any report?

Wasn't this just a useless gesture, doing all of this stuff on microfilm?

A. Ranger was paying for this and they kept wanting this work done and they kept thinking through April that they were going to get a report.

*   *   *

Q. Mr. Suttle, Exhibit 221-030 is a memorandum in Mr. Brown's handwriting entitled "Memo Regarding Possible Fraud," and dated January 18, 1972.

Can you tell me whether you have ever seen this document before?

A. Yes, sir.

Q. Can you tell me when you first saw it?

A. To the best of my knowledge, it was in April 1973.

Mr. Sachnoff: I am going to mark as Exhibit 221-032 a document entitled "Ranger—Equity Funding," dated January 28, 1972, a handwritten document in Mr. Brown's handwriting. (*Ed. note: not reproduced*)

Mr. Sachnoff:

Q. Mr. Suttle, have you ever seen this document before?

A. Yes, sir.

Q. Can you tell me when you first saw it?

A. No, I really can't. This type of memo, I may have seen it at that time rather than in April of 1973 but I can't say definitely.

Q. Do you know whether this meeting took place?

A. I remember the meeting.

Q. Did you attend this meeting?

A. Yes, sir.

Q. Yes, you did, because it says, "Mr. Suttle and Mr. Brown gave status report."

Can you recall what Mr. Vann's and Mr. Rathbun's reactions were to your status report on the EFLIC special work; what did they say?

A. Part of the discussion was that they were concerned about getting the work done, getting whatever records we needed to complete it and give a report. Mr. Rathbun wanted to know, "What do you need to finish this work? I will contact Equity and get it for you."

That was part of the status thing.

Q. Did you tell Mr. Rathbun what you thought you needed to permit Peat to finish its report?

A. Yes, sir. I am not sure how much of that is in here, but we had a discussion about this auditing microfilm. We had quite a difference of opinion. He could not understand why I was not willing to go ahead and do all of this work with microfilm and give him a report. He insisted that he was going to get it. He said, "We will get it in here and why don't you go ahead and do all of the checking that you would do and see if you can't work it out."

We agreed to go ahead and let Howard—I think Howard did most of the checking and I don't know what Krenzke did. I said at that time, "Go ahead and do it but I am not going to give you any assurance that I will give you a report."

At that time I told him what I had previously told Mr. Brown, because of the limitations on the scope and because I was not there to get the feel of being on the premises of an audit, that if something was wrong they would look back in hindsight and say, "There were signs that something was wrong," and that is why I did not want to complete this work using microfilm and give him a report.

*   *   *

Q. Was there any discussion at this meeting about the possibility of bogus or fictitious policies being ceded to Ranger by EFLIC?

A. Only to the extent that I have stated from my standpoint of audit procedures. As I recall, I told Mr. Rathbun we had found nothing that indicated to us that there was any fraud. I had not seen anything that was a fradulent document, at least to me. I told him that and I told him the reason why I wanted to do all of this other work, what I just said a moment ago, from an independent audit standpoint. There are things that you do.

                                        Exhibit 221-030
                                        Memo of John Brown. PMM Los Angeles
                                        9-3-71
                                        (typed from handwritten exhibit)

Memo regarding possible fraud.

9/30/71

Outlined below are my reasons for believing that there is not fraudulent insuring of fictitious policyholders of Equity Funding Life Insurance Company:

1. Senior and RNL representative have found no material exceptions or pattern of exceptions which are unresolved and could have a material adverse effect upon the financial position of RNL.

2. Senior and RNL representative have worked directly with Equity Funding chief financial office vice president and reinsurance coordinator and their other clerical personnel. At no time was a true suspicion of collusion or fraud felt.

3. We have been furnished for our files micro-fiche copies of the complete policyholders files which we tested. Our review of such files has not indicated or suspicioned any falsified information within the files.

4. Equity Funding provides reinsurance (co-insurance) contracts with other confirms. RNL receives first priority under the contracts. Our testing has revealed no evidence of adverse selection.

5. Volume of business forces Equity Funding into such a reinsurance program or they endanger their surplus from viewpoint of state insurance examiner -- not enough surplus for retained in force (risk). If life company underwriting were to cease, the major sales tool for the sale of mutual funds would also cease.

6. By end of each policy year, Equity Funding will have (not legible) to RNL equal to that RNL originally paid to Equity Funding, net of lapses in the interim. Lapses are controlled by minimum persistence clauses (85%) within the reinsurance contract.

7. Claims are being filed, reviewed and paid by RNL,s direct (last word not legible)

Q. In Item 3 of the report Mr. Brown writes: "Don't want to do more such work in future. Just finish this and then let H & S"—I presume that is Haskins & Sells?

A. Yes.

Q. —". . . H & S personnel or Howard and internal audit people do the work. Risk is too great when consider the limited amount of test work we perform."

Did anybody contact the Haskins & Sells people as a result of this meeting?

A. No.

Q. You didn't contact them?

A. No, we had no reason to.

Mr. Woodland: The question that you asked Mr. Sachnoff, does it ask if anyone at Peat, Marwick contacted Haskins & Sells?

Mr. Sachnoff: Anybody. If anybody, as a result of this memorandum, contacted them.

Q. Did anybody, either someone at Peat, Marwick or someone at Ranger, contact Haskins & Sells?

A. I thought you were talking about Peat, Marwick. To my knowledge, no one did but I do not know, of course, about Ranger.

Q. Item 4 in the report that you and Mr. Brown gave says:

"Found no evidence to base suspicion on. Just that delays and high level of people we must work with didn't ring true."

What did you mean by that?

A. I don't remember making such a comment. That does not sound like something I would say.

This is Brown's way of summarizing our discussion at the meeting. I think it gets back to the recap of the things that happened. They were supposed to have everything ready for us and when we got our we had delays and we finally would get the records and we were going along good and then all of a sudden they stop the work. It was this type of thing and that is what we were talking about. These are things that happen in

hindsight, if something turns out to be wrong some day you say that you should have been aware that there was a red flag.

That was part of this discussion that I just went through as to why I wanted to come back out here and do work in the client's office.

*   *   *

Q. What was the next thing that happened after this meeting in connection with the EFLIC-Ranger report?

A. I can't specifically say. Krenzke and Brown and, I guess, Howard got these records in, the ones that they wanted.

Q. Which records were those, sir?

A. Whatever it was they needed, the cash receipts and so forth. They got the microfilm in. I would assume that Gene Howard probably did most of that test work, rather than Krenzke. I did not get very involved with this because I had more or less decided that I was not going to issue a report. They could go ahead and check and see if they could find out from what they were doing. I don't remember getting very involved at that point.

Q. What happened to the project after that?

They got the documents and the information that they requested, it came it; is that right?

A. Apparently they did the check and, I think, there is a report in there that, apparently, Mr. Krenzke or somebody drafted up that I never saw because I never had any idea of issuing a report. I never reviewed it. I told Mr. Brown to put the papers in the file and I was not going to issue a report.

Q. You did not spend much time on this matter after the meeting?

A. That is why I did not see a lot of these documents until 1973, because I did not review these papers as I would have done if I would have issued a report.

*   *   *

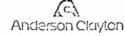

Anderson Clayton
P. O. Box 2533   Houston, Texas 77001   (713) 224-6641

November 20, 1972

Mr. Rex Davis
Ranger Insurance
Houston, Texas

Dear Rex:

I am enclosing a copy of the tentative budget of the time
proposed by Seidman & Seidman in connection with the audit of the
accounting records of Equity Funding.

This budget seems high to me, especially since some of
this work must be done in connection with their regular year-
end examination of Equity Funding.

I shall appreciate any ideas you may have on this subject.

Yours very truly,

W. W. Vann

mn
Enc.

c.c. W. E. Suttle ✓ — Would appreciate any suggestions you might have
concerning the budget.

THE FINAL DAYS

The thin fabric of the Equity Funding fraud endured for years, but the ultimate disintegration came precipitously. During the week of March 19–23, EFCA stock fell from 25 to 18⅞ on a volume of 835,000 shares (with 7,925,000 total shares outstanding). On the following Monday, March 26, 1973, volume reached 768,000 for the day (or 10% of the total shares outstanding) as the price fell another three points. *The Wall Street Journal* ran the first of what was to become a long series of articles about Equity Funding on the next day, May 27, indicating that questions were being raised about the company (article reproduced here). Over 300,000 shares traded that day, as the price fell another three points.

The next morning, Stanley Goldblum sent an inter-office memorandum to the Company's managers (reproduced here) assuring them that EFCA had never been "more sound or more profitable", as *The Wall Street Journal* carried a story echoing these comments. Nevertheless, The New York Stock Exchange suspended trading of EFCA shares that day.

The scent of fraud showed in the next day's *Wall Street Journal,* which described "an intensified audit" by the insurance examiners of three states. Of course, by then it was too late for shareholders who had not taken part in the hectic trading of the last few days.

Early reports of the fraud emphasized its computer implications, much to apparent chagrin of two of Equity Funding's computer people. On April 11, they issued their own press release, protesting the idea that the fraud stemmed from the computer or its programmers. Largely ignored at the time, as later discoveries showed, their protests were correct.

The Wall Street Journal, March 27, 1973

Equity Funding Stock Falls Amid Rumors About a Unit

By a WALL STREET JOURNAL *Staff Reporter*

LOS ANGELES—Recent heavy selling of the stock of *Equity Funding Corp. of America* has been accompanied by rumors that questions have been raised about the operations of Equity Funding Life Insurance Co., a subsidiary chartered in Illinois and headquartered here.

Equity Funding common slid $2.25 yesterday to close at $17, as the New York Stock Exchange's most active stock on a turnover of 768,400 shares. The stock has closed as high as $37.25 earlier this year.

The questions center on the accuracy of the subsidiary's reported statements of new policies written and total insurance in force. In a statement yesterday, Stanley Goldblum, chairman and president of Equity Funding, declined to give the nature of the rumors but acknowledged that they wre circulating in the financial community. He said they were without foundation and that the company was "taking steps" to prevent their further spread.

Examiners from the Illinois and California departments of insurance have been auditing the books of the subsidiary for more than a week, but both departments say that the procedure is a routine triennial audit, for which the company was overdue. Sources in both departments confirmed that they heard the rumors about the alleged irregularities.

EQUITY FUNDING CORPORATION OF AMERICA

INTER-OFFICE COMMUNICATION   **Please use a separate letter for each subject**

To___ EFCA Department Heads, Managers and General Agents _____ Dept._____

From___ Stanley Goldblum _____ Office_____ Dept._____

Subject_ Current Situation _____ Date__ March 28, 1973 _____

Copy to :

In this difficult moment for the company, I want to be sure that everyone connected with EFCA is fully aware of developments regarding our stock.

First of all, let me assure you that EFCA is financially strong and that operating and sales results warrant full confidence in Equity Funding's continued progress.

The current crisis relates exclusively to the company's stock. The SEC has suspended trading in our securities until April 6 to protect shareholders against possible further price drops. Our common stock had been under the heaviest selling pressure in five years as a result of a wave of irresponsible rumors circulated in the financial community. The facts in the matter are outlined in the attached statement read late yesterday to Dow Jones and other news services.

What the statement could not express is my deep and personal concern over the impact of all this on our home office and field associates, particularly those who own EFCA stock or hold well-deserved stock options. You can be sure that the disappointment and possible hardship you may be feeling because of the price drop in our stock is shared by everyone in management.

All of us have built this company together, and I am sure we will weather the storm together. It is ironic that, in spite of the crisis in our stock, our company has never been more sound or more profitable, and our marketing strength has never been greater. The weeks ahead will be difficult times, but I am confident that, once these problems have been resolved, we will continue to grow and prosper as we have without interruption for over a decade.

Please communicate the content of this letter and attached news release to the members of your department, branch or agency. If you have any questions, please feel free to call any of our senior home office or field management people.

The Wall Street Journal, March 29, 1973

Equity Funding Rebuts Rumor That Unit Made Inaccurate Statements

Concern Orders Expanded Audit Of Life Insurance Subsidiary To Confirm Reported Results

By a WALL STREET JOURNAL *Staff Reporter*

LOS ANGELES—*Equity Funding Corp. of America,* whose stock was halted in trading on the New York Stock Exchange yesterday, said there isn't any basis for rumors circulating in the financial community about the accuracy of statements by its life insurance subsidiary, Equity Funding Life Insurance Co.

The company also announced that it had ordered its independent auditors, Seidman & Seidman, to perform an expanded audit of the subsidiary "in response to the rumors which have led to extraordinary activity" in the company's stock. Equity Funding was trading at $14.375 prior to the halt, off $2.625 from Monday's close.

The company said the rumors relate to the accuracy of statements concerning the amount of life insurance sold and in force as reported by the subsidiary in previous years. The concern added that it knows of no basis for these rumors.

Equity said "these rumors furthermore suggest a connection between these allegations and the routine examination of our subsidiary currently being conducted by the Illinois, California and Mississippi department of insurance. This is entirely without basis in fact."

Equity stated that the examination of its subsidiary, "which has been in progress for the past three weeks, is the previously scheduled regular triennial examination normal for all insurance companies and in fact required by the state insurance regulations." The company said "no findings have been issued in connection with the state examination."

"We are confident," the company added, "that the voluntary inquiry being performed by our independent auditors and the triennial examination currently in progress will confirm our previously reported financial and insurance results." Equity also said it asked the Securities and Exchange Commission and the Big Board to extend the time for filing and publishing the company's annual report until the auditors have completed their work.

The company announced it intends to initiate a program for the purchase of up to one million shares of its common in the open market to take advantage of the current price of the stock.

Equity's chairman and president, Stanley Goldblum, said he had "no comment" on reports that Loews Corp. is buying a large position in Equity stock.

The Wall Street Journal, March 29, 1973

SEC Halts Trading in Equity Funding Corp. As It Begins Study of Firm, Insurance Unit

By WILLIAM E. BLUNDELL
Staff Reporter of THE WALL STREET JOURNAL

LOS ANGELES—A full-scale investigation of *Equity Funding Corp.* and a subsidiary, Equity Funding Life Insurance Co., has been launched by the Securities and Exchange Commission. At the same time, state insurance departments are widening their own audit of the subsidiary's books.

The launching of the formal SEC investigation accompanied the suspension yesterday of trading in the company's securities by the SEC until April 6. The New York Stock Exchange had halted trading Tuesday.

By then, the price of Equity Funding common had been hammered down from an opening of $24.87 on the Big Board March 19, to $14.37. Volume was heavy and big blocks of stock changed hands.

Several big institutional investors are believed to have dumped their holdings of Equity Funding on rumors about the life insurance subsidiary. During the heavy trading period, the company at first said it didn't know of any internal reason for the sell-off, but it later acknowledged the existence of rumors. Stanley Goldblum, Equity's chairman and president, declined to say what they were but declared they were without foundation.

The SEC won't comment, but it is known that the staff of its western regional office in Los Angeles has begun an extensive investigation of the case, centering on rumors about the accuracy of the subsidiary's reports of new insurance sold and total insurance in force. As do many other life companies, Equity Funding Life reinsures with other companies a sizable amount of the business it writes, getting cash in return. It is understood that this portion of Equity Life's business is under special scrutiny.

At the same time, an intensified audit of the subsidiary's books is being carried on by examiners from the insurance departments of Mississippi, California and Illinois. Illinois is leading the examination, as Equity Funding Life is incorporated there, though it is headquartered in Los Angeles.

Equity Funding has characterized the examination as a "routine" triennial audit. The life insurance unit was overdue by a year or more for such an examination, due to a backlog of work in the Illinois department.

Though the Illinois department declines to comment, insurance sources note that the audit it ordered was a surprise audit, an unusual practice in the ordinary triennial. Also, it is believed that the Illinois examiners are conducting a more extensive audit than is usually done. The examiners know of the rumors.

Though the Illinois department declines to comment, insurance sources note that the audit it ordered was a surprise audit, an unusual practice in the ordinary triennial. Also, it is believed that the Illinois examiners are conducting a more extensive audit than is usually done. The examiners know of the rumors.

Mr. Goldblum of Equity Funding wasn't immediately available for comment on the latest developments. But Rodney Loeb, general counsel for Equity Funding, said the company stands on its prior statement that it doesn't know of any foundation for the rumors. He noted that Equity's independent auditors, Seidman & Seidman, have begun an expanded audit of their own on the subsidiary's books at the company's request.

"If this expanded audit shows something, we would be the most surprised guys in the world," said Mr. Loeb. As previously announced, Equity Funding has asked the SEC and the Big Board to extend the time for filing and publishing the company's annual report until Seidman & Seidman can finish its work. Mr. Loeb also said that the company, alarmed by the rumors, had contacted the SEC in Washington on its own initiative. A meeting of company officials and SEC western region staffers is scheduled for tomorrow.

Contact: Frank Hyman   893-4990   FOR IMMEDIATE RELEASE
            Bob McGindley 823-3081

Los Angeles, April 11, 1973 --------------------------------

"PEOPLE FRAUD" -- NOT "COMPUTER FRAUD" SAY EQUITY FUNDING

CORPORATION COMPUTER PROFESSIONALS

"Credit for a highly sophisticated computer fraud not ours,"

says Frank Hyman, manager of systems and programming. "I didn't

do it and I resent the implication," says Bob McGindley, systems

manager.

Calling this scandal "the largest computer fraud ever perpetrated"

is incorrect and unjust, say these two computer specialists.

Previous examples of computer frauds involved using a computer

to "talk to" a competitor's computer for the purpose of stealing

proprietary information; using a computer terminal to fraudently

misdirect the property of another company for one's personal

advantage; taking small amounts of other persons' interest or

income and diverting them to the account of the programmer or

his accomplice. In all of the above computer frauds, the

system was intentionally designed to do something illegal.

This was not the case in the Data Processing Department at

Equity Funding.

                        - more -

- 2 -

The responsibility of the Data Processing Department at Equity Funding was to process data exactly as it was received from other departments, and not to pass judgement on its validity. This was done in all cases.

Great emphasis was put on the balancing and control of computer systems. It was considered a primary part of design criteria and they did their best to instill these philosophies upon all members of their staff. To the best of anyone's knowledge, all systems had sufficient controls within them to correctly process all data received.

As the story of Equity Funding unfolds, it becomes obvious that they were receiving "garbage in", which was accounted for in a highly sophisticated manner, and were producing "garbage out". Unfortunately, this garbage was created beyond the control of the data processing organization. If any mistake was made, it was in assuming that legitimate data was being received.

The alleged fraud at Equity Funding Life Insurance Corporation could have been performed through the use of manual techniques.

- more -

- 3 -

The major contribution of the computer was that it lent an air
of authenticity to otherwise bogus data. Anyone unfamiliar
with the computer will tend to accept a computer report as
Gospel, when in reality, it is no more accurate than the person
supplying the information to the computer.

The discovery of fraud at Equity Funding was particularly
frustrating to both Mr. Hyman, formerly a consultant and past
director of the EDP Auditors Association, and Mr. McGindley,
a former internal auditor for a leading financial institution.
They stated that, "We tried to generate interest a few years
ago in expanded audits utilizing both accounting and data
processing expertise, with no success. The situation we now
find ourselves in proves the validity of our theories."

With the continual reference to this as a computer fraud,
the reputations of not only the Equity Funding data processing
staff, but the entire computer industry is being maligned.

-- 30 --

THE FRAUD AND HOW IT WORKED

Notes on the Report

The full text portion of the *Report of the Trustee* has been reproduced here. The original report also includes reproductions of the consolidated financial statements from the published annual reports of Equity Funding for 1964 through 1971. In order to provide more details for a longer period, we have instead reproduced, in the last section of this volume, financial materials taken from several sources including annual reports, interim reports, and prospectuses.

The footnotes in the trustee's report that refer to Appendix B are to the annual report financial statements of the year mentioned in the text. The same information can be found in the materials at the end of this volume, which are presented in chronological order.

Footnotes in the *Report of the Trustee* that refer to "Report of the Trustee" are to an earlier report, which is not reproduced here.

Unfortunately, it is difficult to duplicate most of the trustee's computations since almost all are based in part on figures which are not readily available. For example, the figure of $2,382,000 is cited on page 27 in the explanation for column (A) of the table found on that page. The $2,382,000 represents the January 1, 1964, amount of premiums financed on so-called old programs. It can be derived by referring to page 11 of a prospectus dated December 14, 1964, where a table provides the amount of premiums financed in each of the years 1960 through 1963. The amounts (not including the amount in the column for nine months ended 9-30-64) total to $2,381,970, which rounded is the number used by the trustee.

The amount for premiums on terminated programs, given by the trustee as $468,000 in the

same example, cannot be derived from the same source. The difference is apparently because terminations occur at any time. The table in that prospectus was prepared in late 1964 and shows a total of $531,769 for terminations, presumably reflecting terminations that occurred in 1964 on earlier programs. One assumes that the trustee had data with an early 1964 cutoff.

The continuous change in the terminations amount can be noted by reference to the reproduced page 11 of a May 12, 1965, prospectus, with the same table. The premiums financed for 1960 through 1963 are the same figures and total to $2,381,970. However, terminations for the *same* years now total $550,291, since the prospectus covers a period three months later than the earlier documents. (*Note:* The row "Amount of Annual Premiums Involved in Terminations" shows a cross total of $350,291. This was an apparent *misprint* of the total, which adds to $550,291, based on the items.)

Some amounts are easier to trace. The trustee's table on page 43 gives "Funded loans receivable" and "Notes payable" at the end of 1964 as $6,682,076 and $5,975,585, respectively. These amounts will be found in the December 31, 1964, balance sheet of EFCA.

Unfortunately, even this table (on p. 43 of the trustee's report) provides some problems. The computed "Maximum bogus income" figures for the years 1964 through 1967 are derived as described on the same page. The 1968 "Maximum," if computed as stated by the trustee, would be $9,677,000 instead of the $6,879,000 shown in the table. No explanation is given.

FILED

REPORT OF THE TRUSTEE

of

Equity Funding Corporation of America

Pursuant to Section 167 (3)
of The Bankruptcy Act
[11 U.S.C. §567(3)]

ROBERT M. LOEFFLER
Trustee

O'MELVENY & MYERS
Of Counsel

October 31, 1974

TABLE OF CONTENTS

i

Chapter	Page

iii

United States District Court
Central District of California

In the Matter — of — EQUITY FUNDING CORPORATION OF AMERICA *Debtor*	**IN PROCEEDINGS FOR THE REORGANIZATION OF A CORPORATION** No. 73-03467 **REPORT UNDER SECTION 167(3)**

To The Honorable Harry Pregerson, Judge of the United States District Court for the Central District of California:

ROBERT M. LOEFFLER, Trustee of EQUITY FUNDING CORPORATION OF AMERICA, the above named Debtor, in the Debtor's Chapter X proceeding under the Bankruptcy Act [11 U.S.C. §501 et. seq.], hereby renders his report to this Court pursuant to Section 167(3) of the Bankruptcy Act [11 U.S.C. §567 (3)] and the Order of this Court dated as of April 5, 1973, based upon the facts ascertained by him pertaining to fraud, misconduct, mismanagement and irregularities, and to causes of action which might be available to the Debtor's estate.

PART ONE

INTRODUCTION

This report is made by the Trustee in reorganization of Equity Funding Corporation of America ("EFCA" or "the Company") in compliance with Section 167(3) of the Bankruptcy Act, which requires the Trustee to report to the reorganization court:

> ". . . any facts ascertained by him pertaining to fraud, misconduct, mismanagement and irregularities, and to any causes of action available to the estate."

The requirements of Section 167(3) are of peculiar significance to the EFCA reorganization because of the widespread fraud perpetrated by some of the Company's managers and employees. The ensuing paragraphs of this introduction will describe the scope of the Trustee's investigation into these matters. The body of the report will describe the major areas of fraud, misconduct, mismanagement and irregularities at EFCA, and the final part will draw some conclusions. The report as a whole sets forth facts pertaining to causes of action available to the estate. For obvious reasons, it does not discuss the merits of suits that have already been filed by the Trustee or that may hereafter be filed, nor the legal analysis that the Trustee's counsel has made with relation thereto. These are matters that will come out as such suits are prosecuted in the courts.

The Trustee's investigation focused primarily upon facts which might give rise to actionable claims on behalf of the EFCA estate. However, because the EFCA fraud challenged so many assumptions which underlie business and regulatory practices in this country, the question, "How did it happen?" was thought to be of more than academic interest. Accordingly, the Trustee felt a special responsibility in this case to report the story of the EFCA fraud in some detail, although financial and practical limitations precluded an exhaustive report.

Since possible future litigation was a major purpose of the investigation, an effort was made to develop evidence that would be admissible in court. It is believed that this report is based on such evidence. The extraordinary duration of the fraud and the incredible variety of irregularities involved made the task of finding such evidence a formidable one, as will readily appear from a reading of the report.

The first steps of the investigation were taken immediately after the Trustee was appointed. Files and other documents which had been maintained by the former officers of EFCA who resigned upon disclosure of the fraud were collected, inventoried and, except for purely personal items which were released to their owners, placed under the custodianship of representatives of the Trustee. In the succeeding months, these and literally tens of thousands of other corporate documents were reviewed to determine whether they might be of assistance in piecing together the story of the fraud.

The task was unusually difficult because EFCA's books and records were in a chaotic condition when the Trustee took over the Company. Many records may have been lost with the passage of time, and there was ample opportunity for others to have been destroyed during the last hectic days prior to the collapse, or before. Consequently, enormous amounts of time were required simply to find tangible evidence from which reliable financial data could be reconstructed. Moreover, even such tangible evidence sometimes made no sense and was disbelieved at first. Only gradually, as other pieces of the puzzle fell into place, was such evidence integrated into a whole picture of the fraud.

In addition to scrutinizing the voluminous files and records at EFCA, representatives of the Trustee obtained documents from various public agencies and from outside entities with whom the Company had maintained business and professional relationships, including banks, auditors and law firms which had rendered services to the Company in the past. These materials were studied and analyzed in detail.

Witness interviews constituted a second major source of information. In the early stages of the investigation, counsel and other representatives of the Trustee participated in a number of unrecorded interviews of some of the EFCA conspirators in order to acquire a working knowledge of the mechanics, entities and individuals involved. This information was supplemented by a review of over 10,000 pages of recorded testimony taken by various govern-

3

ment investigators from more than 90 witnesses, and by numerous additional unrecorded interviews. Thereafter, the Trustee's attorneys conducted their own recorded depositions and interviews of 20 key individuals, including many fraud participants who had entered pleas of guilty to federal indictments filed against them. The transcripts of these interviews comprise more than 3,000 pages. While these interviews and testimony were important sources of information for this report, they created their own problems in analysis because of frequent inconsistencies and apparent conflicts.

Substantial accounting analysis performed in connection with the Trustee's inquiry helped to resolve many of these problems. A review of the work papers from past audits of EFCA and its subsidiaries, coupled with a study of available books and ledgers, provided indispensable information regarding the consolidated operations of EFCA and the manner in which the fraud was perpetrated. A decision was made not to attempt a complete re-audit of the Company's operations during its entire corporate lifetime, and not to seek to comprehensively trace the cash which flowed in and out of the Company. Such undertakings would have required an enormous expenditure of funds, and it is not at all certain that they could have been successfully completed, given the state of EFCA's books and records and the high probability of difficulty in obtaining satisfactory information from independent sources. Nevertheless, in the course of their examination of EFCA and its subsidiaries, the Trustee's accountants followed critical areas of the fraud back to their apparent origins. In addition, tests of cash receipts and disbursements were made for some periods on a sampling basis.

Representatives of the Trustee also conducted a limited investigation in Europe in an effort to obtain information concerning the foreign companies involved in the EFCA fraud, and to locate possible assets belonging to the Company.

As information was developed from each of these sources, it was evaluated with an eye toward identifying and explaining the major themes in the evolution of the fraud. Often, newly acquired information caused a reassessment of previously held beliefs and required the investigation of fresh clues or the renewal and redirection of prior searches. Eventually, however, it was possible

4

to reconstruct a basic chronology of the EFCA fraud which was consistent with the large body of knowledge acquired during months of investigation. Once a reasonably secure understanding of those events was developed, an analysis of the resulting legal implications was undertaken so that an informed judgment could be made in regard to pursuing potential causes of action on behalf of the estate.

The investigation is continuing. Efforts to interview other individuals who might possess relevant information are even now under way, as are efforts to obtain additional documentary evidence from outside sources. In this connection, for example, it should be noted that the Trustee has not secured the cooperation of Stanley Goldblum, former President and Chief Executive Officer of EFCA. His testimony and other data will doubtless be obtained in the course of litigating the Trustee's claims and in other related litigation.

Because the investigation has not yet been completed, this report cannot be considered definitive. It is submitted now, however, so as to be available for consideration in connection with the Trustee's proposed plan of reorganization for EFCA. And, although the ongoing investigation may strengthen or possibly alter some of the observations and conclusions which follow, the Trustee believes that this report is not only timely but also accurate and sufficiently complete to serve the purposes sought to be achieved.

PART TWO

THE FRAUD AT EQUITY FUNDING

I. OVERVIEW AND SUMMARY

When the shocking news of the problems at EFCA first came to the public's attention in April 1973, the fraud at the Company was almost a decade old. In the months which have elapsed since those initial revelations, much has been written about the fraud and its history. Despite all of the commentary, three basic points remain obscured.

First, the fraud at EFCA was essentially a *securities* fraud. While much attention has been focused on the insurance aspects — especially the manufacture of bogus policies — that activity was merely one part of a much larger stock fraud that began at or before the time of EFCA's first public offering in 1964. This scheme appears to have been initially motivated and then sustained throughout the decade of its existence by an obsessive desire on the part of its participants to inflate and keep aloft the market price of EFCA's common stock. It is not incidental that the originators of the conspiracy were also the major holders of the Company's stock, for one result of the fraud was their personal enrichment. It may well be, however, that as time went on pride and vanity played as great a motivating role as greed for many of the participants.

Second, theft and embezzlement seem to have been a relatively small part of the fraud.* Most of the so-called "missing" assets never in fact existed or were dissipated in the Company's continuing operating losses.

Third, the fraud was relatively unsophisticated in both design and execution. It was neither comprehensively planned nor systematically developed. Rather, its various individual elements were created on an ad hoc basis, as need dictated or opportunity presented itself, and little attempt was ever made to integrate these various elements with one another. In order to coherently describe the fraud,

---

* The thefts and embezzlements known to the Trustee are described at pages 129-133.

6

this report has attempted to order and structure its elements into a number of broad categories. But this organized presentation really belies the true helter-skelter, hand-to-mouth nature of the fraud.

Moreover, notwithstanding some publicized accounts to the contrary, the fraud was not the brainchild of computer-age financial wizards. It was to a great extent simply a pencil fraud, perpetrated by means of bogus manual accounting entries, with virtually no support for those entries in many cases. That the fraud persisted undetected for so long is attributable to the audacity and luck of its perpetrators and, just as importantly, to the glaring failure of the Company's auditors to perform properly the obligations which they had undertaken.

The EFCA fraud was carried out principally by inflating the Company's reported earnings, largely through recording non-existent commission income in EFCA's books and records.* This practice appears to have begun at least as early as 1964, in anticipation of EFCA's first public offering of common stock, and to have continued on an increasing scale until the fraud was discovered in early 1973. Since the majority of bogus income was booked in connection with the Company's funding business, that aspect of the EFCA fraud is referred to in this report as the "funding fraud."** (It should be noted, however, that nothing about the funding business made it inherently subject to fraud.)

The basic concept of the funding fraud is easily grasped. The bulk of EFCA's real income during the early period of the Company's history derived from commissions earned on sales of "Equity Funding Programs," a combination of mutual fund shares and life insurance policies which EFCA helped to pioneer. Beginning at least with the first known bogus entries in 1964, and each year thereafter until the Company's collapse in 1973, the amount of commission in-

---

*Appendix B to this report contains reproductions of the consolidated financial statements for EFCA and its subsidiaries which were published in annual reports to shareholders from 1964 to 1971. The annual report for 1972 was at the printer when the fraud was discovered and, accordingly, a reproduction of a printer's proof of the financial statements for that year is also included.

**See "The Funding Fraud," beginning at page 13.

7

come which EFCA earned in connection with such sales was inflated in the Company's financial statements. Over the years, the amount of bogus income reported by this means alone totalled in excess of $85 million.

The funding fraud had a number of attributes which made it particularly attractive as a method for reporting bogus income, not the least of which was its operational simplicity. It required only manual entries in the Company's books and records to produce the precise amounts of earnings inflation desired. No effort was made to provide underlying documentation to back up the entries, nor was any attempt made to conform EFCA's individual funding customer accounts to the fictitious entries in the books and records. Hence, the funding fraud was easily perpetrated by a small group of people, and this minimized the risk of its discovery.

Through 1967, the funding fraud appears to have been sufficient to boost the earnings of EFCA to the level desired by those managing the scheme. Despite its more attractive attributes, however, the funding fraud had an inherent characteristic which limited its usefulness as a means of inflating income. Because of the manner in which EFCA's funding programs operated and were accounted for on the Company's books, each dollar of bogus income produced through the funding fraud resulted in a dollar increase in an asset called "funded loans receivable," representing amounts supposedly borrowed by customers and ultimately due for repayment to the Company.* EFCA's management hardly objected to an increase in the Company's reported assets. But as the inflation of funded loans receivable increased, it became more and more difficult to support the patently excessive figures to the satisfaction of even EFCA's easily-satisfied auditors. Moreover, while the funding fraud made EFCA appear to be more profitable than it really was and made it appear to hold larger assets than it really held, it did not supply any cash to the Company. As time went on, EFCA's cash needs became severe, most notably because of continued operating losses.

---

* See "The Equity Funding Concept," at pages 13-14, and "Accounting Treatment for EFCA's Funding Program," at pages 18-23, for a more comprehensive explanation of EFCA's funding business and the accounting therefor.

Beginning around 1968, as a result of these problems, the EFCA fraud broadened beyond the simple device of funding account over-statements and inflation of commission income. One device employed by the conspirators was designed to help ease the cash needs of the Company, and also to reduce the burgeoning funded loans asset and thereby permit the reporting of still more fictitious income through the funding fraud. This device involved borrowing funds without recording the amounts borrowed as liabilities on the Company's books. Sometimes this was done simply by not recording the sources of the funds at all, and on other occasions by incredibly complicated bogus transactions which wound their way through numerous subsidiaries, foreign and domestic. However it was done, the borrowed funds were applied to reduce the funded loans asset as though Equity Funding Program participants had retired their loans by cash payments. The conspirators referred to funds brought into the Company in this manner as "free credits."

The expansion of the EFCA fraud after 1968 involved not only "free credits" but a diverse variety of other frauds, some simple and some complicated. For example, a sham sale of supposedly valuable future commissions, which EFCA owned, to a foreign shell controlled by the conspirators resulted in the inflation of income by $17.2 million in 1969. Because many of these schemes in some manner concerned foreign transactions and subsidiaries with which the Company purported to be involved from 1968 to 1970, this period in the history of the fraud is characterized in this report as its "foreign phase."*

Ultimately, these various schemes proved insufficient to generate the amount of bogus income desired by the conspirators. An "insurance phase" of the fraud developed to fill this void.** The fictitious record of growth which resulted from the funding overstatements had facilitated expansion of the Company's operations through acquisitions financed by a series of debt offerings and by inflated EFCA stock.† As a result, EFCA was transformed from a

* See "The Foreign Phase of the Fraud," beginning at page 45.
** See "The Insurance Phase of the Fraud," beginning at page 77.
† The period of acquisition is chronicled in Report of the Trustee of Equity Funding Corporation of America pursuant to Section 167(1) of the Bankruptcy Act (Feb. 22, 1974) (hereafter "Report of the Trustee") at pages 7-12.

9

simple marketing organization into a life insurance-based conglomerate. Most important among EFCA's insurance subsidiaries was Equity Funding Life Insurance Company ("EFLIC"), acquired in late 1967. A major part of EFLIC's insurance business involved "reinsurance" — in effect, the resale of insurance policies to a second insurance company. It was through EFLIC's reinsurance operations that the conspirators perpetrated the most celebrated aspect of the EFCA fraud.

The integration of EFLIC's reinsurance operations into the EFCA fraud evolved in stages. In 1968, EFCA negotiated a release from the terms of an exclusive sales agreement it had with Pennsylvania Life Insurance Company ("PLC") in order to permit EFCA to market insurance policies underwritten by EFLIC. To secure the release, EFCA committed itself to reinsure a large amount of insurance with PLC over a three-year period. Early in 1968, it became clear that EFCA would not be able to fulfill that commitment through its regular business, a prospect which was disturbing to EFCA's management for a number of reasons. To solve this problem the Company decided to issue what it termed a "special class" of insurance, consisting of policies issued to its agents and employees on which it paid all or part of the first year premium. These policies were reinsured with PLC, but the nature of the business was not disclosed.

"Special class" insurance was followed in 1969 by the implementation of a new scheme to help EFLIC meet its reinsurance commitments and "production goals" set by the conspirators. Pending business — that is, applied-for insurance which still required approval by the underwriting department and payment by the applicant — was posted on the Company's books as if it were in-force and paid-up. This pending business was reinsured with other companies, despite the recognition that much of it would never legitimately become effective.

The Company had difficulty with PLC because of the high lapse rates on the "special class" business which had been reinsured. To avoid a suspiciously high lapse rate on reinsured pending policies, the conspirators arranged for the Company to pay renewal premiums on that portion of the pending business which never became

10

effective. It was but a short step from this to the outright creation of wholly bogus policies, a step that was taken the following year.

The conspirators began in 1970 to record wholly fictitious insurance in order to lend an illusion of production to the Company's operations, and then to reinsure those policies in order to generate needed cash. This practice continued through 1971 and 1972 at an increasing pace. The conspirators thus found a device which they hoped could assist the funding fraud in augmenting the Company's reported earnings on a sustained basis.

But the insurance phase of the fraud created monumental difficulties. The most immediate of these was a serious cash flow problem. Under the Company's reinsurance arrangements, EFLIC received a significant cash payment from its reinsurers at the time policies were reinsured. In succeeding years, however, EFLIC was required to forward to the reinsurers the renewal premiums it received from policyholders. In the case of the bogus policies, of course, there were no policyholders. Consequently, the Company had to pay these renewal premiums itself. The conspirators tried to meet this cash need by reinsuring more bogus policies, but this only made next year's cash flow problem worse. Thus, in 1972 EFLIC had a negative cash flow of $1.7 million in connection with its bogus reinsurance operation.

A second difficulty resulted from the manner in which insurance sales were accounted for on the Company's books. EFCA's general insurance agency subsidiary, EFC-Cal, earned commissions on the sales of EFLIC policies, and received the insurance premiums paid in connection with these policies. The premium amounts which EFC-Cal owed EFLIC, after its commissions were deducted, were reflected in an "inter-company account" between the two subsidiaries. Fictitious insurance resulted in a growing imbalance in this inter-company account because premium amounts purportedly due to EFLIC from bogus business were recorded on EFLIC's books but not on those of EFC-Cal. To cope with this problem, the conspirators had to create more and more fictitious assets.

The conspirators were still grappling with these problems when their house of cards collapsed in March and April of 1973. The col-

11

lapse was by then inevitable, a reality which the perpetrators of the fraud refused to face. Even as the fraud came apart at its seams, they tried to respond to the situation with further intrigue and deceit, but their time had at last run out.

In the end, the results of the fraud were massive. From 1964 through 1972, at least $143 million in fictitious pre-tax income was reported in the Company's financial statements.* During the same period, the total net earnings reported by EFCA amounted to just over $76 million. Although the Company thus was never actually profitable, it appeared to flourish and its securities attracted thousands of investors. The story of the fraud at Equity Funding, which has had tragic consequences for many, is told in greater detail in the following chapters of this report.

* See Report of the Trustee at page 38.

12

II. THE FUNDING FRAUD

The program from which EFCA took its name played a predominant role in the fraud from start to finish. This chapter begins with a description of the "equity funding" concept, a brief history of the equity funding program at EFCA and an explanation of the basic accounting treatment applicable to it. Then, after describing the origins and development of the funding fraud, the chapter concludes with an assessment of its overall magnitude.

A. Evolution of EFCA's Funding Program.

(1) THE EQUITY FUNDING CONCEPT.

EFCA began as an independent sales company which marketed mutual fund shares and life insurance policies, primarily to middle-income families. It vigorously promoted a package of these products known as the "Equity Funding Program," which was based on the British "life funding" concept. This concept involves borrowing on mutual fund shares to purchase life insurance in the hope that the income on and appreciation of the mutual fund shares will exceed the interest cost of the borrowing and pay for at least a portion of the insurance premiums.

In a typical Equity Funding Program, the participant undertook to purchase a life insurance policy and to invest in mutual fund shares over a 10-year period. The participant paid cash for the mutual fund shares. EFCA paid his life insurance premiums, recording the payment as a loan to the participant and retaining the mutual fund shares as collateral to secure the loan. In essence, the equity in the participant's mutual fund investment was used to finance ("fund") his purchase of an insurance policy. Hence, the package was called an "equity funding" program, and the loan itself a "funded loan." As the renewal premium on the insurance policy and interest on the funded loan became due each year, the loan was increased to cover these costs. At the same time, the participant purchased additional mutual fund shares in an amount at least sufficient to secure the increased loan.

Upon termination of the program, the participant repaid his loan by direct cash payment, by application of the proceeds from the sale of a sufficient number of his mutual fund shares, by applica-

13

tion of the cash surrender value of his life insurance policy, if any, or by any combination of these methods. If at the end of the program the value of the participant's mutual fund shares had increased as hoped, the appreciation would have reduced the effective cost of his insurance policy or, ideally, paid for the policy entirely.

In theory, the equity funding concept could be applied to any periodic purchase; for example, the purchase of a car or home. And, of course, any individual could purchase mutual fund shares on a regular basis and pledge them as collateral to secure loans with which to pay the premiums on a life insurance policy. EFCA's funding program provided financing for its participants, together with a package of administrative services which made it easier to use the funding concept. The long-term success of this concept depended upon steady increases in the value of the pledged mutual fund shares which, in turn, required a generally rising stock market.

(2) A BRIEF HISTORY OF EFCA'S FUNDING PROGRAM.

EFCA grew from the amalgam of two small securities and insurance marketing organizations. In the late 1950's, Gordon C. McCormick developed and sold his own funding program, and Stanley Goldblum ran a small insurance agency. In 1959, they combined their organizations and made plans to expand their funding program sales through a new corporation, "Tongor Corporation of America." McCormick became dissatisfied with the developing plans for Tongor and did not become a stockholder of the new corporation, which soon changed its name to "Equity Funding Corporation of America."

Three other men joined Goldblum in the venture, and each of the four received an equal, one-fourth interest in Tongor. Those other than Goldblum were: Raymond Platt, who had been the manager of McCormick's San Francisco office; Eugene Cuthbertson, the owner of a small securities firm; and Michael Riordan, a Keystone mutual fund representative. In return for their stock in the new corporation, the owners contributed a small amount of cash and full ownership of two insurance general agencies and one securities broker-dealer. From the beginning, Goldblum and Riordan ran the operation: Goldblum as President and Chairman of the Executive

14

Committee, and Riordan as Executive Vice President and Chairman of the Board. Platt and Cuthbertson later left the Company, selling most of their stock to Goldblum and Riordan.

From 1960 to 1966, the Company remained essentially a marketing organization selling life insurance, mutual funds and funding programs combining the two. EFCA's individual agents were licensed to sell insurance through marketing subsidiaries which acted as general agents for a handful of insurance companies. The primary insurance general agency was Equity Funding Corporation of California ("EFC-Cal"). Other subsidiaries were used in states such as New York which required incorporated insurance agencies to be domestic corporations. EFCA agents also were licensed to sell mutual fund shares through Equity Funding Securities Corporation ("EFSC"), the Company's broker-dealer subsidiary. EFSC had selling agreements with the underwriters of numerous mutual funds. For the most part, however, Keystone Custodian Funds were used in connection with EFCA's funding programs. The sale of such programs accounted for the biggest share of the Company's business during these years.

EFCA's revenues from the sale of funding programs consisted of commissions on the sale of the life insurance policies, commissions on the sale of the mutual fund shares and interest paid by program participants on their funded loans. In addition, some small service fees were charged to participants. EFCA's expenses in connection with the funding programs consisted of commissions paid to agents, the cost of maintaining a marketing organization, the cost of administering the funding programs and interest on such borrowings as EFCA made to support the program.

Prior to 1963, EFCA financed the funded loans for its funding programs (hereafter called "EQU" or "Old Programs") through demand or short-term commercial bank borrowings approximately equal in amount to the aggregate outstanding amount of its funded loans. As security for its loans to participants, EFCA required each program participant to sign an agreement which gave the Company power to sell his shares if he defaulted under the program, and to apply the proceeds against any outstanding balance on his funded loan. The shares themselves were placed in escrow.

15

Operating on this basis, the Company made a modest, but promising start. In May 1962, however, the Securities and Exchange Commission ("SEC") concluded that funding programs constituted investment contracts and, as such, were subject to registration as securities under the federal Securities Act of 1933. As a result, few additional Old Programs were sold after May 1962. However, EFCA continued to advance renewal premiums for established Old Programs, and program participants continued to purchase mutual fund shares as needed to secure these advances.

Most of the Company's efforts between June 1962 and October 1963 were directed toward designing a new funding program for registration under the 1933 Act. On October 21, 1963, EFCA's registration statement for "Programs for the Acquisition of Mutual Fund Shares and Life Insurance" was declared effective by the SEC, and the Company resumed selling funding programs under which the Company made direct loans to participants for premium payments as it had under the Old Programs. In lieu of merely recording these loans as advances, as had been done under the Old Programs, they were evidenced by a series of notes. At the commencement of a program, a one-year note was signed by the participant equal to the amount of his first year premium plus the first year's interest thereon.* This note was secured by the mutual fund shares purchased by the participant. Each year thereafter during the ten-year term of the program, as the annual premium on the insurance policy became due, the Company made a new loan to the participant, taking in return a new note equal to the next annual premium, plus the aggregate amount of the past years' loans, plus the advance interest for the coming year on the total. At all times, the participant was required to maintain as collateral mutual fund shares worth a specified amount greater than the face amount of his note.** If at any time the redemption value of the participant's shares dropped below the required level, EFCA was authorized to terminate the program unless the participant either purchased additional shares or paid down his loan.

---

*From 1963 to 1972, the effective rate of interest on such notes generally ranged from 6% to 10%. For programs commenced after August 31, 1969, interest was accrued at the end of each year instead of in advance, in part as a result of changes in Federal Reserve Board regulations.

**See Report of the Trustee at pages 25-27.

16

The new funding programs (hereafter called "Custodial Programs") were designed to permit the Company to obtain financing from outside lenders on the security of the participants' notes. To accomplish this, EFCA entered into four "Custodial Collateral Note Agreements" with New England Merchants National Bank ("NEMB") as custodian bank. Under these agreements, EFCA delivered the participants' notes and mutual fund shares to NEMB, and NEMB agreed to hold them in four separate pools as collateral security for EFCA borrowings from outside lenders. These lenders advanced funds to EFCA upon the receipt from EFCA of Custodial Collateral Notes in the amount of the borrowing and a certificate by NEMB that the collateral in the pool that secured the note was sufficient. Although EFCA subsequently reported to the contrary in its financial statements and prospectuses,* the aggregate notes receivable from the program participants never significantly exceeded the aggregate amount borrowed by EFCA from outside financial institutions through the sale of Custodial Collateral Notes.

From 1963 to 1967, the Company reported steady growth — primarily attributed to its funding business.** Then in 1967, EFCA embarked on a program, described in an earlier report by the Trustee,† of acquiring companies whose products could be sold in place of or in addition to the products of unaffiliated companies. Three proprietary insurance companies were added from 1967 to 1972, and the underwriting of insurance ultimately replaced funding as the mainstay of EFCA's reported business. Nevertheless, as the following table demonstrates, funding remained a significant and ever increasing source of reported income.

---

* See page 42.

** See Appendix B at pages 155-182.

† See Report of the Trustee at pages 7-12.

17

REPORTED GROWTH OF FUNDING BUSINESS°
(1961-1972)

	Total Gross Income	Commission and Interest Income from Funding°°	Percent of Gross Income from Funding	Funded Programs Sold	Funded Loans Out-standing†
1961	$ 1,765,947	$ 1,452,823	82%	2,309	$ 1,490,483
1962	1,836,260	1,479,118	81	2,180	3,337,271
1963	1,324,852	739,864	56	371	4,912,340
1964	2,869,200	1,492,348	52	682	6,913,699
1965	5,363,348	2,693,499	50	1,525	10,372,710
1966	7,486,812	3,904,565	52	2,763	16,477,869
1967	11,178,943	5,343,710	48	3,912	25,094,811
1968	19,179,117	9,306,093	49	5,783	36,311,037
1969	45,571,643	15,238,875	33	9,354	51,188,119
1970	60,912,874	18,559,100	30	11,139	63,324,413
1971	130,951,000	22,280,560	17	13,813	88,616,000
1972	152,601,000	—	—	—	117,715,000

B. Accounting Treatment for EFCA's Funding Program.

The mechanics of the funding fraud are more easily appreciated if one understands how a funding program should have been recorded in the Company's books and records. Hence, this section attempts to provide a simple lesson in funding program accounting. After an introduction to the subsidiaries involved in the Company's funding business, the section traces the relevant accounting for a hypothetical Equity Funding Program into a consolidated statement of earnings for such a program. Although this discussion sets out the proper accounting treatment, it should be borne in mind that, because of poor systems and record-keeping at EFCA, even legitimate transactions were not always correctly recorded.

EFCA was organized as a holding company. Its funding business was actually conducted through wholly-owned operating subsi-

---

° Figures shown for 1961 to 1971 were reported in EFCA prospectuses. Figures for 1972 are taken from printer's proof of 1972 annual report. See Appendix B at page 227. Other 1972 figures not available.

°° Includes gross commission income from both securities and insurance sales.

† Combined figures for "Old" and "Custodial" Programs.

18

diaries.* To understand the funding fraud, only two of these subsidiaries are important: EFSC (the securities broker-dealer), through which sales of mutual fund shares to program participants were effected; and EFC-Cal (one of the insurance general agencies), through which the great bulk of funding program insurance sales was made.

EFCA earned commission income from the sale of funding programs through both EFSC and EFC-Cal. On mutual fund sales, EFSC received a dealer's commission equal generally to 7% of the offering price, 50% of which went to the individual selling agent (on sales of affiliated funds, the agent's share was 60%). On insurance sales, EFC-Cal earned a commission which varied according to the type of policy and riders attached thereto, but which for the most part equaled 100% of the first year's premium and 10% of all renewal premiums for the second through tenth years. Out of its gross commissions, EFC-Cal paid the individual sales representative commissions usually equal to 50% of the first year's premium and 5% of all renewal premiums.

Interest income on loans made to program participants to pay premiums ("funded loans") was entered on the books of EFC-Cal, as was the interest expense on the borrowings made by EFCA to finance such loans. The interest rates charged to program participants on funded loans ranged from 6% to 10%, depending on the year and the state in which the funding program was purchased. At the same time, EFCA incurred interest charges of from 4½% to 10% on its own borrowings.

The following discussion illustrates how income from funding and related expenses were reported on EFCA's financial statements by following the steps which would have been involved in the purchase of a single $25,000 life insurance policy through an EFCA funding program. Since the annual premium on such a policy was $356, an initial investment of $1,000 in mutual fund shares was required to enroll in such a program.** In addition, this hypo-

---

*Since EFCA's corporate structure changed over the years, the mechanics described in this section are not entirely accurate for every period of the Company's development. Nevertheless, the description given should serve the purpose for which it is intended in this report.

**An initial investment requirement of 250% is assumed, and the figure is rounded-off to an even $1,000.

19

thetical example assumes the purchase of non-affiliated products, and a yearly investment in mutual fund shares of $1,000 over the life of the program. Lastly, the following commission and interest rates are assumed: A 7% brokerage commission on the sale of the mutual fund shares, half of which went to the individual agent who made the sale; an agency commission on the sale of the insurance policy equal to 100% of the first year's premium and 10% of all renewals, half of which also went to the individual agent; an interest rate of 7% charged to the participant on the annual funded loans made to him by the Company, and a rate of 6½% incurred on borrowings maintained by EFCA to finance such loans.

When such a funding program was sold, the Company received $1,000 in cash to buy the participant's mutual fund shares. Of this amount, $70 (7% of $1,000) was retained by EFCA and recorded on the books of EFSC as securities commission income and as an increase in cash; $35 was paid out to the individual selling agent and recorded as an increase in commission expense and a reduction in cash. Thus, after the initial payment, EFSC's books showed commission income from the transaction of $70; $35 of which was paid out as a commission expense and $35 of which was retained as cash. The remaining $930 was paid to the mutual fund distributor to purchase the participant's shares.

At the same time, steps were taken to purchase the participant's life insurance policy. The Company advanced the participant's $356 premium to the life insurance company, recording this advance on EFC-Cal's books as an increase in funded loans receivable and a reduction of cash. Simultaneously, $356 (100% of the first year premium) was recorded on EFC-Cal's books as insurance commission income and as an increase in cash. This represented EFC-Cal's commission from the insurance company. Since the two cash entries cancelled each other out, the net effect on EFC-Cal's books in the first year was thus to record commission income of $356 and an increase in funded loans receivable of the same amount.

Upon the initiation of such a hypothetical program, entries were also made on EFC-Cal's books to record $25 of "interest income" (7% of $356, due as interest from the customer in the first year on his

20

funded loan) and to increase the funded loans receivable in that amount.* EFC-Cal also recorded $23 of "interest expense" (6½% of the $356 which EFCA borrowed to finance the funded loan). Finally, $178 (50% of $356) was paid out to the individual selling agent as his commission, and was recorded on EFC-Cal's books as "commission expense" and as an equivalent reduction in the cash account.

On a consolidated basis, a single sale of this hypothetical funding program resulted in first year income of $451 ($70 from securities commissions, $356 from insurance commissions and $25 from interest); and expenses of $236 ($35 to securities commissions, $178 to insurance commissions and $23 to interest). Assuming no other expenses,** this single program sale thus generated consolidated net earnings of $215 for EFCA in the first year.

In the second through tenth years, additional purchases of mutual fund shares and payments of insurance renewal premiums were accounted for in the same manner, except that insurance commission income was recorded as $36 (10% of the renewal premium of $356), and insurance commission expense was recorded as $18 (50% of the renewal commission). Of course, interest income increased, because each year there was added to the principal of the loan an additional premium plus the interest charged during preceding years. By the same token, when EFCA borrowed money to fund the loans, interest expense also increased.

---

*Up until September 1969, interest was recorded on funded loans each year in advance. Thereafter, it was recorded at the end of each year. See note at page 16.

**Expenses such as the cost of maintaining the sales and funding operations and general corporate costs are not included in the hypothetical example.

Taken all together, if this were the only business done by EFCA over a two-year period, the sale and renewal of a single such hypothetical funding program had the following effects on EFCA's consolidated statements of earnings.

HYPOTHETICAL CONSOLIDATED STATEMENT OF EARNINGS

	Year Ended December 31	
	1st Year	2nd Year
Income		
Securities Commission	$ 70	$ 70
Insurance Commission	356	36
Interest on Funded Loans	25	52
Total Income	$451	$158
Expenses		
Agent's Commission on Securities	$ 35	$35
Agent's Commission on Insurance	178	18
Interest on Custodial Collateral Notes	23	48
Total Expenses	$236	$101
Net Earnings Before Taxes	$215	$ 57

The aggregate amount of funded loans made to program participants, together with the interest earned on such loans, was reported as an asset called "Funded Loans and Accounts Receivable" on EFCA's consolidated balance sheet. This asset grew each year as premium loans to program participants were increased to cover accrued interest and annual renewal premiums due, and as funded loans were made to new program participants. Conversely, whenever participants terminated their programs, funded loans made to such participants were paid off and the asset was reduced. The amounts which EFCA borrowed to finance premium loans made to program participants, together with the accrued interest on such borrowings, appeared as liabilities on the balance sheet. In the aggregate, these borrowings were referred to as "Custodial Collateral Notes Payable." Thus, in the hypothetical example, at the end of the first year Funded Loans and Accounts Receivable would have been carried at $381 (insurance premium of $356, plus first year interest of $25); and at the end of the second year at $789 (first year loan, plus renewal premium of $356 and second year interest of $52). These balances

22

would have been offset by Custodial Collateral Notes Payable and accrued interest of substantially the same amount.*

As will be seen from the following narrative, the main thrust of the funding fraud involved the systematic and simultaneous inflation of commission income and funded loans receivable in the Company's books and records.

C. A Funding Fraud Narrative.

The statistics reporting the growth of EFCA's funding business were a fraud. They were the product of a pervasive conspiracy to inflate the Company's reported earnings by overstating the volume and scope of its operations. All told, more than $85 million of bogus income was generated from fraudulent funding entries. A fraud of this magnitude, of course, was not accomplished in a single stroke. Indeed, it apparently began with or before the Company's first public offering and grew steadily over the following decade. In the process, indications of the fraud multiplied on the Company's books and records. Nevertheless, year after year EFCA's auditors continued, inexplicably, to certify the inflated financial statements.

(1) THE EARLY YEARS (1964-67).

In 1964, New York Securities Co. underwrote a small public offering of 100,000 shares of EFCA's stock at a price of $6 per share. With the development of a public market for its stock, the Company's earnings became a subject of intense concern to the handful of executives who until then were its only shareholders. A good earnings record would increase the value of the stock and thereby enrich the conspirators, who held large amounts of stock and who received more through the years as bonuses. Furthermore, inflated reported earnings and assets made it possible for EFCA to acquire other companies in exchange for its stock, and to borrow money with which to make other acquisitions and finance the Company's operations, which lost huge amounts each year.** Based upon the available evidence, it appears that these factors motivated the fraud.

* From 1964 to 1967, the Company reported separate figures for EQU Programs. In those years, the EQU asset was called "Loans Receivable from Clients for Premium Loans," and the liability was called "Notes Payable on Clients Premiums Loans." See, for example, the 1967 financial statements in Appendix B at pages 178-179.

** For a listing of the borrowings, see Report of the Trustee at pages 13-14. For a description of the acquisitions, see Report of the Trustee at pages 7-12.

Late in 1964, Goldblum told Jerome Evans, the Company's Treasurer, that he should increase EFCA's reported earnings for 1964 above the amount reflected on the Company's books and records at the time. According to Evans, Goldblum said that arrangements were being made for EFCA to participate in commissions earned by brokerage houses from various securities transactions. Goldblum gave no details, but he assured Evans that through these arrangements EFCA would soon receive "reciprocal commissions" of $300,000 to $400,000. Goldblum told Evans that, in order to give the truest picture of EFCA's performance for the year and to push the price of the Company's stock as high as possible, this income should be accrued in 1964. However, supposedly because it was improper for the Company to receive reciprocal commissions, Goldblum told Evans they would have to be disguised in EFCA's financial statements. He suggested that this be done by reporting the reciprocals as commission income with an accompanying increase in the EQU funded loans receivable account.

The so-called "reciprocal" brokerage commission arrangements to which Goldblum attributed EFCA's increased income were once a common practice in the securities business. The varieties of such reciprocal arrangements were legion. Under one not unusual arrangement, the manager of a mutual fund would direct a securities broker executing transactions on a stock exchange for the mutual fund's portfolio to "give-up" a portion of the brokerage commission on such transactions to a sales dealer who sold the fund's shares, or to another entity designated by that dealer. These commissions were called "customer directed give-ups." They were permitted by stock exchange rules until December 1968, provided the recipient of the "give-up" was a stock exchange member. The purpose of the practice was to encourage the mutual fund dealer who received the "give-up" to sell more shares of such funds. Exchange members generally were willing to "give up" a substantial percentage of their commissions — which were relatively high on large orders at that time due to the absence of meaningful volume discounts — in order to encourage placement of more business with them by the fund.

As a mutual fund sales organization, EFCA (through EFSC) was the indirect beneficiary of some customer directed "give-ups," chiefly from Keystone Custodian Funds which made up the bulk of

24

the Company's mutual fund sales. In 1967, for example, according to representations made by Riordan to the SEC, Keystone directed commissions aggregating $366,060 to several exchange member firms at the request of EFCA. These "give-ups" were apparently directed to the recipients as compensation for various financial services which they purportedly had performed for EFCA. Since no EFCA subsidiary was a member of any stock exchange prior to late 1969, the Company could not itself have received any amount of "reciprocal" or "give-up" income — let alone the amount indicated to Evans by Goldblum.*

Acting on Goldblum's instructions, Evans made an entry directly into the EFC-Cal general ledger to accrue the supposed reciprocal commission income. The entry was dated December 31, 1964, and showed a credit to commission income of $361,984.97 and a corresponding increase in the EQU funded loans receivable account. The amount of the entry was furnished by Goldblum, but so far as can be ascertained, it had no support whatever in the underlying records of the Company. In any event, as a result, EFCA's reported pre-tax earnings and assets for 1964 were overstated to at least this extent.** This entry by Evans was probably the first reflection of the fraud on EFCA's books.

Several months later when Evans prepared EFCA's unaudited first quarter interim statement for 1965, the Company still had not received any reciprocal commissions. Evans asked Goldblum about the status of the brokerage arrangements and was told that they were still being worked out, but that the money definitely would be received. In fact, Goldblum added, more reciprocal commission income should be accrued in the first quarter of that year because EFCA had generated more mutual fund sales. Again Goldblum supplied the amount, and Evans increased income and EQU funded loans receivable on the interim statement.

Thereafter, Evans made periodic entries in EFC-Cal's books and records to inflate income and EQU funded loans receivable,†

---

* The terms "reciprocal" and "give-up" were sometimes used interchangeably to describe such commissions, despite their different technical meanings.

** See Appendix B at page 155.

† The corresponding account for Custodial Programs (programs sold after October 1963) does not appear to have been tampered with until 1968. See pages 29-35.

posting the cumulative amount of the overstatements to the general ledger at various intervals. This procedure was followed until he left the Company in early 1969. At first, Goldblum gave Evans the precise amount for these increases. Later, however, Goldblum supplied Evans with an inflated earnings per share figure — still attributing the overstatement to "reciprocals." Evans was instructed to make whatever increases were necessary to support the inflated earnings per share figure. Throughout this period, the phony entries made by Evans appear to have been completely unsupported by any detail in the records of EFCA or its subsidiaries. As time passed and the purported "reciprocals" were never received, Evans realized there was a problem, but he continued to assist in the overstatement of the Company's earnings and assets.

Although the Company had stopped selling Old Programs in 1963, some annual increase in the EQU funded loans receivable account was to be expected thereafter from normal renewals and the addition of interest. However, due to Evans' entries, the receivable increased from 1963 to 1967 at an average annual rate that was greater than 40%. This extraordinary rate of increase should have appeared suspect to anyone who studied EFCA's financial statements closely during these early years. The following analysis, based on figures publicly reported by the Company, including reported figures for terminations (which were surely understated), indicates that the maximum amount to which EQU funded loans receivable could have grown by 1967 was in the neighborhood of $13 million, whereas the Company actually reported a figure in excess of $19.5 million for that year.

ANALYSIS OF MAXIMUM POSSIBLE GROWTH
IN FUNDED LOANS RECEIVABLE
FOR "OLD PROGRAMS"
VERSUS REPORTED GROWTH°
1964-67

	A	B	C	D	E	F	G	H	
Year	Annual Premiums In Force	Premiums Terminated	Maximum Premiums Financed	Funded Loans Outstanding At Beginning	Less Terminations	Maximum Funded Loans Refinanced	Interest	Maximum Funded Loans Receivable	Funded Loans Receivable Reported
1963									4,913,000
1964	1,914,000	74,000	1,840,000	4,913,000	191,000	4,722,000	394,000	6,956,000	6,682,000
1965	1,840,000	66,000	1,774,000	6,956,000	250,000	6,706,000	551,000	9,031,000	9,211,000
1966	1,774,000	62,000	1,712,000	9,031,000	316,000	8,715,000	704,000	11,131,000	13,777,000
1967	1,712,000	67,000	1,645,000	11,131,000	434,000	10,697,000	926,000	13,268,000	19,512,000

° In this table, the "Maximum Funded Loans Receivable" (Column H) for each year is determined by adding together the "Maximum Premiums Financed" (Column C), "Maximum Funded Loans Refinanced" (Column F) and "Interest" (Column G). The process is more fully explained in the notes to each column which follow:

(A) *"Annual Premiums in Force."* This figure represents the maximum amount of annual premiums due on Old Programs in force at the beginning of the year indicated. The annual premiums for all Old Programs sold (including additional insurance purchased by Old Program participants through 1967) totalled $2,382,000, while the premium amounts of terminated programs totalled $468,000. Hence, at the beginning of 1964, "Annual Premiums in Force" equalled $1,914,000. For each year thereafter, the "Annual Premiums in Force" is determined by subtracting the amount of "Premiums Terminated" in the previous year.

(B) *"Premiums Terminated."* This represents the annual premium amounts of Old Programs terminated during the year indicated. The figure is based on Company representations, and is probably well below the true amount.

(C) *"Maximum Premiums Financed."* This represents the maximum amount of annual renewal premiums financed during the year indicated, and is arrived at by subtracting Column B from Column A.

(D) *"Funded Loans Outstanding at Beginning."* This is the maximum amount of funded loans receivable for Old Programs on the Company's books at the beginning of each year. The 1964 figure is based on the Company's financial statements as of December 31, 1963. See Appendix B at page 156.

(E) *"Less Terminations."* This is an estimate of the portion of the Funded Loans Receivable which is attributable to Old Programs termi-

27

It appears that Riordan (who headed EFCA's sales organization) was one of the original architects of the funding fraud. He also frequently acted as a spokesman for management when EFCA's reported figures were questioned. For example, Riordan told a stock analyst at a 1967 breakfast meeting in New York that the Company received reciprocal commissions which it reported in its annual earnings statements as securities commission income. Later, in December 1968, Riordan confided in a conversation with another EFCA officer that the Company was reporting a higher amount of income than was reflected in its internal records. Riordan conceded that reciprocals received by the Company accounted for only a small part of the difference, but justified reporting the higher income figures on the basis that the Company's underlying books and records were incomplete and did not reflect what he believed to be the full magnitude of actual sales. Although such explanations seem to have been accepted at the time, it is now clear that they were false.

The falsity of these figures should have been discovered by the Company's auditors, Wolfson Weiner & Company, a small independent firm of certified public accountants which was retained from 1961 on to conduct annual audits of and render opinions on EFCA's

---

(footnote continued from page 27)

nated during the year indicated. The figure is based on the percentage of in force programs which were terminated during the year (Column B as a percentage of Column A). The percentages for the years indicated are as follows: 1964, 3.9%; 1965, 3.6%; 1966, 3.5%; 1967, 3.9%. This percentage is then applied to the funded loans receivable outstanding at the beginning of the year to determine the approximate amount by which funded loans receivable were reduced as a result of terminations. The estimate is undoubtedly low because (i) termination figures for each year are probably understated, and (ii) terminations usually consisted of older programs which accounted for a greater percentage of funded loans receivable than their annual premium amounts would indicate.

(F) *"Maximum Funded Loans Refinanced."* This represents the maximum amount of funded loans refinanced each year and is determined by subtracting Column E from Column D.

(G) *"Interest."* This is an estimate of the maximum amount of interest which the Company could have earned on loans to participants under the Old Programs. It is arrived at by applying the interest rate charged during the year to the sum of the renewal premiums financed that year (Column C) and the funded loans refinanced (Column F). The interest rates used were as follows: 1964, 6.0%; 1965, 6.5%; 1966, 6.75%; 1967, 7.5%.

financial statements. Evans' bogus entries had a cumulative effect upon the Company's books and records which should have been obvious to the auditors. Each such entry widened the gap between the Company's general ledger balance for EQU funded loans receivable and the underlying detail support. However, work papers of Wolfson Weiner for audits conducted from 1964 to 1967 contain almost nothing to support the figures for EQU funded loans receivable reported by EFCA in these years. According to Evans, whenever the auditors requested additional detail to support the inflated balance, he was able to stall them off to the last minute and then refer them to Goldblum. In all such cases, Wolfson Weiner closed the audit without further inquiry after a conference with EFCA's President.

(2) Transition (1968-69).

Michael Riordan was killed by a mudslide at his home in January 1969, just as the audit for the year ending December 31, 1968 was getting underway. Evans, sobered by a heart attack he had suffered the previous autumn, was fed up with what he was doing. Riordan's death appears to have been the last straw. Not wanting to go through another audit, Evans packed his bags and — without telling anyone at EFCA — went for a 6-week drive across the country. He never came back to the Company. EFCA thus lost two of its top executives at the start of 1969.

(a) *The 1968 Audit.*

The 1968 audit appears to have been the first occasion when anyone connected with Wolfson Weiner sought back up detail to support all of the Company's funded loans receivable balance. Probably because the audit fell in the midst of a turnover of management, the conspirators experienced considerable difficulty in attempting to supply that detail.

When Evans left, John Pennish (an EFCA Vice President who had been the former President and principal stockholder of the first proprietary insurance company acquired by the Company*) asked John Templeton (whom Pennish hired as EFCA's Controller in October 1968) to take over responsibilities within the Company for the

---
* The Presidential Life Insurance Company of America ("Presidential"), later renamed Equity Funding Life Insurance Company ("EFLIC").

audit. Prior to that time, all of the Company's books had been kept by Evans, and Templeton had never even seen them. To his dismay, the 1968 general ledger for EFC-Cal could not be found. However, the problem seemed solved when Wolfson Weiner agreed to accept a reconstructed ledger starting from an unaudited trial balance as of September 30, 1968.

In financial statements for prior years, separate figures had been reported annually for EQU Programs and Custodial Programs. Supposedly to simplify EFCA's financial statements, it was decided to combine the figures for the two programs in the 1968 statements. It became Templeton's job to start with separate figures on the September 30 trial balance and, using basic documents from the last three months of the year, to reconstruct a combined year-end figure for the two categories of programs. By this process he arrived at a figure in the neighborhood of $36 million — an increase of about $11 million over the total of figures reported for year-end 1967.* But Templeton was unable to provide detail support for this figure. Accordingly, Harry Watkins, the accountant who was coordinating the 1968 audit for Wolfson Weiner, decided that confirmations from 100% of EFCA's funding program participants should be obtained. Watkins was a temporary Wolfson Weiner employee who only worked on the 1967 and 1968 EFCA audits. It is noteworthy that he seems to have been the first Wolfson Weiner representative to press for underlying detail to support the funded loans receivable asset.

For the purpose of obtaining confirmations, Watkins requested a listing of participants from the Company. Templeton made arrangements to obtain the listing from EFCA's newly established data processing system, which purportedly contained records for all of the Company's funded programs. After extensive work and several tries, data processing personnel were able to generate a computer print-out of EQU and Custodial Program participants showing a combined balance of only about $7.6 million for all funded loans outstanding. Templeton could not understand the discrepancy between this figure and his reconstructed trial balance figure of $36 million, so he went to Goldblum for an explanation.

According to Templeton, Goldblum attributed the difference to reciprocal commissions which he claimed Evans had accrued through

---

* See Appendix B at page 178.

increases in the funded loans receivable account. As he had to Evans, Goldblum explained to Templeton that "reciprocals" (he called them "recips") could not be separately disclosed in EFCA's financial statements. Templeton argued that Evans' prior entries should be explained to Wolfson Weiner so they would accept the reconstructed balance, but Goldblum disagreed and instructed his Controller to find another way to complete the audit.

Acting on Goldblum's instructions, Templeton added some terminated programs to the computer print-out, increasing the total to about $15.4 million, and gave it to Watkins for confirmation. Evidently, requests for confirmation were mailed to some of the names on the print-out during March 1969 and, as a result of the return the auditors received, they reduced Templeton's figure of $15.4 million to about $11 million. However, it appears that less than one-third of the requests for confirmation were answered and, based upon the work papers for the 1968 audit, substantial questions are raised as to whether the validity of even the $11 million figure was established.

This left a discrepancy of $25 million between the reconstructed general ledger amount and the "confirmed" $11 million figure. In late March 1969, a meeting was held to consider the problem, attended by Templeton, Marvin Lichtig (the Wolfson Weiner junior partner in charge of the audit), Watkins and his junior assistant. According to Watkins, after he reported the results of the confirmation program, Templeton or Lichtig asked if the procedure included new business "in the pipeline." Watkins said no, and Lichtig suggested a figure for such business which surprised Watkins because of its size. No other explanation for the discrepancy was given, and the meeting ended.

After this meeting, Lichtig reassigned Watkins to another EFCA project and personally took over the audit. A second meeting was then held, attended by Goldblum, Lichtig and Julian Weiner (the Wolfson Weiner senior partner responsible for the EFCA account). According to Lichtig, he informed Goldblum that there was no detail to support EFCA's figure for funded loans receivable. In response, Goldblum told the auditors — possibly for the first time — the story about Evans' entries to accrue "reciprocals" by increasing fund-

31

ed loans receivable. He said that Riordan had kept track of the Company's "recips," and was the only person who knew the total amount of them. Because of Riordan's death, Goldblum said, the Company was having some difficulty in collecting the money. But he pointed to $10 million of cash received up to that point in 1969, stating that this money represented payment in part of "recips" earned in 1968 or earlier and that he was trying to collect more. He promised to have Templeton prepare a schedule of the "recip" money already collected so Lichtig could use it as support for the 1968 funded loans receivable. No one asked why EFCA's books did not show similar cash receipts in earlier years as payment of "recips."

According to Templeton, after this meeting Lichtig told him the "recips" were okay, and that the auditors would not disclose them as a separate item. Goldblum then directed Templeton to prepare a schedule for Lichtig to support the entire reconstructed funded loans receivable balance. Templeton actually prepared two such schedules, the first showing a total of $36,176,614, and the second a total of $35,383,622. The second schedule appears in the 1968 audit work papers as the only apparent support for the $36,311,037 ultimately reported by EFCA in its 1968 financial statements as "Funded Loans and Accounts Receivable."* Nowhere does anything appear in the work papers to explain the discrepancy between the totals in Templeton's two schedules and the total reported in the 1968 financial statements.

Templeton's second schedule, upon which the auditors evidently relied in certifying the amount of funded loans receivable, lists several items in addition to the $11 million supposedly confirmed by Watkins. As support for the funded loan balance, those items ranged from the dubious to the patently improper. Two of the items on the schedule (together totaling more than one million dollars) appear to represent new funded loans and liquidations being processed by EFCA's funding department, and are without any detail support in the work papers. A third item, in the amount of $2,115,000, is completely unrelated to Funded Loans and Accounts Receivable, as de-

---

* See Appendix B at page 184.

fined in the notes to the statements, but nothing is said therein to disclose its inclusion.*

Still another item on the schedule purports to be the dollar value of collateral held by EFCA arising from closed funded loans, which is "estimated" to be worth $6,672,337. According to Templeton, while trying to teach himself about EFCA's funding business one night, he reviewed 390 funding program files and found that in seven cases the collateral was still outstanding although the client's loan had been closed. Templeton brought this situation to Lichtig's attention during the 1968 audit. Although his data admittedly were not based upon a valid sampling technique, Templeton calculated on a separate schedule the rate of such closed loans as a percent of all cases, and arrived at 18% (instead of 1.8% which was the correct result of dividing seven by 390). After estimating the total amount of available funding program collateral, he multiplied this figure by 18% and thereby purported to determine that EFCA held mutual fund shares from closed loans worth $6,672,337, and included this figure as support for the funded loans receivable balance on the schedule he gave to the auditors.

It cannot be determined from available records why or if the Company continued to hold mutual fund shares from closed loans. Nor is it clear how such shares could have been thought in any event to provide support for funded loans receivable. The shares pledged as collateral, of course, belonged to the respective program participants, except for so much of their value as would be necessary upon closing an account to pay off the participant's loan. To the extent that, prior to actual sale of the shares, loans were discharged on the basis of the value of pledged collateral, offsetting bookkeeping entries should have resulted in reclassifying these shares to other accounts. For these reasons alone, it seems totally improper for the

---

* The third item is described in the auditors' schedule as "Equity Resources Loans." EFCA formed an oil and gas limited partnership in July 1968 ("ERLP 68"). Equity Resources Corporation, a wholly-owned EFCA subsidiary, was the general partner of ERLP 68. EFCA sold 250 units of this partnership during the year at $10,000 per unit. Of the $2.5 million of units sold, EFCA financed the purchase of $2,115,000 of units through five-year loans made by EFC-Cal at 7½% interest. More than $850,000 of these loans were made to EFCA officers and directors. The full amount of these loans apparently was included in the 1968 figure for Funded Loans and Accounts Receivable.

auditors to have relied upon mutual fund shares retained by EFCA
as support for the funded loans receivable account.

Whatever the basis for the auditors' reliance upon this collateral,
there is no evidence of any attempt to count or otherwise verify
whether EFCA really held mutual fund shares worth $6,672,337, or
any other amount. Moreover, the figure on Templeton's schedule was
plainly erroneous. That figure was derived from various calculations.
But the data from which calculations were made were not a valid
statistical sample, and the arithmetic itself was obviously fallacious.
Indeed, a schedule of "open items" found in the audit work papers
indicates that the auditors discovered the miscalculation — but
neglected to correct it.

The final item on Templeton's schedule — amounting to about
$13.5 million — was described as "collections of recip monies in
1969." Even had "recips" in this amount been received by the
Company in 1969, it would have been wrong to use these
receipts as support for the funded loans receivable account at year-
end 1968. For one thing, there is the obvious problem of mislabeling.
More fundamentally, it would have been improper to accrue such
income; recipients had no legally enforceable right to reciprocal commissions because payments were completely at the will of the particular broker involved. Accordingly, any such commissions should
have been reported as income only when actually received and not
accrued in advance of receipt.

Furthermore, this item in the schedule was implausible on its
face. First, an incredibly large volume of securities sales would
have been necessary to generate $13.5 million of reciprocal broker-
age commissions. Second, as previously mentioned,* "give ups"
could be sent only to stock exchange member firms. Since neither
EFCA nor any of its subsidiaries was a member of a stock exchange
during this period in early 1969, the Company could not properly
have received reciprocal commission income.

Notwithstanding these reasons for suspicion, the auditors failed
to verify the "recips" purportedly received by EFCA. Lichtig claims

*See page 24.

that a member of the Wolfson Weiner audit staff checked the "recip" amounts shown on Templeton's schedules against the cash journal. However, a schedule of "open items" found in the audit work papers suggests that no such check was made. And even if the cash journal showed that the amounts on Templeton's schedule had actually been received, some effort should have been made to verify that they were indeed reciprocal commissions received. The astonishing fact is that all $13.5 million came from unrecorded EFCA borrowings. The following table compares the purported "recip monies" shown on Templeton's schedule with the proceeds from loans discovered during the Trustee's investigation.

Date*	Templeton "Recip" Amounts	Proceeds from Borrowings	Lender
1/ 9/69	$1,961,250	$1,961,250	Neuwirth
1/14/69	113,668	113,668	Merban
1/18/69	96,000	96,000	Merban
1/24/69	222,529	222,529	Merban
1/27/69	1,988,334	1,988,334	First Jersey Bank
2/13/69	4,533,480	4,533,480	LRI
2/17/69	4,535,195	4,535,195	LRI

In summary, EFCA reported a combined figure of more than $36 million for Funded Loans and Accounts Receivable in its 1968 financial statements.** Although this item alone accounted for 46% of the Company's reported assets for the year, it is virtually without detail support in the 1968 audit work papers. At best, Wolfson Weiner could only confirm a balance of about $11 million of funded loans outstanding to program participants. Of the remaining $25 million, $13.5 million was supposed to be, but obviously was not, reciprocal commissions, more than $3 million was completely without detail support or wholly unrelated, and about $6.7 million was "verified" through a combination of invalid auditing procedures and errors in arithmetic.

---

* These dates appear on Templeton's schedules and, with immaterial variations, on relevant loan documents as well.

** See Appendix B at page 184.

(b) *Personnel Changes.*

According to Templeton, throughout the 1968 audit he complained to Pennish about the problems he was having with the funded loans receivable. Templeton went to Pennish because he respected him and hoped for some help. He told his boss that there was a large discrepancy between the general ledger balance and the underlying detail, but got little sympathy. By the close of the audit, Templeton had reached the conclusion that the 1968 financial statements were not good enough to release to the public. He informed no one of his decision until, in the presence of a roomful of EFCA officials and attorneys, he refused to sign a Form S-1 containing the financials for filing with the SEC. Templeton recalls that when asked to explain his conduct he said he was unable to describe what was wrong. So he was ushered out of the room, and Pennish signed the Form S-1 in his place.

About a week after Templeton refused to sign the Form S-1 he was summoned to Goldblum's office. Templeton told Goldblum he thought there was fraud at the Company. Goldblum responded to this statement by asking Templeton if he was going to settle down and work. Templeton recalls that he exclaimed "No, effective now!" and walked out of the office. Later in the day, he was called back. This time Goldblum offered the Controller a substantial sum to stay and help fix EFCA's problems. After thinking it over, Templeton asked for a larger sum in immediate cash, plus stock options and additional money to exercise them. Goldblum agreed. After talking with his wife, however, Templeton had a change of heart and decided to quit. He wrote a note of resignation, left it on Goldblum's desk late at night and never went back to EFCA.

With Riordan, Evans and Templeton gone, EFCA was sorely in need of new management personnel by the middle of 1969. Pennish assumed some of the management burden, but he was evidently aware of enough irregularities to conclude that he did not want to sign any more financial documents. Apparently for this reason, Lichtig was hired from Wolfson Weiner to be the Company's Treasurer. Lichtig was replaced at Wolfson Weiner by Sol Block, who supervised all of the remaining EFCA audits.

Around the same time, Samuel B. Lowell was hired to replace Templeton as Controller. Lowell recruited Michael Sultan to be his assistant. In October 1969, while reviewing the 1968 audit work papers which he found in Lichtig's office, Lowell came across Templeton's funded loans schedules. His suspicions were aroused and he went to Goldblum for an explanation. Once again Goldblum told the "recip" story he previously had related to Evans, Templeton, Lichtig and Weiner. He asked Lowell to help conceal the "true" source of EFCA's purported "recip" income. After thinking it over for a weekend, Lowell agreed. Thereafter, Lowell learned about the rest of the fraud, and, aided by Sultan, he became one of the most active participants in the conspiracy.

By the end of the year, Pennish seems to have been told a good deal about the fraud by Fred Levin (a Pennish protege from Presidential who assumed responsibility for EFCA's insurance operations), who in turn had learned about it from Lowell. Following a trip to Europe paid for in part by EFCA, Pennish exercised his valuable EFCA stock options and left the Company. Thereafter, Lowell and Levin (who became executive vice presidents and directors) joined Goldblum as captains of the EFCA fraud — assisted by a crew that increased in size as the fraud grew and diversified.

(c) *"Free Credits" and Related Devices.*

Beginning perhaps as early as 1968 and certainly by 1969, the conspirators adopted a device they called the "free credit." Although the conspirators did not use this term with a high degree of definition, the explanation which follows appears closest to the sense in which it was commonly used, and will be the sense in which the term is hereafter used in this report. The device was really quite simple. As the conspirators increased EFCA's borrowings, they often concealed the source of the cash so that it did not appear on EFCA's books as a liability. Rather, it was recorded on the books of EFC-Cal as a reduction ("credit") to funded loans receivable, as though program participants had reduced their loans by cash payments in the amount recorded. The credit to the funded loans receivable account was the "free credit." Occasionally, "free credits" were also recorded without any receipt of actual cash through fraudulent entries that created the appearance of cash receipts.*

---

* See, for example, discussions of such entries at pages 71 and 74-75.

37

The purpose and effect of these "free credits" was to reduce the funded loans receivable account, which had been and continued to be inflated in the course of the funding fraud, to a balance which more closely approached the underlying accounting detail. In addition, because they reduced funded loans receivable, "free credits" restored some leeway to the conspirators to create more bogus income by again increasing the receivable. Of course, the use of the "free credit" device created problems of its own. The borrowed money had to be repaid some day and, when it was, it became necessary to disguise or cover up the repayment since the loan was not recorded on the Company's books. This was done by making still other unrecorded borrowings, or by other fraudulent devices that will be described later in this report.

Many of the borrowings that were used to produce "free credits" were effectuated through EFCA's foreign subsidiaries and are described in the next chapter. The practice started in October 1968, however, when EFCA began to place short-term unsecured dollar and Swiss franc notes pursuant to arrangements made with Dishy, Easton & Co. (a small New York brokerage house with whom the Company and certain of its executives did a great deal of business). Minutes for a meeting of EFCA's Board on November 8, 1968 show the directors authorized up to $25 million of such notes. At least 18 were placed in 1968, each for a term of six months or less. Although some were repaid during the year, it appears that $1.6 million of them were outstanding at year-end but not reported as a liability in EFCA's 1968 financial statements. It is reasonable to assume that at least this amount was applied as a "free credit" to some asset account, but it is impossible to know for certain because the relevant records have been lost or destroyed.

The accountants' work papers for the 1968 audit contain numerous references to the notes placed by Dishy Easton during that year. Most notable is a December 30, 1968 memorandum from Goldblum to Evans which specifically describes two of the notes outstanding at year-end. Notwithstanding these references, there is no evidence of any attempt by the auditors to obtain from Dishy Easton, nor indeed from EFCA, a list of such notes placed during 1968 or any other relevant information about them.

During 1969, Dishy Easton continued to place EFCA's unsecured notes, as it had done in 1968. A number of the 1969 borrowings showed up on Templeton's schedule of "recip monies" during the 1968 audit. Some were subsequently recorded by the Company as liabilities in a notes payable account. Others were not so recorded and, instead, were used as "free credits" and were fraudently recorded as "collections" of funded loans receivable. By this means, the funded loans receivable account was reduced by at least $14 million.

Although many of the unsecured notes placed during 1969 matured and were repaid before December 31 of that year, unrecorded notes to Loeb, Rhoades International Inc. ("LRI") and Dow Banking Corporation ("Dow") totalling almost $14 million were outstanding at year-end. Schedules found in the auditors' 1969 work papers describe some of the notes which were repaid during that year, but do not include the LRI and Dow notes. Again, however, the work papers contain no evidence of an attempt to obtain information from Dishy Easton concerning any of the borrowings arranged through that firm. Such information, if obtained from Dishy Easton and properly analyzed, would have revealed the undisclosed LRI and Dow liabilities. Thus, the auditors should have found that the "recip monies" on Templeton's schedule were in fact unrecorded loans and, as a result, that EFCA's 1968 financial statements contained material misrepresentations.

Also in 1969, some $17.2 million of bogus income was generated through a variation on the funding fraud. Entries were made in that year to accrue commission income that was expected in the future from ongoing mutual fund contractual plans. These future commissions were recorded as an asset, and combined with funded loans receivable in EFCA's 1969 financial statements. This accounting treatment was improper for the reasons explained below, and to justify it the conspiracy fabricated a bogus sale of the purported asset.*

---

* See page 66.

(3) THE FINAL PHASES (1970-73).

After 1969, the funding fraud became even simpler. More entries were made to book fictitious "commission income" in the Company's general ledger with a resulting increase in funded loans receivable. Initially, these entries were made in lump sums at the end of each quarter — often in round numbers and always without detail support. Early in the foreign phase of the fraud,* the bogus income booked through these entries was attributed to undescribed foreign operations in England, France, Germany and Italy. After June 1970, however, the entries were simply made without explanation. Beginning in mid-1970, to help avoid the obvious questions which might be raised by quarterly lump sum entries, the overstatements were made on an irregular basis. From two to four such entries were made each month and, in addition, larger entries were made as needed to bring income up to a level consonant with the conspirators' earnings goals.

In addition to bogus commission income, bogus "interest income" was also booked. Initially, "interest" was recorded in lump sums of $200,000 or $300,000 — some of which was undoubtedly legitimate, but none of which was supported by detail. Beginning in March 1971, however, an attempt was made to compute plausible estimates of interest based upon EFCA's reported funded loans receivable. The conspirators applied the current interest rate to the inflated funded receivable balance on the general ledger, and monthly "interest" entries were made to record this amount. The amount of the overstatements made in this manner is not presently known.

At the same time, the conspirators also needed to show a level of expenses reasonably commensurate with the amount of EFCA's reported funding business because, if the reported funding business had been real, the Company would have paid a percentage of its commission income to its individual sales agents. However, if the conspirators merely increased EFCA's "Agents Commission Expense" account, EFCA's net income would have been reduced and the purpose of the fraud defeated. Therefore, the conspirators reclassified a portion of the real administrative operating expenses incurred by the Company as "Agents Commission Expense." This practice had the added advantage of lowering reported operating expenses, and

---

* See page 45.

40

thereby helped to foster the Company's reputation as an "efficient" sales operation.

The most remarkable feature of the funding fraud is that, for practical purposes, it was accomplished by manual book-keeping entries which were almost entirely without underlying documentation. Although the Company kept case files for all of its legitimate funding program participants, at no time were any such files created to support the fictitious funding business. Only legitimate commission income from the sale of mutual funds was recorded on EFSC's books. And only legitimate funding program records were maintained in EFCA's computer system. Thus, when a print-out was needed during the 1972 audit to support the bogus funded loans receivable, a legitimate computer tape was simply repeated a sufficient number of times to reach the desired balance.

Moreover, only the most haphazard attempt was made to coordinate the steps of the funding fraud into one coherent whole. For example, after EFLIC policies began to be used in funding programs, entries on EFC-Cal's books to record bogus premium loans and commission income were completely unrelated to the entries made on EFLIC's books to record bogus premium income and commission expense. During the fraud's insurance phase, such slipshod management created problems for the conspirators which grew more difficult with each passing year.* As a result, it was only a matter of time before one of these many loose ends would have unraveled the whole fraud. The amazing thing is that the fraud persisted as long as it did. In the end the collapse was brought about, not because of the remarkably disorganized and unsystematic character of the fraud, but by a disgruntled former conspirator turned informant.**

D. **An Estimate of the Magnitude of the Funding Fraud.**

Reconstructing accurate statistics to determine the magnitude of overstatement in EFCA's financial statements has been a most difficult task. For one thing, the Company's books and records for the years prior to its collapse were always — and still are — in relative disarray. Indeed, it appears that EFCA never had proper ac-

---

* See page 93.
**See pages 106-107.

counting control over its funding operations. As a result, probably no one during this time could have satisfied himself from internal records alone that the funding business was accurately reported, even if no fraudulent entries had been made. Hence, the exact amount of bogus entries has not yet been determined for each year of the fraud. Based upon known facts, however, it has been possible to make a reasonably accurate estimate of the annual magnitude of the funding fraud.

First of all, it appears that EFCA correctly reported the amount of notes payable on funded loans (both EQU and Custodial) throughout its history. Indeed, prior to 1964, the Company did not base its legitimate funded loans receivable balances upon basic records; instead it assumed they were equal to the amount of notes payable on funded loans which it knew to be outstanding. Thus, even though at any one time there must have been some amount of funded loans not yet financed with an outside lender, EFCA's financial statements from 1960 to 1963 show funded loans receivable exactly equal to notes payable on funded loans.*

Beginning in 1964, however, the financial statements report more EQU funded loans receivable than notes payable on such loans. It appears that this change was brought about by Evans' bogus income entries, which inflated EQU funded loans receivable above the corresponding note payable balance. To conceal these entries, the fraud participants invented the fiction that the growing difference was "held by EFCA."**

In truth, although EFCA always held some amount of funded loans which had not yet been financed through an outside lender, the evidence is clear that the amount could not have been more than 25% of the reported figure — and probably was far less. Thus, between 75% and 100% of the amount of EQU funded loans purportedly held by EFCA were bogus and, since the bogus funded loans

---

* See, for example, the figures for 1963 which were reported in the 1964 financial statements, at pages 156-157 of Appendix B.

** See, for example, note 5 at page 159 of Appendix B.

receivable resulted from bogus income entries, between 75% and 100% of the yearly increase in the amount of loans reported as held by EFCA approximates the fictitious income generated in that year. Although the EQU and Custodial Program figures were combined in 1968, it is still possible to use this same analysis to estimate the range of fraudulent income generated in that year. These figures are summarized in the following table.

ESTIMATED BOGUS INCOME FROM FUNDING FRAUD (1964-1968)

Year	Reported Funded Loans Receivable*	Reported Notes Payable*	Difference "Held by EFCA"*	Percent "Held by EFCA"	Maximum Bogus Income	Minimum Bogus Income**
1964	$ 6,682,076	$ 5,975,585	$ 706,491	10.6%	$ 706,000	$ 361,000
1965	9,210,597	7,079,599	2,130,998	23.1%	1,425,000	1,068,000
1966	13,776,971	7,439,599	6,337,372	46.0%	4,206,000	3,155,000
1967	19,512,475	8,443,194	11,069,281	56.7%	4,732,000	3,549,000
1968	36,311,037	15,564,629	20,746,408	57.1%	6,870,000	5,152,000

After 1968, the difference between reported funded loans receivable and funded notes payable ceases to be a good barometer for the amount of annual bogus income, among other reasons because the funded loans receivable account was reduced from time to time by "free credits" to keep its balance plausible. Nevertheless, because the Company's books and records after 1968 are more complete, it has been possible — with the assistance of some of the fraud participants — to estimate the magnitude of the falsifications directly from the records themselves. Thus, based upon the available evidence it appears that at least $17.2 million in bogus income from the funding fraud was reported in 1969; $15.6 million in 1970; $17.9 million in 1971; $21 million in 1972; and $1.8 million in the first two months of 1973.

---

*Figures shown are taken from financial statements in EFCA's annual reports. See Appendix B, beginning at page 155. Figures for 1964 to 1967 are for Old Programs only. Figures for 1968 are the reported combination of Old Programs and Custodial Programs.

**The minimum shown for 1964 is based upon available records and testimony. See page 25.

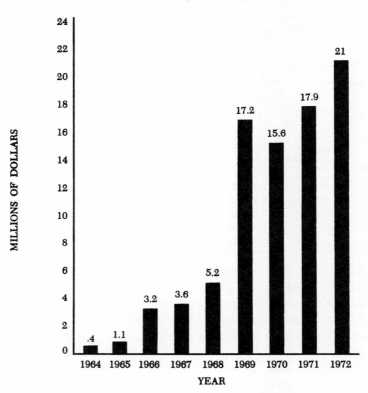

SUMMARY OF ESTIMATED BOGUS INCOME FROM FUNDING FRAUD*
(1964-1972)

From the foregoing, it should be apparent that funding provided a convenient device by which to inflate EFCA's reported earnings. The funding fraud enabled the conspirators to increase pre-tax income and assets dollar-for-dollar with no offsetting "expense". Whenever the asset got too large, it was reduced by a "free credit" and the conspirators were ready to go again. Nevertheless, as the following chapters will demonstrate, even this convenient fraud device was inadequate to meet the grandiose objectives of the EFCA conspiracy. New devices had to be found, and they increased the risk of eventual exposure of the fraud because they required the participation of an increasing number of people.

---

* Probable minimum amounts shown for 1964 to 1968.

44

III. THE FOREIGN PHASE OF THE FRAUD

The conspirators began to establish foreign subsidiaries in 1968. The multifarious and bizarre adventures in which they caused these subsidiaries to engage served but one rational function — to advance and conceal the fraud by recording bogus income and by raising money through unrecorded loans which were used as "free credits." Otherwise, the activities of EFCA's foreign subsidiaries were largely unrelated to the usual business of the Company and, at best, they served only a limited legitimate purpose. Moreover, their exotic and involved nature suggests that some of EFCA's managers — most notably those actively engaged in the fraud — became entranced by a romantic self-image as captains of international business and finance.

The first part of this chapter will relate the beginning of the foreign adventures and will attempt to convey some of their flavor. After describing how phony entries on the books of the foreign finance subsidiaries aided in the overall fraud, it will devote some attention to an absurd foray into the pasta business in Italy. Finally, it will explore the role of two foreign shell companies in concealing the funding fraud.

A. Overview of EFCA's Foreign Activities.

Although some thought may have been given to overseas marketing operations, significant steps toward involvements abroad were first taken in the finance area. In August 1968, Equity Funding Corporation International (later renamed EQF Capital, Inc.) was organized. EQF Capital, Inc. was originally intended to be an overseas financing vehicle, but ultimately became a holding company for other subsidiaries involved in overseas financing.

Two actions taken by EFCA's directors at their November 1968 meeting proved to be important in the foreign area.* First, the directors authorized a multi-million dollar underwriting of convertible subordinated guaranteed debentures to be offered in Europe (a "Eurodollar" offering) to obtain financing for proposed foreign operations of the Company. The authorizing resolution contem-

---

* At this same meeting the Board also authorized up to $25 million of unsecured dollar and Swiss franc notes. See page 38.

plated creation of a Netherlands Antilles subsidiary,* Equity Funding Capital Corporation N.V. ("EFCC-NV"), to issue and sell the debentures through an underwriting group managed by New York Securities Co., Banque de Paris et des Pays-Bas and Banca Commerciale Italianna.

Second, the directors authorized the acquisition of 50% of the stock of Bishops Bank (a Bahamian bank organized by Dishy Easton, Riordan and others in 1965).** Goldblum advised the Board that the remaining shareholders desired to keep their stock with the understanding that after additional capital contributions by EFCA, their ownership interest would be reduced to approximately 5%.

Following its incorporation under the laws of the Netherlands Antilles in December 1968, EFCC-NV issued stock to EQF Capital, Inc. which thereby became its 100% parent. A 25 million Eurodollar offering was successfully made through EFCC-NV, and on February 6, 1969, the net proceeds were credited to an account opened for EFCC-NV at Franklin National Bank. On Goldblum's instructions, all but a fraction of the proceeds were transferred immediately to EFCA accounts. In May 1969, EFCA used $3,080,000 of the proceeds to acquire 95.4% of the stock of Bishops Bank in the name of EFCC-NV.† In this manner, EFCA gained two offshore financing vehicles which served a variety of purposes in the foreign phase of the fraud.

About this time, Yura Arkus-Duntov (Executive Vice President — Investment Management Operations, and an EFCA director)

---

* Many domestic corporations have used a Netherlands Antilles subsidiary to borrow capital, primarily because of the tax benefits conferred by the United States-Netherlands Antilles Tax Convention. Upon meeting certain requirements, interest payments made by a domestic parent through its offshore subsidiary to foreign lenders are exempt from U.S. withholding tax (normally 30%) under the convention. This can be a significant advantage in securing favorable terms from foreign lenders.

** This was not a new development. The Company had considered purchasing the bank as early as 1966, when Goldblum and Riordan were among its largest stockholders.

† The minority interest was acquired by EFCA in December 1971. The balance of the offering was used for a variety of operating purposes.

introduced his fellow executives to Joseph G. Golan, who thereafter played a major role in the Company's international activities. Golan was born in Alexandria, Egypt, but grew up in Palestine. After serving in the Haganah underground in Egypt during Israel's war of independence, Golan studied at the University of Paris where he met a number of African nationals who later became leaders of that continent's emerging nations. By virtue of his contacts and an economics background, Golan was able to establish a number of projects in these nations financed by European and American capital. His principal operations were conducted through Bedec International S.A. ("Bedec"), a Liechtenstein company which he organized in 1965.

In April 1969, Golan was invited to Los Angeles to meet Goldblum and other EFCA executives. Evidently, the men got along well because Golan went to work immediately for EFCA on a handshake. In September 1969, EQF Capital, Inc. acquired all of the outstanding shares of Bedec in exchange for EFCA stock. At about the same time, EFCA organized Economic Development Corporation ("EDC") under the laws of Delaware to replace Bedec as the primary international operating company.

Golan immediately involved EFCA in a host of ongoing and proposed projects. Perhaps the most significant among these involved formation of an Italian subsidiary, Equity Immobiliare Industriale S.p.A. ("EII"), and the acquisition of Molini e Pastificio Pantanella S.p.A. ("Pantanella").* Other projects included mining concessions in Zambia (copper) and Equatorial Guinea (gold); cattle feed lots in Senegal, Madagascar and the Ivory Coast; a ceramic factory in Cameroon; and, at various times, proposed banks and hotels in all of these places. By December 1969, Golan had established offices for EDC and its affiliates in New York; Rome; Abidjan, Ivory Coast; Dakar, Senegal; and Yaounde, Cameroon.

Most of these schemes had scant logical relationship to EFCA's traditional domestic lines of business. It is noteworthy, for example, that in all of this international wheeling-and-dealing no serious attempt appears to have been made to market funding programs abroad. (The closest EFCA came was to establish an unprofitable

---

* See page 56.

offshore mutual fund, based in Panama.) Few of the schemes even proceeded beyond the formative stages, and none of them ever amounted to anything. Hence, the conclusion seems justified that EFCA's foreign escapades entailed an investment of executive time and Company funds that was greatly disproportionate to their real business worth.

Golan also assisted in the secret acquisition of two shell companies: Etablissement Grandson ("Grandson"), a Liechtenstein company; and Compania de Estudios y Asuntos, S.A. ("Estudios"), a Panamanian company. No one at EFCA other than the conspirators appears to have known about these secret acquisitions. Neither of these companies engaged in legitimate business operations, but both were used by the conspirators in fraudulent accounting transactions which are described later in this chapter. In fact, the most conspicuous characteristic of a good part of EFCA's foreign activities was that they provided opportunities and vehicles with which to further the fraud.

48

The following chart summarizes EFCA's international structure at its high-water mark in 1970:

EFCA FOREIGN STRUCTURE

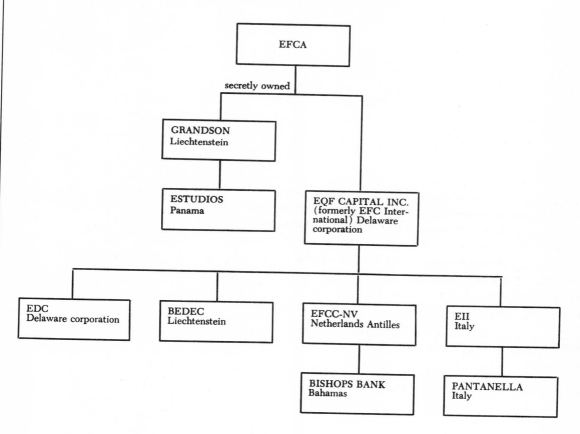

B. **The Offshore Finance Subsidiaries.**

Throughout the life of the conspiracy, EFCA had a voracious appetite for cash, and it borrowed heavily. Prior to 1968, virtually all of EFCA's borrowings were from domestic lenders. In 1968, as EFCA's cash needs grew, the Company turned to overseas money markets for more financing.

At the outset, Dishy Easton played a central role in obtaining foreign capital for EFCA. Pursuant to arrangements described earlier in this report,* Dishy Easton placed more than $20 million of unsecured short and long-term EFCA notes in 1968 and 1969, at least $11 million of which were placed with European lenders. In addition, short-term borrowings of over $7.6 million were arranged for EFCA during this period through Bishops Bank.

Many of these borrowings do not appear to have been properly recorded by EFCA as liabilities at the time. Instead, their proceeds were taken as "free credits" to funded loans receivable. This was done, for example, with the proceeds of a pair of borrowings from LRI in February 1969.** The addition of EFCC-NV and Bishops Bank created further opportunities for fraud in EFCA's financing activities.

(1) MORE ABOUT EFCC-NV.

(a) *A Conduit for "Free Credits."*

In 1969, Dishy Easton's role in obtaining financing for the Company diminished, and the conspirators assumed most of the note placement function themselves. The practice of using such borrowings as "free credits" was continued, and EFCC-NV was made to play an important role. By way of illustration, Goldblum and Lowell arranged to place EFCC-NV notes in the total amount of 20 million Swiss francs (about $4.6 million) through Dow Banking Corporation ("Dow") in December 1969. The notes were guaranteed by EFCA, and were due for payment on December 10, 1970. On the closing date, Dow transferred $4.6 million to various banks at the

---

* See pages 38-39.
** See Pages 39 and 73-74.

direction of EFCA, and EFCA gave a promissory note (signed by Lowell) to EFCC-NV for the entire amount of the proceeds.

Although clearly outstanding as of year-end 1969, the loan was unreported in EFCA's consolidated balance sheet for that year. Rather, when the cash was received, Sultan, acting on Lowell's instructions, made a journal entry crediting the entire amount of the loan proceeds to funded loans receivable, as though participants had paid that amount on their loans — another "free credit." Thus, a practice that began with the proceeds from notes placed by Dishy Easton in late 1968 and early 1969 was continued by the conspirators after they developed their own international banking contacts.

(b) The "Call Account" at Bishops Bank.

EFCC-NV and Bishops Bank each set up what was essentially an inter-company account to record day-to-day activity between them. Bishops treated this account as an interest-bearing "deposit" by EFCC-NV which could be withdrawn ("called") at any time. Hence, the account was referred to as the "call account." Bishops reported the balance of the call account on its financial statements as a deposit liability, while EFCC-NV reported the balance as a cash asset. Obviously the two should have balanced at all times, but they did not.

The imbalance occurred because EFCC-NV inflated the call account from time to time to cover up other bogus transactions. For example, when the unreported Dow notes were paid in 1970, it was necessary to record the outflow of the money, but this could not be recorded as a payment on notes that had never been entered on the books as a liability. As a partial solution to the problem, EFCC-NV recorded $1.6 million of this cash outflow as an increase to the call account.* In another series of related entries, the call account was inflated by approximately $500,000 to facilitate an equivalent reduction of other bogus asset accounts.

No corresponding entries were made on Bishops' books during the year and, consequently, the call account balance on EFCC-NV's

---

* The remaining $3 million was recorded by charging EFCC-NV's intercompany account with EFC-Cal.

books exceeded the balance on the books of its bank subsidiary by $2.1 million. In order to adjust this imbalance, Sultan made a journal entry at the end of 1970 to record the $2.1 million overstatement on EFCC-NV's books as an additional investment in Bishops, thus, in effect, turning the overstatement into "goodwill." It is not known how the appearance of such "goodwill" on EFCC-NV's books — more than a year after it acquired Bishops — was explained by the conspirators to EFCA's auditors.

(c) *The Account at Banque Jordaan.*

In 1969, EFCC-NV opened a U.S. dollar investment account at Banque Jordaan (Paris). The first deposit was made around March 1969, and was in the neighborhood of $100,000. The account was used for a short while to speculate in assorted U.S. securities, including EFCC-NV's own Eurodollar debentures. After reaching a high of some $132,000 in April, the balance tailed off rapidly and the last activity in the account appears to have taken place in October 1969. Bank statements from that point forward reported an unchanged balance of $57,847.46.

Nevertheless, at year-end 1969, EFCA recorded a transaction that attributed at least $1.5 million to this account. In June 1969, "adjusting" journal entries had been made on EFCA's books to record fictitious income of $1.5 million and a corresponding increase in an investment account. At the end of the year, entries were made to reduce this investment account by $1.5 million and, correspondingly, to increase an account that purported to record arbitrage transactions made by EFCA through Dishy Easton. This adjustment was accompanied by a notation that it was made "to transfer investments in Banque Jordaan-Paris."

Wolfson Weiner's 1969 audit work papers contain a letter from Banque Jordaan acknowledging a balance of only $57,847.46 in EFCC-NV's name. There is nothing in the work papers to support the $1.5 million of investments which were supposedly maintained at that bank. According to Lowell, Julian Weiner knew that the asset was inflated, and the following year he insisted upon some documentation for Wolfson Weiner's files. For this purpose, Weiner gave Lowell a blank confirmation form and, on Lowell's instructions, Sultan prepared a forged letter of confirmation from Banque Jordaan for

52

the 1970 audit work papers. After the audit, the conspirators concluded that this relatively minor deception was not worth the trouble it caused. Consequently, in June 1971 the entire bogus amount was written off and balanced by an arbitrary increase in an "accrued commissions" account.

(2) FRAUD AT BISHOPS BANK

Until early 1971, Bishops Bank's main activity was to obtain financing for EFCA. However, because Bishops was an unconsolidated subsidiary audited by a different accounting firm, the bank's books were also a convenient place for the conspirators to record bogus assets which had been created to generate fictitious income on EFCA's books. Thus, at least two bogus notes receivable were placed on Bishops' books in 1970. Each appears to have resulted from entries made on EFCA's books to record fictitious income.

(a) *The Wangerhof Note.*

The first of these bogus notes, in the amount of $2 million, was manufactured as part of a phony sale of future commissions described later in this chapter.* In brief, the conspirators funneled $2 million through Bishops as part of arrangements made to create the appearance of a down payment needed for the sham transaction. To conceal this ruse, the cash was recorded as a loan to "Dr Heinrich Wangerhof" (a fictitious name invented by Goldblum and Lowell) and was set up on the bank's books as a note receivable in that name.

(b) *The EII Note.*

The second bogus note was purportedly issued by EFCA's Italian subsidiary, Equity Immobiliare Industriale S.p.A. ("EII"). Sometime in December, 1970 Goldblum instructed Golan to sign a $3 million promissory note on behalf of EII, dated December 4, 1970 and payable to Bishops Bank on December 1, 1971. Golan claims Goldblum told him at the time that demand deposits of that amount would be made available to EII at Bishops for operating purposes. Lowell says, however, that Golan was aware no loan was to be made and that he simply signed the note at Goldblum's request. In any event, the bank immediately recorded the EII note as a

---

* See pages 66-72.

receivable and showed the note as a $3 million asset on its year-end 1970 balance sheet, despite the fact that no funds were made available to EII at Bishops. Golan did not record the note to the bank as a payable on the books of EII and, it did not appear as a liability on EII's year-end 1970 balance sheet.

The EII note appears to have been put on Bishops' books as part of a plan to conceal earlier fraudulent entries on EFCA's books. Journal entries by Sultan in March 1970 created fictitious income for EFCA of approximately $3 million by recording an asset he called "securities and investments in Italy." Subsequent journal entries first reclassified this bogus asset as an "investment in [Pantanella] subsidiary," then as an "arbitrage" investment and finally took it off EFCA's books altogether. The $3 million bogus EII note appeared on Bishop's books as an asset concurrently with the disappearance of the "arbitrage" investment from EFCA's books. It therefore seems reasonable to conclude that the former was related to and intended to replace the latter, perhaps by ostensibly reflecting proceeds of a purported disposition of the "arbitrage" investment.

The relevant journal entries have not been found, but correspondence in EFCA's files suggests that the bogus EII note was then transferred to Bishops Bank in exchange for a legitimate asset. Bishops held $3.5 million of Custodial Collateral Notes, which were cancelled by EFCA in early December 1970 to release the underlying collateral. According to correspondence between EFCA and Bishops personnel, the bogus $3 million EII note was entered on the bank's books to replace $3 million of the Custodial Collateral Notes. Bishops was told to record the remaining $500,000 as a draw down of the EFCC-NV call account.

(c) The Cover-Up of the Phony Notes.

The two bogus receivables (the Wangerhof and EII notes) were undetected during the audit of Bishops' books for the year 1970. According to Roger Coe, who took over as President of Bishops in March 1971, the bank's auditors (Tait, Weller & Clark) had difficulty confirming the $2 million receivable with Wangerhof. Upon inquiry, Coe was advised by Lowell that Goldblum had given instructions not to pursue the matter. No explanation was given to Coe for the

Wangerhof loan. At the same time, Tait also attempted to confirm the $3 million EII note. According to Lowell, Tait was finally furnished with a letter, signed by Golan, fraudulently confirming both notes.

After the audit was closed, Coe objected to carrying both the Wangerhof and the EII loans on Bishops' books, and asked that they be taken off by EFCA. In October 1971, the EII note was eliminated from the bank's books. Although the exact method of removal is not yet known, it can be surmised. Just before year-end 1971, EFCC-NV's call account with Bishops was out of balance by a little more than $3 million, *i.e.*, EFCC-NV recorded a receivable of $3 million more than the payable recorded by Bishops. At year end, this imbalance disappeared. Therefore, it is reasonable to conclude that the EII note was "transferred" from Bishops to EFCC-NV, thereby "solving" two problems: The note was taken off Bishops' books as an asset, thus satisfying Coe, and added to EFCC-NV's assets, thereby permitting a writedown in the call account without any overall reduction of recorded assets.*

The fictitious Wangerhof note was taken off Bishops' books in December 1971 and never reappeared anywhere. Nevertheless, total assets of EFCA and subsidiaries were not affected because of other entries — some bogus — which were made at that time. The Wangerhof note was recorded as paid on Bishop's books through the transfer of $2 million in cash from EFCA to Bishops. EFCA, however, recorded the payment as an investment in commercial paper, which in fact was nonexistent.

Lowell demanded that Coe provide a confirmation from Bishops of a non-existent commercial paper sale to EFCA in return for removing the Wangerhof note from Bishops' books. Lowell told Coe that EFCA needed the confirmation temporarily because it was having trouble collecting from Wangerhof, but that payment was expected shortly. Accordingly, Bishops supplied Sultan

---

* The call account imbalance was corrected by journal entries made on Bishops' books by Sultan on December 29 to record purchases of $3.2 million of fictitious commercial paper. See page 95. It is not unlikely that $3 million of these entries were made to balance the transfer of the EII note to EFCC-NV.

with a confirmation which represented that $2 million in notes of
Apatinska Tekstilna Industrijia ("APATEX"), a Yugoslavian manufacturing firm, had been purchased by Bishops for EFCA as of
December 14, 1971. The confirmation was bogus, inasmuch as no
such purchase was made.

An interesting sidelight of this transaction involved the recording of a fictitious interest payment to Bishops on the Wangerhof note.
At the time EFCA transferred the $2 million to Bishops in replace-
ment of the note, the Company was in the process of securing another
20 million Swiss franc loan from Dow through Bishops. When the
proceeds of that loan were received, Bishops withheld some $240,000
which it recorded as payment of interest on the Wangerhof note. The
remaining proceeds were remitted to EFCC-NV. In recording the new
Dow borrowing, however, EFCC-NV capitalized the missing $240,000
as an additional loan financing cost to be amortized over the life of the
loan.

C. The Pantanella Transactions.

Out of the incredible hodgepodge of deals Golan brought to
EFCA, the one involving acquisition of an Italian pasta company
named Molini e Pastificio Pantanella S.p.A. ("Pantanella") is most
noteworthy. It illustrates three characteristics of EFCA's top executives: (i) their fascination with international wheeling-and-dealing;
(ii) their talent for mismanagement; and (iii) the lengths to which
they would go to further the fraud in even a small way.

Pantanella was brought to Golan's attention early in 1969 by an
acquaintance who represented the owners of approximately 93%
of the company's stock: The Special Administration of the Holy See
("Holy See"), which manages the Vatican's real estate holdings in
Italy; and Assicurazioni Generali ("Generali"), a large Italian insurance company.* (Collectively the Holy See and Generali are referred
to in this report as "the AG Group.") Despite gross sales from 1964
to 1968 averaging $9.3 million per year, Pantanella had begun to lose
money. More importantly, the company had debt in the neighborhood
of $8 million and was badly in need of financial reorganization.

---

* The other 7% was publicly held and traded on the Rome stock exchange.

56

Although the AG Group had used its influence to obtain interim financing to keep Pantanella afloat, it recognized that many of its workers would have to be dismissed in order to make the operation profitable. Because it did not wish to suffer the repercussions of laying off any significant part of the work force, the AG Group had decided to sell Pantanella. To encourage the sale, it was willing to help a new owner obtain additional financing.

Goldblum and Herbert Glaser, Executive Vice President in charge of EFCA's international activities, traveled to Rome in October 1969 to get the acquisition talks with the AG Group under way. Golan retained the law firm of Pavia & Harcourt ("the Pavia firm") to assist in the talks and, during the next five months, on-again-off-again negotiations produced a variety of acquisition schemes. By early April 1970, the negotiations had focused on the deal that was ultimately consummated. During the remainder of the month and into May, Glaser, Golan and lawyers from the Pavia firm worked with representatives of the AG Group over a draft agreement. Finally, on May 11 Goldblum and Lowell left for Europe to conclude the transaction, and on May 20 the final purchase agreements were executed in Geneva, Switzerland. The documents designated newly-formed EII as the purchaser of the AG Group's Pantanella stock for the nominal price of 10 million lira ($16,000). The AG Group promised to help EFCA obtain a six-year loan of $5 million at a favorable interest rate, and to advance directly to EFCA another 750 million lira (approximately $1.2 million) almost immediately. All of this money was to be used for the pasta company's reorganization. The advance money was to be treated as an interest-free loan and repaid to the AG Group if EFCA sold its Pantanella stock before the end of 1985. Otherwise, the funds were to be repaid in that year after certain adjustments.

This arrangement presented EFCA with the opportunity to earn legitimate profits in the rehabilitation of Pantanella. Its outdated factory was located in the heart of Rome on land valued at $6.4 million. Glaser thought EFCA might relocate the operation in an industrial area outside of Rome, tear down the old factory, and build income-producing structures which, because of their choice location, could be sold at a profit. These opportunities were never developed, however, because for Goldblum and Lowell the primary purpose of the transaction was to lay hands on the easy money that the AG Group was to provide. Steps were immediately taken to achieve this purpose.

In June 1970, the AG Group advanced $1.2 million (in U.S. dollars) to EFCA as promised in the Geneva agreements. The advance money was deposited in an EFCA bank account at Chase Manhattan Bank (London), and was recorded by Sultan on EFC-Cal's books, not as a liability to the AG Group, but instead as a "free credit" to funded loans receivable. Moreover, rather than immediately contributing the money to Pantanella as required, the conspirators invested it in Eurodollars for a month, and then transferred the $1.2 million to Banca Nazionale del Lavoro (Rome), where it was pledged as collateral for a loan of an equivalent amount in lira to EII. (The pledge was made in U.S. dollars so the collateral could be exported from Italy when the loan was repaid without violating Italian currency regulations which made it illegal to take lira out of the country.) The proceeds of the loan apparently were transferred to Pantanella in August 1970.

In the meantime, evidently with the help of the AG Group, arrangements were made for a $5 million loan at 6% interest from Efibanca Ente Finanziario Interbancario S.p.A. ("Efibanca"). The transaction was structured as a loan to EII, guaranteed by both EFCA and EFLIC. Under the extraordinary terms of these "guarantees," EFCA and EFLIC actually appear to have become the real borrowers from Efibanca. Each company irrevocably and unconditionally assumed the primary obligation for the full principal and interest of the Efibanca loan to EII, without any requirement of notice or presentment to the Italian subsidiary.

The final loan agreement was signed in Rome by Golan (for EII) and initialed by Glaser (for EFCA) in the first week of September 1970, and Efibanca credited EII's bank account with $5 million of lira. On September 8, $1.2 million of lira was transferred from EII's account to Banca Nazionale del Lavoro (Rome) to repay the earlier loan from that bank, and thereby release the $1.2 million of U.S. dollars held on deposit as collateral. When released, the amount on deposit was transferred to an EFCA account in Rome and, eventually, to another EFCA account in Los Angeles. These funds were never recorded as a liability on EFCA's books, having already been applied to reduce the funded loans receivable account, as previously noted. Shortly thereafter, another $400,000 was transferred to Pantanella from EII's bank account, leaving $3.4 million of the original $5 million loan from Efibanca in that account.

Thus $1.2 million of the funds earmarked for Pantanella was in EFCA's control, $1.6 million had gone to Pantanella and $3.4 million remained in EII's Italian bank account. Steps were immediately taken to move the latter amount to EFCA. Because the Efibanca loan had been made in lira, some means had to be found to evade Italian currency regulations. Lowell says that he and Goldblum considered using someone from the Italian underworld to move the lira to Switzerland where they could be changed into U.S. dollars. The fee for such a service was so high, however, that it would have negated the advantage of the cheap loan. Instead, Lowell found a circuitous route to remove the funds from Italy.

The $3.4 million was transferred to a "special account" opened by Golan in EII's name at Banca Unione (Milan). The Banca Unione deposit then was pledged as collateral to secure a loan of the same amount to EFCA from Amincor Bank AG (Zurich). Pursuant to arrangements made by Lowell, the $3.4 million loaned by Amincor was transferred to an EFCA bank account in Los Angeles on September 30. Thus, all told, $4.6 million in cash, intended under the agreement with the AG Group for Pantanella's rehabilitation, went to EFCA in Los Angeles.

Following the acquisition, Golan was placed in charge of Pantanella and, for a variety of reasons, the situation deteriorated steadily. Golan closed down part of the plant, laying off 120 workers and precipitating a crisis with the trade union involved. Disaster was averted temporarily when the Italian government agreed to pay the workers out of a special fund. But in late December 1970, the situation turned from bad to worse and Arkus-Duntov was sent to Rome to assess EFCA's options. Arkus-Duntov concluded almost immediately that the only solution was for EFCA to sell Pantanella as soon as possible. Several months of tortuous negotiations followed before EFCA was finally able to withdraw from the pasta business by disposing of EII and its subsidiary for a nominal consideration.

In the process, EFCA and some of its executives became involved in local criminal investigations into the Pantanella debacle. Consequently, additional lawyers had to be hired, and more of the Company's executive resources were diverted to Italy.

Arkus-Duntov also insisted that arrangements be made to repay the Efibanca loan of $5 million, and this of course caused EFCA still more trouble. Lowell and Sultan arranged for EFC-Cal to borrow $5 million from First National City Bank of New York. About $1.6 million of this was paid directly to Efibanca to reduce the $5 million loan. The balance — about $3.4 million — was paid to Amincor to discharge Amincor's loan to EFCA in that amount and thereby release the pledge of the deposit at Banca Unione. That deposit was then used to repay the remaining $3.4 million of the Efibanca loan. In all of this, it does not appear that Pantanella made any contribution to the repayment of the Efibanca loan, although as previously indicated Pantanella had received $400,000 of the proceeds of this loan. This amount thus became one of the costs to EFCA of this disastrous transaction. Moreover, Amincor withheld about $67,000 as a penalty for prepayment of the loan to EFCA, and Efibanca claimed another $17,000 for prepayment of its loan. Thus, on top of everything else, EFCA had to pay about $84,000 in prepayment penalties to get out of Pantanella.

The premature repayment had other effects as well. Only the $3.4 million borrowed from Amincor was recorded on EFCA's books as a liability at the time the Company was forced to make the $5 million repayment to Efibanca. When the payment was made, the $1.6 million in cash used to pay the unrecorded portion of the liability was reclassified to a cash suspense account. A month later, that amount was again reclassified as a bogus account receivable. At the end of 1971, the bogus receivable was taken off the books as part of a series of fraudulent entries made to record a sale of future profits from EFCA's casualty insurance business which had the additional result of generating $800,000 of bogus income.

Thus the Pantanella adventure finally came to an end. It seems quite clearly to have been a mistake from start to finish. As a possible legitimate business deal it had some marginal potential, but it bore no rational relationship to the remainder of EFCA's business

60

and, accordingly, was fraught with the risks attendant upon such a venture in a foreign country. And these risks were greatly escalated since the apparent prime object of the transaction — the proceeds of a cheap loan — could be accomplished only if EFCA chose to ignore the terms of its agreements with the AG Group and Italian currency regulations. Even as a step in the ongoing fraud, Pantanella was a failure. It required an enormous expenditure of executive time to set up in the first place; it ultimately had to be unwound because of the unexpected but predictable collapse of Pantanella; and its unwinding consumed additional executive time, cost money, and required the recording of even more bogus transactions.

D. **Estudios and Grandson.**

Two foreign companies covertly acquired by EFCA in 1970 played a prominent part in the fraud. One was a Liechtenstein entity named Etablissement Grandson ("Grandson"), which had been organized by Golan in 1969 for his personal use. Early in 1970, in discussions with Goldblum, Golan agreed to sell Grandson and thereafter made arrangements to transfer ownership in the company to EFCA. Evidence of ownership of a Liechtenstein etablissement is a document similar to a deed which may be transferred simply by assignment. No public record of such a transfer is necessary, and none was made in this instance. Indeed, the transaction appears to have been known only to the conspirators and the manager of the bank in Geneva where Grandson's bank account was maintained and its certificate of ownership was held for safekeeping.

The other foreign company was Compania de Estudios y Asuntos, S.A. ("Estudios"), an inactive Panamanian company originally organized by the Pavia firm, which first came to EFCA's attention during the Pantanella negotiations. At one point in those negotiations an agreement was drafted which provided for the transfer of Pantanella to Estudios. This plan was ultimately discarded but Estudios was not forgotten, and in April 1970 Lowell instructed Golan to arrange to purchase Estudios. The arrangement negotiated with the Pavia firm by Golan contemplated that Grandson would be the purchaser, and ownership of Estudios was formally transferred to Grandson in May 1970.

61

Thus did EFCA come secretly to own a Liechtenstein etablissement that in turn owned a Panamanian company, both of which
almost immediately were put to use in furtherance of the fraud.

(1) ESTUDIOS AND THE TRAIL COMMISSIONS.

On April 1, 1969, EFCA acquired from Bernard Cornfeld's
Investors Overseas Services Ltd., S.A. ("IOS"), substantially all
of the domestic assets of Investors Planning Corporation of America
("IPC"). EFCA gave IOS an aggregate consideration of $10.2
million, consisting of $6.3 million in cash, notes totaling $2 million
and 26,830 shares of EFCA stock which then had a total market value
of about $1.9 million.

The IPC deal supposedly helped EFCA in several ways. First,
EFCA acquired the IPC sales force, which was reported to consist of
29 sales offices in 21 states (mostly in the East), and more than 2,000
sales representatives. Second, EFCA gained another proprietary
mutual fund through the acquisition of a wholly-owned subsidiary
of IPC, which was that fund's investment adviser. Lastly, IPC was
the sponsor and distributor of contractual plans for the accumulation
of mutual fund shares, and some 150,000 of these plan accounts were
supposed to be outstanding at the time. They provided more grist
for the EFCA fraud mill.

(a) *The Value of the Contractual Plans.*

IPC sponsored and distributed contractual plans to purchase
shares in four mutual funds. Two types of systematic contractual
plans were offered. The first contemplated that the participant
would make periodic investment payments of a specified amount
per month. Although the plan was predicated on the assumption
that the participant would continue the plan for a 12½ year period,
thus making 150 monthly payments, the plan could be terminated
by the participant at any time. The second type of systematic plan
was identical to the first, except for the addition of a plan-completion
life insurance feature. In the event of the participant's death prior
to completion of the contemplated 150 payments, the unpaid balance
of his payments was made in a lump sum by the plan's insurance
carriers under a renewable term group life insurance policy.* Either

---

* This discussion applies equally to insured and non-insured plans.

plan could be used to purchase shares of any of the four different funds.

Both types of plans provided for the collection of charges by IPC out of the payments the participant made into the plan. In total, these charges were to be 8.75% of the participant's total anticipated investment into the plan over its lifetime. However, 50% of the total charge — called a "creation and sales charge" — was to be deducted in equal amounts from the first 13 monthly payments. The other 50% was to be deducted from the remaining 137 monthly payments in equal amounts known as "trail commissions." Twenty percent of the charges deducted under these plans was paid to the individual agent who sold the plan. And, of course, if the participant terminated the plan at any time, the collection of monthly charges stopped.

By way of example, a plan providing for monthly payments of $50 each would anticipate a total investment of $7,500. The total sales charge would be $656.25, half of which would be deducted from the first 13 payments at the rate of approximately $25 per payment, and the other half of which would be deducted as a trail commission from the remaining 137 payments at the rate of approximately $2.42 per payment. The total amount of commissions payable over the life of such a plan to the agent who sold it would be $131.25.

Trail commissions were the valuable part of the contractual plan business. When EFCA acquired IPC, it acquired the right to continue to deduct these charges from the monthly payments being made under the then outstanding approximately 150,000 contractual plans. In contemplation of the acquisition, a study was made in October 1968, based on historical data, to determine how much the trail commissions would be worth to EFCA over the next ten-year period. The study projected the number of plans EFCA could expect the participants to continue over the ensuing ten-year period. It then calculated the annual trail commissions that would be received from the four funds and reduced those figures by an estimated 25% commission payout (to individual sales agents). The results were summarized in a report to Goldblum in December 1968. It showed that EFCA could expect to receive "net trail commissions" over the next ten years of about

63

$7.9 million. Discounted by two different methods to their present value, the net trail commissions were figured to be worth no more than $3 million to $5 million as of December 1968. Nevertheless, by an elaborate ruse, the anticipated receipt of these trail commissions was used by the conspirators to justify entries made to record $17.2 million of current income in 1969.

(b) *Treatment of the Trail Commissions.*

During the course of the year 1969, the conspirators recorded at least $16 million of bogus funding income, which correspondingly inflated the funded loans receivable account. The trail commissions were seen as a means of providing support for these bogus entries. The first step in the process was to attribute a value to the future income anticipated from the trail commissions. The next step was to attribute a part of the bogus funded loan entries to the value of this future income and to do so in a manner which made it appear that accrued income from trail commissions had been included in the Company's commission income and funded loans receivable accounts right along.

This idea evidently originated with EFCA's auditors. It will be recalled that, during the 1968 audit, the auditors permitted $13.5 million of reported funded loans receivable to be supported by reciprocal commissions supposedly accrued in or before 1968 and supposedly received in early 1969. Templeton claims he pointed out to Lichtig (the Wolfson Weiner junior partner in charge of the 1968 audit) that, with the receipt of the cash payments in early 1969 (which were in fact loan proceeds rather than reciprocal commissions), there would be a $13.5 million reduction in the funded loans receivable account (and a corresponding increase in the cash account) in the first interim report for 1969. He expressed concern that this would raise questions in the mind of anyone reading that report. Templeton says Lichtig reassured him by explaining that the trail commissions EFCA had acquired in the IPC acquisition would be combined with funded loans receivable in 1969 so that the drop would not be evident. This step was not in fact taken when the deal closed. Instead, the problem foreseen by Templeton was averted

64

by recording $16 million more of bogus funding income, with a corresponding fictitious increase in the funded loans receivable account.

The idea was recalled later in the year, however. According to Lowell, the plan for the treatment of the trail commissions, as well as a supposed accounting rationale for the plan, were worked out in several meetings he and Goldblum had with Julian Weiner just prior to the 1969 audit.

Wolfson Weiner accountants working on the audit under Weiner and Sol Block were told that the $16 million of bogus entries made during the year represented periodic estimates of the trail commissions expected from the IPC deal, and that these estimates had been booked in this manner until enough data were gathered to make a final determination of the value of the trails. In November and December, it was said, entries had been made to reclassify the trail commissions from the funded loans receivable account to a contractuals receivable account newly set up on EFC-Cal's books for this purpose. Supposedly when the value of the trails had been finally computed, it was found to be about $17.2 million, so a year-end adjusting entry had been made to increase the new asset by $1.2 million and to accrue that additional amount of commission income.

This explanation would lead one to expect that $16 million should have been transferred out of the funded loans receivable account into the contractuals receivable account, and that an additional entry of $1.2 million should have been made in the contractuals receivable account and the commission income account. Actually, it did not occur this way. The table on page 71 shows that contractuals receivable of $17,874,290 were recorded, along with commissions payable of $4,560,655, so that the net asset added by these entries was $13,313,635. Consequently, net trail commissions should have accounted for only about $13.3 million of commission income — not $17.2 million. Furthermore, funded loans receivable were not written down by $16 million, but rather by $12,017,477, leaving $3,982,523 still unsupported.

Computations prepared by the conspirators to substantiate the value placed on the trail commissions for Wolfson Weiner's 1969 audit work papers seem to tie in more closely with the actual entries in the accounting records. According to these computations, "gross trail commissions" were projected of about $17.9 million.* Reducing this figure by an estimated $4.6 million of commissions payable, "net trail commissions" were projected of about $13.3 million. No mention was made of EFCA's December 1968 study projecting "net trail commissions" of only $7.9 million with a present value of from $3 million to $5 million, although Weiner evidently was given a copy of the study. Indeed, the conspirators made no effort to adjust their computations for any of the factors that had been considered in the December 1968 report.

On their face, the computations were unreasonable, because it was obvious they neglected to correct for liquidations or lapses on an historical basis, and because the net trail commission figure was not discounted to present value. Even more importantly, because a participant could quit his plan at any time, ultimate realization of any of the trail commissions was uncertain. Nevertheless, Goldblum, Lowell and Weiner planned to accrue the entire projected amount of income by capitalizing the trails. When Sol Block complained to Weiner that the rationale proposed for this treatment was too weak to "protect" Wolfson Weiner, however, a new plan was devised. Goldblum, Lowell and Weiner decided upon a "sale" of the trails.

(c) *The Sham Sale.*

On Friday evening, May 8, 1970, Goldblum instructed Loeb to draft a contract for sale of the trail commissions to an unnamed European buyer, after indicating that he and Lowell were leaving for Europe on the following Monday and that they needed the contract to take with them. Loeb and another attorney spent the weekend preparing the necessary documents. On Monday morning, Loeb sent the final draft to Goldblum under cover of a memo indicating that the contract was ready except for dollar amounts and the name of the purchaser, which information Loeb did not have. Goldblum and Lowell left for Europe later that day to close the Pantanella acquisition.

---

* Some $600,000 was included to represent "first year" commissions expected in 1970. Such commissions would appear by definition to be irrelevant to a computation of "trail commissions". The computations contain no explanation for including this sum.

When Goldblum and Lowell returned from Europe, Loeb learned that Estudios (which he believed to be an independent party) would be the purchaser of the trail commissions. Loeb incorporated this and other revisions made in Goldblum's handwriting on a marked-up draft, and presented the President with a clean copy on May 28, 1970. The final version provided for Estudios to purchase "net trail commissions"* from contractual plans to acquire shares of three of the four EFCA mutual funds for $13.5 million, which was to be paid $5 million in cash, due immediately upon execution of the agreement, and the balance in promissory notes due from 1970 to 1978. Net trail commissions collected during each year were first to be applied against the note due on December 31 of that year. Any excess was to be applied against the remaining notes as they matured. If sufficient trail commissions were not collected to satisfy any one of these promissory notes, then Estudios was liable for any amount remaining due. The notes themselves were non-interest bearing.

The actual purchase agreement was dated May 19 and signed by Goldblum for EFCA and by "Alphonso Perez da Silva" (another fictitious person invented by Goldblum and Lowell) for Estudios. The notes also purported to be signed by Perez da Silva. According to Lowell, Golan signed the fictitious name on each of the documents in his presence at Goldblum's request. Although all of them bear the seal of Compania de Estudios y Asuntos— with the correct spelling of "Asuntos" — in every case the company name was misspelled as "Assuntas" above the signature of the non-existent Perez da Silva.

Minutes for the May 29, 1970 meeting of EFCA's directors report that the Board voted unanimously for a resolution to authorize the $13.5 million agreement with Estudios. In fact, nothing at all appears to have been said about Estudios at the May 29 Board meeting, and the "resolution" was added to the minutes as an afterthought by EFCA's legal staff. Nevertheless, the minutes were approved unani-

---

* "Net trail commissions" were defined as all trail commissions to be collected by EFCA on plans sold prior to December 31, 1969, less 25% representing the approximate amount of commissions payable and less an administrative handling fee of 3% for collecting and transmitting the trail commissions.

mously as written without discussion at the next meeting of the Board on July 29. There is no evidence that the Board considered the Estudios transaction on any other occasion.

In July 1970, a journal entry was made to increase the contractuals receivable amount to an even $18 million, adding about $265,000 of commission income in the process. The entry appears to have been made as an adjustment to conform the books to the terms of the Estudios purchase agreement, inasmuch as $18 million less 25% of that amount (estimated commissions payable) equals the $13.5 million purchase price for the net trails. No other entry was made to adjust the contractuals receivable to reflect the Estudios deal.

A $5 million down payment was due upon execution of the agreement, but no payment was arranged at that time. The conspirators finally made arrangements for a bogus down payment in September. First, Goldblum instructed Loeb to prepare documents necessary to change the manner of payment of the purchase price and the amount of the down payment under the Estudios contract. Pursuant to Goldblum's instructions, Loeb prepared an Amendment No. One to the purchase agreement (and related documents) to reduce the down payment from $5 to $2 million, and to provide for a tenth promissory note in the amount of $3 million to make up the difference. These documents were given to Goldblum on September 18.

Amendment No. One provided for payment of the $2 million "concurrently with the execution" of the amendment. The down payment in fact was made by EFCA to itself. First, $2 million was transferred from EFCA to an EFCC-NV account at United California Bank. Then on October 14, Sultan sent that amount from the EFCC-NV account to a Bishops Bank account at Franklin National Bank. Both Bishops and EFCC-NV correctly recorded this transfer as an increase in the call account.* On the same date, instructions were given to Franklin National Bank to charge the Bishops account for $2 million, and wire transfer that amount to Chase Manhattan Bank, as U.S. correspondent bank for Cifico Bank, Ltd. (Geneva) to the credit of Etablissement Grandson. Finally, on October 21 the $2 million was transferred back to the United States, where it was

---

* See page 51.

received by EFCA and recorded in the intercompany account with EFC-Cal as the down payment from Estudios required under Amendment No. One.

The transfer of $2 million from Bishops Bank to Cifico Bank, Ltd. (Geneva) is what gave rise to the note in that amount from the fictitious "Dr. Heinrich Wangerhof" described earlier in this report.* The transfer was intially set up on Bishops' books as a $2 million fictitious note receivable from Grandson — and then reclassified as a loan to the fictitious Dr. Wangerhof. It will be recalled that this bogus note remained on the bank's books until December 1971, when it was taken off in exchange for a fraudulent confirmation showing a $2 million purchase of APATEX commercial paper for EFCA.

The entire down payment round-robin is summarized by the following chart.

---

* See pages 53-56.

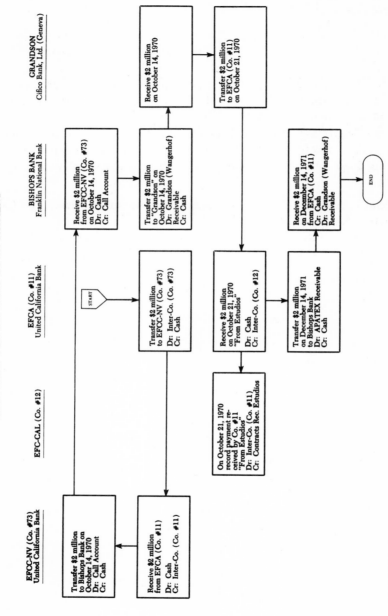

CASH FLOW FOR ESTUDIOS DOWN PAYMENT*

* This and the other flow charts in this report show the relevant journal entries actually made on the books of the companies involved. The accounting terms "debit" (abbreviated "Dr.") and "credit" (abbreviated "Cr.") are used in these charts for accuracy, although they have not been used elsewhere in the report in order to make the text as readable as possible.

70

The ultimate effect of the series of fraudulent entries was increased by related entries made on EFC-Cal's books later in the year. In October the commissions payable were wiped out altogether by the simple device of a journal entry transfer of the balance in that account to a reserve for bad debts. Then in November, the reserve for bad debts balance was recorded as a "free credit" to funded loans receivable. Thus, when all entries related to the trails are combined, the bottom-line effect was a $17.5 million inflation of income and a small decrease in funded loans receivable.

The following table reflects the accounting entries that are described above.

SUMMARY OF 1969-70 TRAIL COMMISSION ENTRIES*
(EFC-Cal)

Date	Contractuals Receivable	Funded Loans Receivable	Commissions Payable	Commission Income**
June 1969	$	$ 4,000,000	$	$ 4,000,000
Sept. 1969		3,500,000		3,500,000
Oct. 1969		2,000,000		2,000,000
Nov. 1969 ...		3,000,000		3,000,000
Nov. 1969 ...	7,424,509	(7,424,509)		
Dec. 1969		3,500,000		3,500,000
Dec. 1969	560,152	(217,593)	342,559	
Dec. 1969	2,441,964		2,441,964	
Dec. 1969 ...	5,853,982	(4,375,375)	1,478,607	
Dec. 1969 ...	1,593,683		367,525	1,226,158
Year-end 1969	$17,874,290	$ 3,982,523	$ 4,630,655	$ 17,226,158
July 1970	125,710		(138,474)	264,184
Oct. 1970			(4,492,180)	
Nov. 1970		(4,492,180)		
Year-end 1970	$18,000,000	$ (509,657)	—0—	$ 17,490,342

Subsequent monthly entries had the cumulative effect of reducing the contractuals receivable balance to about $12.6 million as of March 31, 1973, a decrease of $5.4 million, while recording only $2.7 million of trail commissions as received over that period. These entries purported to record the amount of actual trail commissions received by EFC-Cal, and the Company's year-to-year accounting

---

* Figures in parentheses are reductions; other figures are increases.
** Combines securities and insurance commission income.

with Estudios. In fact, they appear to have done neither. Among other things, they booked almost one million dollars to funded loans receivable, despite having no legitimate relationship to that account.

(d) *Evaluation of Accounting Treatment.*

The conspirators' use of the trail commissions was not an end in itself. It was an attempt to cover up the ongoing funding fraud. As before, the conspirators had inflated commission income and funded loans receivable to create the impression of ever-increasing earnings and business activity. The recording of the trail commissions was merely a device to support those inflated figures.

Taken all together, the accounting treatment given to the trail commissions was obviously improper for several reasons. For one thing, although the auditors justified $13.3 million of income and asset figures on the basis of the trail commissions, the public never knew that. In EFCA's 1969 financial statements the contractuals receivable were lumped together with the funded loans receivable as "Funded Loans and Accounts Receivable." Note 2 to the balance sheet purported to disclose the combination of these unrelated assets by explaining that Funded Loans and Accounts Receivable represented the amount clients owed as a result of "the various Equity Funding Programs offered by the Company, *and net contracts receivable.*"* The conspirators thus got their cake and ate it too. By including the contractuals receivable in Funded Loans and Accounts Receivable, without adequately disclosing the nature of this asset or the fact that it was included, they were able to sustain an appearance of growth for EFCA's funding business, generating $17.2 million of funding fraud income for 1969. And they were able to do so while increasing the discrepancy between the funded loans receivable balance and its underlying detail by only $3.9 million.

Second, EFCA was thereby permitted to accrue an enormous amount of income in a single year from an uncertain source of revenue. The fact that the trails were purportedly sold in 1970 should not have affected the accounting treatment given to them in 1969. The books for 1969 should have been closed as of December 31, almost four months before the conspirators even conceived of the bogus trails contract.

---

* See Appendix B at page 199.

72

Additionally, absent solid verification of the purchaser's ability to pay — to insure a true transfer of the economic risk — accrual of income from the transaction should not have been considered in any year. A receivable from a company whose financial condition was unknown was no more certain of realization than the trail commissions themselves. In any event, the amount recorded should have been discounted to present value because the purchaser's notes were non-interest bearing.

A separate and equally fundamental objection derives from the fact that at the time of the 1969 audit the value of the trail commissions was already reflected as an asset on EFCA's books. The purchase price paid by EFCA for IPC was approximately $8 million greater than the value of the tangible assets acquired. The difference was undoubtedly attributable to the value of the trail commissions and the IPC sales force, and was thereafter carried as goodwill on EFCA's consolidated balance sheet. Consequently, apart from everything else, the sale of the trail commissions should have been treated as the sale of an asset, with the sales price being applied to reduce the purchased goodwill and, at the same time, to set up an appropriate receivable. As a matter of basic accounting principles, the transaction should not have generated income.

Lastly, the reduction of Funded Loans and Accounts Receivable which took place in connection with the treatment given to the contractuals receivable should have been cause for serious concern to the auditors. This is especially so given the fact that most of the reported balance for funded loans receivable had to be supported in the 1968 audit by reference to a variety of unrelated items. Thus, despite the fact that funding was supposed to be the mainstay of EFCA's business, for at least two years in succession the funded loan asset ostensibly consisted in large part of something quite different from what it purported to be.

(2) THE GRANDSON TRANSACTIONS.

Like Estudios, Etablissement Grandson (EFCA's secret Liechtenstein subsidiary) was a mere shell used by the conspirators to further the EFCA fraud during its foreign phase. Among other things, Grandson was used to cover up part of the funding fraud in connection with a pair of 3-year unsecured Swiss franc note placements arranged in February 1969 by Dishy Easton through Loeb,

Rhoades International, Inc. ("LRI"), an international investment broker. Pursuant to these placements, EFCA received proceeds of about $9 million which were improperly recorded on EFCA's books as "free credits" to funded loans receivable, instead of as notes payable to LRI.* Consequently, the LRI debt obligations did not appear on EFCA's 1969 financial statements.

Having successfully accomplished this deception in 1969, presumably nothing further was required to conceal the LRI liabilities until 1972, when the notes matured. However, in June 1970 LRI discovered that its notes were not on EFCA's balance sheet, and representatives of LRI came to Los Angeles where they confronted Goldblum and Lowell with the omission. According to Lowell, Goldblum told them that the loan proceeds had been used to make funded loans to clients and, thus, that EFCA's auditors had insisted upon including the LRI notes with the rest of the company's notes payable for funded loans. After Goldblum left the meeting, the still skeptical LRI people questioned Lowell further and he assured them Wolfson Weiner would confirm Goldblum's explanation. Then, as soon as the LRI representatives left his office, Lowell called Julian Weiner to alert him to an inquiry and to tell him what to say.

As a result of this episode, the conspirators decided to put the LRI notes on EFCA's books. At Goldblum's direction, Sultan made an entry to record the $9 million of notes payable by setting up a bogus Swiss franc receivable from Grandson. According to Lowell, two promissory notes were prepared by the conspirators to support the bogus Grandson receivable because Sol Block wanted documentation for Wolfson Weiner's files. The bogus notes were typed on a letterhead for Grandson (misspelled "Granson"), and purported to be executed by the fictitious Dr. Heinrich Wangerhof, as Managing Director of the etablissement. Wangerhof's name was signed by Goldblum on the notes, which were identical to the LRI notes in all material particulars. Both sets of notes were unsecured and had the same face amounts and dates of maturity. Unlike the LRI notes, however, the Grandson notes were non-interest bearing.

There is no evidence that any cash was ever transferred to Grandson. However, additional activity was recorded in the Grand-

---

* The proceeds of these notes were also used to support the balance of Funded Loans and Accounts Receivable reported by EFCA in 1968. See table at page 35.

son account receivable during the rest of 1970 to further the funding fraud. The account was reduced about $2 million by creating other bogus assets on EFCA's books, the largest of which was entitled "Exploration Costs." Then later in the year the original balance of the Grandson receivable was restored by an entry which, at the same time, reduced funded loans receivable by $2 million. Thus, taken all together, the net result of the activity in the Grandson account — coupled with the original treatment of the LRI notes in February 1969 — was to record fraudulent "free credits" to funded loans receivable of about $11 million by creating bogus assets of the same amount.

Work papers for the 1970 audit contain copies of both bogus Grandson notes, as well as letters from Wolfson Weiner to the etablissement seeking to confirm each of them. Another letter appears in the work papers purporting to acknowledge one of the notes, but there is nothing to indicate whether a similar reply was obtained for the other. The reply, signed by Golan, is on a Grandson letterhead (correctly spelled) and confirms that the Grandson receivable was unsecured and non-interest bearing.

According to Levin, the interest-free feature of the notes was explained to the auditors as a commission to Grandson for acting as broker in the sale of the trail commissions to Estudios.* Assuming this explanation to be true — and it was not — then the entry made to record the Grandson notes was still wrong for at least two reasons. First, because they were non-interest bearing, the Grandson notes should have been recorded at their discounted present value, instead of at their face amount. Second, because the Estudios sale was recorded as a completed transaction in 1969, the difference between present value and face amount of the Grandson notes should have been booked as a commission expense in connection with the sale at the time it was supposedly made.

Although they were dated to mature in February 1972, the bogus Grandson notes were still on EFCA's books in April 1973 when the Company collapsed. A schedule found in the 1972 audit work papers correctly describes the delinquent notes — including their dates of maturity — but nothing appears in any of the papers to indicate why they were considered collectible and not reserved

---

* See pages 66-72.

or written off as uncollectible bad debts. The auditors' conduct is all the more puzzling because there is no information in any of the work papers as to the financial condition of Grandson or the nature of its business. Thus, as in the case of Estudios, it is impossible to see how the auditors could have determined that this unknown foreign company had the ability to pay a $9 million unsecured debt to EFCA.

IV. THE INSURANCE PHASE OF THE FRAUD

The importance of international activities to the continuing vitality of the fraud declined steadily as EFCA withdrew from its foreign entanglements. During this period, insurance emerged as the backbone of the Company's business and — although funding remained the mainstay of the fraud — an insurance phase of the conspiracy developed as well. This chapter will begin with a brief history of EFCA's insurance operations, turn next to a description of the insurance fraud, and conclude with consideration of some difficulties this last phase of the fraud created for the conspirators.

A. Evolution of EFCA's Insurance Operations.

(1) THE MARKETING PERIOD (1960-67).

It has been noted above that EFCA began as a marketing organization, selling shares of non-affiliated mutual funds and life insurance underwritten by non-proprietary insurance companies. The Company's life insurance sales during this period were effected primarily through wholly-owned sales subsidiaries, of which EFC-Cal was the most significant. From 1960 to June 1963, EFC-Cal was licensed as a non-exclusive general agent for Citizens Life Insurance Company of New York and for Pennsylvania Life Insurance Company, the life insurance subsidiary of Santa Monica-based Pennsylvania Life Company (herein jointly "PLC").

In June 1963, EFCA and its insurance sales subsidiaries entered into agreements with PLC under which EFCA became the exclusive general agent of PLC for the sale of life insurance policies in connection with Equity Funding Programs in all but two states. With limited exceptions, EFCA agreed not to sell policies underwritten by companies other than PLC. In exchange, PLC agreed not to appoint any other agent whose primary business was the sale of life insurance in connection with funding programs. These agreements ran until December 31, 1968, and were terminable thereafter on six months notice by either party. They ultimately bore the seeds of the insurance phase of the fraud.

During the marketing period, EFCA earned commission income on the policies sold through EFC-Cal. Prior to June 1963, the gross commissions earned under the Company's licensing agreements with

77

PLC and Citizens Life Insurance Company of New York amounted to approximately 100% of all first year premiums and approximately 11% of all renewal premiums. Under the 1963 agency agreement with PLC, the commission schedule was similar. For most policies sold, commissions amounted to 100% of first year premiums and 10% or 11% of renewal premiums for the succeeding ten years.

Out of these gross commissions, EFC-Cal paid a commission expense to the individual agents who actually sold the policies which ranged from 30% to 50% of the first year premium, and was approximately 4% of renewal premiums. Thus, the accounting for EFCA's insurance operations during the marketing period was relatively simple: EFC-Cal recorded gross income in the form of commissions and, after paying part of these commissions out to individual agents as an expense, retained the remainder as net insurance commissions earned.

In October 1965, as an inducement to continue marketing PLC policies, PLC granted to EFCA an option to purchase 7,500 shares of its common stock at $12.63 per share (100% of the fair market value of the stock on the date of the grant). The option was exercisable from October 11, 1968 through October 10, 1970, but only if at the time of the exercise EFCA was actively engaged in the sale of insurance underwritten by PLC. This stock option became increasingly valuable in succeeding years, and proved to be more and more significant in the relationship between EFCA and PLC.

In 1968, major revisions made in the PLC agency agreement drastically changed the character of EFCA's insurance operations. The pressure for change stemmed from the fact that in the life insurance industry, the selling end of the business is the least profitable. Greater income is realized from the volume of in-force life insurance on a company's books, which produces renewal premiums with no selling expense and minimal agent commission premiums after the year of sale. EFCA's management evidently realized that so long as the Company remained a mere marketing organization, it would never grow into an insurance business of major proportions. As a result, management eventually decided to abandon the pure marketing status and to develop a "proprietary" role for the Company's insurance operations.

78

(2) THE REINSURANCE PERIOD (1968-73).

As a first step in the conversion to a proprietary insurance operation, in October 1967 EFCA acquired a small Illinois-domiciled company, Presidential Life Insurance Company of America ("Presidential"), whose name was later changed to Equity Funding Life Insurance Company ("EFLIC"). In October 1971, EFCA acquired all of the stock of Bankers National Life Insurance Company ("Bankers"), a New Jersey corporation. Then in June 1972, EFCA acquired Northern Life Insurance Company ("Northern"), a Washington corporation. The insurance operations of Bankers and Northern were not involved in the EFCA fraud, although Northern's stock was the focal point of one of its last episodes.* EFLIC, however, became the center of the insurance phase of the fraud.

In order to utilize Presidential in a proprietary insurance role, EFCA had to obtain a modification of the 1963 agency agreement with PLC. Under the terms of that agreement (which was terminable after 1968), EFCA was prohibited from utilizing other than PLC policies in connection with its funding program. To induce PLC to accept a modification, EFCA's management decided to offer to "coinsure"** with PLC an agreed-upon amount of insurance underwritten by Presidential. Based upon internal projections of the volume of business which Presidential could expect to underwrite, EFCA's management formulated a coinsurance proposal and undertook negotiations with PLC. Agreement was reached in January 1968.

The 1968 modifications took the form of two major agreements. The first was a mutual release from the exclusivity provision of the 1963 agency agreement. The release allowed EFCA and its subsidiaries to sell life insurance policies in any state on behalf of Presidential in connection with the Company's funding program. At the same time, PLC was given the right to engage in funding operations apart from EFCA. The release further provided that EFCA was to cause Presidential to enter into a coinsurance agreement with PLC.

---

* See page 109.
** "Coinsurance," often called "reinsurance," is explained at pages 80-82. The terms are commonly used interchangeably, although they have distinct technical meanings. See generally Thompson, *Reinsurance* (3d ed. 1951). With the exception of the agreement with PLC (which was designated a "coinsurance" agreement), the term "reinsurance" generally was used in EFCA's public reports. The same usage is adopted in this report.

The coinsurance agreement required Presidential to transfer ("cede") to PLC a total of $250 million in face amount of insurance over a three year period in accordance with the following schedule: In 1968, 80% of the total face amount of Presidential policies issued and paid for were to be ceded to PLC, up to $125 million in face amount; in 1969, 66⅔%, up to $75 million in face amount; and in 1970, again 66⅔%, but up to $50 million in face amount. In meeting this quota, Presidential was to be given credit for any PLC policies sold by EFCA agents. On the other hand, if the quota was not met in any given year, a deficit was to be carried over to the following year — and so on — until a total of $250 million in face amount of life insurance was ceded to PLC. Lastly, the PLC stock option granted in 1965 was modified to provide for exercise only if Presidential was not in default of the quota at the time of exercise.

Beginning only months after the PLC Coinsurance Agreement, Presidential entered into a series of reinsurance treaties with a number of other insurance companies, including Connecticut General Life Insurance Company, Sierra Life Insurance Company, Ranger National Life Insurance Company, United Presidential Life Insurance Company, Phoenix Mutual Life Insurance Company, Great Southern Life Insurance Company, and Kentucky Central Life Insurance Company. As indicated by the following table, EFLIC reinsured most of its reported new business at least through 1971.

REPORTED EFLIC REINSURANCE STATISTICS° (1969 – 1971)			
Year	Face Amount of Insurance Reinsured	Per Cent of New Business Reinsured	Reinsurance Considerations Received
1969	$239,000,000	90%	$2,343,000
1970	$435,000,000	60%	$4,374,000
1971	$625,000,000	50%	$5,747,000

In a typical reinsurance transaction, the underwriting company and the reinsurer enter into an agreement (called a "treaty") based upon a projection of the amount of profit expected over the life of a

---

° These figures were reported in the registration statement for EFCA's common stock dated May 24, 1972.

80

block of the underwriting company's policies, discounted to present value. Under such a treaty, a portion or all of the policies are ceded by the underwriting company (usually referred to as "the ceding company") to the reinsurer, which thereafter assumes some of the risk on these policies and the responsibility for setting up adequate policy reserves for the assumed risk.

The ceding company generally remains responsible for administration of the reinsured policies. The ceding company collects the annual premiums from its policyholders on the ceded business, and, depending upon the portion of risk assumed, pays them over to the reinsurer. In the first year that a policy is reinsured, the reinsurer pays to the ceding company a fee ("reinsurance consideration"), which is expressed as a percentage of the premiums for that year (generally from 100% to 190%). This represents the ceding company's profit share plus reimbursement for policy acquisition costs. In succeeding years, renewal premiums are paid over to the reinsurer in the same manner, but the ceding company no longer receives such a large consideration. Instead, a relatively small percentage (generally from 10% to 20%) is returned for administration expenses.

Under state regulatory accounting methods ("statutory accounting"), policy acquisition costs must be treated as expenses of the underwriting company in the year of a policy sale. Since such costs exceed first year premiums on new insurance policies, new business results in a large initial loss for the underwriting company. Thus, although a new insurance company ultimately can expect significant earnings from underwriting, such a company rarely has sufficient net worth to satisfy statutory requirements in its start-up years without additional contributions to capital or reinsurance of some new business.

Reinsurance provides legitimate assistance to a new insurance company in several significant ways. First, the reinsurance consideration received by the company includes both a share of the ultimate profit anticipated from the reinsured business and a reimbursement of its policy acquisition costs. Hence, the new company is able to report underwriting earnings right from the beginning. Second, reinsurance generates immediate cash for the new enterprise. It should be noted, however, that a company which reinsures all or a substantial portion of its business must sell more and more insurance each year in order to show growth in reported earnings, because such a company does not build a profitable base of in-force policies.

Sometimes such an arrangement may amount to a financing mechanism. A "buy back" provision may give the ceding company the right to reacquire its reinsured policies after a certain number of years. Thus, in economic terms, reinsurance may amount to a loan to the ceding company — secured by the future cash stream of renewal premiums from the reinsured business — for which the ceding company pays a "loan fee" in the form of part of the premiums.

Presumably, if the new company retained its reinsurance considerations and invested its cash wisely, it eventually would be able to satisfy statutory net worth requirements on its own without reinsurance. From that point forward, the company would enjoy the full benefit of the underwriting income generated from its in-force insurance. EFCA claimed that EFLIC was relying less and less on reinsurance as the years passed, thereby suggesting that it was reaching the point where its insurance operation could stand on its own. Indeed, the Company asserted that, beginning in 1972, EFLIC intended to retain the bulk of its new business and to deemphasize the role of reinsurance in its operations. However, long before that point reinsurance by EFLIC — like funding — had become an important device in the EFCA fraud and, as will appear from the following discussion, the cash flow consequences of this device left the conspirators no choice but to reinsure ever increasing amounts of EFLIC's purported new business.

B. The Role of Insurance in the Fraud.

With this brief summary of the evolution of EFCA's insurance operations as background, it is now possible to discuss the part of the fraud that has received the greatest public attention — its insurance phase. Through the first two phases of the EFCA fraud, the funding fraud device provided a relatively convenient means of inflating earnings because it enabled the conspirators to generate fictitious income by making simple one-step entries in the Company's books and records. Despite its relative convenience, however, the funding fraud created a problem because it resulted in permanent inflation of a balance sheet asset, funded loans receivable.

82

Although "free credits" were used periodically to reduce funded loans receivable, thereby making it possible to generate more bogus income, there was a limit to the credibility of the funding fraud. When the stock market went sour in 1970, the limit was reached. It no longer appeared plausible for funding overstatements to generate the full amount of income desired to reach the earnings goals set by the fraud participants. Casting about for another effective device to sustain EFCA's amazing but fraudulent earnings record, the conspirators eventually settled upon insurance.

(1) An Insurance Fraud Narrative.

Fictitious reinsurance seems to have emerged almost by accident as a complement to the funding fraud. The 1968 Coinsurance Agreement with PLC required Presidential to cede $250 million in face amount of insurance to PLC over a three-year period, or write that amount directly with PLC, beginning with $125 million in 1968. EFCA's management had projected production of $200-250 million in face amount of insurance by Presidential in 1968, with a 15% annual increase thereafter. Thus, the PLC agreement appeared easy to satisfy.

The projection of Presidential's 1968 production, however, proved wholly unrealistic. As of May 31st, EFCA's agents had written only $56 million face amount of insurance, only $9 million of which consisted of Presidential policies (the remainder being PLC policies marketed by EFCA's sales force). Hence, it became evident to EFCA's management that the Company was in trouble. They had made an unrealistic commitment in order to break the exclusive PLC sales agreement and had tied the now valuable PLC stock option to that commitment. Furthermore, if it became known in the industry that EFCA failed to meet its PLC commitment, prospects would diminish for favorable reinsurance agreements with other companies. Both these factors in turn promised adversely to affect EFCA's earnings and, consequently, the market performance of its stock.

In the face of such a prospect, at the suggestion of John Pennish, then President of Presidential, it was decided that a "special class" of insurance would be offered to EFCA agents and employees and reinsured with PLC. Some or all of the first year's premium was forgiven on this "special class" of insurance. It was possible to do

83

this without cost to EFCA, because no first year premiums had to be paid to PLC on the coinsured policies (EFC-Cal's commission on those policies was at least 100% of the first year premium) and no commission expense had to be paid to individual agents. Although EFCA thereby lost the forgiven premium income, "special class" insurance would make it possible to meet the PLC quota for 1968. On the other hand, such policies could be expected to have a high lapse rate in the second year when the employees would have to pay the premiums themselves to keep the policies in force. Hence, while "special class" insurance eased the short-term problem, it created new long-term problems.

"Special class" insurance — coded in the Company's records as "Department 94" business — was vigorously promoted by circulars to EFCA employees and agents as part of an active solicitation campaign by management. Apparently such insurance was initially offered with a 50% premium forgiveness, but when the response proved insufficient to meet Presidential's scheduled commitment to PLC, the Company forgave the entire premium and issued the policy "free." Competitions were arranged between departments to encourage personnel to sign up for as big a policy amount as possible and, as a result, many employees bought high face amount policies with premiums much greater than they could afford. Although the precise amount of "special class" insurance issued in 1968 is not known, former Company executives estimate the face amount to have been from $30 to $50 million, virtually all of which was ceded to PLC to meet the 1968 quota.

EFCA exercised the PLC stock option in October 1968, as soon as it became exercisable by its terms, although some doubt remained at PLC as to Presidential's ability to fulfill the 1968 quota by year-end. PLC was paid $94,725 (per the terms of the 1965 option), and because of stock splits, EFCA received 25,000 shares of PLC stock in return. By December 1968, the market value of these shares was in excess of $1 million over the option price of the stock. Despite the fact that it had not sold or otherwise disposed of the PLC stock, EFCA reported the full amount of this excess as income in its 1968 financial statements.

84

It appears that additional "special class" insurance was issued in 1969 and 1970. More significantly, 1969 witnessed the adoption of an even more ominous step toward the insurance phase of the fraud. As year-end approached, top officers of the Company who were involved in the conspiracy concluded that they could not meet either the PLC quota or target earnings figures for that year without some further "assistance." To solve this dilemma, Fred Levin devised what he called the "pending business caper." Pending business (insurance for which applications had been received but which had neither been approved by the underwriting department nor paid for by the applicant) would be posted on the Company's records as if it were in-force and paid up. This practice was adopted despite the recognition that a material portion of such business normally never becomes effective.

To handle the mechanics of the pending business caper, Levin recruited the assistance of others at EFLIC, including Arthur Lewis, Lloyd Edens, James Smith and Frank Majerus. The mechanics decided upon were relatively simple: Entries would be made in the applicable premium receivable and commission payable accounts on EFLIC's books as if the policyholder had already paid his initial premium. Although the necessary increase in policy reserves was also calculated and inflated accordingly, the various other expenses incident to placing an insurance policy in force — expenses for underwriting, administration, and medical and credit reports — were not increased.

Estimates of the amount of pending business reported as placed in force in 1969 vary, but range from $350,000 to $750,000 in premium income. This pending business was more than enough to satisfy the 1969 PLC quota, and the remainder was ceded to other reinsurers in order to generate cash. EFLIC's treaties with these other reinsurers provided for relatively high first year reinsurance considerations, ranging up to 190% of the initial premium. Thus, although EFLIC received no premiums from insureds on that portion of pending business which was not ultimately placed in-force, the Company was able to generate cash of up to 90% of the first year premium amount by reinsuring such pending policies.

By the end of 1969, the long-term problems created by these short-term solutions began to emerge. The renewal premiums had fallen due on much of the "special class" insurance which the Company had earlier issued to its employees and coinsured with PLC and were about to fall due on the balance. As was to be expected, a large percentage of the individuals who received such policies free for the first year decided not to renew their policies when it came time for them to pay the second year premium. Consequently, although many "special class" recipients chose to keep their insurance by paying the second year premium, an inordinate amount of the business lapsed. As a result of such high lapse rates, PLC became aware of the "special class" nature of the business ceded to it and negotiated an additional $40 million in face amount of insurance to compensate for the lapsed policies.

The Company faced a similar problem on pending business which it had booked as in-force and reinsured with other companies. Since a significant portion of such business was never legitimately placed in-force, the resulting lapse rate would surely alert the victim reinsurer — just as the high lapse rate on "special class" business had alerted PLC. To avoid this problem, the conspirators decided that when the time came to pay over second year renewal premiums on the reinsured pending business, the Company itself would pay the renewal premium amounts on a portion of the pending policies that had not by then been placed in-force and thereby artificially maintain an acceptable lapse rate. To keep track of such business and assure that policyholder communications were not mailed for it, the pending business kept in force in this manner was coded "Department 65." Thus, the pending business caper led the conspirators to maintain in-force policies which, while they originated with legitimate policy applications, were in fact fictitious. It was but a short step to the point of creating and reinsuring policies which were bogus from their inception.

The final step was taken in the summer of 1970. By that time, it was clear to EFCA's management that the year was turning out to be a disastrous one for the Company. The move to glamorous new headquarters in Century City (dubbed the "Taj Mahal") had been expensive, as had the implementation of new computer systems. In addition, legitimate production was down. The sales force of newly-acquired Investors Planning Corporation ("IPC"), on which EFCA had pinned great hopes, proved to be a great disappointment. Most of IPC's salesmen were trained to sell mutual funds, and few had any experience in selling insurance. Consequently, many were unable to grasp the essential marketing points for selling funding programs. More importantly, the great majority of the IPC salesmen immediately left the organization after the acquisition and never sold for EFCA at all. Lastly, the general slump in the stock market and in the nation's economy made it difficult to sell new funding programs and resulted in a significant increase in both voluntary and involuntary liquidations of existing funding programs.

By the second quarter of 1970, EFCA's common stock, which had soared to more than $80 per share in 1969, hit bottom at close to $12. That was the signal to the Company's stock price-conscious management that something had to be done. The solution — to create and reinsure wholly bogus insurance business — was generated in a series of discussions involving at least Goldblum, Levin, Smith, Arthur Lewis and Edens. According to Levin, it was thought that the plan would serve two purposes: Creation of the business would lend an illusion of production to the Company's operations, and reinsurance of the bogus business would generate needed working capital. In this manner, the Company could obtain cash to pay premiums on lapsed business and also report a suitable amount of "income" while the conspirators searched for an "ultimate" solution to EFCA's growing problems.

The "Y business," as the bogus insurance was internally known, was considered by the conspirators to be simply an extension of the earlier pending business caper. The basic mechanics for the program, again worked out by EFLIC's executives, were similar. To begin, the conspirators simply created "new" policies from existing legitimate policies in the in-force file by changing the policy number and increasing the face amount and premium for each policy by a factor of 1.8. In 1970, $5.5 million of non-existent premium income and appropriate phony figures for commissions and policy reserves were posted to EFLIC's books as they had been earlier in connection with the pending business caper.

87

When a portion of this bogus business (between one-third and one-half of all reported business in 1970) was reinsured later in the year, detail support was created only as needed. Initially, only computer detail was developed: Computer tapes were produced listing the non-existent "insured's" age, sex, policy number, premium and risk coverage. The tapes for bogus business usually consisted of simple repetitions of the detail for legitimate policies already on the computer. It was relatively easy to reproduce such detail because even legitimate runs did not generally list policyholder names and addresses. As had been done earlier with lapsed business on which EFCA paid premiums, the wholly non-existent business was given a special code on the computer tapes ("Department 99") to insure that such policies did not get routed to EFLIC's policy service department for billing.

The amount of bogus business increased in 1971. Up to $10 million in fictitious new premium income was recorded in that year on the books of EFLIC, which for the first time appeared in EFCA's financial statements as a consolidated subsidiary.* To generate fraudulent detail for the 1971 bogus business, the conspirators used legitimate records from newly-acquired Bankers as a source of data — just as they had used legitimate EFLIC data the previous year. In addition, Levin concluded early in the year that it would be necessary to have at least some bogus policyholder files to evidence the non-existent business. At first such files were created on an ad hoc basis by a few Company executives and managers at "fraud parties" lasting well into the night. In April, however, as the creation of bogus business increased, the conspirators concluded that at least 20,000 to 50,000 files would be needed and that they would have to be made up on a more organized basis. To house the bogus file factory, a small office was rented in May 1971 on Maple Drive in Beverly Hills. The conspirators had often attributed some of EFLIC's bogus "sales" to a "mass marketing" operation which was purportedly conducted by direct mail. The Maple Drive facility was said to house this "mass marketing" operation.

The Maple Drive office was managed first by Richard Gardenier and then by Mark Lewis, younger brother of EFLIC Vice President

---

* See Appendix B at page 215.

Arthur Lewis. It operated on an intermittent basis through early 1973. The clerical staff at the office was supplied with lists of common male and female forenames as well as blank credit and medical reports, together with sample information to be typed on the forms. Armed with such tools, Lewis' staff created policyholder files from scratch: Names of "policyholders" were invented, and imaginary credit and health reports written. As needed, the conspirators ordered files, and the staff of the Maple Drive office filled the order.

The recording and reinsurance of bogus insurance continued into 1972 at a stepped-up pace. At least $14,667,000 in fictitious premium income was recorded on EFLIC's books during that year. Thus, although much of the business reinsured in 1970 was legitimate, by 1971 the mix was heavily weighted on the bogus side, as the following table demonstrates.

PERCENTAGE OF BOGUS INSURANCE*
(1970-1972)

Reinsurer	1970	1971	1972
PLC	.3%	—	—
United Presidential	7.4	89.5%	—
Phoenix Mutual	100.0	89.8	—
Ranger	.3	85.5	94.0%
Great Southern	—	100.0	100.0
Kentucky General	—	100.0	100.0

As an offshoot of the reinsurance fraud, the Company also obtained additional revenue from reinsurers by filing claims for death benefits on some of the bogus policies. One can predict with certainty that at least some portion of any large group of real policyholders will die each year. Therefore, in order to maintain appearances, it was necessary for the conspirators to "kill off" a number of the non-existent policyholders they had created, and in the process to file false death claims. Since a large portion of the bogus policies which EFLIC had reinsured were created by duplicating the vital

---

* This table indicates the percentages of fictitious insurance ceded in the first year pursuant to treaties with the reinsurers named. The percentages shown were calculated based upon premium amounts.

statistics of actual EFLIC and Bankers policyholders, the death of a "real" policyholder presented the opportunity to file a death claim on the bogus counterpart of the legitimate policy, or on a bogus policy with similar vital statistics.

The conspirators began by filing a few such claims in 1971, depositing the moneys received in EFLIC accounts. The false death claim scheme did not get under way on a large scale, however, until the summer of 1972 when Goldblum and Levin discovered that a number of ambitious EFLIC officers had been filing false death claims and misappropriating the proceeds for themselves.* When these activities came to light, rather than discharging the individuals involved, Levin put them to work supervising an expanded false death claim operation on behalf of the Company. All told, the conspirators ran up a total of 26 false death claims with reinsurers which netted $1,175,171. Of this amount, $1,031,269 went into Company accounts. The remaining $143,902 enriched the embezzlers personally before discovery of their scheme. Four reinsurers — Phoenix Mutual ($359,746), Kentucky Central ($277,225), Great Southern ($340,200) and Ranger ($198,000) — were the victims of the bogus death claim activity, which continued through March 1973.

If the EFCA fraud had not been uncovered, the false death claim scheme would undoubtedly have escalated to far greater proportions. According to Levin, he had proposed that $7-10 million be obtained by means of such claims during 1973. After some discussion, Arthur Lewis and others at EFLIC involved in the fraud convinced Levin that $10 million was unrealistic. A goal of $3-5 million in false death claims was settled upon instead. EFCA's collapse in April, however, cut short the false death claim scheme in its infancy.

(2) PROBLEMS CREATED BY THE INSURANCE PHASE.

Once fictitious insurance assumed an important part in the EFCA conspiracy, it was just a matter of time before the fraud collapsed. On the one hand, reinsurance of non-existent insurance policies created a cash flow problem which increased geometrically with each passing year. On the other hand, the practice of recording premium income from such policies created a growing imbalance in inter-

---

* See discussion of the "Cookie Jar Caper" at pages 129-131.

company accounts which was only concealed by creating more and more fictitious assets. Ultimately, the house of cards had to fall.

(a) *The Cash Flow Problem.*

It has already been observed that a company which reinsures all or a substantial portion of its business must sell more and more insurance each year in order to show growth in reported earnings.* In EFLIC's case, where many of the policies reinsured were phony, the increase in non-existent "sales" needed to show growth in income created a cash drain because EFLIC had to pay renewal premiums to the reinsurers of its bogus policies. This problem could not be solved by allowing the bogus business to lapse because a number of EFLIC's reinsurance treaties guaranteed a persistency rate for some period, and because high lapse rates might have alerted the reinsurers to the fraud. Thus, the scheme inevitably required the creation and reinsurance of an ever increasing number of bogus policies.

Transactions pursuant to the 1970 reinsurance treaty with Phoenix Mutual will illustrate the cash flow problem thus created. In 1970, as a result of the cession of bogus insurance to Phoenix Mutual, EFLIC received approximately $1.4 million in reinsurance considerations. In 1971, however, EFLIC had to pay out to Phoenix Mutual almost $1.4 million in "renewal premiums" on those non-existent policies, and in 1972 another $1.2 million. Hence, by the end of 1972 EFLIC had already a negative cash flow of $1.2 million on the bogus policies ceded under that treaty. To obtain that cash, EFLIC had to reinsure even more fictitious policies, which in turn created additional cash flow problems in succeeding years.

As the table below indicates, by 1972 EFLIC had a negative net cash flow of some $1.7 million in connection with the bogus business which it had reinsured. In other words, the total amount received as reinsurance consideration on bogus policies was about $1.7 million less than the aggregate amount of renewal premiums which had to be paid on bogus policies ceded in prior years. The problem could only become geometrically worse as time passed. As the conspirators reinsured greater amounts of fictitious business to solve their immediate problem, they increased the magnitude of next year's

---

* See pages 81-82.

problem. Thus, once the first step down the path of fictitious reinsurance had been taken, the fraud was destined to increase exponentially each year until it reached an unmanageable level.

NET CASH FLOW BETWEEN EFLIC AND REINSURERS ATTRIBUTABLE TO BOGUS POLICIES*
(1970-1972)

Reinsurance Cession	1970	1971	1972
1969 Cessions			
PLC	$ (7,369)	$ (24,299)	$ (32,646)
Conn. General	(15,932)	(28,702)	(38,321)
Ranger (1st)	0	0	(8,699)
Ranger (2nd)	(3,355)	(61,495)	(53,673)
United Presidential	(2,593)	(2,959)	(3,458)
1970 Cessions			
Ranger	8,296	(777,368)	(1,013,794)
United Presidential	21,750	(117,760)	(153,395)
Phoenix Mutual	1,400,010	(1,392,405)	(1,197,479)
1971 Cessions			
Ranger		2,242,518	(2,293,291)
United Presidential		179,200	(236,529)
Phoenix Mutual		897,607	(972,245)
Great Southern		900,602	(770,477)
Kentucky Central		1,215,235	(1,036,630)
1972 Cessions			
Ranger			3,597,736
Great Southern			900,190
Kentucky Central			1,620,440
YEARLY NET CASH FLOW	$1,400,807	$3,030,174	$(1,692,271)

Some of the conspirators — Levin and Edens among them — considered at times utilizing the "buy back" provision in EFLIC's reinsurance treaties as a possible way out of the problem.** However, for a number of reasons, this solution was never seriously entertained by the fraud participants. To begin with, a company which reinsures business with the intention of later repurchasing it may not properly

---

* Cessions shown were made pursuant to treaties with the reinsurers identified. The table does not include false death claim amounts. Parentheses indicate negative cash flow.

** See page 82.

92

record the reinsurance consideration received in a treaty year as "current income." Resort to the "buy back" provisions therefore would have created a serious risk of depriving EFLIC of a principal benefit of the insurance fraud scheme.

Even more importantly, as indicated above, by 1972 EFLIC was experiencing a serious cash flow problem in connection with its bogus reinsurance. The conspirators tried to alleviate this problem by entering into new bogus reinsurance deals each year. Since repurchase rights on ceded business could not be exercised for a number of years after such treaties were made, EFLIC faced enormous cash flow problems for the foreseeable future. To contemplate repurchase of fictitious business as an ultimate solution meant accepting the prospect that EFLIC would have to stop creating and reinsuring bogus policies. In turn, EFLIC would have to increase its legitimate sales considerably, and not report the resulting revenue from those sales.

In short, every means of resolving the problem that the conspirators considered would have reduced EFCA's reported earnings. According to Levin, whenever such a solution was proposed, Goldblum rejected it categorically. Reported production and earnings had to continue to increase each year, he insisted, or EFCA's loans would be called and the price of its stock would tumble. As EFCA's major stockholder, Goldblum would not stand for any proposal which produced such a result. Thus, at the time of EFCA's collapse, the conspirators had yet to conceive of a solution to the cash flow difficulties brought about by their bogus reinsurance scheme, and it is highly doubtful that any solution existed.

(b) *The Inter-Company Accounts Problem.*

A second side-effect of fictitious insurance also proved to be a problem. No cash passed between EFC-Cal (the general agency) and EFLIC at the time of a legitimate policy sale. Instead, entries were made on EFLIC's books in the inter-company account with EFCA to record premiums due from the sale as a receivable to EFLIC, and commissions due EFC-Cal as a payable to EFCA.* No

---

* There was no separate inter-company account between EFLIC and EFC-Cal. Entries made on EFCA's books to record commissions receivable due from EFLIC thus had to be adjusted indirectly, through EFCA's inter-company account with EFC-Cal.

entries were made on EFCA's books until year-end, when its inter-company account with EFLIC was adjusted and closed out by appropriate cash transfers to EFLIC.

In the case of fictitious insurance transactions, this procedure created no problem during the year in which a bogus policy was first recorded as "sold," but in succeeding years it created an imbalance in the inter-company accounts between EFLIC and EFCA which could not be adjusted at year-end in the normal manner. In the first year of fictitious policies, the receivable recorded by EFLIC for fictitious premium income due from EFC-Cal was offset on EFLIC's books by fictitious commissions payable to EFCA (100% of the first year premium) for the alleged "sales" made by EFC-Cal. In the second and succeeding years, however, there were no commissions payable to offset against the premiums due because EFC-Cal did not receive a renewal commission on EFLIC business. Since EFCA never recorded a corresponding payable due to EFLIC, the fictitious premium receivable thus continued to grow in EFLIC's inter-company account without any counterbalance on EFCA's books.

By year-end 1971, the imbalance was approximately $16 million and had become a major problem for the conspirators. According to Sultan, the problem was discussed at several meetings attended by him, Goldblum, Levin, Edens, Smith and Arthur Lewis. Lowell was kept abreast of these developments by Sultan. Ultimately, it was decided that the imbalance could not be corrected on EFLIC's books without assistance from EFCA.

The plan finally adopted to solve the problem was formulated by Goldblum at a meeting with Sultan. According to Sultan, Goldblum's plan called for EFCA to transfer $16 million in cash to EFLIC from the proceeds of a public debenture offering in December 1971. EFLIC recorded this cash as a pay down of the inter-company receivable due from EFCA, but EFCA recorded the transfer differently. Sultan intercepted the bank memoranda to EFCA confirming the transfer. In their place, he substituted fraudulent bank charge advices and confirmations to evidence fictitious commercial paper purchases by EFCA in the same amount. Thus, the conspirators

94

decided to transfer cash from EFCA to cover for EFLIC's fraudulent overstatement of premium income and, in turn, to conceal this cover-up by recording a fictitious asset on the parent's books.

These steps were taken in anticipation of the 1971 audit of EFCA, which early in 1972 came to be the responsibility of Seidman & Seidman, a national firm of certified public accountants which combined practices with the Los Angeles office of Wolfson Weiner in February 1972. Under the terms of the agreement entered into between the two firms, the former employees of the Los Angeles office of Wolfson Weiner became employees of Seidman. Thereafter, the personnel who previously had performed accounting services for EFCA and certain of its subsidiaries under the name of Wolfson Weiner continued to perform the same services for these companies under the name of Seidman & Seidman — including the 1971 audit then in progress.

The conspirators planned to have the fictitious commercial paper "mature" near the close of the 1971 audit and to record an appropriate cash receipt at that time, to "prove" to Seidman auditors that the bogus 1971 investment in commercial paper was real. It appears that this ploy worked. In February 1972, non-existent commercial paper in the amount of about $19.2 million was recorded as having been redeemed.* To support the fictitious redemption, about $14.3 million in cash was returned from EFLIC, which recorded the transfer on its books as an advance to EFCA and thereby restored almost the full amount of the previous year's inter-company imbalance on EFLIC's books. The proceeds of a $4.9 million loan from Dow Banking Corporation to EFCC-NV were diverted to the parent company to make up the remainder of the bogus transaction.** For good measure, the

---

* On or about December 29, 1971, the conspirators had created an additional $3.2 million of fictitious commercial paper by crediting the EFCC-NV inter-company account for that amount. See page 55.

** A valid journal entry, dated February 18, 1972, was prepared to record cash coming in to EFCA and a payable to EFCC-NV. However, a fraudulent journal entry, dated February 22, was substituted to show the receipt of cash as a redemption of commercial paper. On its books, EFCC-NV properly recorded the Dow loan as an inter-company charge to EFCA and a credit to notes payable. This treatment resulted in an imbalance in the inter-company accounts with EFCC-NV which was eliminated in July 1972,

95

conspirators even recognized interest income of $177,000 in connection with the redemption.

This series of transactions took advantage of the fact that different accounting firms were retained to audit EFCA and EFLIC: Seidman for the former and Haskins & Sells for the latter. As of December 31, 1971, EFLIC's books showed only a negligible receivable due from EFCA in the inter-company account. Consequently, Haskins auditors were not prompted to look beyond the confirmation of that amount which they received from Sultan. At that same point in time, EFCA's books showed fictitious commercial paper which Seidman auditors were not prompted to confirm, supposedly because the bogus investment had "matured" and cash had been received. Of course, had Haskins coordinated with Seidman, or vice versa, such a transparent shell game would not have been possible.

The sequence is summarized in the following chart.

(footnote continued from previous page)

when the conspirators recorded cash received from PLC (representing reserves for policies ceded by that company to EFLIC in a coinsurance transaction) as a credit against the inter-company payable to EFCC-NV. The conspirators concealed this misappropriation by treating the PLC policies as new business requiring very small reserves.

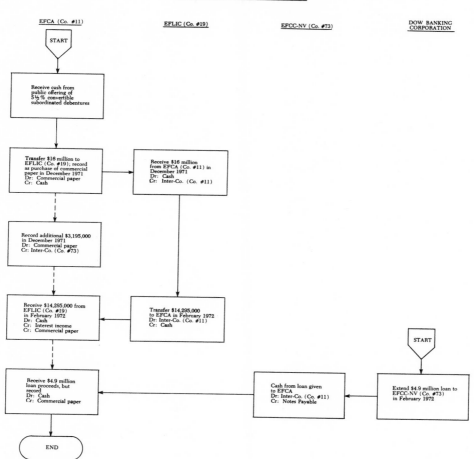

1971 FICTITIOUS COMMERCIAL PAPER

EFCA (Co. #11)   EFLIC (Co. #19)   EFCC-NV (Co. #73)   DOW BANKING CORPORATION

START

Receive cash from
public offering of
5½% convertible
subordinated debentures

Transfer $16 million to
EFLIC (Co. #19); record
as purchase of commercial
paper in December 1971
Dr: Commercial paper
Cr: Cash

Receive $16 million
from EFCA (Co. #11) in
December 1971
Dr: Cash
Cr: Inter-Co. (Co. #11)

Record additional $3,195,000
in December 1971
Dr: Commercial paper
Cr: Inter-Co. (Co. #73)

Receive $14,295,000 from
EFLIC (Co. #19)
in February 1972
Dr: Cash
Cr: Interest income
Cr: Commercial paper

Transfer $14,295,000
to EFCA in February 1972
Dr: Inter-Co. (Co. #11)
Cr: Cash

START

Receive $4.9 million
loan proceeds, but
record
Dr: Cash
Cr: Commercial paper

Cash from loan given
to EFCA
Dr: Inter-Co. (Co. #11)
Cr: Notes Payable

Extend $4.9 million loan to
EFCC-NV (Co. #73)
in February 1972

END

97

The creation of fictitious commercial paper at year-end 1971 helped the conspirators survive another audit, but it did not solve the underlying problem. When EFLIC returned $14.3 million to EFCA to support the bogus redemption, the inter-company imbalance was almost fully restored. The situation was aggravated by improper entries made in inter-company accounts with other subsidiaries.* Indeed, the account between EFCA and EFLIC got so hopelessly out of balance that each company carried an unbalanced receivable due from the other. On EFLIC's books, the unbalanced receivable purportedly due from EFCA evidently had grown to about $24 million. At the same time, it appears that EFCA's books showed an $8 million unbalanced receivable purportedly due from EFLIC. These receivables could not be offset because neither company's books showed corresponding payables.

Another round of meetings attended by Goldblum, Levin, Sultan, Edens, Smith and Arthur Lewis took place to decide what to do. Again Sultan kept Lowell advised as to the problem. One solution proposed in these meetings involved the sale of several large annuities (face amounts of $100,000 or more) with lives of 10 years or more, purportedly issued by EFCA's life insurance subsidiaries. Normal accounting for such annuities would require the seller to establish a reserve against which to charge periodic payments over the life of the annuity. The conspirators proposed to conceal all such annuity sales and to set up no such reserves, however, and instead to apply the proceeds of annuities sold against the inter-company account. In this manner, the imbalance might be narrowed and perhaps eventually eliminated. Moreover, although there would be inadequate reserves for the annuities, that problem could be deferred for some time because of their long life.

Some steps were taken to implement this plan. On Levin's instructions, Sultan opened two bank accounts at United California Bank to process funds received from the scheme, and annuities were printed. In addition, Levin and others had discussions with several union representatives in an attempt to interest their pension funds in purchasing large annuities. These discussions produced no results, however, and it appears that the scheme was dropped after the sale of only one annuity.

---

* See, for example, the note at pages 95-96.

After the annuity scheme failed, the conspirators decided to try bogus bonds to solve the problem. A great deal of time was spent attempting to obtain proper materials. Smith obtained specimens from which to determine the format and quality of paper and printing of legitimate bonds. Edens and Arthur Lewis visited a large financial printer in Los Angeles to learn how bonds are printed. Edens developed a portfolio of bogus bonds which listed the names of issuers, amounts, due dates and interest rates. Gary Beckerman was assigned the task of finding the highest quality paper available.

Sultan, Arthur Lewis and Beckerman coordinated the preparation of paste-ups for the face and back sides of several styles of bonds. Goldblum kept close tabs on the process, and after the paste-ups were sent to outside typesetters for proofs, he ordered changes in the text which interfered with the printer's time schedule. On at least one occasion, Goldblum also criticized the grade of paper being used, and said he would try to get a better grade. However, no better grade was obtained and at least some of the bogus bonds apparently were printed on the paper obtained by Beckerman.

The plan was to use the bogus bonds to cover the $24 million imbalance on EFLIC's books. It was contemplated that the bonds would be placed in a safe deposit box at American National Bank & Trust Co. in Chicago, Illinois ("American National Bank"), where they would be inspected by the auditors. EFLIC had legitimate business with American National Bank and it was chosen for that reason. The conspirators planned to use a safe deposit box, instead of a custody account, to avoid having to obtain a bank confirmation of the existence of the bonds. Ultimately it was decided, however, that the bogus bonds were not good enough to pass an audit and should not be used. Most of the bonds were burned by the conspirators in the last hectic days when discovery of the fraud appeared certain.

The final plan developed by the conspirators involved establishing a fictitious custodian account for $24 million of bonds at a nonexistent branch office of American National Bank. Levin was in New York when the decision was made. He recalls that Goldblum telephoned him in New York and gave him instructions to go to Chicago on his way back to Los Angeles and open an office using a name very close to that of American National Bank & Trust Co.

99

Levin did so and leased office space in the name of "American National Trust." He also made arrangements for a caretaker to accept mail at the fictitious branch. From time to time thereafter, fraud participants sent letters addressed to "American National Bank" at the mail drop address to accustom post office employees to delivering mail so addressed to the bogus location.

A print-out of the bogus bond portfolio was prepared on EFCA's System/3 computer, and was given to Seidman & Seidman during the 1972 audit to support purchases of $24 million of the bonds at American National Bank. When the auditors also requested a direct bank confirmation for the bogus bonds, a request for confirmation was prepared, addressed to the fictitious branch office and given to them for mailing. Collins went to Chicago to receive it at the phony American National Bank branch. Nothing was received for a period of several days, causing great consternation among the conspirators who feared that the post office had delivered the request to the real American National Bank & Trust Co. However, they later learned that a Seidman & Seidman accountant simply forgot to mail the confirmation request. Collins returned to Los Angeles, and James Banks replaced him in Chicago. When the auditors' confirmation finally arrived at the mail drop, Banks apparently signed and returned it to them in Los Angeles. In this manner, the conspirators concealed the $24 million imbalance in the inter-company account on EFLIC's books at year-end 1972.

The $8 million receivable due from EFLIC on EFCA's books was taken care of by fictitious EFCA purchases of commercial paper in that amount. After another conversation with Goldblum and on his instructions, Sultan arranged a series of round-robin cash transfers to support the bogus buys.

First, on December 22, 1972, Sultan caused Bankers and Northern each to transfer $2 million to EFLIC. Bankers and Northern both properly recorded these transfers. EFLIC made no entry and instead transferred the aggregate amount of $4 million to EFCA, which recorded the receipt of the funds as a reduction in the inter-company receivable from EFLIC. Sultan then used the $4 million for a legitimate EFCA purchase of commercial paper through United California Bank, and properly recorded the transactions. The

100

commercial paper was scheduled to mature on December 26, but the conspirators created false documents which gave the investment a maturity of March 26, 1973. When the paper was redeemed on December 26, it was recorded on EFCA's books as the receipt of additional cash from EFLIC, thus eliminating the rest of the inter-company receivable due from EFLIC.

Subsequently, Sultan used the $4 million received from redemption of the real commercial paper to pay back the funds originally received from Bankers and Northern, both of which again properly recorded the transfers. However, these transfers were recorded on EFCA's books as the purchase through American National Bank of $4 million more of commercial paper, instead of as a repayment to Bankers and Northern. The entire round-robin is summarized by the following chart.

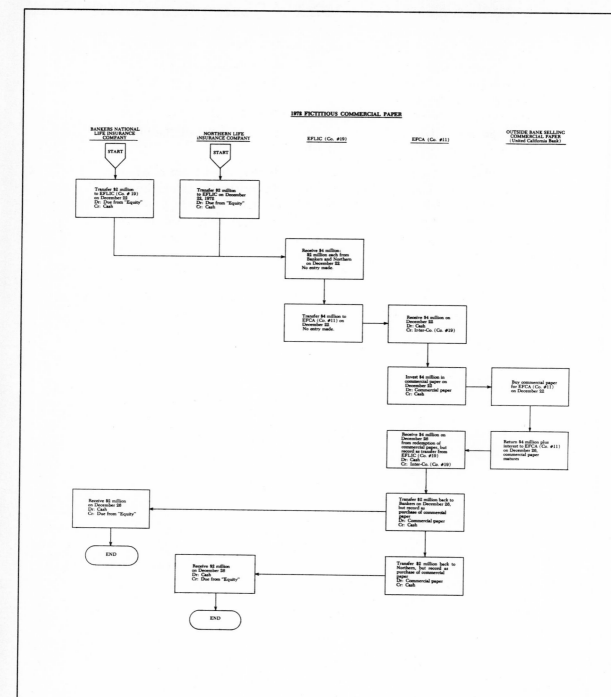

1972 FICTITIOUS COMMERCIAL PAPER

In anticipation of a possible effort by Seidman & Seidman to confirm the transaction with United California Bank, documentation was prepared showing a wire transfer of funds to American National Bank to purchase commercial paper to be held in safekeeping. Thus, if necessary, the bogus branch ploy could be used a second time to obtain a bank confirmation. The precaution was unnecessary, however, because the auditors apparently made no attempt to confirm the existence of the commercial paper.

Thus, an even bigger inter-company imbalance was concealed at year-end 1972. Again, however, the root problem remained.

V. THE LAST DAYS

In early 1973, only months before the collapse of the Company, EFCA's management believed it had reasons for optimism about the future. For one, the conspirators had come through another year-end audit unscathed. They had anticipated many of the questions which the auditors asked and, as before, the explanations which they concocted were accepted. Second, the transformation of the Company from a funding program sales organization into a proprietary insurance conglomerate had been successfully completed. EFCA now referred to itself as "a life insurance-based financial services company". Third, the Company was preparing to issue its 1972 Annual Report reflecting its best year ever. A glowing press release on March 12th would chronicle EFCA's supposed recent accomplishments, with Goldblum announcing a 17% increase in earnings over the previous year and record sales of life insurance by the Company's subsidiaries.

Despite such optimistic notes, however, a serious and dangerous situation remained: The very nature of the insurance fraud meant that it was growing in almost geometric proportions; more and more cash was required to pay renewal premiums on reinsured false policies; and the imbalance in the inter-company accounts was increasing. In short, the Company was like a time bomb.

Without warning, on March 12th the Illinois Insurance Commission sent examiners into EFLIC for an intensive audit. The time bomb was triggered. There had been no time for the conspirators to prepare, and the events now moved too fast to be managed. By the end of the month, the explosion had occurred and the Company was being purged of the fraud and its perpetrators. This chapter chronicles those last dramatic days.

A. Project Z Meetings.

Beginning in mid-1972, some of the conspirators met on an irregular basis to attempt to deal with problems caused by the fraud. These "Project Z" meetings, as they were termed by some of the participants, were attended generally by Goldblum, Levin, Capo, Edens, Arthur Lewis, Smith and Sultan (Lowell came to the 1973 meetings only occasionally). At the meetings, the younger members of the conspiracy, pragmatically concerned about the magnitude of the fraud, pressed for what they saw as a way out. According to records these conspirators were keeping, operating losses had actually *increased* in 1971 and 1972, despite expansion and acquisitions by the Company. They argued that the only way to eliminate the phony insurance and bogus assets was to stop the artificial increases in corporate growth by reporting "flat earnings" for a while. Earnings would have to be reported at the same level as for the prior year and no additional phony assets could be booked, while at the same time real sales would have to be dramatically increased but not reported. This action was to be coupled with the institution of a new cost control system and drastic cost reductions, hopefully to create real profits. However, Goldblum flatly rejected such proposals. A leveling of reported earnings would adversely affect the market price of EFCA's common stock, a prospect he would not entertain.

Project Z therefore came ultimately to focus on two less sweeping ideas which it was thought would help alleviate some of the pressure building up as a result of the fraud. First, a cost-cutting program was inaugurated by notifying department heads that a 20% reduction would have to be made in all departmental budgets. Every department was reviewed with respect to personnel and overhead expenses. At the same time, an effort was supposedly instituted to reduce expense accounts and eliminate the use of first-class air travel and limousines.

The second idea involved a new fraudulent device conceived by Levin and Goldblum — the unrecorded annuities scheme.* The Company would sell several large annuities, take in the cash but not record its receipt and use the proceeds to reduce the imbalance in the intercompany account with EFLIC. Together with the burgeoning "false death claim scheme,"** the annuities scheme was supposed to provide cash to help divert some of the increasing fraud burden from the funding and insurance areas.

Neither of these programs progressed very far. Executives who were not involved in the fraud resisted the proposed cost-cuts in their

---

* See page 98.
** See pages 89-90.

departments, and the annuities scheme proved to be a flop. In retrospect, it seems clear that Project Z was a futile effort, for there was no "way out" for the conspirators. There were no steps which could have been taken to eliminate or significantly reduce the cumulative effects of a decade of deceit.

B. **The Gathering Storm.**

On March 8, 1973, the last regular EFCA board meeting was held in New York City. All nine directors were present, plus general counsel Rodney Loeb. Spirits were high and the outlook for the Company was excellent. It is indicative of the upbeat mood that the directors considered raising the dividend on the Company's common stock, but finally settled on staying at the 10 cents per share declared the prior year. Four days after the meeting, EFCA issued a glowing press release to report "record earnings from operations at $2.81 per share, up from $2.45 per share for 1971." According to the release, Goldblum said consolidated net income rose to $22,617,000 in 1972, a 17% increase over 1971 earnings of $19,332,000. This enthusiastic statement painted the rosiest of corporate pictures only three weeks before the Company filed a petition in bankruptcy.

The debacle was triggered the same day the press release was issued. Examiners from the Illinois Insurance Department arrived unexpectedly at EFLIC to audit the subsidiary's books. This audit was the result of growing rumors of fraud at EFCA which originated with Ronald Secrist, a former employee of EFLIC and Bankers.* On March 6, Secrist had telephoned the Deputy Superintendent of the New York State Insurance Department and said that he had certain information that might be of interest to the Department. He requested an appointment the following day. On March 7, Secrist arrived at the Department offices and told an almost unbelievable story. He alleged that for several years Equity Funding Life Insurance Company had been padding its in-force life insurance with fictitious

---

*Secrist went to work for EFLIC in 1970 as Assistant Vice President. He was transferred to Bankers on December 31, 1971, and on January 1, 1973 he was transferred back to EFCA. Personnel records show that Secrist was terminated effective March 15, 1973 "due to overstaffing."

policies, and that this bogus business had been reinsured with other companies.

Upon hearing Secrist's story, the New York officials relayed the allegations to the Chief Examiner of the California Department of Insurance, Christy Armstrong. The California officials, in turn, notified the Los Angeles office of the SEC, and then the Illinois Insurance Department, which shared regulatory responsibilities for EFLIC with California. By March 9, officials from the two states had concluded that a special examination of the insurance company should be conducted, disguised as a routine triennial audit by the Illinois Insurance Department so as not to unduly alarm the conspirators. The Illinois examiners were to arrive at the Company the following Monday, March 12, and the California examiners would follow a few days later as would be normal for such an examination.

The appearance of the Illinois examiners, however, greatly upset the conspirators. Goldblum called Levin, who had remained in New York after the EFCA board meeting, to tell him that the examiners were on the premises. Levin knew from his earlier experience working for the Illinois Department of Insurance that among the procedures employed in this examination would be a physical examination of EFLIC's assets. Thus, Levin feared the examiners would discover that $24 million of EFLIC's reported assets were non-existent bonds. Before returning to Los Angeles, he called up friends in the Illinois Insurance Department to ask them to postpone the examination, but to no avail.

EFCA's management then engaged John Bolton, a former deputy insurance commissioner in Illinois, to try to postpone the Illinois examination, ostensibly because EFCA was in the midst of a pending acquisition of another insurance company. Bolton contacted Richards Barger, a Los Angeles attorney and former Commissioner of the California Department of Insurance, to ask him to undertake similar efforts with the California Department. When Barger contacted the Los Angeles office of the Department to request postponement, he was told that Maury Rouble was supervising the California examination and that it could not be postponed. Barger did not press further. To him, the fact that Rouble had been assigned to the case meant that something serious was involved, and that the audit was not routine.

When the Illinois examiners arrived at EFCA's headquarters, they were given a room on the 28th floor. To find out what the examiners were looking for and what they were finding, a plan was developed by Goldblum and Banks to equip the room with electronic surveillance devices. On the evening of March 14, Collins and Banks, with the help of two experts, made the first of a series of installations of eavesdropping equipment. Partly as a result of information which the conspirators received through these listening devices, they took countermoves to attempt to hide the fraud from the examiners. The first problem they attempted to deal with was EFLIC's non-existent reported assets.

The $24 million in bonds purportedly held in the EFLIC custodian account at the American National Bank & Trust Company in Chicago presented the most pressing problem. When the Illinois examiners first sought to confirm the existence of these bonds, they were supplied with the bogus confirmation which Seidman & Seidman had accepted.* Since Illinois examiners would be aware that branch banking was not permitted in Illinois, the confirmation had been altered to reflect the proper bank address rather than the address of the bogus branch in Highland Park. As expected, however, the examiners announced their intention to go beyond this confirmation and send one of their people to count the bonds personally. To solve this problem, Goldblum apparently wanted to utilize the counterfeit bonds which had been printed, but others persuaded him that they were not of sufficient quality to stand scrutiny. A new explanation had to be quickly devised to explain why the bonds were no longer in the bank.

The new story to be given to the Illinois examiners was that at some time after December 31, 1972, the $24 million in bonds had been used in three different transactions. The conspirators planned to tell the examiners that part of the bonds had been transferred to EFCA, which held all of EFLIC's stock, as payment of a $3.4 million dividend to the parent; that $5.5 million had been used to purchase

---

* See page 100.

certificates of deposit; and that EFLIC had used the remainder to purchase 80% of the stock of Northern Life Insurance Company from EFCA for approximately $15.7 million.

The purported Northern stock transaction required the most effort to document. Levin and Smith arranged to make appropriate alterations in company records. On March 16, Smith directed Bill Raff, an EFCA attorney, to prepare drafts of two back-dated agreements, as well as new Northern stock certificates, to document the purported purchase by EFLIC of 80% of Northern's stock in a two-step transaction: 40% on February 5 and 40% on March 5.* Raff was told that First National City Bank of New York ("FNCB"), which held a certificate representing 100% of the stock of Northern as collateral under a 1972 Revolving Credit Agreement, had agreed to the transfer. The two certificates created to represent the 80% of Northern stock were then placed in an EFLIC safe deposit box. Levin next retrieved the already outstanding 100% certificate on March 23 by persuading his friend at FNCB, Hugh Brewer, to exchange it for a 20% certificate. Levin explained to Brewer that EFLIC could save $700,000 in taxes if it acquired 80% of Northern.**

In order to convince the Illinois examiners that the $5.5 million certificates of deposit had been purchased before their arrival, the conspirators determined that it would be necessary to go into the secondary market and purchase certificates issued before March 12. At either Sultan's or Goldblum's request, Dishy Easton purchased the needed certificates in bearer form. It appears that Dishy Easton was also asked to supply an undated confirmation of this purchase, which the conspirators planned to fill in with a false date. The certificates were delivered to Goldblum's office on March 19. On March 21, they were placed for safe-keeping at Wells Fargo Bank in Century City, where they were found by the California and Illinois Insurance Departments on March 30.

---

* The transaction supposedly was set up in two steps to circumvent the Washington Holding Company Act requirement that a transfer of control of a domiciliary insurer must be approved by the Washington Department of Insurance.

** See Report on Trustee's Draft Proposed Plan of Reorganization (May 17, 1974) at pages 29-37 for a detailed chronology of the facts relating to the Northern certificates.

The conspirators also took steps to make it difficult for the examiners to discover the bogus insurance policies. The week the examiners arrived, Arthur Lewis, Smith, Edens, Banks and Collins met to plot their course of action. They instructed William Gootnick, a Company Vice President in charge of computer operations, to run the Company's master computer tape through the computer and scramble all of the code numbers which identified the bogus business, and then to replace the hard copy records of insurance business with a completely new set showing the scrambled code numbers. Gootnick had his staff perform the task. Gootnick was also instructed to destroy any evidence of the bogus business in the Company's computer tape library, but later the conspirators decided merely to change the tape log (the listing of information in EFCA's computer tape library). A member of Gootnick's staff carried out this instruction as well.*

All these efforts proved unavailing, however, because of the accelerating pace of events outside the Company. Between March 19 and March 27, rumors on Wall Street of fraud at EFCA began to significantly affect trading in the Company's stock. These rumors were based on information Secrist had given to Raymond Dirks, an insurance analyst with the New York brokerage firm of Delafield Childs Inc. Secrist had called Dirks the same day he met with New York officials and, by the end of the week, had told him the story of the fraud at EFLIC. Dirks proceeded to investigate the allegations. During the week of March 19, he came to Los Angeles and met with former EFLIC employees who confirmed many of Secrist's charges. Then on March 21, Dirks met with Goldblum and Levin and questioned them about the fraud allegations. Both flatly denied that there was any truth to the stories of phony insurance at EFLIC, and they arranged for other Company officers — Smith, Lewis and Edens — to join in the denials.

In the interim, Dirks evidently told some of his institutional clients about the Secrist allegations, because while Dirks was in Los Angeles investigating, rumors in New York circulated wildly. The same day that Dirks interrogated Goldblum and Levin, EFCA's general counsel, Rodney Loeb received a call from Yura Arkus-

---

* A couple of days later, Gootnick apparently had second thoughts about his actions and had his staff restore the tape log to its original form.

Duntov and Lawrence Williams (of EFCA's legal staff) in New York. They told Loeb of rumors circulating there that the Company had issued large quantities of nonexistent life insurance. Loeb conveyed this information to Goldblum and told him that an inter-office memo concerning the rumors was being typed. Goldblum scoffed at the story and told Loeb to destroy all copies of his memo. Loeb did not do so.

While the rumors gathered steam, EFCA's stock became a volume leader on the New York Stock Exchange and its price declined steadily. On Thursday, March 22, Goldblum and Levin flew to New York City. Goldblum delivered an address the next day at the Institutional Investors Conference, and then met with New York Stock Exchange officials to try to squelch the rumors and reassure the market. But when trading opened the following Monday, EFCA was the volume leader with 768,400 shares traded. The price had dropped from $28 per share on March 6 to $16 per share on March 26.

Goldblum was back in Los Angeles at the start of the next week trying to grasp control of the rapidly deteriorating situation. This was to be the last week that he and the other conspirators would run the Company, and they were coming to realize that the game was nearly up. On Monday, March 26, representatives of Seidman & Seidman, which had just completed its annual audit of EFCA, met with Goldblum and Loeb. Goldblum claimed he was unaware of any irregularities in the insurance operations, but at Loeb's insistence Seidman & Seidman was directed to reopen an extended audit of EFLIC to determine if the Dirks rumors were true. Coupled with the Illinois and California Insurance Departments' examinations and inquiries from the New York Stock Exchange and the SEC, the Seidman & Seidman audit made it a hectic period at Company headquarters.

On March 27, the rumors of phony insurance business on EFCA's books grew stronger. The Company issued a press release denying the allegations and announcing its intention to purchase one million shares of EFCA stock on the open market "to take advantage of the currently depressed price of the company's stock." But frenzied trading and rapid price deterioration continued. At 12:45 EST, the New York Stock Exchange halted all trading in EFCA stock.

111

The stock exchange action shook the Company and its employees. Their suspicions aroused by the halt in trading, attorney Bill Raff and two other EFLIC employees began their own secret investigation of the rumors of bogus policies. Bill Gootnick, the Vice President who had helped to conceal some of the computer tape evidence, came to Goldblum and told him that he wanted no more of the fraud and planned to quit. Goldblum asked Gootnick to stay on as a favor to him until Friday because "something magic" was going to happen on that day, and maybe everything would be okay. Gootnick agreed to stay.

An Executive Planning Committee meeting was called for the same afternoon to discuss the situation. At the meeting, Goldblum, Levin, Lowell, Lichtig, Arkus-Duntov, Glaser, Loeb and Williams were present. No one at the meeting seemed to comprehend what was happening to the Company. One theory was that the stock was being manipulated downward so that someone could accumulate shares and gain control. Whenever the suggestion was made that the rumors could be true, it was rejected. The prevailing theory was that there might always exist some minor larceny in the Company of which these officers were unaware, but that it would be impossible to have false life insurance policies. After all, the premiums would have to be paid and reserves kept for false policies, so it made no sense.

Finally, Glaser directly asked Goldblum, Levin and Lowell whether there was any substance to the Dirks rumors. Lowell denied knowing anything about the fraud. Levin characterized the allegations made by Dirks as "bizarre" and denied the charges vehemently. According to him, the Company's problems were all a result of charges being made by a disgruntled employee who only had particles of knowledge. Goldblum's response, however, was not as reassuring. He simply said that anything was possible and that certain events could have occurred without his knowledge. Consequently, it was agreed that the legal department, under the supervision of Williams, would conduct an internal investigation and work in conjunction with the Seidman & Seidman audit team.

Although the conspirators kept a cool facade, their actions behind the scenes indicated that they knew discovery of the fraud was imminent. A number of meetings were held to consider what was going to happen to the Company and to the fraud participants, whether to hire attorneys, and who would pay the legal fees. In addition, plans were developed for several of the conspirators to flee the country. Levin, Lowell and Goldblum discussed leaving, and Levin suggested that they take the recently purchased $5.5 million certificates of deposit to finance their exile. Lowell agreed with Levin's plan, but Goldblum declined because he feared that his wife would refuse to leave with him.

Having decided to run, Levin went to the Wells Fargo Bank on March 28, and removed the certificates from the EFLIC safe deposit box. He gave Lowell half, and Lowell began making phone calls to contacts in Argentina, Europe and the Bahamas to determine the marketability of the certificates abroad. A day later, however, Levin had a change of heart and abandoned his plan. He persuaded Lowell to give back the certificates by claiming that he would attempt to negotiate them. On March 30, Levin returned the certificates to the manager at Wells Fargo Bank, who placed them in an EFLIC safe-keeping account.

While the conspirators considered running away, the pace of events quickened. On March 27, Larry Baker, Chief Deputy Commissioner of the California Insurance Department, got a call from SEC officials relaying information received from an informer at Equity Funding. The informer revealed that alterations had been made on computer tapes the prior weekend, and that many tapes were being erased at that moment. The information was relayed to the examiners at the Company offices who moved to stop further erasures.

The following day, Wednesday, March 28, the SEC suspended trading of all EFCA securities on all public markets and demanded that Goldblum, Levin, Lowell, Smith, Edens and Arthur Lewis give testimony at the Los Angeles office of the SEC and also sign affidavits swearing there was no phony insurance on the Company's books. The end was at hand.

C. **Collapse**.

The final chapter of the EFCA fraud began on Thursday, March 29. At the Company, the day started with an impromptu meeting in Levin's office at which Goldblum, Levin, Loeb and Milton Kroll, an attorney from the Washington, D.C. law firm which handled EFCA's SEC work, were present. Goldblum wondered aloud whether he should have his own legal counsel. Kroll advised against it at this stage, since he felt it would imply that Goldblum had something to hide. The subject of the affidavits requested by the SEC also came up, and Goldblum indicated a reluctance to sign one. There was some discussion of the inflexibility of the written word in an affidavit, and Kroll explained that each man would have an opportunity to give testimony at the SEC the next day in addition to his affidavit.

A little before noon, Loeb was notified that Frank Rothman, a Los Angeles attorney, was on his way to see him. Kroll was present in Loeb's office when Rothman entered. Rothman announced that he had been with Goldblum for the previous two hours, and had been engaged to represent him. He said he had heard a story from Goldblum, Levin and Lowell that he could only describe as "incredible." Rothman had recommended that Levin and Lowell immediately hire their own legal counsel and had advised Goldblum not to sign any affidavit for the SEC. Further, Rothman announced that Goldblum would not go to the SEC the next day to give any testimony. Loeb said he thought that if Goldblum did not appear voluntarily, the SEC would simply issue a subpoena. Rothman's response was that if his client was subpoenaed to testify, he would invoke his Fifth Amendment privilege. Kroll and Loeb then pointed out what such a move would mean for the Company. They felt the SEC would certainly ask that a receiver be appointed and the investigation of the Company would continue. Rothman said he had discussed such ramifications with his client.

Loeb was now firmly convinced that the rumors of fraud were true and that Goldblum was involved. As Secretary of EFCA, Loeb arranged to call a special meeting of the Board of Directors for the week-end.

Goldblum and Glaser then joined Kroll, Rothman and Loeb in Loeb's office. Loeb recited to Glaser the announcements that Rothman had just made about his client's refusal to testify and about the decisions of Lowell and Levin to retain their own counsel. Glaser excitedly told Goldblum that his refusal to sign an affidavit would ruin the employees and the shareholders of the Company and bring incredible hardship to everyone involved. Goldblum was solemn. He persisted in his refusal to testify and indicated he would follow his attorney's advice. Glaser told him that he would have to infer that the rumors were true if Goldblum would not deny them. Goldblum refused to talk about it any further. Goldblum then left the group and walked back down the hall to his own office with Glaser following behind. In Goldblum's office, Glaser begged him to disclose what he knew and sign an affidavit. Goldblum stalled for time, saying he would talk to somebody about it. He added that someday Glaser would find out he was innocent.

That same afternoon, Loeb received a call from Bill Raff who, with other EFLIC employees investigating the fraud, had discovered "hard evidence" of bogus insurance. Raff wanted to arrange a meeting with Loeb. Instead, Loeb arranged for Raff to meet that evening with representatives from Seidman & Seidman at the hotel where Milton Kroll was staying. The meeting lasted well into the morning hours. Raff's group revealed to the auditors not only evidence of fictitious insurance, but also the operation at Maple Drive.

On the morning of Friday, March 30, Larry Baker of the California Department of Insurance, who had by then learned of Raff's findings, went to the Los Angeles office of the SEC with Seidman & Seidman representatives to share with them the latest discoveries. Following that meeting, Baker met with a representative of the California Attorney General's office to decide what steps could be taken to prevent the destruction of records and the flight of persons possibly involved in the fraud. Earlier that day, Baker had learned of Levin's removal of the certificates of deposit from the Wells Fargo safe deposit box, and he feared that further assets would be taken and possibly spirited out of the country. The California examiners had also observed Collins and Symonds removing records from the Maple Drive office and loading them in a truck. Something had to be done fast. The officials concluded that the situation was an appropriate one in which to exercise the summary seizure procedures provided for under Section 1013 of the California Insurance Code.

115

While the seizure order was being drafted, a Department attorney called the branch manager of Wells Fargo Bank, informed him of the pending seizure and told him not to let any EFLIC assets go out. The seizure order was served on the bank a short while later.

At 5:30 p.m., Baker and Ed Germann of the Department arrived at the Company offices and went immediately to the sixth floor, where EFLIC was headquartered. They served everyone they could find with copies of the order and asked all employees to leave the premises. The Company's auditors, Seidman & Seidman, had a very large crew on the premises implementing security at the request of the SEC. Baker informed the auditors of what was happening and went over the procedures that were to be put into effect. The locks on EFLIC's doors were changed and armed security guards were posted. Although the California Insurance Department had jurisdiction only over EFLIC, and not EFCA, Baker decided that since he could not tell which operations were attributable to which entity, he would, for the time being, exercise control over all Company operations. During the rest of the evening, Baker took statements from any of the officers willing to talk about the Company's operations and what they knew of the fraud. At 4:00 a.m., Baker ended his eventful day and left the premises.

At 7 a.m. the next morning, a Saturday, Baker returned. As he entered the parking garage at EFCA's offices, he noticed a Rolls Royce pulling into the space marked "Fred Levin." As Levin and his attorney got out of the car, Baker introduced himself and asked Levin to accompany him to the 28th floor. When they arrived at the executive suite, they encountered the California Insurance Commissioner talking with Goldblum. Levin and Goldblum were then formally served with a copy of the seizure order. Goldblum was hostile. He fumed that the seizure was a big mistake, and that the Department was interfering with the right of the Company's salesmen to earn a living. Baker cut Goldblum's speech off, and informed him and Levin of their Fifth Amendment rights. Having done so, Baker began to question the two concerning the whereabouts of EFLIC's assets. Levin's attorney intervened, however, and the conversation ended.

116

That afternoon, various meetings were underway. A number of EFCA officers and directors were meeting with representatives of the SEC and Seidman & Seidman to discuss the crisis. Baker, at this point suspicious of everyone in EFCA's management, left that meeting after a short while. He next met with Raff and the other Company employees who had uncovered some aspects of the fraud at EFLIC. The group again outlined what they had learned of bogus insurance, the Maple Drive operation, the Northern stock transfer, and the "Cookie Jar Caper." Meanwhile, at the insistence of director Robert Bowie, Seidman & Seidman conducted a telephone survey of a sample of supposed EFLIC policyholders. Of 82 listed policyholders, only 6 of the 35 reached by telephone confirmed that they owned the policies attributed to them. The survey gave those concerned some idea of the magnitude of the fraud at EFLIC.

On Sunday, April 1, a special meeting of the EFCA Board of Directors commenced at 4:15 p.m. All the members of the board were in attendance, including Stanley Goldblum, Herbert Glaser, Fred Levin, Samuel Lowell, Judson Sayre, Gale Livingston, Nelson Loud, Robert Bowie and Yura Arkus-Duntov. The following individuals also attended: Rodney Loeb, Lawrence Williams, and John Schneider, all members of EFCA's legal department; Richards Barger; Stuart Buchalter and Jerry Nemer of the law firm of Buchalter, Nemer, Fields & Savitch, specialists in insolvency law who had been retained by Loeb; and Milton Kroll and Peter Panarites of Freedman, Levy, Kroll & Symonds.

The meeting was called to order and presided over by Rodney Loeb. After relating the chronology of events which led up to the special board meeting, he repeated the allegations raised by Dirks and summarized some of the evidence thus far discovered which tended to show that EFLIC had manufactured life insurance policies and that these policies had been sold to a number of reinsurers. (As of this time, the funding and other frauds described in this report were still undiscovered.) Next, Stuart Buchalter summarized his discussions with the SEC, indicating that the SEC had concluded that an enormous number of false insurance policies were on EFLIC's books, and that a number of other purported assets were of questionable validity. Buchalter advised the directors that the SEC was

117

demanding that Goldblum, Levin and Lowell resign as officers and directors, and that the Company terminate Smith, Arthur Lewis, Edens, Collins, Banks and Symonds. Before any more details of the SEC's fraud investigation were revealed, the directors requested that Lowell, Goldblum and Levin resign and leave the premises.

Before leaving, however, the three officers insisted that their services were necessary to run the Company. They agreed they would resign, but said they were willing to act as consultants for a fee in order to help save the Company. This suggestion was immediately rebuffed by Bowie, who insisted that the Company was in no position to contract with these men, and that any such discussion should be deferred until later. The three then requested severance pay. Goldblum argued that, "Even the lowest clerk gets severance pay. I've been with the company thirteen years." Again, Bowie replied that this was not a subject for discussion.

Goldblum and Levin then left the room. Lowell stayed behind to make a statement to the assembled group. He said that while he had "played games with numbers" and capitalized certain expense items, he was not involved in the phony insurance operation. Bowie again cut off Lowell's speech, saying this was not the time for such a statement and asking Lowell to leave the room, so that the meeting could continue.

Prior to the meeting, EFCA's legal department had prepared letters of resignation for the three officers. Goldblum signed his before leaving the premises, but Levin and Lowell indicated they would not sign before speaking with their lawyers. After the three exited, the meeting continued for four more hours and concluded after accountants from Seidman & Seidman reported their findings regarding bogus policies to the directors.

Baker, meanwhile, spent Sunday reviewing Company files and speaking with two former EFLIC employees who had been involved in the fraud — Allan Greene and Allan Venuziou. Greene explained to Baker how the bogus policies were created and reinsured, and how the false policy numbers were scrambled on the computer. More importantly, he confirmed that a number of present EFLIC employees were involved in the conspiracy: Levin, Sultan, Collins, Capo, Symonds, and Arthur and Mark Lewis.

On Monday April 2, the general public first learned of the fraud when an article by William Blundell appeared that morning on the front page of the Wall Street Journal. The article caused an immediate panic among EFCA's employees, creditors and stockholders, and among EFLIC's reinsurers and policyholders. When EFCA's doors opened on Monday, the Company was in a state of upheaval. Employees arriving that morning were greeted by security guards who screened them on entry. The guards had pictures of each of the known conspirators and orders not to let them enter the premises unescorted. When Collins, Edens, Banks, Smith, and Arthur Lewis arrived, Baker told them to go up to Rodney Loeb's office. Loeb had been authorized by the Board of Directors to terminate anyone connected with the fraud. When the group arrived at Loeb's office, they were fired at one time. Upon being terminated, Lewis offered his consultant services for $200 a day. Loeb replied that if the window were open, he would throw him out. Later that day, Michael Sultan was also fired by Loeb, when the SEC informed him that evidence of Sultan's complicity had been discovered.

The special meeting of the Board of Directors was reconvened that afternoon. Present were Bowie, Livingston, Sayre, Glaser, Loud, Arkus-Duntov, Loeb, Williams, Buchalter and Brian Manion, attorney for director Gale Livingston. Glaser presided over the meeting, and the main topic for discussion was the complaint to be filed the next day by the SEC charging EFCA with fraud and violations of other federal securities laws. The Board had to decide if it would consent to a permanent injunction drafted by the SEC which enjoined EFCA from future fraudulent acts, provided a plan of operation under which Glaser was to be interim manager, and appointed Touche Ross & Co. to audit the Company's financial statements.

Earlier that day, Glaser and Williams spent several hours at the SEC discussing what provisions would be included in the injunction. At the Board meeting, some directors objected to the language of the SEC's complaint. They were told that unless they agreed, the SEC would move immediately to seek a receivership under which the management of the corporation would be turned over to the SEC and the courts. Following extensive discussion for several hours, the directors finally agreed to approve the proposed decree. After voting the approval, and almost as an afterthought, the directors took one final

119

step. They authorized the filing of a petition under Chapter X of the Bankruptcy Act if it was later deemed to be appropriate by the SEC and the federal District Court.

On April 3, the four banks participating in the Revolving Credit Agreement declared their loans in default and due. They then purportedly offset approximately $8 million of EFCA's deposits against amounts owed to the banks by EFCA under the agreement. Other banks offset another $2 million of EFCA funds. These funds represented the principal cash resources available to operate the Company. As a result of these offsets and other problems, a decision was made to file the petition for protection under Chapter X of the Bankruptcy Act. The petition was filed and approved on April 5, 1973.

The decade of fraud at EFCA had come to an end.

PART THREE
REWARDS TO THE FRAUD PARTICIPANTS

As described more fully in the following section of this report,* the fraud at Equity Funding does not appear to have been motivated by a desire on the part of the conspirators to provide a cover for large scale embezzlement. The primary purpose of the fraud, rather, was to cause EFCA to appear to flourish, and thereby to inflate the value of its stock.

At the same time, however, a closely associated object of the conspiracy was the personal enrichment of its members. This goal was furthered in various ways. At the very top, of course, Goldblum and Riordan, who had obtained many thousands of shares of stock at very little cost prior to 1964, realized huge profits through subsequent dividends and from stock sales. It is believed that Goldblum gained more than $5 million from trading in EFCA stock over the years. Similarly, Riordan is believed to have obtained well over one million dollars from sales of EFCA stock prior to his death in 1969. Most of Riordan's remaining shares were sold by his executors when the stock was near its peak and brought in excess of $18 million.

Others entered the conspiracy when it was too late to obtain organizing shares. They nonetheless benefitted from the fraud because it provided them with prestigious and exceptionally well-paid positions. In this respect, membership in the conspiracy was in several important instances the passkey to responsible jobs and increased compensation at EFCA, including sizeable stock bonuses. Finally, the effects of the fraud permitted many of the participants to live in the luxurious corporate style afforded to executives of a high-flying "go-go" company with a "glamor" stock.

But to many conspirators these substantial and ostensibly legitimate rewards proved inadequate. The contagion of deceit at work within the fraud conspiracy, probably fueled by the heady atmosphere of conspicuous corporate success, created a climate in which it became perhaps inevitable that certain of the participants would find it natural to steal from the Company. Stealing was easy because the conspirators purposely avoided normal accounting controls in those parts of EFCA's operations that were involved in the fraud.

---

* See pages 134-137.

In some cases, this theft took the form of recurring expense account padding and petty frauds to exploit purported "fringe benefits." Such abuses occurred at every level of the conspiracy. In other instances, participants at the middle-management level turned to out-and-out embezzlement. Both types of looting, at least so much as thus far discovered, were trivial in comparison with the dimensions of the corporate fraud. But they were far more widespread and systematic than the occasional internal cheating which can afflict any institution. In short, within the circle of fraud participants at EFCA, and thus in key positions throughout the Company, there seems to have been a thoroughgoing breakdown of common restraint and morality.

I. CONSPIRATORS ON THE PAYROLL

EFCA's management enjoyed a feeling of substantial accomplishment and was optimistic about the future of the Company. Its officers (both those who knew about the fraud and those who were unsuspecting) felt they were responsible for the reported revenues and profits of the corporation, and they expected to be rewarded for their evident success. And rewards did flow from the Company, in the form of salaries, stock bonuses and other benefits.

Executive compensation at EFCA was generous. In 1971 and 1972 Goldblum's annual salary alone was $100,000, and in 1973 he raised it to $125,000.* Lowell and Levin each received annual salaries of $70,000 in 1971 and $80,000 in 1972. But salaries were only a part of the executive compensation package at EFCA. Indeed, in the final years, salaries came to reflect less than half the total compensation to top officers. This was due primarily to the Company's Stock Bonus Plan.

Bonuses were proposed by Goldblum in 1970 to supplement the salaries of top executives. This proposal was prompted by disappointment with prior stock option plans, which had failed to accomplish their purpose when the price of EFCA's stock, after peaking in mid-1969, followed the downward turn of the rest of the market in 1970. As a result, the market price was well below the exercise price of many of the options previously granted.

---

* Ironically, this raise occurred at about the same time Goldblum was telling all department heads that a 20% cost reduction had to be effected within the Company for 1973. See page 105.

122

The bonus concept went through several forms before finally being implemented. An EFCA prospectus dated August 20, 1970 announced generally that "subject to the approval of stockholders, management has adopted an Executive Compensation Plan for the benefit of its executive officers." That proposed plan, however, met with stiff opposition from various quarters and it was abandoned before it could be submitted to the shareholders. Several of the participating underwriters of a forthcoming debenture offering reacted unfavorably to provisions of the plan, disclosure of which would have been necessary in the prospectus for the debentures. Robert Bowie, one of EFCA's outside directors, also expressed concern about various aspects of the plan, specifically the maximum amount of bonus payable to each executive, the procedure for administering the plan, and the method for evaluating the performance of the recipient.

The Executive Compensation Plan was redrafted several times and finally was given a more democratic sounding name, the Employees Stock Bonus Plan. Under this version, all company employees were eligible to participate and awards were to be made in EFCA common stock. Each recipient was to be credited with a number of units, each unit consisting of four shares of stock. The stock was then to be issued in four equal annual installments, provided the employee stayed with the Company over the four-year period. This plan had several advantages. Its structure resulted in camouflaging the extraordinary value of the individual awards in prospectuses and other public reports. Bonuses were reported in terms of "Plan Units," but never in dollar amounts. In addition, since the awards were made in EFCA common stock, there was no drain on the Company's cash position.

Goldblum's persistence in getting a bonus plan succeeded. The Employees Stock Bonus Plan was adopted by EFCA's Board of Directors on December 28, 1970, and approved by the shareholders on May 23, 1971. Bowie again raised some criticism, this time about the size of the grants which could be made and their possibly repetitive nature. The actual operation of the plan showed that Bowie's reservations were well taken. During the first year, awards were made only to the president and the seven executive vice presidents of EFCA. In 1972 these same top officers were repeat recipients, and five of the eight were then receiving more in bonuses for the year than they were in salary. In fact, for Goldblum and three executive vice presidents, stock received under the plan was worth more than twice their 1972 salaries. The total compensation that year of the three top conspirators, as indicated in the following table, is believed to have been at or in excess of the maximum level for top executives of other financial services companies reporting comparable gross revenues.

TOTAL 1972 COMPENSATION FOR TOP CONSPIRATORS				
Name	Position	Salary	Stock Bonus*	Total 1972 Compensation
STANLEY GOLDBLUM	President, Chairman of the Board	$100,000	$204,063	$304,063
FRED LEVIN	Executive Vice President — Insurance Operations & Marketing	80,000	163,250	243,250
SAMUEL LOWELL	Executive Vice President — Corporate Operations & Finance	80,000	163,250	243,250

The stock bonus shares were registered under the federal securities laws and could be sold immediately. During 1972, each of these three executives received substantial proceeds from the sale of EFCA stock. Goldblum sold shares worth $670,000; Lowell, almost $200,000; and Levin, $110,000. Other shares were used as collateral for large personal loans.

At the executive vice president level, among the officers not involved in the fraud only Herbert Glaser came close to the top three in his total compensation. At the middle-management level as well, the fraud participants tended to be more generously remunerated than others. This was attributable partly to the procedure by which stock bonuses were awarded. At year-end department heads recommended employees whom they felt were deserving. Goldblum, Lowell and Levin then met to discuss these recommendations and decide how many shares of stock each person should be given. The

---

* The value of bonus stock is determined according to the market value of EFCA stock on the date or dates the respective shares were originally granted.

124

list of proposed recipients was next reviewed by the stock bonus plan administrative committee, consisting of Goldblum, Arkus-Duntov, Loud and Livingston. Occasionally the committee made minor changes, but most of the grants on the list, especially those to middle and lower-level employees, were approved automatically. Since decisions on awards were thus effectively made by the fraud's architects, the plan could be used to satisfy and reward those involved in the conspiracy. That it was so used is illustrated by the soaring increases in compensation granted to six young executives in sensitive positions who were significantly involved in furthering the fraud. These figures are set out in the following table. During 1972 and 1973, the total compensation of EFCA's other vice presidents was lower, and in most cases very substantially lower.

TOTAL COMPENSATION FOR SELECTED MIDDLE-MANAGEMENT CONSPIRATORS (1971-73)

Name and Position	1971	1972	1973*	
MICHAEL E. SULTAN Vice President and Corporate Controller (Born 2-13-43)	$ 26,833 $ 26,833 –0–	$ 62,463 $ 38,750 $ 23,713	$118,250 $ 45,000 $ 73,250	Total Annual Salary Stock Bonus
JAMES C. SMITH, JR. Vice President — Insurance Operations (Born 11-12-37)	$ 28,500 $ 28,500 –0–	$ 62,465 $ 38,743 $ 23,713	$118,250 $ 45,000 $ 73,250	Total Annual Salary Stock Bonus
DAVID J. CAPO Vice President — Investment Operations (Born 3-3-44)	$ 23,750 $ 23,750 –0–	$ 46,313 $ 29,375 $ 16,938	$ 82,613 $ 35,000 $ 47,613	Total Annual Salary Stock Bonus
ARTHUR LEWIS Vice President — Actuary (Born 1-10-43)	$ 23,417 $ 23,417 –0–	$ 47,106 $ 30,168 $ 16,938	$ 81,282 $ 35,004 $ 46,278	Total Annual Salary Stock Bonus
LLOYD EDENS Vice President — Agent Services (Born 10-29-42)	$ 23,417 $ 23,417 –0–	$ 47,106 $ 30,168 $ 16,938	$ 81,282 $ 35,004 $ 46,278	Total Annual Salary Stock Bonus
LAWRENCE COLLINS Assistant Vice President — Insurance Operations (Born 11-19-39)	$ 20,500 $ 20,500 –0–	$ 36,263 $ 26,100 $ 10,163	$ 66,625 $ 30,000 $ 36,625	Total Annual Salary Stock Bonus

* These individuals were terminated on or about April 1, 1973. The salary amounts shown for 1973 are what each man would have received if he had been employed the entire year. For each year, the value of bonus shares is determined according to the market value of EFCA shares on dates the shares were granted.

125

In addition to salaries and bonuses, of course, there were other perquisites of office for EFCA's management. These fringe benefits included, among other things, monthly auto allowances of from $125 to $300, and regular tax shelter investment opportunities through EFCA-sponsored limited partnerships. Certain of the conspirators, moreover, received interest-free loans from the Company to pay the withholding tax on their stock bonus shares. Finally, in the realm of ego gratification, it is worth noting that EFCA's executives conducted business in fabulously plush surroundings. In October 1969, the Company moved its head office to five leased floors at 1900 Avenue of the Stars in Century City. The offices of the president and other high executives were situated on the top floor and had a miles-wide view of Beverly Hills and Los Angeles. No expense was spared in furnishings or decor for these quarters. Goldblum's office, for instance, was an opulently furnished suite, complete with fireplace, reception area, kitchen and bathroom. There were other lavish touches on the top floor. For example, company practice was for the president and all the executive vice presidents to meet daily in the richly appointed EFCA board room for luncheon prepared by Goldblum's personal cook.

In short, then, EFCA's officers were handsomely rewarded by the Company. They were exceedingly well-compensated. And they benefitted from the creature comforts and the prestige which came from being executives of a company which was at some pains to cultivate the indicia and symbols of corporate affluence. But for many of the fraud participants these seemingly ample rewards were not enough. Knowing that Equity Funding and its reported financial condition and performance were fraudulent to the core, these men thought nothing of augmenting their personal income by outright or thinly disguised peculation.

II. SELF-DEALING SCHEMES

A. The "Fringe Benefits."

Certain of the self-dealing schemes at EFCA were thought of as "fringe benefits" by the fraud participants. Some of the transactions which fall into this category involved creation of new company benefits while others were abuses of already existing benefit

126

programs. One of the new benefits invented was the "entertainment allowance." In 1972, Goldblum initiated monthly cash grants for himself, Lowell and Levin. These appear to have had nothing to do with company entertainment expenses, but were simply Goldblum's response to a demand by Lowell and Levin for a raise as extra reward for the risk they were incurring by furthering the fraud. Goldblum determined that Lowell and Levin should receive $1,000 per month in addition to their other compensation, and that $3,000 per month would be an appropriate amount for himself.

Other fraud participants increased their fringe benefits by charging their medical bills to EFLIC. All insurance companies, of course, regularly pay for the medical examinations required of life insurance policy applicants. This practice at EFLIC was used by several fraud participants as a cover for submission to the Company of medical bills for themselves and members of their families. Arthur Lewis approved such bills submitted by Lowell, James Banks, Collins, Edens and Mark Lewis, and EFLIC checks were issued to pay the named physicians. The medical services thus paid for by EFLIC from 1969 to 1973 ran the gamut and included x-rays, laboratory tests, dermatology, gynecological services, dental work, new eye glasses, allergy testing and psychiatric treatment.

In the category of abusing existing legitimate benefits are a number of petty defalcations relating to expense vouchers used to reimburse employees for money spent while purportedly on EFCA business. Some conspirators generated additional cash for themselves by submitting inflated or wholly false expense vouchers. One executive made a practice of charging the Company twice for his travel expenses. His habit was to charge all travel expenses on a credit card, and upon returning from a trip to submit an expense voucher for reimbursement of these expenses. Ultimately, he also submitted the bill from the credit card company for payment by EFCA. This double reimbursement was often claimed for first class travel on totally non-business excursions.

In the area of automobile expenses, one executive had two leased cars, one paid for by EFCA and the other by EFLIC. Another officer at EFLIC drove a car leased by the Company for which all expenses were paid. Then to get additional cash, he filed expense vouchers to be reimbursed for the cost of repairs, maintenance and gas for the car, although these were never personal out-of-pocket expenses. Since the executive approving this double payment was also a fraud participant, the expense vouchers were honored. Another vice president loaned his gas credit card to his girl friend, also a company employee. She charged her gasoline on his credit card, signed his name, and later submitted the invoices on his expense reports so that she could be reimbursed by the Company.

One other EFCA fringe benefit which some fraud perpetrators sought to corrupt was the qualified stock option plan. In late 1972, one middle-level conspirator complained to an EFCA officer that he felt he was entitled to more compensation because of his contribution to the fraud. He was unhappy because he had not received any stock bonuses, but he did have several stock options granted at various prices. Knowing the ease with which corporate records could be altered at EFCA, he persuaded the officer to modify the records of his stock option grants so as to facilitate exercise of the options out of sequence and the reporting of what should have been ordinary income as capital gains for tax purposes. Later, others heard of this scheme and made similar demands for their option records to be changed.

The Company paid for some luxuries for all executives, but the fraud participants were as inventive and dishonest in this area as in others. A myriad of personal expenses were charged to the Company by officers, including first class vacations to Hawaii, Mexico, South America and Tahiti, rented Rolls Royce limousines for social occasions, and substantial quantities of stereo equipment and television sets. One executive had a girl friend in New York whose apartment was furnished for $2,000 at EFCA's expense. Another officer had the Company pay the bill for his divorce.

During EFCA's last days, some of the fraud conspirators made a final grasp at company funds. In late March 1973, Goldblum, Lowell and Levin drew "advances" on their salaries and entertainment allowances before their employment was terminated. Goldblum drew $4,000 and Lowell $2,573 as salary advances. Lowell also drew an advance of $9,000, purportedly his entertainment allowance for the rest of the year. Goldblum and Levin drew one month advances on their entertainment allowances. And James Smith drew an unaccounted for advance of $1,200 before departing.

After Goldblum was fired, much controversy ensued between him and the Company over the ownership of a number of items of furniture in his office, including an old-fashioned telescope valued at more than $1,200 which he said was a gift from his wife, and a painting over the mantel for which he said he personally had paid $10,000 and which he also claimed belonged to him. Invoices from Equity Funding's accounting department showed that in fact the Company had paid for each of these items, and Goldblum's demands were rejected. The benefits flowing to the fraud conspirators had finally stopped.

B. Theft and Embezzlement at the Company.

The corrupt atmosphere at EFCA spawned a number of personal misappropriation schemes. At least four such intrigues have been uncovered to date. The largest of these has been previously referred to in the discussion of the false death claim scheme, and involved the theft of over $600,000 by a number of EFLIC officers during 1971-72. Two other embezzlement schemes perpetrated by lower level EFLIC employees — one involving the payment of excessive agent commissions and the other bogus cash surrender payments — netted approximately $16,000 and $12,000 respectively. And a fourth scheme, only recently uncovered, involved the theft of at least $77,000 during 1971-72 by means of fictitious funding program liquidations.

(1) THE "COOKIE JAR CAPER."

Between July 1971 and August 1972, four EFLIC officers — James Banks, David Capo, Arthur Lewis and Lloyd Edens — misappropriated approximately $616,000 through a variety of related stratagems which have become known as the "Cookie Jar Caper." Almost $144,000 was taken from reinsurers in a personal version of the false death claim scheme already described.* Another $220,000 was embezzled by filing false death claims directly with EFLIC. The remaining sums were taken by purloining $199,000 worth of legitimate checks sent to EFLIC, almost $47,000 in checks drawn on EFSC accounts, and another $6,000 worth of checks from EFCA

---

* See pages 89-90.

accounts. The great bulk of these stolen funds went to James Banks, who began the thievery in the summer of 1971.

On July 27, 1971, Banks walked into the Century City office of United Savings and Loan and opened an account in the name of a "Mrs. Anne Wood," with Banks (ostensibly her "brother") holding power of attorney over the account. That same day, Banks deposited into the account a $15,000 EFLIC check, which represented payment of a death claim on a fictitious EFLIC policy to the non-existent Mrs. Wood who appeared as the beneficiary. After drawing all of the funds out of the account, Banks closed it one month later. He repeated this same procedure a number of times in succeeding months to embezzle further sums from EFLIC by means of fictitious death claims.

In early 1972, Lewis, Edens and Capo discovered Banks' scheme. Rather than exposing Banks, however, they joined him. Their joint misappropriations were perpetrated through a variant of the previous modus operandi. On February 3rd, they opened a corporate account at Union Bank in the name of Bankers National Life Insurance Company. Lewis and Edens were the authorized signators on the account, into which over $53,000 was deposited. Six EFCA checks, each for just under $1,000 and each made payable to Bankers, were deposited between February and April of 1972. A seventh check made payable to Bankers for a similar amount, this one from an EFSC account, was deposited in April. The bulk of the funds in this account, however, derived from a $46,000 check drawn on a valid EFSC account by Capo in June 1972. Capo also withdrew most of the money from this "Bankers" account.

The false corporate bank account procedure was repeated when Banks opened an account at Wells Fargo Bank on February 25, 1972 in the name of EFLIC. It was through this "EFLIC" account that most of the stolen funds were funnelled, including a $58,000 check from Phoenix Mutual Life Insurance Company to EFLIC representing a mortality adjustment due under the reinsurance agreement between the two companies, as well as two bogus death claim checks from reinsurers for $63,000 and $81,000. Virtually all of the money in this account appears to have been withdrawn by Banks and diverted to three bank accounts which he opened in Toronto, Canada in 1972.

130

A third fictitious corporate account was opened by the embezzlers in June 1972, only two months before discovery of their scheme, at Security Pacific National Bank in Century City. It was an "EFLIC" account used as the depository of approximately $118,000. The bulk of this money derived from two checks sent to EFLIC from reinsurers as repayment of valid death claims paid by EFLIC to the beneficiaries of policies which had been reinsured. Again, the withdrawals from this account were made mostly by James Banks.

On August 15, 1972 Lewis was told to come to Fred Levin's office. When he arrived, Goldblum and Smith were waiting with Levin. The misappropriation scheme had been uncovered. The four individuals involved in the thefts were not fired, however. Instead, they were made to promise to repay over a two-year period all of the money they had taken. To help them make the repayments, Edens, Lewis and Capo were given substantial added compensation from the Company in the form of stock bonus awards.* The embezzlers were further assured that neither the auditors nor the authorities would be told anything about their misdeeds, and were enlisted to coordinate the filing of false death claims for the benefit of the Company.

The extent to which the four repaid the moneys they had taken is not fully known, nor is it clear whether the full scope of their thefts (especially those of Banks) had been discovered by higher-ups. The only repayment which has yet been substantiated is a $20,000 payment by Banks on August 24, 1972 in the form of a cashier's check from a Toronto bank. Edens and Lewis have asserted that they each repaid about $30,000 (purportedly half of what they had taken), a claim with which Levin concurs. In addition, approximately $102,000 remaining in two of the accounts opened by Banks to facilitate the thefts was confiscated by the Company management at the time of discovery and returned to EFLIC.

(2) OTHER EMBEZZLEMENTS.

A different type of embezzlement scheme was executed in 1972 by three EFLIC employees working in the commissions department, Robert Gibson, Otis Poole and Ronald Gordon, younger brother of Stanley Goldblum. These three individuals devised a means of

---

* See page 125.

131

causing the EFCA computer to issue unauthorized commission checks to them each month. The idea originated with Gordon, a registered representative, who approached Gibson, the manager of EFLIC's commission department, and convinced him to issue phony checks from the commissions department which the two men would split. The plan worked so well that Gibson then approached Poole, another registered representative, and asked if he would like to join in the practice.

The scheme was uncovered in February 1973 during a routine comparison of actual commission earnings with checks made payable to agents. The matter was reported to Stanley Goldblum and Fred Levin, who decided to keep the three on the payroll. Each man signed a promissory note to pay back the amount that was taken: for Poole that amount was $2,472.05, for Gordon, $5,778.75 and for Gibson, $8,250.60. Poole paid the full amount of his note to the Company on May 11, 1973. Gibson paid only $125 against his note, and Gordon has as yet made no payments.

In still another scheme, William Symonds, an EFLIC employee involved in the larger fraud, changed computer records to indicate that all premiums were paid to date for certain policies which had actually lapsed. Symonds then attempted to siphon off for himself the apparent cash surrender value of these policies. He did this by filing a forged request to surrender the cash value of the policy in the insured's name. Symonds then intercepted the EFLIC checks for the cash value before they were mailed. Although a number of lapsed policy records were changed, only two cash surrender checks, totaling $11,565.39, actually went to Symonds. The moneys thus embezzled were deposited in savings accounts opened by Symonds in the name of the insureds. In late March 1973, as discovery of the larger EFCA fraud was imminent, evidence of Symonds' embezzlements came to the attention of Banks and Smith. Symonds was forced to return to EFLIC all of the funds he had taken, which he did on March 29th.

A fourth embezzlement scheme has been recently uncovered. This one involved the issuance of checks to fictitious funding program customers purportedly representing the excess proceeds from the sale of the customer's mutual fund shares upon liquidation of his account. To obtain such fraudulent checks, a funding program account in the process of liquidation was first located. A duplicate check request for the proceeds due the customer under that account was then submitted, using the proper account number but substituting a fictitious name. Under company procedures, such check requests were then routed to a particular individual for approval. That individual is believed to have been the person behind this thievery scheme. He approved the check request, intercepted the check when it was issued, and later destroyed some or all of the internal documentation for the transaction.

To date, three such fraudulent liquidation checks — totaling more than $77,000 — have been discovered. The checks were issued in late 1971 and early 1972, at the same time the "Cookie Jar Caper" was underway. Although the two schemes do not appear to have been perpetrated by the same people, the individual apparently involved in the newly-discovered scheme was an employee who stumbled upon evidence of the "Cookie Jar Caper." In addition to exacting over $1,000 for his silence about those thefts, he apparently decided to embark upon his own embezzlement caper.

In retrospect the factors which motivated the increasing personal fraud and thievery at Equity Funding are reasonably clear. As the scope of the corporate fraud widened and the number of participants increased, there was a growing likelihood of discovery by the authorities. This steadily increasing risk seems to have prompted the escalation of demands on the corporate treasury made by certain of the fraud conspirators, particularly those on the middle-management level who were not as well compensated as Goldblum, Levin and Lowell. Thus, as the fraud grew, so too did the climate of personal moral decay.

PART FOUR

CONCLUSIONS

I. SETTING THE RECORD STRAIGHT

In the wake of the highly publicized EFCA scandal, a number of misconceptions about the fraud appear to have gained wide acceptance. Hence, there may be some value at the outset of this final chapter in specifically setting the record straight with respect to three such misconceptions.

A. **EFCA Was Not a Corporate Giant Looted by Insiders.**

The most frequently asked question about the EFCA fraud probably is, "Where did all the money go?" This question rests upon two assumptions: (1) that EFCA was a prosperous corporate giant with substantial real income and assets; and (2) that the fraud consisted of stealing huge amounts of those sums. Both assumptions appear to be incorrect.

First, it is now known that EFCA never was a true corporate giant. When the fraud was discovered, EFCA proved to be a "paper giant." While several of its subsidiaries had value and were untainted by the fraud, as an overall matter the Company's reported statistics were mostly a fraud. Simply put, EFCA never had the assets it reported; never had the revenues; never had the sales; never had the net worth; and never made the profits. Thus, despite all of its acquisitions, the Company appears to have always been relatively small, devoid of equity, and totally unprofitable.

It is now apparent that EFCA sustained operating losses for years in its home office, insurance and marketing operations, and probably in the financing of its funding business as well. On a consolidated basis, deficits from the Company's losing operations clearly exceeded total earnings from its few profitable subsidiaries. Moreover, the most profitable subsidiaries were but recently acquired: Bankers in 1971 and Northern in 1972.

Thus, it appears that the only way EFCA was able to report any net earnings at all was through the fraud. As the following table demonstrates, from 1964 to 1972 the Company reported net earnings of $76 million. During the same years, the fraud generated at least $143 million of bogus income,* more than $114 million of which came from funding and insurance. Without this bogus income, EFCA undoubtedly would have reported a loss in every year of its operations and, for all years taken together, it would have reported aggregate net operating losses in the millions of dollars.

COMPARISON OF ESTIMATED BOGUS FUNDING AND INSURANCE INCOME TO REPORTED NET EARNINGS°° (1964-1972)

	Bogus Funding Income	Bogus Insurance Income	Minimum Gross Income From Fraud	Reported Consolidated Earnings†
1964	$ 361,000	$ 0	$ 361,000	$ 389,467
1965	1,068,000	0	1,068,000	795,944
1966	3,155,000	0	3,155,000	1,177,355
1967	3,549,000	0	3,549,000	2,530,380
1968	5,152,000	0	5,152,000	7,825,857
1969	17,200,000	350,000	17,550,000	10,911,632
1970	15,600,000	4,000,000	19,600,000	11,715,625
1971	17,900,000	10,000,000	27,900,000	18,192,000
1972	21,000,000	14,667,000	35,667,000	22,617,000
TOTAL	$85,345,000	$29,017,000	$114,412,000	$76,155,260

It should be noted that this table shows only the estimated amounts of bogus income from funding and insurance. A sizeable amount of other bogus income was generated over the course of the fraud through a grab-bag of accounting "dirty tricks" which have not been fully explained in this report because of their relative insignificance. Some examples are briefly described later in this chapter.††

From the foregoing, it should be apparent that the first assumption underlying the myth of the looted giant is false: There was no real giant to loot. It also appears that the second assumption is false. Despite the fact that large amounts of cash did come in to EFCA

---

* See Report of Trustee at page 38.
°° Figures shown are estimated minimum amounts.
† See financial statements in Appendix B, beginning at page 155.
†† See page 140.

through borrowings, no evidence has yet been found that the conspirators drained the Company's treasury. It is probable that substantially all of the cash left over after paying off loans and making acquisitions was exhausted by operating losses, although the amount of these losses cannot be determined because of the dismal state of the Company's records. With the exception of the three-quarters of a million dollars in embezzlements and peccadillos reported in Part Three of this report,* it does not appear that there was significant looting. This is not to say that the conspirators were not enriched by the fraud. They received generous emoluments, and the ringleaders realized hundreds of thousands and, in two instances, millions of dollars in wrongful profits from stock sales.** But they do not appear to have dipped directly into the till for large sums.

This conclusion is supported by all of the available evidence. First, the Trustee's lawyers and accountants have scrutinized EFCA's books and records in painstaking detail over the past year and a half. A large share of this enormous amount of time was spent on a balance sheet audit as of April 5, 1973, the results of which have already been reported by the Trustee.† Equally large amounts of time have been spent studying available historical records maintained by the Company and its former auditors, and reviewing the hundreds of files maintained by the conspirators themselves.

Throughout this intensive search, a special effort has been made to look for clues of looting. For example, sample tests of cash receipts and disbursements were made for selected periods of the Company's operations. In addition, some individual transactions have been analyzed for hints of theft. Although many questions are raised by the records, none appear to point in the direction of massive looting by the conspirators.

Evidence taken from more than 100 witnesses —including many of the fraud participants themselves—also buttresses this conclusion. The Trustee's lawyers have taken or reviewed testimony from most of the key conspirators. In addition, dozens of other persons who might know of such looting if it in fact took place have been inter-

---

* See pages 129-133.
** See pages 121-126.
† See generally, Report of the Trustee.

viewed. None of this evidence indicates that any substantial sums of money were embezzled from the Company other than as described in this report. Of course, the possibility of substantial theft remains, especially in view of the unlikelihood that a conspirator guilty of looting would admit to it and the impossibility of determining the actual cash flow in and out of EFCA over the years. Consequently, the Trustee intends to pursue this possibility in the context of contemplated litigation and otherwise. Based upon presently available information, however, it does not appear that the EFCA fraud involved large-scale looting of the sort imagined by those who ask where all the money went.

B. The Fraud Was Not a Brilliant Computer Fraud.

A great deal has been written about the EFCA fraud. Much of the literature seems to characterize the fraud as the brilliant brain-child of "with-it" business and computer wizards. As a result, many readers may have the impression that the EFCA fraud was carefully planned and executed with a high level of precision and sophistication which baffled the world until it was finally discovered in April 1973. Nothing could be farther from the truth than this misconception.

First, EFCA appears never to have had people experienced in management at its top executive level. The four founders, for example, were all salesmen by background. Two of these men — Michael Riordan and Stanley Goldblum—dominated the management of EFCA as long as they were associated with it. Neither had any experience in business outside of sales before they started the Company. With a few exceptions, other "top executives" tended to be either lower-level accountants or lawyers — none of whom had significant business experience prior to the time they were put in charge of EFCA. Thus, Jerome Evans had a variety of bookkeeping jobs prior to becoming the chief financial officer of the Company, but it is safe to say that he never managed more than a handful of people before he was put in charge of EFCA's operations. Samuel Lowell, while he worked at one time for a big-eight accounting firm, also seems to have had no prior management background. Fred Levin was a lawyer with the Illinois Insurance Department when he was hired by Presidential, and he too had little or no executive experience before assuming a major management role at EFCA. Furthermore,

137

the top managers — who tended to be the top fraud participants — were primarily assisted in running both EFCA and the fraud by a growing corps of vice presidents in their 20's and early 30's most of whom also do not appear to have held any previous management positions. In short, the majority of EFCA's managers appear to have been inexperienced men, lacking in seasoned business judgment, who played at high finance — and failed miserably in the process.

Not only did these men fail at running the Company; in fact, they did not run the fraud any better. As this report demonstrates, there simply was no "grand scheme." Every step of this fraud was jerry-built — one misstep requiring another more complicated misstep to conceal all that had gone before. It is true that the conspirators can sometimes be credited for a degree of inventiveness in extricating themselves from near hopeless situations. On the whole, however, their helter-skelter, hand-to-mouth efforts demonstrate a striking lack of analytical insight and forethought. Indeed, some of the devices used to further or conceal the fraud are totally devoid of economic sense and seem to be in almost open defiance of generally accepted accounting principles and auditing standards. For example, although the conspirators were creating bogus income both from the insurance operation and from funding, they never figured out how to effectively coordinate the steps of the fraud. This failure created growing imbalances in inter-company accounts which might have been eliminated by effective administration and a degree of farsightedness. Moreover, from the outset, no one appears ever to have given serious thought to a way out of the scheme.

Oddly enough, the slipshod character of much of the fraud may be a reflection of the attitude of some conspirators who appear to have looked upon the fraud as a game. The curious flippancy of the conspirators is illustrated by a sheet of game instructions given to Samuel Lowell by Arthur Lewis which was found in a Lowell file entitled "Kudos." This document explains how to play "Sam-O-Wits." The "player" is instructed to reply to questions concerning EFCA's financial statements by saying, "That was caused by a . . .," followed by his choice of one word from each of three columns on the sheet. The "player" is admonished to "emphasize the third word" and, if asked to explain in greater detail, he is told to "comment that the

138

subject is so complex and technical that it took two years to understand it." The three columns are as follows:

Column 1	Column 2	Column 3
Complicated	Phase III	Adjustment
Complex	Commission	Reinstatement
Preliminary	Persistency	Provision
Convoluted	Morbidity	Experience
Favorable	Recapture	Retrocession
Mature	Actuarial	Fluctuation
Consolidated	Non-Refund	Ruling

Least of all was this a modern "computer" fraud. The computer did not even contain complete records for EFCA's legitimate business — let alone the fraud. For example, the critical records for the Company's legitimate funding business were kept on microfiche, and were dealt with entirely by hand. The only record for funding business kept on the computer was an inventory of funding accounts. Entries to book fictitious income were made by manual additions to the books and records in total disregard of the Company's computer print-outs. And in insurance, although reams of print-outs were created to support the fraud, there was little or no underlying detail for these print-outs. Hence, while the computer may have generated a paper "screen" for some aspects of the fraud, in fact the role it played was no bigger or more complicated than that played by the Company's adding machines.

C. The Fraud Was Not an Insurance Fraud.

Probably because they were discovered first, the insurance aspects of the EFCA fraud have received the most publicity, and the scandal has frequently been characterized as an insurance fraud. However, as this report has shown, the insurance activity was merely one particular phase of a much larger stock fraud that began at or before the time of EFCA's first public offering in 1964. The fraud was designed to pump up the value of the Company's stock by systematically inflating EFCA's reported earnings through every means available to the conspirators.

The funding and insurance devices contributed the most bogus income to EFCA's reported earnings, and thus had the biggest impact upon the Company's earnings. Although this report has focused upon these revenue-inflation devices, many others were used as well to keep EFCA's stock flying high. For example, in 1968 — in addition to the estimated $5.5 million of bogus funding income recorded — approximately $3 million of bogus revenue was generated by recording as income in that year the difference between market value and cost of various securities, even though these securities were still held by the Company and had not been sold. Another oft-used trick involved the "sale" of future income from some aspect of EFCA's business **for** a promissory note which was to be paid-off out of that income as it was received. In several instances, although the "sale" amounted to a mere financing arrangement, the full amount of the note was improperly recorded as income in the year of the transaction. Another ploy involved overstating the percentage of completion on real estate projects in order to recognize a greater amount of income than was proper. Still another device involved improperly recognizing more than $1 million of income earned by a recently acquired subsidiary, despite the fact that the acquisition was rescinded during the year the income was recognized.

The list of bogus income creating devices is a long one, and all the examples may not yet be known. The point is that all of these devices had as their goal the fraudulent inflation of the market price of EFCA's common stock. Hence, as this report has tried to demonstrate, the primary impact of the fraud was upon holders of EFCA securities and others who were misled by the Company's fraudulent financial statements. There was no impact upon its insurance policyholders — and relatively little impact upon EFLIC's reinsurers. Thus, insurance was merely the last phase of what should now be seen as a classic stock fraud.

II. HOW DID THE FRAUD LAST SO LONG?

If the EFCA fraud was truly as haphazard and disconnected as it has been portrayed in this report, then it is legitimate to ask how it persisted for a decade without detection. Obviously a number of factors contributed to the longevity of the conspiracy. Foremost, of course, were the lies, audacity and luck of the ringleaders. Of almost equal importance was the surprising ability of the originators of the fraud to recruit new participants over the years. Closely related was the moral blindness of those participants, including several who helped execute the scheme and then left the Company, but remained silent. It is noteworthy that in the end, the fraud was undone by the spite of a former conspirator who had been terminated, not by anyone's conscience pangs.

The foregoing factors explain how the conspiracy was sustained for so long from within the Company. Responsibility for failing to detect the fraud rests primarily with the accounting firms retained to certify the financial condition of EFCA and its subsidiaries. As this report makes clear, the fraud took place "on paper" — in the books and records of the Company and some of its subsidiaries. Aside from the perpetrators themselves, only the auditors, as part of their annual examinations, had regular opportunities to review these books and records. In the Trustee's judgment, had the auditors properly discharged their obligations, the fraud would have been caught years ago.

A. The Parent's Auditors.

From 1961 to 1970, EFCA and most of its subsidiaries were audited by Wolfson Weiner. There is strong evidence that several of the accountants in charge of these audits were aware of or suspected the fraud and cooperated in its concealment. Such a conclusion seems irresistible to the Trustee if only because Wolfson Weiner's performance was so manifestly incompetent for so many years as to be inexplicable on any other basis.

First, EFCA's books and records were a literal mess over the entire life of the fraud, and it seems reasonably clear that the Company never had adequate internal controls in many areas, including its funding operations. Thus, it is difficult to see how Wolfson Weiner performed any audits at all. Had the auditors done their job by requiring management to maintain orderly records and to develop adequate control procedures as a condition of annual certification, it would have been impossible to get the funding fraud off the ground.

Equally important, Wolfson Weiner failed in numerous respects to conduct its examinations in accordance with generally accepted

141

auditing standards. The omissions and errors were legion, and many examples are recounted in the body of this report. Four prominent instances will serve to illustrate this essential point: Evans' first bogus commission entry in 1964;* Templeton's problems with funded loans receivable in 1968;** the treatment of the net trail commissions in 1969;† and the patently inadequate support for funded loans at year end 1972.†† Substantial income was booked or justified in each instance virtually without supporting detail and on the strength of inherently unacceptable explanations. Reasonable tests of EFCA's accounting records and other auditing procedures necessary in the circumstances should have exposed the impropriety of these and many other improper entries and thereby exposed the fraud.

After Seidman & Seidman combined practices with the Los Angeles office of Wolfson Weiner, the audits for EFCA and most of its subsidiaries in 1971 and 1972 were performed by that firm. But the change was in name only. After the combination of practices the same people were left in control of the EFCA audit and apparently no Seidman representative reviewed their performance. Hence, the imprimatur of Seidman & Seidman on EFCA's financial statements did not signify any notable change in underlying procedures. It is not surprising, therefore, that the 1971 and 1972 EFCA audits were also conducted incompetently.

The 1972 audit by Seidman was especially deficient because only on that occasion did a single accounting firm audit each aspect of the funding operation. As has been explained elsewhere in this report, the funding operation consisted of four basic activities: sale of programs, financing, purchase of mutual fund shares and issuance of insurance. These activities were conducted in three entities: EFC-Cal, EFSC and EFLIC. The various accounting aspects of the funding fraud at these three companies were not integrated with each other. A single bogus transaction could not be traced through the books and records of the respective entities involved, because no effort was made by the conspirators to develop mutually consistent documentary

---

* See page 25.
** See pages 29-35.
† See pages 64-73.
†† See page 41.

support. Thus, for example, on the books of EFLIC, journal entries were made to record fictitious insurance premium income in an inter-company account as a receivable due from EFC-Cal, and bogus files were developed at EFLIC as needed to support this fictitious income. On EFC-Cal's books, however, no corresponding entries were made to show premiums payable to EFLIC.

Through 1971, Wolfson Weiner (later Seidman & Seidman) examined the books of EFC-Cal and EFSC, while Haskins & Sells examined the books of EFLIC. Numerous improper entries should have been discerned by a careful auditor from the books of EFC-Cal and EFSC alone. When in 1972 Seidman & Seidman audited EFLIC, as well as EFC-Cal and EFSC, the funding fraud ought to have been nearly self-revealing, because of the obvious inconsistencies between the books and records of the three companies. Evidently, however, the accountants from Seidman & Seidman who examined EFLIC's books did not coordinate their work with personnel who audited the parent and other subsidiaries (who were mostly former Wolfson Weiner accountants). In any event, the discrepancies were either not discovered or ignored.

B. **EFLIC's Auditors.**

From 1968 to 1971, EFLIC was audited by Haskins & Sells. The body of this report does not contain as much information about these audits as it does about those performed by Wolfson Weiner and Seidman & Seidman. This is primarily a function of the fact that EFLIC has been under the joint conservatorship of the Departments of Insurance of the States of California and Illinois, and not under the direct jurisdiction of the Trustee. Moreover, thus far the Trustee's counsel has not had the same access to testimony by Haskins & Sells' accountants or to work papers for audits conducted by that firm. Enough is known, however, to suggest that Haskins must share significant responsibility for the persistence of the fraud at Equity Funding.

It is by now obvious that the fraud was not merely an insurance scandal. However, the fact remains that a massive fraud was perpetrated on the books of EFLIC, the Company's primary insurance subsidiary. More than $2 billion in face amount of bogus policies were reinsured by EFLIC, and almost $30 million of fictitious premium and other income was reported by that company. For a number of reasons it appears to the Trustee that Haskins & Sells should have detected sufficient evidence of this aspect of the fraud to have prompted its discovery.

For one thing, Haskins & Sells did not adequately check the procedures by which information was generated through EFLIC's data processing system. Very heavy reliance for information about EFLIC's operations was placed on print-outs and similar data produced by the Company's computers. Nevertheless, Haskins & Sells failed to review the internal controls of the computer installation. These controls were in fact weak or non-existent, a condition which made it possible for special print-outs which merged legitimate and bogus information to be prepared for the auditors.

In the Trustee's judgment, this failure was a serious omission. However, the most fundamental shortcoming in Haskins & Sells' performance was its nearly complete dependence upon information from internal EFLIC sources. It failed to obtain verification of this information either from the books and records of affiliated companies or from third parties.

Normally accountants auditing an insurance company have primary source records readily available from which to correlate reported data concerning premiums, insurance in-force and commissions paid. In a proper audit, tests are made to determine that all this information ties together and is internally consistent. Haskins & Sells did not have primary source records from which to perform such tests at EFLIC because records of both premiums earned and commissions paid to agents were kept by EFC-Cal, a separate entity. In these circumstances, EFLIC was not auditable apart from some reasonable verification of the premium and commission information furnished by its affiliate. Haskins & Sells should have tested EFC-Cal's records showing premium receipts, or the generation of premiums through funding, and commission payments to EFC-Cal salesmen. Had the auditors done so, they would have found glaring discrepancies which should have prompted discovery of the fraud.

Nor did Haskins & Sells confirm insurance in-force directly with purported policyholders. Such confirmations were called for in

EFLIC's case. Under principles of statutory accounting, policies are carried on the balance sheet of an underwriting company as a reserve liability. There would be limited, if any, reason for such a company to inflate the amount of in-force policies on its books since that would increase its liabilities. Under such circumstances, it might be argued there is no need to confirm the amount of insurance in-force.

However, where a company reinsures a substantial portion of its business, the situation is materially different. The ceding company generates income from such business, while the reinsurer assumes the reserve liability. Hence, even a statutory reporting company has an incentive to overstate the amount of its in-force insurance when it reinsures much of its business. Where such a company converts from statutory accounting to generally accepted accounting principles ("GAAP"), the incentive is all the greater. This is so because GAAP accounting results in the accrual of income from policies at the same time reserves are set up. EFLIC began large-scale reinsurance in 1969 and converted to GAAP accounting in 1971. Thus, for both these reasons Haskins & Sells should have confirmed the amount of insurance the company claimed to be in-force. Such confirmation was even more vital in EFLIC's case in view of the absence of any testing by the auditors of primary source documents for EFLIC's principal income and expense items.

III. A FINAL POSTSCRIPT

Literally hundreds of persons and firms had business relations with EFCA during the life of the fraud. To a varying degree, they all had some opportunity to observe the real workings of the Company. Others, including government regulators and investment analysts, had an ongoing professional interest in the Company's performance and presumably had regular occasion to review EFCA's financial statements. All these individuals and entities had at least a chance to spot clues of the scandal. Without intending to prejudge questions of legal duty, the Trustee does not find it surprising that no one did so.

Although it is now evident that there were some discrepancies in EFCA's financial statements over the years, only someone examining the statements thoroughly, regularly and with a critical eye would have found them. And only someone with an exceedingly skeptical bent of mind would have then inferred massive fraud. Such an inference would have been hostile to the presumption of good faith and honest-dealing which customarily prevails in American business practice. To the Trustee, that presumption, though sometimes grievously abused, is probably indispensable to a vigorous and productive economy.

When the scandal broke, lawsuits were filed all over the country naming as defendants nearly every person and company or institution that appeared to have had any significant contact with EFCA or its subsidiaries. Most of these lawsuits were filed when few of the facts were known and are evidently premised upon the assumption that these parties either knew or should have known about the fraud. Based upon the available evidence, this reaction seems to the Trustee unjustified. It appears rather that the banks, underwriters, reinsurers and others named in many of these lawsuits probably could only have discovered the fraud at EFCA by blind luck.

The same probably can be said of most of EFCA's Board of Directors. During the better part of the fraud years, EFCA's outside directors included a Harvard professor, a senior partner of a New York investment banking firm, and two experienced business executives—all of whom appear to have played active roles as directors of the Company. Based upon present information, however, there is nothing to indicate that any of these outside directors knew about the fraud. And, of course, they clearly had nothing to do with its discovery. Whether these men should have discovered the fraud depends upon one's view of the role directors should or realistically can be expected to play in the affairs of a large, publicly held corporation engaged in complex business activity, as was EFCA.

To the Trustee it seems unrealistic to expect directors to exercise the detailed oversight necessary to discover frauds perpetrated by determined and unprincipled executives. First, outside directors normally cannot make the major time commitment which such oversight would require. They are active in other pursuits and, indeed, are retained as directors because of the experience and judgment gained by reason of their principal activities. Moreover, outside directors rarely have substantial experience with the business of the

146

company upon whose board they have been asked to sit, since active outsiders with such experience are often precluded from serving as directors by antitrust considerations or conflicts of interest. As a practical matter, even inside directors have scant opportunity to discover an accounting fraud conducted outside of their area of responsibility.

The principal effect of imposing a duty to discover such frauds would probably be to discourage membership on corporate boards. An observation on this question fifty years ago by Judge Learned Hand seems no less apt today:

> "It seems to me too much to say that he [the director] must read the circulars sent out to prospective purchasers and test them against the facts. That was a matter he might properly leave to the officers charged with that duty. He might assume that those who prepared them would not make them fraudulent. To hold otherwise is practically to charge him with detailed supervision of the business, which, consistently carried out, would have taken most of his time. If a director must go so far as that, there will be no directors."*

At a time when many corporations are seeking to diversify their boards of directors with members having a public interest orientation, it seems especially inappropriate to depart from the notion that directors, like investors and others, are entitled to presume that the top management of a public corporation is essentially honest and that its auditors competently perform their duties.

---

* *Barnes v. Andrews*, 298 Fed. 614, 620 (S.D.N.Y. 1924).

APPENDIX A

GLOSSARY OF NAMES

AG GROUP. Collective name for the owners from whom EFCA purchased Pantanella: the Special Administration of the Holy See and Assicurazioni Generali, an Italian insurance company.

AMINCOR. (Amincor Bank, A.G.) Swiss bank which loaned money to EFCA in connection with the Pantanella acquisition.

AMIR, Dov. Vice President—Natural Resources Operations for EFCA from June 1968 until January 1973.

ARKUS-DUNTOV, YURA. EFCA officer and director, 1966-1973; elected to EFCA Board of Directors in January 1969; held offices of Vice President and Executive Vice President — Investment Management for EFCA; also director of Bishops Bank, EFCC-NV and Bankers National Life Insurance Company.

BAKER, LAWRENCE. Chief Deputy Commissioner of the California Insurance Department.

BANKERS. (Bankers National Life Insurance Company) New Jersey-based insurance company acquired by EFCA in October 1971.

BANKS, JAMES. Assistant Secretary and Counsel-Legal for EFLIC, November 1968 to March 1973, and Vice President—Corporate Insurance Operation-Legal for EFCA's insurance group, January to March 1973.

BANQUE JORDAAN. Paris bank at which EFCC-NV maintained accounts.

BECKERMAN, GARY. Assistant to President of EFLIC August 1969 to April 1970, and Director of Advertising and Communications for EFCA, May 1970 to January 1973.

BISHOPS BANK. (Bishops Bank and Trust Co., Ltd.) Bahamian Merchant Bank acquired by EFCA in May 1969.

BLOCK, SOL. Accountant with Wolfson Weiner who assumed responsibility for the EFCA audits after Marvin Lichtig was hired by the Company.

BOWIE, ROBERT. Harvard professor elected to the Board of Directors of EFCA in May 1970.

BREWER, HUGH. Vice President of First National City Bank of New York.

BUCHALTER, STUART. Attorney with the firm of Buchalter, Nemer, Fields and Savitch, Inc., retained as counsel for EFCA in March 1973.

CAPO, DAVID. EFCA Group Controller, October 1969 to December 1970; Director, Securities and Investors Services for EFCA, January 1971 to December 1971; Vice President — Investment Operations for EFCA, January 1972 to February 1973.

COE, ROGER. President and Director of Bishops Bank.

COLLINS, LAWRENCE. EFLIC Vice President from April 1969 to March 1973, and Assistant Vice President — Insurance Operations for EFCA, August 1972 to March 1973.

COMPANIA DE ESTUDIOS Y ASUNTOS, S.A. See "Estudios."

CUTHBERTSON, EUGENE. One of the founders of EFCA; Treasurer of the Company from September 1962 to November 1963; Secretary and Executive Vice President from September 1962 until October 1965.

DIRKS, RAYMOND. Wall Street securities analyst to whom Ronald Secrist told the story of fraudulent insurance at EFLIC in March 1973.

DISHY EASTON. (Dishy, Easton and Co.) New York brokerage firm which performed many financial services for EFCA.

DOW. (Dow Banking Corporation) International banking corporation from which EFCA and its subsidiaries obtained a number of borrowings in 1969, 1971 and 1972.

EDENS, LLOYD. Treasurer of EFLIC from September 1968 to March 1973, and Group Controller and Vice President — Financial Services for EFCA, April 1971 to March 1973.

EFC-CAL. (Equity Funding Corporation of California) EFCA's primary insurance agency subsidiary.

EFCC-NV. (Equity Funding Capital Corporation N.V.) Netherlands Antilles subsidiary used as a financing vehicle by EFCA.

EFIBANCA. (Efibanca Ente Finanziario Interbancario S.p.A.) Italian bank from which EFCA arranged a $5 million loan to EII in connection with the Pantanella acquisition.

EFLIC. (Equity Funding Life Insurance Company) EFCA's primary insurance subsidiary. See "Presidential."

EFSC. (Equity Funding Securities Corporation) EFCA's securities broker-dealer subsidiary.

EII. (Equity Immobiliare Industriale S.p.A.) Italian subsidiary formed by EFCA in 1969.

ESTUDIOS. (Compania de Estudios y Asuntos, S.A.) Panamanian shell corporation secretly acquired by EFCA in May 1970.

ETABLISSEMENT GRANDSON. See "Grandson."

EVANS, JEROME. EFCA Treasurer from November 1963 until February 1969.

GARDENIER, RICHARD. EFLIC employee who helped supervise Maple Drive "mass marketing" office.

GIBSON, ROBERT. EFLIC employee involved in small embezzlement scheme in 1972.

GLASER, HERBERT. EFCA officer and director, 1962-1974; elected to EFCA Board of Directors in September 1962; held offices including Assistant Secretary, Vice President — Legal, and Executive Vice President — Real Estate and International Operations for EFCA; also served on boards of directors of Bishops Bank, EFCC-NV and EFLIC.

GOLAN, JOSEPH. European entrepreneur who helped organize EFCA's foreign operations from 1969 through 1971.

GOLDBLUM, STANLEY. One of the organizers of EFCA; President and member of the EFCA Board of Directors from September 1960 until April 1973, and Chairman of the Board of Directors of EFCA from January 1969 to April 1973; also held positions as officer and/or director of at least 63 subsidiary corporations.

GOOTNICK, WILLIAM. EFCA Vice President in charge of computer operations.

GORDON, RONALD. EFLIC employee involved in a small embezzlement scheme in 1972; younger brother of Stanley Goldblum.

GRANDSON. (Etablissement Grandson) Liechtenstein entity secretly acquired by EFCA in early 1970.

HASKINS & SELLS. Accounting firm which audited EFLIC from 1968 through 1971.

IPC. (Investors Planning Corporation of America) Subsidiary of Bernard Cornfeld's Investors Overseas Services Inc., acquired by EFCA in October 1968.

KROLL, MILTON. Attorney with the Washington, D. C. law firm of Freedman, Levy, Kroll & Simonds, which handled EFCA's securities work.

LEVIN, FRED. Officer and director of EFCA and its subsidiaries from October 1967 until April 1973; elected to EFCA Board of Directors in May 1971; held offices of President of EFLIC, and Executive Vice President—Insurance Operations for EFCA.

LEWIS, ARTHUR. Officer of EFCA and its subsidiaries from April 1969 through March 1973; held the positions of Vice President and Actuary for EFLIC and EFCA's insurance group, and Vice President of Bankers.

LEWIS, MARK. Employee of EFCA and EFLIC who helped manage the Maple Drive "mass marketing" operation.

LICHTIG, MARVIN. Accountant with Wolfson Weiner, who was in charge of EFCA's audits until he became Treasurer and Executive Vice President — Administration for EFCA in May 1969.

LIVINGSTON, GALE. Executive with Litton Industries Inc. who was elected to the Board of Directors of EFCA in May 1971.

LOEB, RODNEY. Vice President — General Counsel and Secretary of EFCA from July 1969 to present.

151

LOUD, NELSON. Former partner of New York Securities Co. who was elected to the Board of Directors of EFCA in January 1965.

LOWELL, SAMUEL. Officer and director of EFCA and its subsidiaries from May 1969 to April 1973; elected to the EFCA Board of Directors in May 1971; held positions of Controller and Executive Vice President — Corporate Operations and Finance for EFCA.

LRI. (Loeb, Rhodes International Inc.) A financial corporation through which EFCA and its subsidiaries arranged a number of borrowings.

MAJERUS, FRANK. EFLIC Controller from March 1969 to November 1971.

McCORMICK, GORDON. Insurance and mutual fund salesman who organized EFCA's predecessor companies.

MOLINI E PASTIFICIO PANTANELLA S.p.A. See "Pantanella."

NEMB. (New England Merchants National Bank of Boston) Bank which acted as custodian pursuant to the agreement under which EFCA's custodial collateral notes were issued.

NEW YORK SECURITIES Co. New York brokerage firm which underwrote most of EFCA's public offerings from 1964 to 1973.

NORTHERN. (Northern Life Insurance Company) Washington-based life insurance company acquired by EFCA in June 1972.

PANTANELLA. (Molini e Pastificio Pantanella S.p.A.) Italian pasta company acquired by EFCA in June 1970.

PAVIA FIRM. (Pavia & Harcourt) Law firm with offices in Rome and New York through which EFCA arranged the Pantanella acquisition, and from which EFCA purchased Estudios.

PENNISH, JOHN. President of The Presidential Life Insurance Company of America who, after the acquisition of that company, became Executive Vice President — Administration of EFCA from August 1968 through October 1969 and Treasurer from April 1969 until May 1969.

PEREZ DA SILVA, ALPHONSO. Apparently fictitious person whose name was signed on behalf of Estudios as part of the bogus trail commissions sale in May 1970.

152

PLC. (Pennsylvania Life Company and its subsidiary Pennsylvania Life Insurance Company) Santa Monica-based insurance company whose policies EFCA sold from 1963 until 1968, prior to the development of its own proprietary insurance operations.

POOLE, OTIS. EFLIC employee involved in a small embezzlement scheme in 1972.

PRESIDENTIAL. (The Presidential Life Insurance Company of America) Illinois insurance company acquired by EFCA in October 1967 and later renamed Equity Funding Life Insurance Company.

RAFF, WILLIAM. Assistant General Counsel for EFCA from July 1971 until June 1973, when he became Corporate Counsel for EFLIC.

RIORDAN, MICHAEL. One of the founders of EFCA and Chairman of the Board of Directors and Executive Vice President of the Company until his death in January 1969.

ROTHMAN, FRANK. Los Angeles attorney retained by Stanley Goldblum in March 1973.

SAYRE, JUDSON. Retired corporate executive, elected to the EFCA Board of Directors in May 1971.

SCHNEIDER, JOHN. Attorney on EFCA's legal staff.

SECRIST, RONALD. Employee with EFCA and its subsidiaries who was terminated in March 1973 and who subsequently revealed the existence of fraud at EFLIC to state authorities and to Raymond Dirks.

SEIDMAN & SEIDMAN. Accounting firm which combined practices with Wolfson Weiner in February 1972 and thereafter became EFCA's auditors.

SMITH, JAMES. Officer of EFCA and its subsidiaries from November 1968 through March 1973; held the positions of Vice President and Actuary of EFLIC, Vice President of Bankers, and Vice President of EFCA.

SULTAN, MICHAEL. EFCA officer from May 1969 through March 1973; held the positions of Assistant Controller, Controller and Vice President of EFCA.

SYMONDS, WILLIAM. Employee of EFCA and its subsidiaries from December 1969 through March 1973; held the positions of Supervisor for Policy Services for EFLIC and Assistant to the Vice President and Actuary of EFCA's insurance group.

TAIT, WELLER & CLARK. Accounting firm which audited Bishops Bank from 1969 through 1971.

TEMPLETON, JOHN. EFCA Controller from October 1968 until April 1969, when he became Assistant Treasurer of the Company, a position which he held for only a short time before resigning.

WANGERHOF, HEINRICH. A fictitious individual who supposedly was Managing Director of Etablissement Grandson.

WATKINS, HARRY. An accountant employed by Wolfson Weiner for work on EFCA audits.

WEINER, JULIAN. A partner at the accounting firms of Wolfson Weiner and, subsequently, at Seidman & Seidman.

WILLIAMS, LAWRENCE. EFCA Associate General Counsel from 1969 through 1974.

WOLFSON WEINER. (Wolfson, Weiner & Company, later renamed Wolfson Weiner, Ratoff & Lapin) The accounting firm which served as auditors for EFCA and certain of its subsidiaries from 1961 through 1971. Wolfson Weiner combined practices with the firm of Seidman & Seidman in February 1972.

PICKING UP THE PIECES

Touche Ross Audits after the Fraud

After the fraud was disclosed, it was necessary to put the pieces back together, quickly. The accounting firm of Touche Ross & Co. was given the job. The following two articles, one written by Norman Grosman, the partner in charge of the engagement and the principal government witness against the Wolfson, Weiner auditors, describe the dimensions of the engagement and the unusual problems encountered.

It is interesting to compare Grosman's comments about the difficulty of accountants doing the kind of interrogation that was necessary in his work, with the problems of auditors discovering fraud, which were demonstrated in the section here on the Peat, Marwick audit of EFLIC.

Behind the Scenes at Equity Funding

by Albert Hudes

On Monday, April 2, Dave Amsterdam, a partner in the Los Angeles office, received a call at 9:15 a.m. at a client's office. The call was from Irwin Buchalter of the law firm of Buchalter, Nemer, Fields & Savitch, a Los Angeles firm specializing in bankruptcy. Buchalter said that his firm had been called in on Friday concerning a conservatorship for Equity Funding Corp. of America, one of the major companies in the insurance industry with a reported $6.5 billion of policies in force. All that Dave Amsterdam knew at that time about the company was that two weeks before, Equity Funding had announced that its earnings for 1972 showed an increase of 17 percent over 1971 and shortly after that the New York Stock Exchange had halted trading in Equity Funding shares. (Later, the proof sheets of the company's unpublished 1972 annual report showed year-end assets at $737 million, stockholders' equity at $243 million, and profits for the year of $22.6 million.)

What Dave could not know was that there was in process a sequence of events which would culminate in a scandal that would rock the financial world.

Buchalter asked Dave if Touche Ross could take on an engagement which would require about 30 people immediately and sketched out the dimensions of the problem. Time was running short and he needed an answer by 4:00 p.m.

Dave discussed Buchalter's request with Robert Dodson, partner in charge of the Los Angeles office, and Norman Grosman, the partner on the Beneficial Standard Insurance Company account. Bob called Managing Partner Russ Palmer, who promised the Los Angeles office any support it needed. After a few more calls and a request for additional information describing the magnitude of the engagement, Buchalter was told Touche Ross could do the job.

Touche Ross was appointed auditors by U.S. Federal Judge Harry Pregerson, in the court's conservatorship of the company. Several days later, on April 5, Equity Funding filed for reorganization under Chapter X of the Federal Bankruptcy Act. Touche Ross was again appointed, even before the trustee was found. An unusual arrangement, but it was deemed necessary because of the need for immediate work to be done, particularly for computer security. The engagement was reconfirmed after the court had appointed Robert Loeffler as trustee. Touche Ross was separately appointed auditors of the subsidiary, Equity Funding Life Insurance Company (EFLIC), by the Illinois and California Insurance Departments, which have conservatorship responsibilities for this company.

Reprinted with permission from *Tempo,* published by Touche Ross & Co., Volume 19, Number 1, 1973. Alberg Hudes is executive editor of *Tempo.*

According to the court order, Touche Ross would be responsible for examining the balance sheet of Equity Funding as of April 5, 1973, the day it went into bankruptcy and performing such other services as needed by the trustee.

Organizing for the Job

As soon as our appointment was confirmed, the first order of business was to staff the job.

Norm Grosman, because of his general background and his experience in the insurance industry, was named partner in charge of the engagement and would devote most of his time to it.

Steve Finney, a partner in the Chicago office, was appointed "cold review" partner. This was a departure from the Touche Ross quality control system where a partner from one office was selected, usually at the end of an engagement, to review the work of another office. Steve was selected from the outset so that he could review the engagement on a continuing basis, including the audit program and other steps in the process of the job. Steve has been averaging about one day a week in Los Angeles on this engagement.

The next step was to set up Touche Ross audit teams to conform with the operations of Equity Funding.

For purposes of creating staff, Equity Funding headquarters activities were defined as follows:

—Parent company.
—Life insurance.
—Insurance general sales agency.
—Cattle.
—Security broker/dealer.
—Real estate.
—Oil and gas.

In addition to the headquarter companies, Equity Funding operations included a sizeable insurance company in Seattle, a savings and loan association in Los Angeles, and a bank in Nassau (Bahamas). This part of the engagement was staffed separately and administered in those locations.

The Touche Ross operation at Equity Funding was divided into two audit groups under Norm Grosman. William Worthen, a manager in the Los Angeles office, was to be in charge of the overall administration of the audit of the parent company and all the Los Angeles companies, with the exception of Equity Funding Life Insurance Company (EFLIC). He would supervise the firm's work at the parent company and at the general insurance agency, which was selling and financing life insurance and mutual funds.

Nelson Gibbs, a partner in the Los Angeles office, was given the responsibility of supervising the Touche Ross operations for EFLIC. Other partners and managers, mostly from the Los Angeles office, would work on the other Equity Funding subsidiaries. *(Continued on facing page.)*

Moonlighting on the Job—or, STRATA by Starlight

The first two weeks at Equity Funding was a period of high tension and drama. Most of the Touche Ross work took place in the computer area, and no one knew exactly what would be happening to the computer operations or to the computer files.

Initially, according to Carl Pabst, a few STRATA-trained people took over custody of the approximately 4,000 computer tapes, trying to learn how the company's computer operations functioned. STRATA is a generalized computer software program, developed by Touche Ross, that allows the auditor to locate, retrieve, and manipulate information in a client's computer files. It was used in the Equity Funding audit more extensively than ever before.

During this first stage, there were two separate and almost conflicting conditions: the establishment and maintenance of adequate security over the computer installation (which operated 24 hours a day) and the attempt to recreate normal computer operations to support on-going company activities. In addition, security procedures had to be established before Equity Funding's systems analysts and programmers could return. (They were not allowed in during this period.) By April 23, the tapes were secured and files needed for on-going operations had been duplicated, so that the Equity Funding people could resume operation on the IBM 370-145.

From then on, the Touche Ross computer audit project team concentrated on developing STRATA applications to support the other audit groups. To do this, it took over the third shift of the computer operations—2:00 a.m. to 8:00 a.m. and weekends. Carl Pabst points out that the STRATA people on loan from other offices rarely saw the sun in sunny California. "This is the only time," Carl said, "that moonlighting was not only approved by the firm, but was programmed."

By early June, the staff had grown to 27 professionals, and management control procedures over EDP STRATA development activities had been established along with new standards for its use and documentation. The work performed was in response to the demands of the other audit groups. STRATA application encompassed seven major areas of work, including EFLIC and several other subsidiaries.

To date, the computer audit project team has completed more than 7,000 man-hours, clocking 1,000 hours of computer time, and generating in excess of 2,000 STRATA programs.

A third unit, the computer audit project team, was organized under Carl A. Pabst, a manager who heads the audit EDP operations in Los Angeles. This group was organized to conform to the two audit groups and functioned as a captive "service" bureau to them.

One of the first activities for the Los Angeles office was the actual business of lining up professionals to staff the jobs. The Los Angeles office, naturally, was the initial source of manpower, and it was able to assign 20 full time and part time people almost immediately. "The Los Angeles office alone could not have met the demands of this engagement," Bob Dodson pointed out, "even if we had had more lead time. Younger staff assistants were fairly easy to get, but assembling experienced seniors was more difficult."

The support promised by Russ Palmer was quickly made available and a call went out to the other offices for qualified people.

Within a short time, a staff of 68 professionals with the necessary qualifications were gathered from 20 Touche Ross offices around the country.

Finding these people was only part of the task of creating a team. Because of the extended duration of the engagement, many wives and families were also involved. And since landlords are sometimes reluctant to sign short leases or take children, housing became a real problem. The Los Angeles office organized a small housing agency, booking rooms at nearby hotels and tracking down houses or apartments where the tenants were willing to sublease. One supervisor found accommodations in an ex-movie mogul's Hollywood mansion.

Scope of the Engagement

Much has been written about Equity Funding and what seems to emerge from the publicity is some real information and some sensational speculation. The purpose of this article is not to add to either the information or to the speculation, but to indicate the nature of the engagement.

The Equity Funding engagement is not a simple bankruptcy. It is complicated since government agencies have been brought into the picture because of the allegations of fraud.

By order of Judge Harry Pregerson, Robert Loeffler was named trustee to take over the operations of Equity Funding for the purpose of reorganizing under Chapter X and rehabilitating the company. EFLIC, the subsidiary in which massive fraud has also been alleged, is being run by J. Carl Osborne, appointed by the Illinois Insurance Department since EFLIC is domiciled in Illinois. (Because EFLIC is headquartered in California, the California Insurance Department is also concerned.)

In addition to the two regulatory agencies, investigatory agencies are concerned with possible fraud: the FBI is involved; the U.S. Attorney is concerned about the possibility of a criminal case against certain officers of the company; the Los Angeles regional office of the SEC is conducting its own inquiry; the Division of Corporate Reorganization under Chapter X bankruptcy proceedings is representing the shareholders; and the Post Office Department is investigating possible mail fraud.

Touche Ross reports directly to the court through the trustee and to the Illinois Insurance Department through its conservator. However, there is extensive cooperation between Touche Ross and the investigatory agencies.

The Engagement Is Underway

"The first two weeks," Norm Grosman said, "were total bedlam." The court determined that Touche Ross should secure the computer room and take physical custody of all tape files. It took two nights and one day to inventory, box, and seal the files. The files were moved out of Equity Funding over Easter weekend and are now secured in a vault accessible to only Touche Ross. After they were moved, the files needed for regular processing had to be duplicated. There could be no erasing on tapes generated before March 30. Files generated after March 30 were also frozen but are being released gradually. "Before we would allow these files to be returned to the company," Norm said, "we had to review the systems documentation to determine which tapes would be required for future audit purposes." Other files were released under a reasonable retention schedule.

The parent company was not an operating company, but it originated a series of major transactions, such as long-term debt borrowings and "special receivables." Each is a case study in itself and the audit work required that Touche Ross carry out "extended" audit procedures to check carefully these transactions. To do this, the staff had to:

—Examine voluminous files and recores.
—Contact people outside the company (the other party to the transaction).
—Interview people still with the company.
—Exchange vital information with investigating agencies.

Extended audit procedures are a necessary feature of this kind of audit. Sampling used in the normal audit is inadequate under circumstances where fraudulent transactions are suspected. Furthermore, the bank statements found in the files cannot be relied upon because they might be fictitious. Photocopies must be obtained from the banks to confirm file copies. Checks must be examined; deposits must be verified; and bank debit and credit memoranda must be reviewed.

The cash/inter-company transactions are being examined on a centralized basis, with the same detail through extended audit procedures, and as an entity since the function operated as an entity.

This philosophy of extended audit procedures was applied with greatest emphasis in operations called General Agencies, which controlled the "funding programs," the combined mutual fund and life insurance sales program. The plan allowed a customer to participate in the program by buying fund shares every year, then borrowing against them to pay the premiums on a life insurance policy. The funding program was for ten years, and at that time, in theory, the customer could sell enough shares to pay off the loans.

There were about 20,000 funded loan accounts on record and each one of these had to be checked individually. These accounts were pulled out of the company's computer files by STRATA. Each account that was identified was sent a confirmation form specially designed to conform to the STRATA confirmation print program, which included pertinent information on each transaction and which requested conformation on the loan balances and mutual fund shares. (The returns were examined individually and those which disagreed with the records were removed.) The confirmation replies were then summarized by STRATA and the updated detail files maintained.

The transfer agents for the mutual funds have been very cooperative and have given the project team their tapes or other information to be compared with STRATA tapes taken from Equity Funding computer files. This arrangement facilitates accuracy and speed in confirming the existence of securities and balances of accounts.

Touche Ross has also been able to confirm the existence of the actual mutual fund shares with the two bank repositories.

Thus, the customer confirms what shares he owns, the transfer agents confirm what shares are registered in the customer's name, and the banks confirm what shares they are holding as collateral.

The audit of the company's cattle operation, Ankony Angus Corp., and tax-shelter partnerships, is well underway and their assets essentially confirmed. In counting cattle, Touche Ross added a new technique to its extended audit procedures. One of the techniques used in making an accurate inventory of cattle, is to photograph them from the air in their feeding areas. A pin prick is made on each face in the photograph; each is marked in red on the reverse side, and then counted. (A far more reliable, safer method than trying to ride among the herds with STRATA reports strapped to saddles, according to one of our auditors who fell from his horse during a roundup.)

Equity Funding operated as its own securities broker dealer, and the audit of this activity was relatively simple since the operation itself was not complex; a mutual fund management company: EFC Management Corp.) operated as a profit center and has already been sold to a New York group.

The audit of the real estate operations of Equity Funding Development Corp. is virtually completed. The physical existence of properties (mostly apartment houses) had to be verified and title reports checked to determine who sold them to the company. A $17 million construction-investment operation in Arizona and California is being run by its previous management. Touche Ross had to review the evaluation of profitability because Equity Funding guaranteed cash flow to investors in the real estate operations.

The oil and gas audit is completed. Equity Funding's operation consisted of participating in some drilling in Ecuador, Ethiopia, and Israel and managing proprietary oil and gas limited partnerships for tax shelter investors.

Equity Funding Life Insurance Company

The insurance business, naturally, represented the bulk of the company's operations and was conducted by EFLIC and two other free standing insurance companies.

The audit for EFLIC is obviously extremely complex, both because of the unusual aspects of the business and because EFLIC is under suspicion of massive fraud.

Touche Ross is not charged with the responsibility for investigating for fraud (this is being done by the federal and state investigatory agencies), but in performing the audit, it must try to separate the fraudulent and valid activities.

EFLIC is still in business. It is not permitted to sell new insurance but is servicing its existing policyholders, under the combined conservatorship of the Illinois and California Insurance Departments. The firm's assignment with EFLIC is threefold:

—To assist EFLIC in developing a list of good "in-force" policies;
—To recreate transactions with reinsurers; and
—To carry out a complete audit as of the date of the conservatorship.

EFLIC reported that it had more than 90,000 policy holders, and Touche Ross is attempting 100 percent confirmation. EFLIC employees were able to make a tentative breakdown of approximately 60,000 "fictitious" policies. About 15,000 policies in the files have no names or addresses for the insured or have incomplete addresses. Of those 60,000 policies thought to be fictitious, about 45,000 confirmations were sent out. A significant number of these were returned from the post office as undeliverable. On the basis of the returns, 20,000 second requests were mailed in mid-August. If these bring in no response, and in light of the evidence and additional computer analysis, the assumption will be made that they are indeed fictitious.

Of the approximately 30,000 policies believed to be "good," confirmations were also mailed on a 100-percent basis. Where there is no response, additional effort is being made for substantiation by matching transactions from other sources.

Vital to EFLIC is the determination of the good in-force policies held by reinsurers. EFLIC had entered into coinsurance agreements with other insurance companies by which the coinsurers would make a substantial payment for the policies and also assume responsibility of setting up reserves to cover them.

Touche Ross has to recreate these reinsurance transactions to determine if they are supported by non-existent policies or good policies.

The financial statement of EFLIC for 1972 listed as its major asset $24.5 million in bonds, almost all of which are assumed to be non-existent; revenues of $32.6 million (which included premiums from non-existent policies and investment income from non-existent bonds); and operating expenses of $27.8 million. Determination of the actual financial condition of EFLIC will have to wait for the completion of the audit. In the meantime, every major inter-company transaction (between EFLIC and the parent company) must be examined. The audit team made a detailed computer analysis of all inter-company and parent company cash transactions. From this analysis, key transactions were selected for outside substantiation.

The massive audit of Equity Funding started six months ago with the examination of the balance sheet as of April 5. It is painstaking, meticulous, and time-consuming effort.

The task will be over soon. The facts will emerge and the company's viability will be determined.

The public in general, and the accounting profession in particular, would be ill-served if it turned away from this engagement without paying attention to the lessons to be learned.

Robert Dodson pointed out that we are operating in a changing environment of audit control and that our traditional assumptions no longer apply. "At one time," he said, "we looked to the division of groups as a protection against fraud.

With the advent of computers, the separation of groups is disappearing and a small group of men, or even one man, can conceive a massive fraud by simple programing devices. This can lead to significant changes in accounting where a computer is involved."

How to Audit a Known Fraud

By Norman C. Grosman

In talking about Equity Funding as a securities fraud, it is necessary to understand that the illegal acts started before the company ever went public in 1964.

From the initiations of the fraud through at least 1969, the procedure was highly simple, took very little time, and involved little effort to cover-up. The basic fraud during this period was achieved through regular accounting entries—increasing both accounts receivable and commission income. It was one accounting entry a month, or one accounting entry a quarter. There was no computer involvement at all.

As the fraud developed, it was expanded into the Equity Funding's insurance operations, through the creation and reinsurance of fictitious insurance policies. Since this required significant detailed support, the use of the computer became important.

But the use of the computer in the Equity Funding operations was still not extensive compared to its use in today's business. While certain fictitious information was maintained on the computer, none of it was inputed on a regular basis. The information that was added to the records was done off-line. It did not involve any special technology, or any unusual programming. It did, however, require a lower level of controls and less systems integration than one would ordinarily expect.

Part of the nature of the fraud was that it had to increase in magnitude in order that the company could show increased earnings. Thus increasing amounts of fictitious income had to be created. The company was in an extremely tight cash position at the time of the discovery of the illegal acts, and it undoubtedly had similar problems in the past as well. This required the continual raising of additional capital and additional borrowings. How much longer all this could have continued is unclear.

When we started our work, senior audit personnel from the California and Illinois insurance departments were already at Equity Funding and had begun their investigation. The SEC

Reprinted with permission from *Tempo*, published by Touche Ross & Co., Volume 22, Number 1, 1976.

was also present, as well as the FBI and the U.S. Post Office.

From the start, we really had two basic objectives in our work as auditors. The first was to help establish the current financial condition of the company; the second was to assist in the fraud investigation.

To ascertain the financial condition of the company, we needed to locate the principal fictitious items and identify what adjustments to the accounts were necessary. This information did not have to be highly accurate, but it was necessary to arrive as quickly as possible at a reasonable picture of the company's financial condition. At the same time, we started on a more complete determination of the financial condition of the company as of the date of the filing of the Chapter X proceedings. In other words, we commended an audit of the company's books as of April 5th, the same day as the reorganization filing, and these two phases were done simultaneously.

Practical Problems of a Fraud Audit

In performing this work, we started out with probably 10 to 15 people, and soon had as many as 70 people working on the engagement. The work in connection with the fraud investigation, the other part of our work, was done over a period of two years. The major effort in the investigatory area was done after the completion of our audit, since it was much more important to determine the current status of the company than what went on in the past.

There are, of course, significant problems in auditing a company following an extensive fraud. Most of the senior financial and management people were no longer with Equity Funding, for example; many of them had been involved in the deceit and were immediately dismissed upon discovery. But because of the pervasiveness of the illegal acts, we were not able to determine immediately which of the people who remained were *not* involved. In other words, who could be trusted.

Obviously, too, the records were in very poor condition. Many of them were not complete. We were also not sure if any records had been destroyed or altered in the last days in an attempt to conceal the fraud—particularly computer files. And still other records contained significant errors.

Because the senior financial and management people had been discharged, we had no one to discuss most of the transactions with. Normally you have people who can tell you the background of a transaction—the nature of it, the details. In this case, there was no one to ask. Many unusual receivables existed on the books that we could get little information on. In other areas of fraud, we were able to reconstruct balances, but we had no one to corroborate the information that we developed.

The trustworthiness of those in the computer department was one of our critical problems. The regulatory people were very much concerned that computer files might be destroyed, which is obviously very easy to do. Because of this, we had to control from the start all computer files that had existed on April 5, the date of the Chapter X proceeding.

Our first step was to duplicate the files as they were requested, so that we could maintain control of the computer files at all times. While the company's data processing people were permitted to continue their operation, they had to request files from us whenever they were needed for processing.

However, I think the most significant problem related to our uncertainty whether we had complete records. As an example, the receivables arising through the insurance funding operation had a balance of approximately $108 million on April 5, 1973, whereas the detailed computer file totalled only $43 million. We knew there was extensive fraud in this area, although we still had no idea of the magnitude. That is, we didn't know whether the data processing files which totalled $43 million were the complete files or not, and it took a significant amount of additional work to establish that. We learned eventually that these were the only valid funding receivables of the company. There were no others.

Another major problem was related to a significant number of large and unusual receivables. The company files and records contained little information on the background of these receivables—how they arose and, more particularly, if they were collectible. As it developed, a number of these receivables were fictitious or resulted from transactions that did not have economic substance. But because we had no one to discuss these receivables with, it took a significant effort to determine their nature and particularly their recoverability.

Still another problem was that there were early indications that certain documents in the company's files—such as bank advices, security advices, and bank statements—were counterfeit or fraudulent. We had no idea of their extent, however, and therefore had to perform extensive verification of internal documents with outside sources. Finally, because we didn't know the extent of the fictitious entries, we had to perform almost 100 per cent verification and analysis of the accounts for long periods of time, usually for the full year of 1972.

Another complication, not really a problem, was the need to coordinate our work with a large number of interested parties, including the insurance departments of Illinois and California, the SEC, the FBI, the US Post Office, and the US Attorney, as well as the trustee and his counsel. Certain of the work was divided up, and it was clear that it should not be duplicated. As an example, Equity Funding showed a receivable from a Liechtenstein company of some $9 million. There was no real information about this transaction in the company's files. The investigation of the status of the company was done by members of the SEC staff. It was not necessary for us to redo this work.

I think the proper approach is to take an initial sampling of transactions. In other words, start out with less than 100 per cent testing in a certain area. But structure the testing so that it can be increased in an organized way after the initial sample is evaluated.

It is also extremely important to maintain communications with all of the investigatory and operating personnel. Unfortunately, people tend to be concerned only with their own responsibility. They do not communicate automatically to others, even though we all could benefit from what is learned by other parties.

For example, at the insurance subsidiary headquartered in Century City, approximately two-thirds of the purported insurance in-force did not exist. The company had created large numbers of fictitious insurance policies, and then reinsured them with other insurance companies. In this situation, the insurance in-force file contained details on the fictitious policies as well as the valid ones. When we started our work we knew that a large percentage of the policies purportedly in-force were not valid, but we did not know which ones they were.

To identify which of the policies in the files were valid, so that regular operations could proceed, the fictitious policies were labeled with special department numbers or billing codes. The state insurance department personnel and company computer people split the in-force file between valid policies and policies based on information provided by former employees who had been involved in the fraud.

The accuracy of the split was not clear, however. The credibility of the people providing the information was suspect. The accuracy with which the computer files were regularly maintained was not clear. Also, there was some indication that in the last days of the fraud, when discovery was imminent, the billing codes and department numbers might have been changed in an attempt to conceal the full extent of the fraud. Because of these reasons, the split needed verification. We concluded that the only valid way to do this would be a 100 per cent confirmation of the in-force file.

This involved extensive computer programming to update

the files. It took probably a month's planning to program the confirmation procedure and to prepare the confirmations. The follow-up and other work took two or three months. We used a STRATA developed computer program, but even so we used about eight people in this confirmation process.

A 100 per cent verification was necessary because the company needed to know which policies to bill premiums to, and which policies were valid if a death claim were filed. The results of the confirmation indicated that the preliminary split was substantially accurate. In retrospect, it might seem 100 per cent verification was unnecessary, but we didn't know when we started just how accurate was that preliminary split based upon department numbers and billing codes. Our decision for the 100 per cent verification was based as much upon the company's operating need for an accurate listing of policies in-force as it was for our audit purposes.

There was another related area in which we did not perform 100 per cent verification. The in-force file contains information about the policy holder necessary to calculate reserves: such as the extent of coverage, the age of the insured, sex, any physical impairment which would require additional reserves. We felt that this file would not require 100 per cent confirmation because, while the in-force file contained a significant number of fictitious policies, we had no indication that other information which would be used to calculate the reserve was inaccurate. Of course, if the sample tests indicated that the information was inaccurate, we could always expand our confirmation.

In normal audits, we confirm relatively limited numbers of balances and transactions. Problems of non-response, although significant, don't present important problems. In the Equity Funding situation, however, problems arose in areas that do not exist in regular audits. For example, in regular audits you don't have to obtain information from outsiders in order to *determine* a balance. You go to the outsider in order to verify a balance which you presume to be correct. In Equity Funding, we had to go to outsiders for the basic information needed to reconstruct the balance.

One surprise to me was that we did not get a significantly higher level of response than we would have received in a normal audit. This became immediately clear in the confirmation of the insurance in-force. Despite all the publicity attendant to the Equity Funding fraud, many people who held valid policies did not answer our confirmation requests. I thought they would be concerned that their policy was properly maintained in the company's records, but that presumption was not correct. We did get a higher level of response than normal, but nowhere near the 100 per cent level. Many people with valid policies simply did not answer our request for confirmation.

As I previously mentioned, we had to support the authenticity of a substantial number of external documents that were maintained in the company's files—because we didn't know whether they were authentic or not. The first impulse was to say that no document in the company's files could be relied upon. Therefore to the extent that the document was an important document, its authenticity would have to be verified with third parties. But that, we soon learned, was not practical. Most third parties are not willing to cooperate in any extensive confirmation process. When this became evident, we carefully screened those documents we wanted authenticated. Even so, it took a number of months for banks to answer us, and other parties were less cooperative.

Many of the third parties had become adversaries during the proceeding. Others were afraid of being sued. And some just did not want to be implicated in any way with Equity Funding.

Of course we had no way to force cooperation. We could have gone to one of the regulatory groups and requested subpoenas, but that would not have provided the timely cooperation we really needed.

There as also a need to discuss the substance of transactions with third parties. Indeed, the best source of information on the nature of a transaction would be the other side. But, our ability to obtain meaningful information was almost nonexistent.

In normal audits, we were used to dealing with a final set of balances. Uncertainties, if any, are limited and clearly defined. In Equity Funding, however, if we chose to wait until that point was reached, we still would not have issued our report. As a result, we balanced the number of unresolved items with the need for getting our a public document that had basically accurate information.

That is why we completed our audit and issued our report with a substantial number of uncertainties left unresolved—far more than one would clearly expect in normal audits. One of the principal areas of uncertainty was in creditor claims. The attorneys and company personnel had started to screen and evaluate such claims only a month or so before our report had to be issued. When we issued the report, we indicated that the claims had not yet been evaluated, nor had their effect been determined. Our conclusion was that while this was an important area, even if the claims had been fully analyzed, there would be no way of knowing the ultimate allowance of claims for as long as a year and a half. So we completed our work and issued our audit in early February, 1974.

The Fraud Investigation

Concerning the fraud investigation, there are some obvious points to make. Probably we all realize them. First of all, we didn't do this investigation alone. I have already referred to the FBI, SEC, the US Attorney, the trustee's attorneys, and the state insurance departments. We were all really part of the team and we each had our strengths and weaknesses.

I think it's also obvious that the training and experience of a CPA doesn't help him very much when doing work of an investigative nature. We have limited experience in questioning people and recording the results of that interrogation. Lawyers are trained to do this all the time.

Much of the fraud investigation goes beyond the mere analysis of numbers and records. It involves taking statements—actually testimony—from a large number of people who were involved or had dealings with the company. This really is not our strong point. What we do best is to understand the financial import of what we see, relating information to the total framework of the company's financial position. We can evaluate the known areas of the fraud and its effects on the company's operation much better than can any of the other parties. We can also provide analyses and summaries of transactions in a much better way than they can. We are always doing these things. Concentrating our efforts where we have such experience is the best way, I think, to coordinate our work with that being done by the other members of the investigatory team.

Another important point is that documentation in this area is different from what we normally consider adequate documentation. Our long experience in documenting audit work is not necessarily adequate in a legal or evidentiary sense. So when we start to develop information, it is very important that we spend time with the lawyers to make sure that we will obtain sufficient detail and sufficient support for it to be used as evidence later.

Roundup and Conclusions

Touche Ross issued a report on the audit of Equity Funding's balance sheet in February, 1974. This ended our major man-hour effort. Since then, we have frequently assisted in the investigatory aspects. The trustee issued a report on the fraud at the end of October, 1974. We participated in the preparation of the report and provided much of the basic financial information in the report. Since then we have assisted the trustee in developing the accounting basis for the reorganized entity, and in developing information and preparing the documents filed during the reorganization process. We have also worked with a large number of lawyers who are handling criminal and civil litigation arising out of the fraud. In fact, the civil litigation will continue after the reorganization. Frankly, the work done after the issuance of our audit report in February, 1974, has been far more varied, far more interesting than was the basic audit work done during 1973.

Probably the most difficult part of the audit work in 1973 was pulling together quickly the number of people necessary to do the work, and then managing a group of that size. In retrospect, the auditing and reporting problems seem less than the management problems of the audit.

Recent work has seemed more interesting because the people-management problem has disappeared and because knowledge of the situation and the facts has become clearer. The passage of time alone has firmed up many of the things that we were uncertain about. Also, the viability of the reorganization plan has become clear. And certainly satisfaction with the work we are doing is greater when it is evident that the company will survive.

What were the major auditing lessons learned as a result of this experience at Equity Funding? Three stand out: One, establish the auditor's role and the role of others as early as possible, so that each can benefit from the other's information and not duplicate each other's work. Two, top priority must be given to the continued operation of the business. Traditional auditing and preparation of reports is not nearly so important as is obtaining valid and accurate information that will enable the business to operate. If all the auditor does is to provide an audit of a financial statement, he hasn't been served the reorganization of the company. And three, do not be limited by traditional audit approaches, which depend on an evaluation of the reliability of records and controls. In a fraud, such controls and validity do not exist in all the company's operations.

What is the status of Equity Funding today?

A plan of reorganization has been approved by all major stockholder credit groups, by the SEC, and by the court. The plan provides for continuing the operations of the insurance companies in New Jersey and Washington which were not involved in the fraud. The reorganization of Equity Funding was completed this spring. The operations will be transferred to the new reorganized entity, which will have an estimated net worth of $80-$90 million. The companies are viable and are presently profitable.

About the author

Norman C. Grosman was the partner responsible for the audit of Equity Funding.

THE AUDITORS CONVICTED

Seven months after the Equity Funding scandal broke, a federal grand jury returned a 105-count indictment naming twenty-two defendants on various charges of conspiracy, securities fraud, mail fraud, filing false documents, and electronic eavesdropping. Nineteen of the twenty-two defendants were former officers or employees of Equity Funding, and all but one entered pleas of guilty prior to trial. The lone exception, Stanley Goldblum, the company's former chairman and president, threw in the towel on the fifth day of his trial and pleaded guilty to five felony counts. In March of 1975, two years after the swindle came to light, Goldblum was fined $20,000 and sentenced to eight years in prison. His underlings received lesser sentences. Goldblum and most of his fellow defendants also faced separate charges in Illinois, home state of Equity Funding's principal life-insurance subsidiary, Equity Funding Life.

The remaining three defendants were the auditors: Julian S. H. Weiner, the audit partner; Marvin A. Lichtig, who left the Wolfson, Weiner firm to join Equity Funding in 1969; and Solomon Block, who succeeded Lichtig as audit manager. The charges against them put Equity Funding in a class by itself as a case of accounting fraud. Previous prosecutions of public accountants for fraud had typically centered on a single audit where the auditors apparently caved in under pressure and acquiesced in improper accounting. Never before had public accountants been charged with knowing complicity in a fraud lasting for years.

The trial of the three auditors began on January 6, 1975, and went on for more than four months. Over the course of that unusually long trial, the prosecution (led by John M. Newman, Jr., an assistant United States attorney) relied on testimony by former executives of Equity Funding, mainly by Sam Lowell, to contend that the auditors had stretched or broken proper accounting principles, disregarded accepted auditing standards, closed their eyes to wrongdoing, and candidly discussed ways to doctor the books. The prosecution also sought to show that the individual defendants had profited handsomely from a sweetheart relationship with Equity Funding and, as evidence the appreciation was mutual, that Goldblum had come to a *quid pro quo* with Seidman & Seidman to leave the Wolfson, Weiner people on the audit.

Julian Weiner, the only defendant to testify, carried the burden of rebuttal. Weiner flatly denied any knowledge of the fraud and minimized the financial rewards of the Equity Funding account. For his part, Weiner testified, he had stood aloof from the audit and instead relied on his staff. In addition, both Weiner and Robert Spencer of Seidman & Seidman denied that anyone had cut a deal with Stanley Goldblum over who was to staff the audit. Weiner's attorney, Harold A. Abeles, attacked the prosecution's case as sheer hindsight. Abeles pressed hard with the accounting profession's traditional position that a routine audit can't be relied on to detect fraud. He sought to deflect the testimony of Norman Grosman, the government's expert witness, by contrasting the exhaustive "fraud audit" by Touche Ross with the limited time and resources available to Weiner and his people.

The jury returned its verdicts on May 20 and found Weiner guilty on ten of ten counts, Lichtig guilty on thirteen of thirteen, and Block guilty on seven of nine. Appeals to these verdicts are pending. District Judge Jesse W. Curtis later sentenced each of the convicted accountants to a two-year suspended term, three months in jail, four years on probation, and two thousand hours of charitable work. Judge Curtis explained the relatively light sentences by noting that initially the auditors were misled by the company, and he did not consider them as culpable as Goldblum and his subordinates at Equity Funding.

The excerpts reproduced here are from the official Reporter's Transcript of Proceedings at the auditors' trial. By volume, these excerpts are a tiny slice from some six thousand pages of trial testimony, not to mention many thousands of additional pages of court exhibits and supporting documents. Though we have tried to include the most salient points established by the prosecution or defense, we necessarily have omitted many important items. In reading the excerpts, one should keep in mind that as a matter of law, none of the lawyers' comments—neither their questions or remarks, nor their opening or closing statements—amounts to evidence: only the sworn testimony. One should also note the disparities and flat-out contradictions among the various witnesses. These were peculiarly the province of the jury.

IN THE UNITED STATES DISTRICT COURT
CENTRAL DISTRICT OF CALIFORNIA
HONORABLE JESSE W. CURTIS, JUDGE PRESIDING

UNITED STATES OF AMERICA,
Plaintiff,
vs.
JULIAN S. H. WEINER, ET AL.,
Defendants.

Case No. CR 13390-JWC

REPORTER'S TRANSCRIPT OF PROCEEDINGS
Place: Los Angeles, California
Date: Monday, January 6, 1975

APPEARANCES:

For the Plaintiff: WILLIAM D. KELLER, United States Attorney By: JOHN M. NEWMAN, JR. WILLIAM J. RATHJE Assistant U.S. Attorneys 1300 U.S. Courthouse 312 North Spring Street Los Angeles, California 90012

For the Defendant Julian S. H. Weiner: HAROLD A. ABELES 315 South Beverly Drive—Suite 300 Beverly Hills, California 90212

For the Defendant Marvin Al Lichtig: RICHARD A. DeSANTIS GUY N. JINKERSON 1901 Avenue of the Stars—Suite 790 Los Angeles, California 90067

For the Defendant Solomon Block: SANDS & MARKOWITZ By: NATHAN MARKOWITZ JUDITH A. GILBERT 6420 Wilshire Boulevard—6th Floor Los Angeles, California 90048

LOS ANGELES, CALIFORNIA,

MONDAY, JANUARY 6, 1975.   2:00 P.M.

(Other court matters.)

The Clerk: No. 13390, U.S.A. v. Weiner, Block, and Lichtig.

Mr. Newman: John Newman and John Rathje present on behalf of the United States Government.

Mr. Markowitz: Nathan Markowitz and Judith A. Gilbert on behalf of Solomon Block.

Mr. DeSantis: Richard A. DeSantis and Guy Jinkerson on behalf of Marvin Lichtig.

Mr. Abeles: Harold Abeles on behalf of Julian Weiner.

(The trial proceeded with various motions for change of venue, suppression of evidence, dismissal, etc. This was followed by jury impanelment proceedings and opening statements. The first opening statement is by Mr. John Newman on behalf of the United States Government.)

Mr. Newman: May it please the court, counsel, and ladies and gentlemen of the jury:

Since the court has told you, my function here for a substantial portion of the afternoon is going to be to tell you what in the Government's view the evidence in this case is going to show.

*   *   *

In the case of Equity Funding Corporation of America, Equity Funding had auditors, and from the early 1960's Equity Funding had an audit firm called Wolfson, Weiner & Company, which later changed its name to Wolfson, Weiner, Ratoff & Lapin when it combined with some other very small accounting firms around the country that had locations other than in Los Angeles. The company when formed had two partners. It had a partner named Philip Wolfson and had a partner, who is one of the defendants in this case over against that wall, Julian Weiner. And he got the Equity Funding account in the early 1960's and performed what was described in the documents that were published as an audit, that is, a hearing on the books and records of Equity Funding.

One of the employees of Wolfson, Weiner, beginning in the early 1960's and continuing up until the middle of 1969 was Marvin Lichtig. Marvin Lichtig is also a defendant in this case. He is sitting at the far left-hand side—far right-hand side as you face it of the defense table.

Marvin Lichtig was in actual charge of the field operations of the Equity Funding audit. He would be there. He would be looking over the workpapers. His responsibilities may have varied slightly from year to year, but by and large during those years he was in charge of the field operations at Equity Funding, supposedly gathering the evidence, looking at the books, corresponding with outside third parties, corresponding with Equity Funding's banks and gathering the appropriate evidence necessary in the hearing to come to a conclusion.

In the middle of 1969, and we will discuss this a little more later, Marvin Lichtig took a job with Equity Funding Corporation of America, the company which he had previously been auditing. He became eventually an executive vice president.

In his stead, in the position, as you might say, the head field man on the audit at Equity Funding Corporation of America was Solomon Block, the third defendant in the trial that we have here today and possibly for the next eight to twelve weeks.

Solomon Block, then, from the middle of 1969 through April 1st of 1973, when the company collapsed, was in that position, essentially the same position that Marvin Lichtig had occupied prior to the time of Mr. Lichtig's taking a job with the company.

Now, in February of 1972 Wolfson, Weiner, Ratoff & Lapin merged into another larger, more substantial and more prestigious accounting firm called Seidman & Seidman. However, the actual people who were in charge of the Equity Funding engagement, that particular client, remained essentially the same with Julian Weiner as a partner on the job and Solomon Block as the person in charge of the audit.

So you will hear throughout the trial references to Wolfson, Weiner and to Seidman & Seidman. Wolfson, Weiner is short for Wolfson, Weiner & Company and Wolfson, Weiner, Ratoff & Lapin, which was essentially the same firm and which audited Equity Funding from the early 1960's through the beginning of 1972. Then Seidman & Seidman, which audited Equity Funding Corporation of America from then on.

You will see evidence about what happened with respect to the report for the year ended 1971 and whether it was actually signed by Seidman & Seidman or Wolfson, Weiner and what the situation was in 1972.

But the point is that there are individuals who are on trial here, not firms, and precisely with whom they are associated is not important, it is the matter of the individuals, their connection with the audit and their responsibility for what happened in this case.

(Newman continued his opening statement with examples of the fraud. Here, he classifies the different accusations against the defendants in accounting and auditing terms, with some vivid examples.)

I am going to give you a few examples of some of the treatment that the auditors gave to various of the accounts throughout the years. As I give you these examples you will see aspects of both the first matter, that is, the bending and breaking of generally accepted accounting principles, and the second, that is, the willingness not to abide by generally accepted auditing standards in terms of gathering evidence and doing verification. The third, that is the willingness to look aside when what was plainly to be seen as a problem reared its head. Fourthly, the actual consultation between the auditors and members of the company concerning problems and how to work on them to make sure that they would not be disclosed.

As an example, during the years 1964 through 1968 from time to time Marvin Lichtig would come to Jerome Evans with difficulties in the audit. Because, naturally, if the Funded Loans that Jerome Evans was saying were there were only in part there could not be any legitimate backup, and legitimate detail supporting who the program holder was, and so forth. He couldn't give any of that legitimate information, any of that information to Marvin Lichtig that was legitimate for bogus, because it simply wasn't there.

From time to time Marvin Lichtig would come to Jerome Evans with problems. Jerome Evans eventually got to the point where he could not answer the problems, and under instructions from Stanley Goldblum Marvin Lichtig would be sent to Stanley Goldblum where he would consult, come back and the problems would either not be there or the questions would not be so tough any more. And where there would be a serious problem and Evans, who was in charge of the books and records, could not answer it at all, when Marvin Lichtig returned the problem had disappeared, a financial statement would eventually get certified.

Now, perhaps one of the primary examples of the manner in which this was handled occurred in 1968 for the audit of 1968. You remember that was the year that John Templeton was present at the company. John Templeton was told by Stanley Goldblum about the purported reciprocals that were in

the Funded Loans account and the account on loans receivable clients. So John Templeton prepared a schedule and that schedule, which had on it about $11,000,000 of genuine funded loans, had on it about $13,000,000 of supposed reciprocals. The evidence is going to show that all of that $13,000,000 were just loan proceeds that Equity Funding had not received, again, as part of any commission-splitting arrangement. It was not income but would eventually have to be paid back. Rather, here it was being reflected as a part of an asset.

He included on that schedule an account computation which reached about six million of collateral supposedly being held by Equity Funding. In fact, there was a mathematical error there which increased that amount by about ten, so that if the figure were true it would be more like around $600,000. And three or four other items which he basically made up and estimated and put on the schedule to reach $35,000,000.

He told Stanley Goldblum that the auditors would have to be notified about the existence of this reciprocal because it could not be hidden, it could not be disguised, he couldn't come up with detailed backup claims that there were $35,000,000 in Funded Loans.

Stanley Goldblum said, "All right. I'll have a meeting." And he called a meeting with Marvin Lichtig and Julian Weiner, two of the defendants who are on trial here today. At that meeting there was a discussion of reciprocals. Following the meeting Marvin Lichtig came down and he said, "Reciprocals are okay, they can be included in Funded Loans and there will be no disclosure."

So that when the financial statement came out that year, and this is one of the major reasons that John Templeton did not sign the registration statement containing these financial statements—when the financial statement came out that year there was a footnote which related to the Funded Loans Receivable and which said, "This is a result of our operations in selling funding programs and the difference between the $35,000,000 and the payables over here are programs held by Equity Funding Corporation of America or one of its subsidiaries."

So that upon looking at that statement you would feel that approximately $35,000,000 were these funded loans, whereas in fact they didn't represent funded loans at all, but represented, according to Goldblum, reciprocals. In fact, if you go behind that they were just merely loan proceeds that the company had received.

(Newman concluded his opening statement with the personal characterizations of the defendants that were to be alluded to throughout the trial. Weiner is a "salesman", for whom Equity Funding was the "shining star in his galaxy". Lichtig is portrayed as essentially a sellout, who owned stock in the company he was auditing and later took a high paid job with the company. Repeated reference is made to Block's lack of a CPA and the favors he took from the company while performing the audit.)

I think now in finishing that it is important to discuss what the evidence is going to show about the motive, the motive for what was being done here.

Wolfson, Weiner, Ratoff & Lapin was a relatively small accounting firm. It was started in about 1957 by Julian Weiner and Phillip Wolfson. As it got additional accounts, its major account became Equity Funding Corporation of America. Equity Funding was the only corporation, the only account it had which was traded on any exchange. It was traded on the granddaddy of them all, the New York Stock Exchange.

A number of the companies that Wolfson, Weiner had were publicly held, they were traded over-the-counter. They were in the status as far as trading is concerned that Equity Funding had been back in the period 1964 to the time it was listed on the American Stock Exchange in 1966. In other words, slightly above a mom and pop oepration but hardly a Goliath. Most of these companies had been ones that Julian Weiner had himself promoted to take public as he had arranged to take Equity Funding public in 1964.

Julian Weiner, who was essentially a salesman, a promoter, getting companies to go public and talking to underwriters and arranging financings, and so forth, to him Equity Funding was the shining star in his galaxy, the major sign of his accomplishment, and that which could be used as a sales item to obtain additional clients.

If Equity Funding did poorly or if Equity Funding collapsed, like in the year ended '68 when all of a sudden it is not Funded Loans, it is $13,000,000 or more of reciprocals that is included in this account, if Equity Funding had collapsed there would go the major selling point that Julian Weiner had, major, big-time operation with which he was associated.

Furthermore, Equity Funding provided by far the largest audit fee that Wolfson, Weiner collected. For instance, in the early 1970's it was collecting, Wolfson & Weiner was, a fee of possibly $300,000 per year from Equity Funding. Its next major audit fee was around $75,000, the next one forty, and the next one twenty-five. So that all those three combined didn't add up to half of what Equity Funding paid to Wolfson, Weiner during this period of time.

Julian Weiner was managing to take out of the partnership by the late 1960's and early 1970's compensation for himself personally of about a hundred thirty to a hundred fifty thousand dollars per year.

One of the major supports for his firm up until the time it merged with Seidman & Seidman was Equity Funding Corporation of America.

Now, in connection with the merger with Seidman & Seidman, the fact Wolfson, Weiner had the account of Equity Funding was a major selling point in the attempt to have Wolfson, Weiner merge with Seidman & Seidman, because they could bring the Equity Funding account along with it to this more prestigious, more major outfit.

However, as the evidence will show, essentially the same people in charge of the Equity Funding account before the merger remained in charge of the Equity Funding account after the merger. There is some correspondence which we will show you indicating that Julian Weiner was the partner that was to remain on the job and Solomon Block was to be the person that would remain involved with the day-to-day paperwork, the field work at Equity Funding in connection with developing the audits.

But Julian Weiner gained in prestige and gained in security by managing to become now a partner in a genuine national accounting firm.

With respect to Marvin Lichtig, in addition to having a relatively nondemanding paper-pushing job doing the Equity Funding audit—and I think the evidence will show that there was a considerable amount of paperwork pushed, but basically it was pushed in circles—in addition to having that job Marvin Lichtig was given certain incentives to remain cooperative.

No. 1, back in about 1965 Jerome Evans gave Marvin Lichtig certain shares of stock in Equity Funding Corporation of America shortly after the public offering, the initial public offering.

So that Marvin Lichtig, while he was an independent auditor supposedly exercising an independent judgment and giving an independent hearing to the financial statements and the supporting data of Equity Funding Corporation of America, was also a stockholder of Equity Funding Corporation of America to the tune of 300 shares. But he couldn't hold these in his own name, so he put these shares in his wife's maiden name. He later sold these shares in 1967 and the proceeds of the sale went into the joint account, the joint bank account held in the name of Marvin Lichtig and his wife, Esther Lichtig, whose maiden name was Esther Borkin.

There was a second transaction in which Jerome Evans gave stock to Marvin Lichtig also, and this occurred in 1968, not too long before the disastrous yearend audit of 1968 in which John Templeton was involved and in which the receipts were discussed with the auditors and in which, for instance, although there was supposedly $35,000,000 worth of Funded Loans, in fact the details showed something about fifteen or even less, and whereas there were supposed commissions receivables that Fred Levin had prepared a memo about, no one ever checked to see whether there were actually these receivables, and on and on and on.

Then the greatest reward that Marvin Lichtig got was that after that audit, after that traumatic experience, when there had to be someone brought into the company who knew something about it, Jerry Evans having flown the coop, Marvin Lichtig was given a job at $40,000 a year as an executive vice president of the company, and treasurer.

He made the entries, as I mentioned, in 1969. Eventually his salary rose to $50,000. He signed the financial statements, signed the registration statements, and so forth, as the chief accounting officer of the company.

With respect to Solomon Block, Solomon Block at no time during the time that he was in charge of the Equity Funding engagement was a certified public accountant. He was a public accountant not certified by the state. He bounced around with several different jobs over the years until he finally found a home with Wolfson, Weiner in 1968.

When Marvin Lichtig went to the company Solomon Block was put on the Equity Funding audit to replace Lichtig. Now, that was a very, very prestigious position, to be the head field man in charge of the audit of a New York Stock Exchange company during the years when Equity Funding was one of the growth companies, one of the go-go companies, the big conglomerate whose earnings were going up and up and up. Block enjoyed the prestige of being in charge of that audit. He also enjoyed getting the continual salary increases. So that by the end of 1972 he was making in excess of $30,000 and was still not a certified public accountant.

Incidentally, he became a certified public accountant shortly after the exposure of the fraud.

In addition, Solomon Block enjoyed certain other things. For instance, the people at the company managed to get his son a job at the company. He got noninterest-bearing loans from Marvin Lichtig, who was now with the company and loaning money to the auditor who was supposedly exercising an independent judgment on the books and records, on the financial statements of Equity Funding. He got a $2,000 loan from Fred Levin, which he hasn't repaid to this day.

And he was, toward the end of '72 and the beginning of '73, while conducting the audit for the year ended 1972, soliciting from the company, from various people, from Sam Lowell, from Fred Levin, and from Michael Sultan, soliciting the offer of a job or talking about the possibility of a job for him comparable to the way that Marvin Lichtig had been given a job after his years of service as an auditor, a supposedly independent auditor of the financial statements.

As I have mentioned on several occasions, in April of 1973, beginning of April of 1973, actually the end of March 1973, because of the rumors the company just fell apart. The major officers of the company were asked to resign and did so. A court-appointed trustee was put in charge of the company and he brought auditors in who were also court-appointed.

Among the things that they found among the items that they wrote off were Funded Loans and accounts receivable of more than $62,000,000. Receivables supposedly related to the contractual plans they wrote off more than $12,000,000. Commercial paper they wrote off more than $8,000,000.

This commissions receivable that had started out back in '68 and had the bogus entry put in in 1970 and then never changed between then and the end of 1972, that was written off, $3,993,266.

There was an account known as Excess Deposits From Bishops Bank, which had also been developed in a conversation between Sam Lowell and Julian Weiner. That was phony and that was written off to the tune of $2,717,538.

There was a supposed receivable from a subsidiary of Pennsylvania Life—well, I am not sure exactly of the name of the company of which it was a sub, but it was related to Pennsylvania Life Insurance Company, now located out in Santa Monica. That receivable was written off and it was in the amount of $2,850,000.

There were certain fictitious exploration costs which were on the books, $1,816,475. There were certain supposed receivables from agents known as Debit Balances, which we will go into in a little bit more detail in the evidence, of $2,153,217.

And the total, over $100,000,000 worth of assets on the books, many of which had been there for substantial periods of time and which had been growing and growing. The total had been growing and growing and growing, where at the beginning of April of 1973, utterly fictitious. And when auditors came in and did an examination and did conduct a hearing, independent of any influence by the company and didn't turn their heads and did apply auditing standards and did apply generally accepted accounting principles, were written off of Equity Funding's books.

That basically is the evidence that the Government will present or an outline of the evidence that the Government will present.

Recall that I said at the beginning that I can't tell it all. Although you have been listening for a long time and it seems like in that period of time maybe I should have been able to tell it all, there are many, many more details of substantial items which will be the subject of evidence at the trial, but will fit into the framework that I have laid for you in my opening remarks.

(Mr. Newman concluded his opening remarks and the trial continued with proceedings on the materiality of false or misleading information. At this point Judge Curtis is speaking to the attorneys.)

The Court: Well, gentlemen, as I understand the law the crime is furnishing material which is materially false. Whether it is materially false is to be measured by what a reasonable person under the circumstances would believe. It does not depend upon whether the person who received it relied on it or not in a criminal action. The crime is furnishing this materially false material.

That will be my holding, therefore, that unless I am convinced to the contrary somewhere along the line, which I think you will probably not be able to do, but I will listen, the evidence as to whether or not the statements made are materially false or not will be received. But I will not permit any further interrogation as to what other materials either the New York Stock Exchange or any of these other agencies relied upon.

We will deal with the material. You can bring in such testimony as you can with respect to whether or not a reasonable person would consider the misrepresentations material.

Mr. Abeles: May I make an inquiry of the court, your Honor?

The Court: Yes.

Mr. Abeles: Wouldn't the fact of whether or not the New York Stock Exchange relied on the document be evidence as to whether or not it is a material fact?

The Court: I don't think so.

Mr. Abeles: All right.

The Court: If they relied on it, that's one thing. They may not have relied on it.

It is the same thing where a person attempts to cash a forged check. He is charged with defrauding the Government. It doesn't make any difference whether the Government is defrauded or not, it is whether the defendant intended to defraud the Government and whether he had the instrumentalities by which he could defraud the Government.

The crime here is furnishing the material. We have to look at the material at the time it is furnished to determine whether it is materially false by a standard which does not depend upon whether the receiving agency looked at it and relied upon it or not.

(One of the early witnesses called was Jerome H. Evans. Mr. Evans was Treasurer of Equity Funding until February, 1969. Here he explains stock transactions with Marvin Lichtig while Lichtig was an auditor for Wolfson Weiner.)

By Mr. Newman:

Q. Would you explain, please, how the stock transactions that you recall that you had with Marvin Lichtig came about, including approximately when and the circumstances of how it arose?

A. Stanley Goldblum, Michael Riordan, and some other parties, I don't know who they were, purchased out all the outstanding shares that were held by Eugene Cuthbertson, who was one of the principals of the company. They paid at the time $7 a share. And I mentioned shortly after the transaction that I was not offered any chance to participate in that deal. Stanley Goldblum said to me that at some later date he would sell me 1,000 shares at that same $7 and that Michael Riordan would also sell me 1,000 shares at that same $7 price. And he said there was no hurry, whenever I was ready they would take care of it.

About two years later I approached Stanley Goldblum and told him I wanted this transaction to take place. And he told me that he would be able to give me the 1,000 shares and Michael Riordan mentioned to me that he could only sell me 500 at the time.

Now, since the time of the original transaction and the time I approached them to buy it there had been a 3-for-2 stock split. So it became that I would purchase 1,500 shares from Stanley Goldblum and 750 from Michael Riordan, still based at that $7 original price.

And they said being that when they purchased they borrowed money to do so, that they were going to charge me interest for the two-year period, which I felt was fair.

At that time I had mentioned the transaction to Marvin Lichtig and he said, "Gee, wouldn't it be nice" if he could participate in the deal.

I went to Stanley Goldblum and mentioned it to him. And he says why don't I sell some of these shares to Marvin Lichtig, which I proceeded to do, which was the original 500 block or 750 shares based on a 3-for-2 stock split. And he paid me the same $7 plus the interest that I had paid for it.

Q. Was the stock selling for $7 at that time?
A. No, it was selling for much more.

(Another witness called as a witness for the Government was Michael Sultan. A C.P.A., he was an officer of Equity Funding Corporation of America from May, 1969 through March, 1973. He held the positions of Assistant Controller, Controller and Vice President.)

Q. During your time, Mr. Sultan, at Equity Funding Corporation of America did you have occasion to make journal entries?
A. Yes, I did.

Q. And did you have occasion to direct others to make journal entries?
A. Yes, I did.

Q. Did you have occasion from time to time to receive instructions from Sam Lowell about journal entries that should be made?
A. Yes.

Q. And did you have occasion during at least a portion of the period you were with the company to receive instructions from Stanley Goldblum concerning journal entries that should be made?
A. Yes.

Q. Now, directing your attention, Mr. Sultan, to approximately the end of the first quarter of 1970, which would be right around the end of March or the beginning of April of 1970, do you recall having a conversation or several conversations with Sam Lowell concerning the making of journal entries relating to so-called reciprocals?
A. Yes, I did.

                    *   *   *

Q. Would you explain, Mr. Sultan, how that conversation came about?
A. Yes. I had been working with Sam Lowell on preparing the first quarter report, and there were certain entries that Sam wanted to be made which consisted of increasing a funded loan and increasing insecurities income or insurance income. And it was explained to me at the time that this was recip, recip meaning monies due the corporation from—I would have to say like kickbacks from mutual funds.

Q. And did you proceed to make some of those entries at that time, Mr. Sultan?
A. Yes, I did.

Q. And did Mr. Lowell tell you the amount in which to make those entries?
A. Yes, he did.

Q. Was anyone else present at this conversation that you had with Sam Lowell?
A. Not that I recall.

                    *   *   *

Q. Mr. Sultan, was that the only such meeting that you had with Sam Lowell in 1970?
A. No.

Q. By such meeting I mean referring to this item of recip, or were there similar meetings subsequently in 1970?
A. Yes, there were other meetings.

Q. Did those meetings fall into the same pattern or were they in a different pattern from the meeting that you had at the end of the first quarter in 1970?

A. They were principally the same, but the explanations were getting a little different.

Q. And what were the explanations in the subsequent meetings?

A. At some point in time, I don't recall whether it was the second quarter of '70 or the third quarter of '70, I had completed the financial statements as far as I could go and went up to Sam Lowell's office, and he had indicated to me that the earnings per share for this particular quarter would have to be such and such, how much income did I have per the financial statements.

And I gave him the financial statements that I had worked up. And he actually made a calculation going backwards, multiplying the earnings per share that he wanted to obtain—attain by the number of shares outstanding, and came up with a net income figure and then determined that—I don't recall the amount, approximately a million or two million dollars was needed in additional recip.

At this time I had realized that recip was something that I felt—or he explained to me we really were not going to collect, but it was a plug to the income statement.

Q. Did you make journal entries based on these subsequent meetings, Mr. Sultan?

A. Yes, I did.

Q. And did those journal entries increase commission income, insurance and commission income securities?

A. Yes, it did.

Q. And did they also increase the asset account funded loans?

A. Yes.

Q. Mr. Sultan, did you have similar meetings in 1971 and 1972 through February of 1973?

A. Yes, I did.

Q. Were the participants in those meetings always the same, that is, you and Sam Lowell or at some point in time was there an evolution of the participants in these meetings?

A. In 1972 I had more contact with Stan Goldblum as it relates to what the earnings per share were to be, and he would discuss with me that—Stan Goldblum would say, "I would like earnings per share to be 42 cents," or some number.

Then at that point in time I would actually go and calculate what the difference between what the company had attained versus what was needed to attain to get to that earnings per share.

                    *   *   *

Q. Mr. Sultan, do these represent genuine asset and income entries?

A. No. These are bogus entries.

Q. Do they have any connection, Mr. Sultan, with the entries that you have testified you were making following your periodic conversations with Sam Lowell and Stan Goldblum?

A. Yes, they do.

Q. What connection is that?

A. These are the entries that were made increasing the funded loan and increasing income.

Q. Mr. Sultan, with respect to genuine entries which would go to funded loans and to commission income and securities income in one form of a journal entry or another, were there some kinds of source documents or back-up material showing what kind of entries should be made and in what amounts?

A. Yes, there was.

Q. What kind of back-up material would that be in general?

A. It would be a computer run.

Q. With respect to the entries which are in Exhibit 204, Mr. Sultan, were there any source documents supporting—I beg your pardon. 204, the exhibit you are looking at. Were there any source documents supporting those entries?

A. No, none whatsoever.

Q. Were there any source documents manufactured to support them?

A. No.

                    *   *   *

Q. Mr. Sultan, did you have occasion while you were working at the company to have dealings with the independent auditors who are supposed to audit Equity Funding's financial statements?

A. Yes.

Q. Did you know the defendant Solomon Block?

A. Yes, I did.

Q. Was he one of the auditors?

A. Yes, he was.

Q. While you were there what position did he hold in relation to the audit?

                    *   *   *

The Witness: He was the manager of the Equity Funding Corporation of America job and with the day-to-day responsibility of supervising the staff of—

*   *   *

Q. Mr. Sultan, were the general ledgers made available to the staff of the independent auditors?

A. Yes.

Q. General ledgers of Equity Funding Corporation of America and its subsidiaries?

A. Yes.

Q. And were the groups of journal entries made available to them?

A. Yes.

Q. Mr. Sultan, did Sol Block ever question you concerning any of the logic behind your bogus entries there to increasing funded loans and increasing securities and insurance commission income?

The Witness: No, he did not.

By Mr. Newman:

Q. Did Mr. Block ever ask you for any of the back-up behind those entries?

A. No, he did not.

Q. Did you ever have any phony back-up ready for him?

A. No, I did not.

(Another witness called by the Government was Al Finci. Finci is a partner in the accounting firm of Seidman & Seidman. He was partner in charge of Beverly Hills office from 1969-1973. Here he discusses some of the discussions he had with Julian Weiner concerning the merger of Wolfson, Weiner into Seidman & Seidman.)

Q. Directing your attention, now, to the date of October 21st of 1971, did you participate in a meeting on that date at which the defendant Julian Weiner was also present?

A. Yes.

Q. Where did that meeting take place?

A. It took place at lunch at Hillcrest Country Club in Los Angeles.

Q. Was there anyone else present at the meeting besides yourself and the defendant Weiner?

A. Yes. Mr. Wolfson, who was a partner of Mr. Weiner, was also present. And Mr. Spencer, who was a partner of Seidman & Seidman was also present.

Q. Was that a business meeting or a social meeting?

A. It was a business meeting.

Q. What was the purpose of the meeting?

A. We discussed the possibilities of the Wolfson, Weiner firm merging with Seidman & Seidman.

Q. Do you recall whether or not at that meeting either Mr. Wolfson or Mr. Weiner indicated why Wolfson, Weiner desired to merge with Seidman & Seidman?

A. Yes.

Q. Who said it and what was said?

A. Well, we had really several discussions that began at that particular meeting that we are describing now.

I do recall that at the initial meeting Mr. Weiner had indicated that he personally was disenchanted with the Wolfson, Weiner, Ratoff & Lapin partnership, well, primarily because of the way that the other partners—the partners outside of Los Angeles—of the Los Angeles office wanted to share profits at least initially, and because of that reason he wanted to merge with another national firm.

Q. At that initial meeting did either Mr. Wolfson or Mr. Weiner indicate who the major clients of Wolfson, Weiner were?

A. They did talk about several of their major clients. They did talk especially about Equity Funding Corporation of America as the most important client of theirs.

Q. Again, at that initial meeting do you recall if either Mr. Wolfson or Mr. Weiner indicated whether or not Wolfson, Weiner had any particular area of expertise?

A. Well, Mr. Weiner talked about his accounting expertise. I don't believe that that was right at that particular meeting. But at some of the subsequent meetings we received from him copies of articles on some technical subjects that he had written for a particular magazine. And he told us about his ability to develop important concepts of accounting for various companies. Again he mentioned Equity Funding in that connection very much.

Both Mr. Wolfson and Mr. Weiner talked about their abilities to obtain clients, generally small-or medium-size companies that were either publicly held or just about ready to become publicly held.

*   *   *

Q. During the meetings at which both you and the defendant Weiner were present, would you tell us, please, what the major topic or topics of conversation were with regard to the proposed merger?

A. Well, I related to you that we were told about

their practice in general and that it consisted primarily of small-and medium-size companies that were publicly held or about to become publicly held.

They did talk a great deal about Equity Funding. They indicated to us that a substantial portion of their fees, approximately 20 percent or so, was coming from Equity Funding, and it was their hope that if they would merge with a larger national firm that they would be able to get additional work from Equity Funding and that these fees could increase substantially and possibly go as high as $500,000 a year.

Q. Do you recall whether or not Mr. Weiner indicated what the annual fees derived from Equity Funding were?

A. Oh, the figure that I recall is approximately $200,000.

Q. Was there any discussion at these meetings about the ability of Wolfson, Weiner to keep Equity Funding as a client after the merger, if a merger took place?

A. Well, we had some concern on that subject, because Equity Funding was the major client of Wolfson, Weiner's firm. We were assured by Mr. Weiner and Mr. Wolfson that they would be retained. They told us about the great loyalty of Equity Funding management toward them, especially because of the great work they had done for them when the company initially went public in helping Equity Funding to sell their concept to the Securities and Exchange Commission.

*   *   *

Q. Mr. Finci, during the period before the agreement was executed do you recall whether or not you discussed with the defendant Weiner how Seidman & Seidman would assign partners to be partners in charge of clients that came as a result of the agreement between Wolfson, Weiner and Seidman & Seidman?

A. Yes, I do recall.

Q. What did you tell the defendant Weiner?

A. We explained to Mr. Weiner and Mr. Wolfson that it was the policy of Seidman & Seidman that every client would be assigned to a particular partner who would be responsible for all engagements in connection with that particular client.

We have also requested that they submit to us the list of their clients and decide among themselves which partner will be responsible for which clients.

Q. When you say which partner, are you referring to either Mr. Wolfson or Mr. Weiner?

A. That is correct.

Q. In other words, did you discuss with the defendant Weiner that either Mr. Wolfson or Mr. Weiner would become a partner in charge of the clients that they brought with them once the agreement was executed?

A. That is correct. That is correct.

Q. Did the defendant Weiner become the partner in charge of any of the clients that were brought to Seidman & Seidman as a result of the executed agreement?

A. Yes.

Q. Was Equity Funding one of those?

A. Yes, it was.

Q. Mr. Finci, prior to the time that the agreement was signed, again, did you discuss with the defendant Weiner what responsibilities, if any, the partner assigned as the partner in charge of a particular client would have for signing, for instance, the auditors' report to the financial statements that would be issued?

A. With respect to that instance, yes, we covered that subject and we notified them that partners in the firm were responsible for signing audit reports or any other reports that went out in the firm name.

Q. Was there any discussion as to whether or not any other member of the auditing staff other than the partner in charge could sign such reports?

A. No. I think it was made very clear, it was definitely made very clear that no one other than a partner was allowed to sign these audit reports or other reports issued by the firm.

Q. Was there any discussion, Mr. Finci, with the defendant Weiner as to what responsibilities, if any, a partner in charge of a particular client would have with respect to review of the audit workpapers relative to that client?

A. Yes. We had discussions with Mr. Weiner and Mr. Wolfson relating to responsibilities of partners, and in discussing audit responsibilties we told them that in our firm it was the responsibility of the partner to see that all of the work was properly done and reviewed and that the partner himself has to have that responsibility.

Q. After the combination of the practices of Wolfson, Weiner and Seidman & Seidman, did the defendant Solomon Block become a Seidman & Seidman employee?

A. Yes.

Q. What position did he have at Seidman & Seidman?
A. He was a principal.
Q. Do you recall whether or not the defendant Block was advised as to what responsibility, if any, a principal at Seidman & Seidman would have?
A. Yes.
Q. What was said to the defendant Block?
A. On February 21st and February 24th Seidman & Seidman held an orientation session for the entire staff on the 21st, and for principals and managers on the 24th, to tell them about responsibilities that they would have at their level, and Mr. Block was present at those meetings.
Q. Mr. Finci, was the defendant Block the principal in charge of any particular client of Seidman & Seidman after the combination?
A. Yes.
Q. What client was that?
A. He was responsible for Equity Funding Corporation of America, another company called Wavecom, and I believe there was another company called Golden Age. There may have been others, but those are the three I recall at the present time.
Q. At the time of the combination of Wolfson, Weiner and Seidman & Seidman practices, sir, was the 1971 audit of Equity Funding completed or was it still in progress?
A. It was still in progress.
Q. In connection with the 1971 audit of Equity Funding, did Seidman & Seidman personnel who were not previously employed by Wolfson and Weiner work on the audit of Equity Funding's books?
A. No.
Q. Again, in connection with that audit was there any review of the audit workpapers of Equity Funding by Seidman & Seidman personnel who had not previously been employed by Wolfson and Winer?
A. No.

(The next witness called was Samuel Lowell, Controller and Executive Vice President of Equity Funding. Lowell discusses numerous examples of the auditors' involvement in the fraud.)

Q. Mr. Lowell, in connection with the preparation of the yearend 1969 financial statements and the preparation of the audited financials, and so forth, did you have occasion to attempt to assemble detailed support for the amount which was to be reported as funded loans receivable?
A. Yes.
Q. Initially, Mr. Lowell, were you able to assemble sufficient detailed support?
A. Initially, no.
Q. By how much did the detailed support fall short?
A. Initially we were probably about fifteen million, no more than that. I think close to it.
Q. In the millions?
A. Pardon?
Q. In the millions?
A. In the millions. Probably $20,000,000, somewhere in that range.
Q. What accounted, Mr. Lowell, for the shortfall?
A. The recip we had booked, Ralph.
Q. What, if anything, did you do in connection with tryint to find some detailed support or locate some detailed support?
A. Well, I went to Stanley Goldblum first and Stanley told me to meet with Julie (Weiner).

* * *

Q. Following that did you meet with the defendant Weiner?
A. Yes, I did.
Q. Do you recall where that meeting took place?
A. It was in my office.
Q. Was that meeting soon after or a long time after the meeting that you had with Stanley?
A. Soon.
Q. Was anyone else there besides you and the defendant Winer?
A. I think just Julie and myself.
Q. Did you have a discussion at that time about the shortfall of detail?
A. Yes, we did.
Q. What, if anything, was said by you and by him?
A. Well, he suggested a variety of things, mainly, one was holding the books open.
Q. What does holding the books open mean, Mr. Lowell?
A. Well, items that you sell in January and February and March you hold the books open and record them as if they had been sold in December of the previous year.
Q. Did Equity Funding Corporation of America ever in fact do that during the years that you were there, Mr. Lowell?
A. Yes, every year.
Q. Now, in doing so did Equity Funding Corporation of America bring into the current

year the expenses associated with the income pulled in from the subsequent year?

A. The expenses?

Q. Yes..

A. No, sir, we were trying to create income, not expense.

Q. Did Mr. Weiner say anything in this meeting concerning whether this had been an historical practice at Equity Funding?

A. He made a statement to the effect that Jerry had always been able to do it this way.

Mr. Abeles: I'm sorry. I can't hear.

The Witness: He made a statement to that effect, something about Jerry had done it this way. Jerry Evans.

*   *   *

Q. Mr. Lowell, directing your attention to approximately the second half of 1970, sometime in the second half of 1970 do you recall having a conversation with the defendant Weiner concerning whether the defendant Block should remain on the Equity Funding audit?

A. Yes.

Q. Can you pin the time down any more than in "the second half of 1970?

A. It was about the time they were going to start coming in to do their work. It was shortly before, actually. Maybe September or October, around there.

Q. Do you recall whether anybody else was present at the conversation?

A. Julie Weiner was present, and Stan Goldblum.

Q. So you and Stan Goldblum and Julian Weiner were there?

A. Yes.

Q. Do you recall where that conversation took place?

A. Stanley's office.

Q. Would you recount, please, to the best of your recollection, what was said?

A. At the meeting?

Q. Yes.

A. Well, we discussed, I guess, the problem of Sol. He was creating a lot of problems for us and was digging into things we didn't want him digging into, sort of thing, and just, you know, being overzealous. We didn't want him on the audit. Julie said that he was the only one in his office suited for the audit. And he used the word "Sol was," and I quote, remember this word "flexible," and was suited for our audit because of that, and there were other topics, too.

Mr. Abeles: Could the witness speak up?

By the Witness:

A. Sorry. There were some other topics. I remember a discussion of the fact that Sol wasn't a CPA. I was concerned about whether that complied with the auditing standards. And Julie indicated we didn't have to be concerned about that because he was a CPA and, you know, he was in charge of the audit and that satisifed the requirement.

I believe at the same meeting there was also some discussion of Sol's possibly having taken a coemployee to Las Vegas.

Mr. Abeles: I'm sorry. I can't hear the witness.

By the Witness:

A. I believe at that meeting there was also a discussion of Sol's having taken a coemployee to Las Vegas and I guess for obvious reasons we were concerned, you know, that anything out of the normal would draw attention to ourselves or our auditors.

By Mr. Newman:

Q. Mr. Lowell, following that conversation did the defendant Block remain on the Equity Funding audit?

A. Yes, he did.

Mr. Newman: Your Honor, may Government's Exhibits 210 and 232 be placed in front of the witness, please? 210 is a journal entry and should be in a thin folder. On the table next to the reporter. *(Exhibits passed to witness.)*

By Mr. Newman:

Q. Mr. Lowell, would you please examine Exhibit 210 and then Exhibit 232-A?

Mr. Lowell, do you recall in late 1970 working on an analysis of Equity Funding Corporation of America's investment in Bishops Bank?

A. Yes.

Q. Do you recall the purpose for which you were working on that analysis?

A. As I recall, in connection with an underwriting prospectus additional information was to be disclosed.

Q. Did you encounter—excuse me.

A. Additional narrative information was to be disclosed in the prospectus. And at the request of, I believe it was, Peter Panarites, as I recall. And in developing that information we found out the figures didn't jibe.

Q. When you say the figures didn't jibe, what do you mean?

A. The figures that we had, the information that we had didn't tie into what we had been showing in the prospectus.

Q. In what respect, Mr. Lowell, did those figures not tie in?

A. One of them was a few million dollars higher than the other.

Q. In connection with that, Mr. Lowell, did you have any discussion with Julian Weiner concerning the problem?

A. After we had analyzed it, yes, we did.

Q. Do you recall how that conversation came about?

A. Well, we found that at least $2,000,000 worth of our error apparently resulted from something that either the auditors and/or Marvin had done. Essentially, a duplicate recording of an investment in Bishops Bank.

Q. When had the error been reflected, Mr. Lowell?

Mr. DeSantis: Your Honor, before that question is answered I will move to strike out unless the witness can testify to who made the error.

The Court: Overruled.

By Mr. Newman:

Q. Had the error been reflected on any previous financial statement?

A. Yes, it had. It had occurred in 1969. Well, we were concerned about it and I didn't want—I thought we were going to have to restate the accounts. And I didn't want it to go through the current year's income, I wanted to adjust the prior year's.

   So I called Julie and set up a meeting in my office, told him about the problem, told him I was concerned, I wanted to run it through retained earnings or something.

Q. When you say run it through retained earnings, does that mean it would go as writeoffs of expense, or what?

A. I wanted him to find some way to bypass the income and expense statement so that it would not show up as an expense. And he said not to worry about it, that that was an audited year and once the year was audied it was closed.

   And then I told him, "Well, in that case I can handle everything, correct all the accounts," as long as Sol and his people didn't get into what the beginning balances were to try and verify it.

Q. Did you work on any journal entries then which would correct the accounts or adjust the accounts?

A. Yes, I did.

*   *   *

Q. Mr. Lowell, would you open Exhibit 230, please. It's a file with a number of documents. And Exhibit 230-D and 230-H. Have you looked at them?

A. Yes, I have.

Q. Do you recall two assets listed on the books at the end of 1970, that is, Equity Funding Corporation of America's books entitled Investment in Banque Jourdaan and Investment in Banco Unione?

A. Yes, I do.

Q. Were those two assets genuine or fictitious?

A. Fictitious.

Q. Do you recall whether during the 1970 audit by Wolfson, Weiner confirmations were provided to the auditors on those two times?

A. Yes, they were.

Q. Were those confirmations genuine or were they fictitious?

A. Fictitious.

Q. Were those confirmations provided at the same time or at different time than each other?

A. They were provided at different times.

Q. Would you explain the circumstances leading up to the providing of the first of the confirmations?

A. By the first you mean Banco Unione?

Q. Well, no, not the first in the file, but the first of the confirmations that was provided to the auditors.

A. As I recall, the first was Banque Jourdaan. It hadn't been classified as cash, it was classified as a, I think, securities investment, or something like that. And they hadn't confirmed it in previous years but this year Sol started a project, he wanted to confirm it. Obviously we didn't want him to confirm it because there was nothing there.

   So I called Julie. And I had a meeting with Julie and told Julie that it related to recip and couldn't be determined, but that if he would give me a blank—he told me he had to have a confirmation. Sol was raising a fuss. So I said, "Give me a blank confirmation and I will make one up for you."

Q. At that time did that meeting terminate?

A. Yes.

Q. How did you go about making up a confirmation?

A. I had Mike Sultan type up a confirmation. They give us a form for it. Then I guess Mike traced the signature—the signature, I think, it's traced, a real signature of somebody who we had correspondence with at that bank at one time, I think. I am not certain of that. But he signed it.

Q. Did he give it back to you?

A. Unione—yes. Jourdaan, he gave back to me.

Q. We are speaking of Jourdaan. Did he give it back to you?

A. Yes.

Q. What if anything did you do with it?

A. Gave it to Julie.

Q. How did that come about?

A. He was in my office for a meeting. I had been holding it in my desk drawer. And I gave him the confirmation. I said, "Here's the confirmation."

Q. Mr. Lowell, is this confirmation on a standard bank confirmation form?

A. Right. It's one of their forms.

Q. Well, when you say "they," who do you mean?

A. Wolfson, Weiner, Ratoff & Lapin. It's a standard form that the accountant has his name printed on.

Q. What about with respect to Banco Unione, Mr. Lowell, do you recall how that confirmation came about to be made?

A. Same type of problem; we had an asset, it was not classified as cash, it was classified elsewhere.

Q. In an investment account?

A. Yes. Sol wanted to confirm it, was putting pressure on. And Julie told me to get him a confirmation. So I told Mickey to make up another confirmation for Banco Unione.

Q. Do you recall where that conversation took place?

A. It was in the men's room, 28th floor.

Q. In the men's room?

A. In the men's room.

Q. Mr. Block—

A. Sorry.

Q. —do you recall about when it took place in the course of the audit?

A. I think it was pretty well cleaned up. Must have been in the very last stages.

Q. Mr. Lowell, what, if anything, was said about the postmark?

A. Sol made some joke about the Italians or Swiss using Los Angeles postmarks on their letters, and I said something to the effect of "Very funny."

Q. Did anything come of that, Mr. Lowell?

A. No, not that I know of.

Q. Mr. Lowell, were those Grandson notes paid off or shown as being paid off in February of 1972 when they were supposed to be?

A. No.

Q. Did they remain on the books of Equity Funding Corporation of America through March of 1973?

A. Yes, they did.

Q. Did you have Mr. Sultan give you back that confirmation?

A. No. I told him to mail it to Julie. And he thought I was out of my mind at the time. I told him just to mail it and not to worry about it.

(The proceedings continued with Lowell explaining the activities related to confirmation of the notes of Establissement Grandson.)

Q. Did you supply notes to the Wolfson, Weiner auditors?

A. Yes, I did.

Q. And did you arrange for a confirmation?

A. Yes, I did.

Q. How did you arrange for a confirmation?

A. We had them mail a confirmation to our bank in Switzerland—not our bank, but a bank we used in Switzerland, and Joe Golan picked them up there at the maildrop and signed them.

Q. And were they returned to the auditors?

A. Yes, when Joe came to the United States he mailed them.

Q. Now, with respect to the confirmation, Mr. Lowell, did you have occasion to have a conversation subsequent to the mailing of the confirmation with the defendant Block concerning the postmark on the envelope which returned the confirmation?

A. Yes, I did.

(As the proceedings continued, Lowell discussed Equity Funding's desire to be audited by a major accounting firm and his discussions with Weiner concerning this matter.)

Q. Do you recall approximately when these discussions began?

A. It should be about the time we went to the New York Stock Exchange. It would be what, October of '70? So it would be before that. I don't remember the fellow's name at the Stock Exchange, but he brought it up when we were sort of having our clearing meetings.

Q. When you say "he" brought it up, was it at a meeting which was attended by various people?

A. You mean the requirement that we get a larger accounting firm?

A. Yes.

Q. Yes.

A. No. As I recall, it came through our underwriter or someone, I don't remember exactly who, now, who came to Stan and I—we were at the Exchange—and told us that one of the "requirements" would be that we get a major accounting firm.

Q. Subsequent thereto did you begin having discussions with the defendant Weiner concerning his combining his practice with a larger accounting firm?

A. Yes. I began to be present at those discussions.

                    *   *   *

Q. Did you have any discussions with Mr. Weiner concerning your experiences with Alexander Grant?

A. Yes.

Q. Would you relate the discussions that you had with Mr. Weiner concerning the possible combination of Wolfson, Weiner with Alexander Grant?

A. Yes. I told Mr. Weiner in Mr. Goldblum's presence that we had had some problems with them as to a fellow, Shelley, who had been a local accountant who had merged with them. He did some work for us on a cattle ranch, as I recall.

Q. Is that on the ones in Colorado?

A. The ranch is located in Colorado, but Shelley did his work in our offices in Los Angeles. And that they told him they wouldn't review the working papers and they wouldn't interfere, and that when he come out to do the work they had had all sorts of people from Chicago looking over his shoulder and, you know, just really giving us a bad time, and that we were very reluctant for him to go with Alexander Grant, and would like to give it a lot more throught.

   Then later he came back. And I think it was Wolf & Company, and Wolf & Company on the surface seemed to be very good because they were very heavy in MAS, management advisory services, and apparently, from what we could find out, Stanley and I, now didn't have much of an auditing team. But Stanley got a very adverse reaction from Wall Street. He called analysts, they didn't like Wolfe & Company.

   So Stanley kind of killed that deal. Then the next one was Seidman & Seidman.

Q. Do you recall when the first discussions came up concerning the possible combination of Wolfson, Weiner with Seidman & Seidman?

A. Very early in 1971, I would say maybe late in 1970.

Q. Pardon me?

A. Possibly late in 1970 or early '71.

Q. Did you participate in some of these discussions?

A. Yes, I did.

Q. Did Stanley Goldblum participate in some of these discussions?

A. Yes, he did.

Q. Prior to the combination of Wolfson, Weiner with Seidman & Seidman were there any discussions with the defendant Weiner concerning who would be in charge of the Equity Funding audit following the combination, if there was to be a combination?

A. Yes.

Q. Do you recall who participated in those discussions?

A. Definitely Stanley and I were there. And I think at least at one of these discussions Phil Wolfson was there.

Q. Was Julian Weiner also present?

A. Also, yes. The discussion was with Julian Weiner.

Q. Was there more than one such discussion?

A. Yes. There was also a discussion where we had people from Seidman & Seidman there.

Q. Prior to the discussions at which Seidman & Seidman were present, Mr. Lowell, would you recount what the conversations were concerning who would or would not be in charge of the Equity Funding audit following the combination?

A. The gist of it was that Julie had assured us that he had been assured by them that he would continue to be on the audit and that we would continue having Sol on the audit. And he says, "There might be changes in the lower level staff."

   And, as I recall, Phil Wolfson reaffirmed this, that this was the case.

Q. With respect to the meeting that took place in which there were Seidman & Seidman personnel also present, do you recall where that meeting took place?

A. Well, it started out in Stanley's office. Stanley Goldblum's office. There was a meeting in my office. And there was a luncheon at a country club on Pico Boulevard. I don't know.

Q. Do you recall who from Equity Funding attended that luncheon?

A. I think I was the only one from Equity Funding.

Q. Do you recall who, if anybody, from Wolfson, Weiner attended that luncheon?

A. Julie was there, I'm certain. I believe Julie was the only one from Wolfson, Weiner.

Q. Do you recall who attended that luncheon from Seidman & Seidman?

A. A fellow named Robert Spencer, Joe DeArmas. I remember Robert Spencer. I think it was Joe DeArmas, or something along that line.

Q. Was there a discussion at that time, Mr. Lowell, concerning whether Seidman & Seidman would be given the audits of Equity Funding Life Insurance Company, Northern Life Insurance Company, and Liberty Savings and Loan?

A. There most certainly was.

Q. Was there a discussion at that time about who would be in charge of the Equity Funding audit?

A. Yes, there was.

Q. Would you recount what the conversation was?

A. Well, the meeting began in Stanley's office. Stanley brought up the topic of our wanting Julie and Sol to continue on the audit and not wanting any change in personnel. And I continued on in the same vein, particularly at the country club luncheon, along the lines of we had a lot of money invested in training them over the years and getting them acquainted with our unusual type of business and that Julie had been—I think it is probably true—one of the major ingredients in the early years of the company in keeping it, you know, going and helping it develop. And that if Seidman & Seidman was going to pur somebody else on the account, then we would just have to think about going to the Big Eight firm, but we would much rather be with Seidman & Seidman if we knew we were going to have the same quality of work that we had with Wolfson, Weiner.

Then the discussion immediately turned to which audits Seidman & Seidman was going to get.

They wanted the insurance company and the savings and loan, and so forth. And I left the meeting, it was my impression that we had an agreement.

Q. Mr. Lowell, for the year 1972 did Seidman & Seidman audit Liberty Savings and Loan?

A. Yes, they did, as I recall.

Q. Did they audit Equity Funding Life Insurance Company?

A. Yes.

Q. Did they audit Northern Life Insurance Company?

A. I think so, but I am not certain.

(After the Government examined Mr. Lowell, Mr. Abeles proceeded to cross-examine him. In this short excerpt, Lowell states that he instructed Mr. Mercado to conceal the fraud from the auditors working on the engagement.)

By Mr. Abeles:

Q. Mr. Lowell, I was asking you yesterday when we stopped—I believe that I had asked you had you instructed Mr. Mercado at the end of 1969 to insert $2 million in the funded loans receivable computer run.

A. Yes. I instructed him to increase the total by $2 million.

Q. And you also told Mr. Mercado, did you not, to conceal that from the auditors?

A. From the people working on the engagement, yes.

(After further cross-examination by Mr. Abeles and other defense attorneys a defendants' exhibit was read. It is a memorandum by Roy J. Horn, a certified public accountant.)

Mr. Markowitz: It is dated April 5, 1973, and it says:

"Super confidential, re: Equity Funding Corporation of America.

"On Friday, March 30, 1973, at approximately 11:45 a.m. I arrived at the office of Samuel B. Lowell for the purpose of meeting with Mr. Lowell to determine the extent of his financial situation and what remedies would be available to get him out of the financial mess that he obviously was in due to the sudden decline of Equity stock prices and Mr. Lowell's excessive borrowings against his Equity stock.

"At the beginning of the meeting I informed Mr. Lowell that I was aware that he had contemplated committing suicide earlier this week and that I was personally very concerned that he might feel that he had more than mere financial problems. I continued by telling him that suicide was no answer whatsoever that no matter how serious his problems were that both he and his family would be far, far better off facing those problems and that I as his personal tax adviser was willing to sit down and do everything legal and reasonable to aid him in resolving those problems. Sam (Mr. Lowell) acknowledged to me that he had more than just financial problems and said that he had to tell somebody something. I urged him to talk the situation over with somebody but pointed out that I was not an attorney and that he did not have a confidential relationship and that I was not willing to lie for anyone and that he had to take that into consideration before he decided to confide in me. Sam acknowledged my comments but stated that he has been finding out how few real friends that he had and that I may have been instrumental in his deciding against suicide earlier this week and that he felt I was a friend.

"Sam then proceeded to inform me that the rumors concerning Equity Funding were not only true but that a far worse situation had actually existed. He continued by stating that Fred Levin has maintained an office of approximately forty people here in Los Angeles preparing phony insurance policies and processing them through the company. Sam indicated that no money was involved in the creation of insurance policies inasmuch as they were taken into the company net of the commissions (which would have been 100 percent on the first year premiums).

"I asked him how they handled the renewal problem.

"Sam stated that Jim Banks would prepare phony death certificates on a number of the policies, that the proceeds collected thereunder would then be paid into the company in lieu of the net premium (net of commission) due on the renewals of the balance of the policies and in this manner they kept the necessary money flowing into the company. He elaborated by stating that they were so well organized that when the auditors sent out the confirmations Lloyd Edens would break into the auditor's office at night and substitute phony confirmations, or that is, confirmations with phony addresses on them which would direct the confirmations to an office in Chicago that a relative of Fred Levin's maintained where the confirmations would be signed and returned, and that Lloyd would once again break into the auditor's locked files and substitute signed confirmations with the addresses contained on the insurance policies so that the auditors were convinced that they were

receiving confirmations on the phony policies.

"I asked Sam who individually were all involved.

"Sam named Fred Levin, Art Lewis, Jim Banks, Lloyd Edens.

*   *   *

"I asked Sam if any of the other officers were involved.

"Sam said he doubted it as Stanley kept most of them 'out.' He doubted that either Herb Glaser or Rodney Loeb know anything as both were too honest to allow anything to go on. He indicated he once distrusted Marvin Lichtig but doubted that he knew anything either. He said he really did not know too many of the details himself.

"Sam further indicated that Stanley should have been aware of what was going on but that he was so happy with the 'earnings' that he never sought to question any more than he absolutely had to.

(The memorandum continues and concludes as follows:)

"This transcript was made on Saturday, March 31st, in the presence of a witness, Richard L. Horn, from notes dictated 'in rough' via a portable tape recorder en route to my office Friday afternoon, March 30th.

"Postscript:

"The above-referred tape and portable tape recorder disappeared or were taken from my office between 2:30 p.m. Saturday and 10:15 a.m. Sunday, April 1. No other articles were missing, however, I had removed all files relating to the above-named individuals on Friday evening.

"The theft of the tape recorder was reported to the West Valley Police Department Monday, April 2, 1973."

(The next witness called by the Government was Norman Grossman. Grossman is a CPA and a partner in the accounting firm of Touche Ross and Company. Touche Ross was the auditor for Equity Funding in bankruptcy appointed by the bankruptcy court. Grossman was given overall responsibility for the audit work.)

Q. Mr. Grossman, did Touche, Ross in fact perform an audit of Equity Funding Corporation of America and its subsidiaries?

A. Yes.

Q. Did that include all of the subsidiaries?

A. All of the subsidiaries except Bankers Life Insurance Company, the New Jersey insurance subsidiary.

Q. By whom if anybody was Bankers audited?

A. Bankers was audited by the firm of Coopers & Lybrand.

Q. Were there other individuals besides you, Mr. Grossman, from Touche, Ross who worked on the audit performed by Touche, Ross?

A. Yes; there were a substantial number of people who worked on the audit. Because of the magnitude of the work and the diversity of the operation, there were certain other partners assigned to specific parts of the company and there were supervisory employees and then field auditors working on the job. My responsibility over the entire work performed by our people.

(Grossman continues his testimony with a discussion of the funded loans.)

We accounted for the loan file to see that there were loan files for those customers—for the funded loans that existed.

We also did this to see if there were other loan files around that related to funded loans that we were not aware of that were not on the list supplied to us.

Upon conclusion of this work we found loan files for substantially all of the funded loans that were in the detail supplied to us.

There were only a few—I think the number was something like four loan files that were in the company's records for loans that we had no record of.

So, in other words, there were no extra loan files around that would indicate that there were a significant number of other funded loans.

Q. With respect—excuse me.

A. The collateral—this collateral confirmation established the same thing. We received no confirmation from either the custodial bank or the mutual fund transfer agents of mutual fund shares for accounts which we didn't have the detail for.

So that also gave us another support for the fact that there were no significant number of funded loans other than the ones that we knew about.

Q. Did you analyze any activity in the general ledger in connection with funded loans?

A. Yes. Because of the significant difference between the general ledger account and the detail that we were supplied and were working with we wanted to get a feeling of what caused this significant difference. Therefore, we analyzed the activity in the general ledger, the control account for the period from February 1, 1970, to April 5, 1973.

In doing so we found significant numbers of unsupported entries.

We accumulated and analyzed these. We then met with a former employee of Equity Funding, Mr. Sultan, and reviewed our findings with him. He confirmed to us that most of the entires for which there was no support were in fact fictitious entries.

So the work here really told us that there was a reason for the difference between the general ledger control and the detailed accounts to exist, that there should be a significant difference between the general ledger and the control because of these unsupported and fictitious entries.

Q. Mr. Grossman, in connection with the approximately four loan files that were not reflected on the computer runs of detail, were those loan files determined to represent legitimate funded loans?

A. Yes.

Q. As a result of Touche, Ross's work on the funded loan receivable account, was any adjustment made in the balance of funded loans receivable?

A. Yes, it was.

Q. How much?

A. $62,305,353 (indicating).

Q. On what grounds, Mr. Grossman, was the adjustment made?

A. The adjustment was made to—so that the general ledger record reflected the amount of the detail funded loans of the company—or the existing funded loans of the company.

The general ledger was brought into agreement with the actual amounts owed to the company.

Q. Now, Mr. Grossman, did that adjustment fall into Category 1 of the adjustments which you mentioned earlier in your testimony?

A. Which is Category 1, Mr. Newman?

Q. Category 1 is the category of fictitious and non-existent assets causing adjustments.

A. Yes, it did.

Q. Do you recall approximately what amount of funded loans receivable was determined to be genuine?

A. Approximately $44 million.

Q. In the course of your audit, Mr. Grossman, moving on now to a different account, did you conduct an examination of an account relating to the so-called client contractual receivable and the Estudios Asuntos transaction?

A. Yes, we did.

Q. As a result of Touche, Ross's work on that item was any balance sheet adjustment made?

A. Yes. The receivable was eliminated from the company's records and that adjustment resulted in the elimination of the receivable of $12,631,434.

Q. On what ground was that asset written off?

A. On the basis that there was no support for the validity of the receivable.

(Mr. Grossman continues with a discussion of other balance sheet items that needed adjustment or elimination. Though not all of the related testimony is included here, the following are some examples of the adjustments. In the first section, Grossman discusses the auditor's responsibility as related to the verification of receivables.)

A. It is an auditor's responsibility to evaluate the collectibility of receivables or the recoverability to the company of its receivables.

To do so—there are many different ways of doing it. Where you have an unsecured amount and it's a large amount you should know something about the ability of the debtor to repay the company. So you have to know something about its financial resources or how the amount is going to be repaid to the company.

Q. As a result of your audit on the notes receivable account, was there an adjustment made with respect to the Grandson note receivable?

A. Yes, it was.

Q. What adjustment was made?

A. The receivable was eliminated. The amount of the receivable on the books was $9,068,390.

Q. Would you explain on what facts and circumstances in more general terms, the ground on which your decision to write it off was based?

A. As to the presence or the status of Estudios at April 5?

Q. You mean Grandson?

A. I am sorry. Grandson at April 5, 1973. We could find nobody to communicate with at Grandson Company. We discussed with Mr. Ogg of the SEC the information he knew as a result of his investigation, and he informed us that to the best of his knowledge or what he had found was that Grandson was just a shell company with no real assets, it was a Liechtenstein organized company, but did not have any real assets or any real substance.

*   *   *

Q. In the course of your audit did you conduct an examination of an account on the books of the parent company, Equity Funding Corporation of America, relating to commercial paper?

A. Yes, we did.

Q. Did you obtain from company personnel a listing of the commercial paper supposedly reflected in that account?

A. Yes.

Q. What, if any, role did such a listing play in your audit?

A. From that listing we confirmed the commercial paper with the banks that were supposed to be holding the commercial paper.

We also after having mailed the confirmation then performed additional procedures.

Q. Is the confirmation of commercial paper with third-party outside sources a procedure which is in accordance with the application of generally accepted auditing standards for normal yearend audits?

A. Confirmation or examination is normal, yes.

Q. When you say "examination," does that mean physical observation?

A. Physical observation of the paper, yes, physical examination.

Q. As a result of your work on the commercial paper account was there any adjustment made in the balance on the books of Equity Funding Corporation of America?

A. Yes. $8,000,000 of commercial paper which did not exist was eliminated from the accounts.

(Mr. Abeles next began his cross-examination of the witness.)

By Mr. Abeles:

Q. Mr. Grossman, in your review of the workpapers and documents did you find any document or audit work prepared by Mr. Julian Weiner?

A. In the company files the only item that I saw that had any reference—it was not prepared by Mr. Weiner. There was an accounting entry made in the Grandson account to bring it back to the $9,000,000 original balance.

The explanation of that entry was "per conversation with Julian Weiner."

We did not examine the workpapers prepared by the Wolfson, Weiner firm in connection with its audit.

*   *   *

Q. Now, sir, the audits are not set up for the purpose of catching internal fraud, primarily, are they, sir?

A. That is correct.

Q. In fact, even the most scrupulous audit won't necessarily pick up fraud where there is a collusion by internal management; isn't that correct, sir?

A. It might not.

Q. Right. And in fact that has even happened to your firm, has it not, sir?

A. Yes, it has.

            *   *   *

Q. Mr. Grossman, you knew of fraudulent documents in Equity Funding Corporation of America, after starting the audit, did you not, sir?

A. We knew of certain of them, yes.

Q. As a matter of fact, this was not a usual audit that you conducted, was it, sir?

A. That is correct.

Q. In fact this was unlike any audit you have ever seen conducted before, was it not, sir?

A. I think in my recollection that is right, yes.

Q. In fact how many men did you have on this audit, sir?

A. Oh, approximately as many as seventy at one time.

Q. Seventy men at one time. In fact your fees for this audit were over $2 million, were they not?

A. That's right.

Q. A company of this size, of the size Equity Funding appeared to be, could not normally afford a $2 million audit, could it?

A. I don't know about afford. It is more—it is a more extensive audit than would normally be performed, yes, if that is what you mean.

Q. No company would willingly agree to an audit of that size, would it, sir?

Mr. Newman: Objection, your Honor. It calls for speculation and conclusion.

The Court: Sustained.

By Mr. Abeles:

Q. In fact you did almost a one hundred percent audit, did you not, sir?

A. In certain areas.

Q. Would you tell the jury what that means?

A. That where we had indications of fraud we did a one hundred percent verification. It might well be the funded loans was one area, the commercial paper would be another area.
In other parts of the audit we started out with the concept of doing a one hundred percent verification, significant verification. This was in some of the outlying or free standing entities, and as we became satisifed that there was no real fraud in those companies we then adjusted our audit procedures to sampling and testing.

Q. Now, it isn't normal to do a one hundred percent audit, is it, sir?

A. No, it is not.

Q. I believe you said it's—

A. It is not normal to examine one hundred percent of the items.

Q. As a matter of fact, under normal circumstances, say on funded loans receivable, if there were no 'other—no indications of fraud five or six percent or a few percent might be sufficient on statistical sampling, mightn't it?

A. Well, I guess it deals with the adequacy—by normal maybe I ought to define what I mean by normal. Normal is a company with adequate controls and no indication of fraud.

Q. All right.

A. That is how I would define normal. If you had those conditions then auditing standards permit testing in your verification process, but you have to make those conclusions.

Q. And the percentage then would become a judgment factor, would it not, sir?

A. Predominantly a judgment.

Q. And even the question of whether the internal controls are adequate is a judgment question also, isn't it, sir?

A. Withih ranges I would say it is a judgment.

            *   *   *

Q. Right. All right, sir. And in addition to—in addition to that you had the benefit of the information being supplied to you by the Securities and Exchange Commission, did you not, sir?

A. We were supplied some information by the Securities and Exchange Commission.

Q. Right. In fact, in many cases where you didn't know if an item was good or bad the Securities and Exchange Commission or the FBI or the law firm of O'Melveny & Myers would tell you "This asset is no good," would they not?

A. In certain of the area, yes, sir.

Q. Fine. And they would tell you that they had conducted extensive investigation, would they not, sir?

A. I am not sure extensive. They had certainly conducted investigations, yes.

Q. So you had the benefit of also all of this help from these other organizations, did you not, sir?

A. Yes.

(Fred Chazan was called as a defense witness. He was employed by Wolfson, Weiner and worked on the Equity Funding audits from 1968-1972.)

Q. Did you at any time see anything that caused you to think there was a fraud or anything wrong at Equity Funding?

A. No.

Q. Did you on any occasion on any audit receive any instructions from Julian Weiner?

A. No.

Q. Did you ever see Mr. Weiner working on the audit for any year?

A. No.

(Another defense witness was Robert Spencer, a partner in the firm of Seidman and Seidman. Here Spencer is testifying about a meeting he had with Samuel Lowell.)

Q. Was there any discussion of the role of Solomon Block at that meeting in connection with the Equity Funding audit?

A. None that I recall.

Q. Was there any discussion of the role of Julian Weiner in connection with the Equity Funding account at that meeting?

A. No; none that I recall.

Q. Was there any request direct or implied that Julian Weiner retain a position he had in connection with Equity Funding accounting?

A. No.

Q. Was there any request direct or implied that Solomon Block remain as the person in charge of the audit at Equity Funding?

A. No.

Q. In any of your conversations with Mr. Lowell did he ever imply directly or indirectly, that is, in any of the conversations in '72, that he wanted Mr. Block to remain in his position in connection with the audit at Equity Funding?

A. I don't recall any.

Q. Did Mr. Lowell at any of the conversations in 1972 suggest directly or indirectly that he wanted Mr. Weiner to continue working in connection with the Equity Funding account?

A. I don't recall any specific reference to that, no.

(Lawrence Berkowitz, an attorney and formerly with the Securities and Exchange Commission,

was called as a defense witness regarding the issue of reciprocal income.)

Q. Has it ever been illegal for a mutual fund retailer—that is a broker-dealer selling mutual funds—to receive reciprocal income? That is, an unaffiliated one who is not connected with the mutual fund to receive reciprocal income in the form of customer-directed give-ups?

A. Absolutely not.

Q. All right.
Now, at no time?

A. At no time has it been illegal. There is absolutely no prohibition in probably thirty to forty thousand pages of text and other materials by the SEC and by the Congress, by the exchanges, ever mentioning the recipient of income as long as that recipient was not affiliated with the fund.

Q. All right. What do you mean by affiliated with the fund?

A. Wasn't the investment adviser to the fund or the broker-dealer, underwriter for the fund or officer or director of the fund itself.

Q. That is, he didn't—wasn't in some kind of position of trust?

A. He wasn't in a fiduciary capacity with the fund—a position of trust. I am sorry.

Q. And did the New York Stock Exchange ever attempt to regulate its members as far as customer directed give-ups after 1941? I mean I know earlier they had.

A. Well, in December of 1968, after a great deal of discussion and after many releases and proposals, the New York Stock Exchange amended Article XV, Section 2A of their Constitution to prohibit customer directed give-ups by members of that Exchange to non-members.

Q. Did that apply to anyone other than a member of the New York Stock Exchange?

A. Couldn't.

Q. All right. Now, is the New York Stock Exchange a governmental body?

A. No, it's not. It has a quasi-regulatory authority under the '34 Act; it's given some status. But its rules are by court decision and otherwise not, certainly, rules of a governmental body.

Q. And only apply to its members?

A. And only apply to its members.

Q. All right. So would its rules apply to a recipient if he were not a member of the Exchange?

A. Oh, absolutely not.

Let me add one thing. The December 5, '68 decision or rule by the Exchange did not stop customer directed give-ups—it did stop what you call customer directed give-ups, but it led to the institutional—now all these retail—the fund brokers and advisers to funds all became members of exchanges. It gave rise to institutional memberships. They could no longer get the commissions back as a non-member of the Exchange, they all became members of the regional exchanges.

Q. At that point it became proper for the mutual funds to get some of this money back themselves, did it not, sir?

A. Yeah, Well, it was always proper to do that if there was a way to do it.

Q. I see. But at that point it became—there developed a way for them to get the money back themselves?

A. It became more practical to do it.

(Probably the most important defense witness, was Julian Weiner, one of the defendants. He was a partner at Wolfson, Weiner, and subsequently at Seidman & Seidman. Here he is questioned about the audit fees and the relative importance of Equity Funding as a client.)

Q. By 1960 what was the dollar volume approximately of Wolfson, Weiner?

A. Perhaps two, three hundred thousand. Perhaps about three hundred thousand dollars a year in volume.

Q. All right. Now, by 1965 what was the dollar volume of Equity Funding—I mean Wolfson, Weiner?

A. I believe it should be at least double that amount.

Q. Around six hundred thousand?

A. That's correct.

Q. By 1965 how big a client was Equity Funding?

A. 1965 I don't think Equity Funding was too large. It was a—I wouldn't consider it one of our major clients at that time.

Q. At that time it was still not one of your major clients; is that correct?

A. That's correct.

Q. All right. By 1971 what were the gross billings of Wolfson, Weiner?

A. I think about a million and a half dollars a year.

Q. About what part of that came from Equity Funding?

A. Oh, approximately fifteen to twenty percent.

Q. I see. Now, incidentally, was the business of Equity Funding as profitable as your other business?

A. No. No, it was not.

Q. Why was that, sir?

A. In order to meet the time pressures of handling that account, Mr. Wolfson would engage per diem personnel which meant paying higher than normal salaries for the same level of staff competence. And, in addition, we would have to put in tremendous hours of overtime on the part of the staff for which we paid them time and a half, but the billing rate to Equity Funding remained the same, on the hourly basis.

*   *   *

Q. Now, Mr. Weiner, as a result of all this work were you and your partner each making substantial incomes by 1969?

A. I believe so, yes.

A. All right. What kind of an income were you and your partner each making in 1969 and '70 and '71.

A. I believed it ranged somewheres from about ninety to a hundred thousand dollars to perhaps a hundred fifty thousand, a hundred forty or a hundred fifty thousand each.

Q. Each. All right. How much of that came from Equity Funding? Well, let's go at it a different way.
Equity Funding's averaged commissions were, income to your firm, were what? Between two hundred, two hundred fifty thousand dollars a year?

A. I think we averaged about $250,000 a year, roughly.

Q. After what time did that—it get up to that figure?

A. I believe, in 1970.

Q. All right. What was your percentage return on that, your net out of that?

A. I think somewhere about 15 or 20 percent net of the gross fees.

(Mr. Weiner continues his testimony with a discussion of his role in the Equity Funding audit.)

Q. Did you or Mr. Wolfson review any of the field work for the period from 1964 through 1971?

A. No, we did not.

Q. Did you review any of the work papers?

A. No, we did not.

Q. Did you supervise the field work?

A. No, we did not.

Q. Did you or Mr. Wolfson, to your knowledge,

ever impress your views on the staff, override the staff on anything?

A. No, we did not.

(Mr. Weiner continues his testimony discussing the merger negotiations with Seidman and Seidman.)

Q. Now, at the end of 1971 at some point did you commence discussions for a merger with Seidman & Seidman?

A. Sometime in the latter part of 1971.

Q. Who were those discussions with, sir?

A. They were with Mr. Finci, who was the head of the L.A. office of Seidman & Seidman; with Mr. Spencer, who was the western regional director at the time of Seidman & Seidman. We also had a meeting with Mr. William Seidman.

Q. I see. Is that the William Seidman who is the economic adviser to President Ford?

A. That's correct.

Q. I see. Was he the head of Seidman & Seidman at that time?

A. He was.

Q. What was said in your discussion with Mr. Seidman?

A. Mr. Seidman's meeting took place, I believe the first week of January in 1972.

Q. Who was present at that meeting, sir?

A. Mr. Seidman, myself, Mr. Spencer, Mr. Finci and Mr. Wolfson.

Q. What was said by each of you in that meeting?

A. I don't recall all the specifics, but I recall the substance of the conversation, the exchange that took place.

Q. What was the substance of the conversation?

A. As of that meeting I was under the impression we had a—

Q. What you told them, not what your impression was.

A. All right. Well, Mr. Seidman had, in effect, and he did most of the talking on behalf of Seidman & Seidman, and he had indicated that he had been advised by Mr. Spencer and Mr. Finci as to the growth of our firm over the years and that he also had been advised that my greatest expertise had been in practiced development, obtaining new clients. And that while I may have had, and may still have technical knowledge and technical expertise, that that can be bought at a very reasonable price and that my talents would be better served if I concentrated on bringing in

business and that's the area that I should concentrate on.

Q. All right. Did you, in fact, enter into a merger with Seidman & Seidman?

A. Yes, we did.

Q. When did you agree to enter into that merger with them?

A. I thought we had reached an argeement by December 31st of 1971, but there was no question that in my mind that we had reached an agreement at the time of that meeting which I believe was roughly January 6th, assuming that you can accept the handshake of Mr. William Seidman as being meaningful.

Q. All right, sir. Were subsequently agreements drawn?

A. Yes, they were. And they just conformed to the agreements that had been shown to us before that period of time.

Q. All right. And you did, in fact, combine the Los Angeles office of your practice with Seidman & Seidman, did you not?

A. That's correct.

* * *

Q. Did you pay any money into Seidman & Seidman?

A. We certainly did.

Q. What did you pay into Seidman & Seidman?

A. In addition to transferring approximately half a million dollars of accounts receivable, we also had to pay in approximately $75,000 of capital which was made up of transferring our equipment plus paying cash into the firm.

Q. Have you received any of that back, sir?

A. No, I have not.

* * *

Q. In 1971 or early 1972 when you combined with Seidman & Seidman did your practice have a value that could be ascribed to a sale?

A. Yes, it did.

Q. Are accounting practices sold from time to time?

A. Yes, they are.

Q. What is the normal formula that is applied to the sale of accounting practices?

A. Depending upon the quality of the practice it would range from, as I recall, somewhere from about one and a half times the annual gross billings to twice the annual gross billings.

Q. Based on that what was the value of your practice at the time of the combination of practice?

Mr. Newman: Objection, your Honor; incompetent.

Mr. Abeles: I thought a man could always testify as to the value of his business, your Honor, and I wanted him to value something he owns and I want to show it for the purpose of showing that he was not trying to make a profit out of this. He was combining. He wasn't trying to take money and run, if he had known something was wrong. He was just trying to—He was combining a practice and he was putting money in. He wasn't trying to take anything out.

Q. Did you have any discussions with Seidman & Seidman about what would happen on review of your audit papers or accounts prior to the merger?

A. Yes, I did.

Q. What discussions did you have?

A. Representations were made to us that they had a quality audit practice and that it was their practice to review the workpapers of the audits on an independent basis and that, in fact, they had a—tried to evaluate our fees to determine whether the fees were sufficient to cover this independent review that they represented that they would be doing on our clients.

Q. To your knowledge, was an independent review conducted of any of your clients by Seidman & Seidman?

A. Pardon?

Q. To your knowledge, was an independent review conducted of the audit of any of your clients by Seidman & Seidman?

A. I believe that Seidman & Seidman had conducted an independent review of certain of our other accounts.

Q. I see. Do you know at this time which ones?

A. One account sticks out. I think Price-Stern-Sloan.

Q. What business were they in, sir?

A. Book publishers.

Q. To your knowledge, did Seidman & Seidman conduct an independent review of the workpapers for the year 1971?

A. Not to my knowledge.

Q. When did you first—Were you ever under the impression that they had?

A. I was always under the impression that they had reviewed the 1971 papers themselves.

Q. When did you first learn that they hadn't?

A. When I visited the U.S. Attorney's Office to start reviewing the workpapers maintained in the Equity Funding depository.

Q. I see. What did you base the fact—your conclusion that they hadn't reviewed them all?

A. I could see nothing in the workpapers that would indicate some type of official marking by a firm such as Seidman & Seidman to indicate that they had reviewed the workpapers.

*   *   *

Q. Mr. Weiner, yesterday we were talking about—I believe you indicated you have no particular recollection as to whether or not you signed any of the annual reports.

Are you saying—or, that is, the annual financial statements. Are you saying by that that you didn't sign any of them?

A. No.

Q. Do you recall if you signed any or not?

A. I don't recall if I signed any.

Q. Would you have signed them if you were asked to?

A. Yes, I would have.

Q. Why was that, sir?

A. I had no reason to feel there was anything wrong with the audits and I had full confidence that during the period Mr. Block was the—in charge of the audit that the work done and the review done by Mr. West under the supervision of Mr. Block was done properly and the same applied to the work done by the staff working under Mr. Lichtig.

And so that had I been asked to sign it, any of the reports, I would have signed them.

Q. All right, sir. But you don't have a specific recollection; is that right?

A. No, I do not.

Q. Do you know if Mr. Block ever signed any of the reports.

A. Not of my own knowledge.

Q. Do you know if Mr. Lichtig signed any particular reports?

A. Not of my own knowledge.

Q. Who at your firm was authorized to sign?

A. Any auditing manager or a partner.

Q. All right. What auditing managers did you have at your firm during the various times?

A. I believe we had a Mr. Stalrit, Mr. Slavin, and then in terms of partners we had—and managers, as the case may be, a Mr. Stein, Mr. Lichtig, Mr. Wolfson and myself, and Mr. Block, Mr. Labow, Mr. Kugler.

Q. I see. And any of—

A. There may be others but I don't recall at this time.

(Here, Weiner relates his knowledge of an IRS audit of Equity Funding during 1968-1970 under the direction of Mr. Coons.)

A. Mr. Coons in one of the later meetings in 1968 had told me that a hearing had been conducted in Washington, and I don't know whether it was—I'm not sure whether it was sponsored by the SEC dealing with the subject of reciprocals. Mr. Riordan had testified before that meeting. The hearing was supposed to have taken place either in—excuse me—1967 or the beginning of '68.

And that the SEC had requested—as a result of Mr. Riordan's testimony the SEC had requested the Internal Revenue Service to do an audit of broker-dealers that were selling mutual funds.

As I recall, Mr. Coons said that it was not limited only to Equity Funding but other broker-dealers were being examined as well.

By Mr. Abeles:

Q. Was he more specific about what they were looking for?
A. Yes. I think he became more specific. If not in meetings in 1968, in a meeting that took place in February of 1969.
Q. Who was present at that meeting?
A. Mr. Goldblum, myself and Mr. Coons.
Q. What was said then, sir?
A. I had finally asked Mr. Coons, "What basically is it that the Internal Revenue Service is looking for?" if he could tell me. Then he had told me that in connection with Mr. Riordan's testimony before the hearing conducted in Washington he had also written a letter to the SEC concerning reciprocals and Equity Funding having received reciprocal income or give-up income, or whichever term was used. And that letter had been submitted by the SEC to the Internal Revenue Service and that he was specifically interested in finding out whether Equity Funding had in fact reported all of the reciprocal income it had received.
Q. Did he indicate whether or not they were trying to find if any officers had received any of that income?
A. Yes. He said that they were interested in that information as well.
Q. Did he indicate to you in any way that reciprocal income was illegal or improper to receive?
A. Not at all.
Q. But he did tell you that he had been referred to you by the SEC?

A. That is correct.
Q. Now, in that connection were the work papers for Equity Funding for certain years turned over to the IRS audit team? They did have an audit team then, didn't they?
A. Yes, they did.
Q. Were the work papers for certain years of Equity Funding turned over?
A. I believe we had been requested to turn over all our work papers to the SEC so they could correlate them with the records of the company.

And my recollection was that we had been asked to turn them over in stages. And they had received our work papers at one time through 1967, and they also had received all of our work papers for the year 1968 after that audit had been completed. I am not sure whether they received 1969 as well.
Q. Now, did IRS ever indicate to you that they found anything wrong in your work papers?
A. No, they did not.
Q. Did they indicate to you that they found any reciprocal income reported that was not received?
A. No, they did not.
Q. Or any reciprocal income received that was not reported?
A. Not at all.
Q. How long did that audit go?
A. I know it started in the middle of 1968. To my recollection the Intelligence Division did not withdraw from the audit until sometime in 1969, then the regular branch of the Internal Revenue Service continued with the audit, I believe, until sometime in 1970 or the latter part of 1970.

(Weiner, being questioned by Mr. Abeles, testifies about income recognition within the context of the audit.)

And I had told him that so as the income belonged to the preceding year that—and the audit, any income received of that nature belonged to the preceding period could be picked up until such time as the audit itself was actually completed.
Q. All right. What was your belief as to the legality of receiving reciprocal income at that time?
A. It was my belief that it was completely proper and legal.
Q. Is that still your belief?
A. Yes, it is.

(Weiner continues with his testimony concerning forged audit confirmations.)

Q. Did Mr. Lowell indicate to you in any way that he or Mr. Sultan were going to forge confirmations?

A. No; he did not. Absolutely not.

Q. Did you have any idea that anything of this nature would be done?

A. Absolutely not.

Q. At my request did you receive the work papers for that year to determine whether or not the work papers make any reference to these confirmations?

A. I did.

Q. Just subsequent to all of this breaking?

A. That's correct.

Q. Did you find any reference in the work papers—what year was this for, incidentally?

A. The year 1970.

Q. In the work papers for the year 1970 did you find any reference that indicates that the staff relied upon those confirmations?

A. I couldn't find any reference that the staff had relied on the confirmations.

In fact, when I did look I noticed that there was a memorandum from myself to Mr. Block attached to a—the confirmation with the Banco Unione, and that memorandum was dated November, 1971, to the effect that in cleaning my desk I had found this on my—on my desk and would he please take care of it or file it or something of that sort.

Q. That was six or seven months after the audit?

A. That's correct.

*   *   *

Q. Did you ever get an objection from anyone at Equity Funding about merging with Alexander Grant?

A. No, we did not.

Q. Did you enter into merger negotiations with any other firm?

A. Yes, we did.

Q. With whom?

A. We met—we were negotiating with Wolf & Company and also with Laventhol & Horvath.

Q. Do you know what caused the negotiations with Wolf & Company to break down, if they did?

A. Actually with Wolf & Company we had come to what I considered to be a—an informal agreement or a meeting of the minds. And I think that they really felt we were too large for them to absorb.

Q. I see. What about with Laventhol, Krekstein, Horvath & Horvath?

A. The negotiations with that firm had started I think, after the negotiations had progressed with Seidman & Seidman. When Mr. Finci and Mr. Spencer had told us—and I think this was in December—that as far as they were concerned—and they had unofficially polled the policy group of Seidman & Seidman and that they had agreed to the merger.

*   *   *

Q. Now, following the merger with Seidman & Seidman—prior to your merger with Seidman & Seidman did you have any discussions with the people at Seidman & Seidman about how you staffed your audits?

A. Yes.

Q. Who did you discuss it with?

A. We had discussions with Mr. Finci, Mr. Spencer and, I believe, with Mr. DeArmas.

Q. What was said by each of you?

A. In effect we told them that our normal staff that we maintained on a permanent basis was not sufficient to handle our yearend workload, that we had to hire per diem personnel to take care of the additional work at yearend and that if they did not do that then they would have to have sufficient personnel to cover the workload.

Q. That is on their own staff?

A. On their own staff.

Q. What did they say in response?

A. They said that they felt they would have that sufficient workload. If not they would then try to get personnel from their other offices to cover it because they felt, they said, it was not their practice to hire per diem personnel for work as a general rule.

Q. What occurred in connection with personnel when the 1971 audit actually commenced?

A. Shortly—as soon as the merger—and that merger took place as of February 1, 1972.

Q. When did Seidman & Seidman start giving you directions and control on the audit?

A. Starting in about February 1, 1972.

Q. I see.

A. From that point on neither Mr. Wolfson nor I had any authority to make any assignments of personnel, to hire any personnel, to do anything without the approval of the Seidman management.

(Mr. Newman began his cross-examination of Julian Weiner and questioned Weiner's approach to income recognition.)

Q. So that, again, let me understand your theory. The theory is that if the premium is collected before the audit is closed and it relates to a receivable as to which all the work had been done prior to yearend, that it can be reflected as a receivable for yearend and as income?

A. I believe so.

Q. But that work has to be done to check it out?

A. That's correct.

Q. It's not possible, is it, to confirm something like this with a customer as of December 31, in this case, 1963, because the customer does not owe the money as of December 31, 1963?

A. I think anything is possible. You can design all types of confirmation forms, but that's the first criterion as to whether or not the cash was received. Whether you go beyond that would depend upon the circumstances existing at the time.

Q. Well, you also have to know, of course, whether all of the work was done in the prior year.

A. That's correct.

Q. Now, in connection with that, Mr. Weiner, wasn't it the policy of Wolfson, Weiner—of you, when working on Equity Funding, and the instructions you gave to Marvin Lichtig, to take in the income for the prior year but not to take in—not to accrue into the prior year the expense?

A. No, it was not.

Q. If that were reflected as an adjusting journal entry then on the income side in the working trial balance there should be a corresponding and related adjusting journal entry for commission expense, should there not.

A. It would depend upon what the figure relates to. If the figure only relates to the net commission receivable and due to the company which it would keep, there might not necessarily be an accrual of the commission expense.

(Here, Newman examines Weiner about certain footnotes to the financial statements)

Q. That Exhibit 16, Mr. Weiner, would you look again at the two footnotes, footnotes 4 and 10?

A. I have looked at both notes now.

Q. Mr. Weiner, was it your understanding at the time that the accounts to which those two notes referred contained nothing but loans from clients on premium loans?

A. Yes, I believe so.

Q. There is certainly nothing in the notes to suggest anything different, is there?

A. That's correct.

Q. Now, with reference to note No. 4 and the last paragraph, you will note that the note indicates that the payable and the receivable are not equal.

A. That's correct.

Q. And that the difference is something over six million dollars.

A. That's correct.

Q. Then the final sentence there is an indication the collateral assigned by clients as security for the notes payable on premium loans reported under other liabilities and the portion held by Equity Funding Corporation of America amounted to approximately $22,900,000.

A. That's correct.

Q. Was it your understanding, Mr. Weiner, that the audit staff, Marvin Lichtig and those working under him, if any, also in that year confirmed the full value of the collateral lying behind the receivable?

A. That would be my understanding.

Q. In fact, there were some words added in that footnote, were there not, from the footnote from the previous year specifically indicating that collateral behind the loans held by the company was included in the figure?

A. Yes. That's correct.

Q. Did Marvin Lichtig at any time discuss with you the change in the presentation of the footnote in that regard?

A. As I say, we have had many discussions and there would be no reason for it to stand out in my mind as to whether he did or not.

Q. Well, the confirmation of the collateral at least in your own view was a pretty important item, was it not?

A. That's correct.

Q. And differences in presentation in the financial statement might affect how bankers or how underwriters might look at that particular item?

A. That's possible.

Q. Mr. Weiner, so that in your opinion it was very important how that was presented? I mean, in your understanding back in 1966.

A. Well, everything is a matter of judgment. I don't think it is so much a matter of necessarily as to whether—how it is presented. I think that the confirmation of the collateral was a significant item and whether it was presented in the footnote or not, I don't know whether that's necessarily of the critical area. I think that it is important and my opinion may not conform to others, but in my judgment as opposed to perhaps others that the confirmation of the collateral was important.

The footnote certainly seems to indicate that the collateral is being confirmed in full.

Q. Now, Mr. Weiner, you never had a discussion with Marvin Lichtig, did you, in which he indicated to you that the collateral figure set forth in these footnotes that we have been looking at was informational only, supplied by the company and that no audit work was done on it?

A. I have absolutely no recollection of any such conversation.

*   *   *

Q. These discussions by and large were of matters less serious than missing assets, weren't they?

A. There was never any discussion of missing assets.

Q. Were these discussions also by and large of matters less serious than missing general ledgers which could not and never were found?

A. To the best of my recollection, there was a discussion, I believe, at one time that after Mr. Evans had left the company that there were records that the company was not able to locate.

I don't think I ever had been advised that these records had in fact never been located. But I do recall being advised at one point that they did have difficulty locating records after Mr. Evans had left.

*   *   *

Q. Now, Mr. Weiner, isn't it a fact that on at least two occasions you received telephone calls from Sam Lowell and at his request got people on your staff out of the computer room at Equity Funding during audits?

A. Out of the computer room during audits?

Q. Out of the computer facility—I'll rephrase the question.

Isn't it a fact that you were informed by Sam Lowell that there were people from the staff of Wolfson, Weiner who had gone into the computer facility for the purpose of doing some audit work?

A. I have absolutely no recollection of that. I don't think we had the personnel who would need to go into the computer room, to my recollection.

*   *   *

Q. Do you recall giving those instructions to Solomon Block while you were with Seidman & Seidman?

A. Yes, I do.

Q. What audit was that for?

A. It was not in connection with an audit. Apparently Mr. Block had arranged for someone from Seidman & Seidman to go into—one of the computer men of Seidman and Seidman to go ahead into the Equity Funding computer and to start trying to work out a program for doing an audit through the computer.

This was in connection with the year—this was in, oh, I believe, the latter part or the latter quarter perhaps of 1972. This was prior to any audit. And I believe the arrangements, to my recollection, had been made between Mr. Block and Mr. Goldblum.

Then I don't recall whether I received the call first from Mr. Lowell or Mr. Goldblum, but either one of the two explained to me that the computer was already backlogged as far as work was concerned, and that if Seidman & Seidman wanted to get into doing an audit via the computer that it was too late in the year to start, because it was going to backlog their work, but as soon as they finished their '72 audit they could send their computer men in then and do the job at that time.

And this was the information conveyed to Mr. Block.

Q. So you instructed Mr. Block to have the man removed, didn't you?

A. Yes. And I also had explained to Mr. Finci of Seidman & Seidman as to what the reason for that was.

Q. And you are saying that had never happened in the past?

A. Not to my knowledge. I have absolutely no recollection.

Q. Would that be the kind of thing you would recall if it had happened?

A. I believe so. But I don't recall having any man on our staff that could understand the operation of the computer to go into the audit of the computer.

Q. You didn't have anyone on your staff who was competent to evaluate the internal controls that were necessary, that were present or absent with respect to Equity Funding's computer operation, did you?

A. That's correct. But that wasn't necessary to do an audit.

Q. Is that your opinion?

A. Oh, Haskins & Sells audited through the computer. They didn't have any greater success.

Q. Do you know what the controls were on the computer with respect to the life insurance company, Mr. Weiner?

A. They must have had tremendous controls since I'm sitting here and not them.

(Here, Weiner testifies his discussions with Sol Block regarding the audit.)

Q. During the 1970 audit or thereafter do you recall whether he told you about the discovery of the $10 million plug in the funded loan receivables run?

A. I have no recollection of him saying anything of that sort.

Q. Do you recall at any time whether he discussed with you whether or not the auditors were fully confirming the collateral lying behind—supposedly lying behind the funded loan receivables?

A. I don't believe there was any discussion of that matter.

Q. Do you ever recall whether he discussed with you whether or not the audit staff was independently calculating the value of the collateral set forth in the funded loan footnote for the years 1969 through 1971?

A. No, I don't think so.

Q. You say you don't recall or—

A. I don't recall.

Q. Do you recall whether he ever discussed with you—What if any work was being done in connection with the commissions receivable account on the books of Equity Funding Corporation of California?

A. No; I have no recollection of him discussing that matter with me.

Q. You don't recall him telling you during the 1971 or 1972 audit that in fact there was a commissions receivable account on the books that hadn't changed for years and for which there was no detail?

A. No; I have no recollection of any such discussion.

Q. Do you recall whether or not he discussed with you what if any work was being done on the commercial paper accounts on the books of Equity Funding Corporation of America?

A. No—no, I have no recollection. Mr. Block didn't—didn't discuss the audit procedures with me as a general rule.

Q. So that, then he didn't discuss with you anything about what if anything was being done on the exploration costs item on the books of the parent?

A. That's correct.

Q. Or on the agents receivable item on the books of Equity Funding Corporation of California?

A. That's correct.

Q. Or the supposed investment in Apatex commercial paper?

A. That's correct.

Q. Or on the notes receivable account which included Establissement Grandson?

A. That's correct.

Q. Or on the footnote with respect to the 1969—

A. I did say that he—I'm sorry. I just want to say this, that he had mentioned to me that there were a number of foreign entities that he had wanted confirmed, and I had without paying any particular attention to the names of what these entities—some of these were entities in bank accounts—that's when I had spoken to Mr. Lowell to try to use his best efforts to contact these entities and arrange for confirmations. I don't know whether those were included or not.

Q. But you don't know what he did in 1971 and 1972 during those audits in connection with the notes receivable account?

A. That's correct.

Q. And you don't know what if any work was done in addition to Establissement Grandson? You don't know what if any work was done in connection with the receivable from Penn General Agencies on the sale of casualty commissions?

A. That's correct.

Q. And you didn't have any consultation with him in connection with the change in wording of the footnote for the 1969 year and the insertion of the word in that contracts receivable?

A. That's correct.

Q. So that he was the highest man on the job in a position of responsibility for Wolfson, Weiner on the Equity Funding job who would have been in a position to make any decision on all those matters?

A. Yes. He would have been in a position. But, as I said, I have had discussions with Mr. Block. But he would have been in position to make decisions, that's correct.

(After all of the witnesses were called, Harold Abeles presented the closing argument on behalf of his client, Julian Weiner.)

As you have heard a number of times in the testimony, as you have heard from various documents read, and from the expert witnesses, auditing is not set up to catch fraud. That is not the purpose of it.

And the point is no matter what auditing procedures were used—there will be much hue and cry as to whether they used standard auditing procedures or not.

That, I may point out, all with hindsight and without direct testimony. Because you will notice that in this long, long case we had one expert, really, on accounting, and that was Mr. Grossman from Touche, Ross.

Now, why in a case of this magnitude is there only one expert called who testifies only to a very narrow area?

Now, we had two experts on reciprocal income. After we brought one in then the prosecution brought one in who agreed with what our expert said on the receipt of reciprocal income not ever being illegal, except, that is, in an unaffiliated situation. Obviously it's illegal if, like the officers of Equity Funding, you steal it from the company that you're working from. If the company is entitled to it, that part is illegal, the stealing of it. But that's like stealing anything else.

In any event, in all of this we have one expert. What does he talk about?

Now, first of all, let's look at this expert. He is a capable man. He comes from the firm of Touche, Ross, which to do the audit at Equity Funding was paid over two million dollars. Now, that's a well-paid expert. But it gives you some idea of what it costs to do this kind of an audit and to catch this sort of thing.

And this expert when he did this had the benefit of, first of all, coming in and knowing the fraud existed, the exact opposite of what the auditors from Wolfson, Weiner and Seidman & Seidman had. He not only had that knowledge, he had the FBI, he had the Securities and Exchange Commission, he had the U.S. Attorney's Office, he had the huge law firm of O'Melveny & Myers, he had the postal inspectors, he had officers of the companies who had been hiding things from the accountants now telling him what they did, or at least part of what they did.

Now, even at this it took Touche, Ross ten and a half months to do the audit, and 70 men, as opposed to seven men for three or four or five months on the other audit, including a couple months of preparatory work before you start the intensive part.

At that they were unable to certify because of the thing. They found things because they had all this help.

Remember they had the power of subpoena, they could force things, they could get information all over the world, they had an unlimited budget.

Now, does Touche, Ross always operate that way? No. As the evidence shows you, Touche, Ross themselves had been taken in a similar fraud on U.S. Financial Corporation.

But, as the prosecutor was quick to jump up and say, "We'll stipulate that no one from Touche, Ross was indicted. Yes, we'll stipulate to that, too."

Touche, Ross is one of the Big Eight firms. No one from Touche, Ross was indicted, I'll say, with phony assets and phony sales to corporations. These are not things that auditing is set up to catch.

The point is the type of thing that happened at Equity Funding, it didn't matter what auditing procedure you used. That was not the reason the fraud went over. The fraud went over because of vast amounts of documentation that all these people involved, the amazing thing is that they could put together such an organization of crooks. And the man responsible for putting it together was Sam Lowell.

Until Sam Lowell came in, Mr. Evans' testimony was it was a two-man fraud, he and Mr. Goldblum. After Mr. Evans left and Mr. Lowell came in Mr. Lowell must have expanded to at least a 200-man fraud, highly complex, using his knowledge of having worked on embezzlements at Haskins & Sells, bringing in his old friends, a lot of them from Haskins & Sells, who were accountants and knew how to fool accountants. They didn't care who the accountants were.

It's ridiculous. They try to say, on the one hand, that Wolfson, Weiner and Seidman & Seidman were in on something. Who did they have auditing Equity Funding Life? Haskins & Sells, not Wolfson, Weiner.

And that is at a point from '69 on where the major part of the income—the phony income is being generated in Equity Funding Life, two billion dollars of phony policies under the direction of Haskins & Sells or under their review.

But I'm giving you this by way of background. Also, understand the people that were fooled. The Federal Reserve Board, which regulates money and currency, they came in, they did their audit and they were fooled.

The IRS, the Internal Revenue, they came in, they did their audit, and they were fooled.

Alexander Grant, who came in to do a review. The prosecution tries to play it both ways. They try to say, on the one hand, that they didn't see the workpapers and on the other hand they say, "Well, some things were taken out of the workpapers so they wouldn't see them." I mean you can't have both. Which is it? Did they see the workpapers? Or if something was taken out of the workpapers, what's the point if they didn't see the workpapers, anyhow?

Besides that, what they are trying to say was taken out is something that the workpapers are only some of the accountants'—that portion of the workpapers—only some of the accountants' reason.

Really, this doesn't affect Mr. Weiner, because he is not involved in that phase of it. But I still have to point this out because they're not saying he took anything out of the workpapers.

But the point is that we know that when Alexander Grant came in they had five or six men in there for two weeks reviewing the books and records of Equity Funding.

Now, remember, workpapers are just the accountants going over and getting confirmations of things that are in the books. Things like how the trail commissions were accrued, that's right in the books. That's in the trial balance, also. You don't need the workpapers for that.

So Alexander Grant was fooled.

Incidentally, whether or not they saw the workpapers—what Mr. Weiner knew, as he testified, all he knew is when they were going in they were going to see the workpapers. But we don't know if they saw them or not, although we didn't have them here to testify whether they did or not. And for a good reason, as I pointed out yesterday, because they had approved these things.

Mr. Weiner, the last thing said to him was they were going to see them.

They fooled Seidman & Seidman. They fooled Haskins & Sells. They fooled the insurance departments, the insurance commissioners of three states, with their rackets. They fooled Peat, Marwick & Mitchell, another Big Eight firm, which handled the reinsurance—that is, Equity Funding Life was selling phony insurance policies to other insurance companies.

So the other insurance companies sent their accountants in. They were fooled. They found some files missing, but not enough to alert them. But enough that they warned Haskins & Sells. But Haskins & Sells did nothing on that.

(Mr. Newman sums up the government's case as follows.)

What is the general thrust of the Government's evidence? Well, I think it is pretty clear it's that there were false financial statements and there were false opinions, that these were filed with various bodies which constituted false filings, and that they were otherwise circulated, that the information got into the hands of people who were likely to make decisions based on that information on whether or not to buy the securities that Equity Funding was peddling every year, to wit, the funding programs which were securities, and the other kinds of securities that came somewhat less often, the stock options registrations, the debenture registrations.

As I told you in my opening statement, the role of the auditors in that regard fell into several different categories. I will quote that opening statement now because I still think that the four different categories that I mentioned are the four different categories into which the conduct of the auditors here falls.

This is a quotation:

"The officers at Equity Funding were assisted in three respects by the treatment which the men who were on trial here and who are responsible for what was done in connection with the examination of the financial statements did. No. 1, as the evidence will show, they were willing to bend and even break the application of generally accepted accounting principles so that the company would be permitted to show itself to be more profitable and in a better condition than it actually was.

"Secondly, the auditors showed themselves willing to completely disregard many, many generally accepted auditing standards in terms of gathering evidence to determine the manner in which these financial statements presented the condition of the company whether it was fair or not.

"Thirdly, they were willing to play the See-No-Evil routine and were willing to turn their heads from what was plainly to be seen as a major problem and a major problem there indicating serious holes in the assets and income of Equity Funding and, indeed, even fraud.

"But that was not enough, because there were times when this bending and breaking and disregarding and See-No-Evil, Hear-No-Evil simply would not carry the day.

"There had to be conferences in which the auditors were notified that something was wrong."

*   *   *

In conclusion let me just say that throughout the trial you have had defense counsel talking here about matters of judgment. This was a matter of judgment, that was a matter of judgment, something else was a matter of judgment. $100,000,000 worth of missing or phony assets was a matter of judgment?

There is only one judgment that the auditors had to make here at any time and that was the judgment whether to be open, honest, and aboveboard in discharging their functions of doing the work and in discharging their function of being the independent check upon management, the independent check upon which the people to whom the financial statements were to be circulated would rely.

They asserted that they had done audits, complete audits and in confirmity with certain standards when they had not. They asserted that financial statements fairly presented the condition of the company when the financial statements had not.

Oftentimes they had substantial indication that serious things were wrong and that items were not pursued. And they failed to make a fair, honest, and open disclosure of significant items that they knew did exist, the supposed reciprocals in '68, the contractuals in '69, as two major examples as the turning points in this case.

(Following the closing statements, Judge Jesse W. Curtis gave his instructions to the jury. Included are a listing of the "counts" and an explanation of them.)

There will be sixteen counts submitted to you for your consideration. The remaining counts in which the defendants have been charged were withdrawn by the Government and have been dismissed, so you need not consider them.

Let us first deal with Counts Six, Ten, Eleven, Twelve, Thirteen and Fourteen, all of which charge similar types of offenses,

violations of the Securities Act of 1933. The portion of that statute which is involved provides:

"It shall be unlawful for any person in the offer or sale of any securities by the use of any means or instruments of transportation or communication in interstate commerce or by the use of the mails, directly or indirectly:

"(1) to employ any device, scheme or artifice to defraud, or

"(2) to obtain money or property by means of any untrue statement of a material fact or any omission to state a material fact necessary in order to make the statements made, in the light of the circumstances under which they were made, not misleading, or

"(3) to engage in any transaction, practice or course of business which oeprates or would operate as a fraud or deceit upon the purchaser."

*   *   *

Count Six charges the mailing of a confirmation of purchase of EFCA debentures to William Wilson on or about December 10, 1970.

Count Thirteen charges the mailing of a similar confirmation to Max Fenten, on or about December 7, 1971.

Count Fourteen also charges the mailing of a similar confirmation to Carol Sobieski on or about December 7, 1971.

Counts Ten through Twelve each charge as the jurisdictional act a mailing related to the merger of EFCA with Bankers National Life Insurance Company. Count Ten alleges a mailing of a letter of Stanley Goldblum and a letter of transmittal to Woodrow and Lela Montroy on or about October 20, 1971.

Count Eleven alleges the mailing of similar kinds of documents to Charles Morris on or about October 20, 1971.

Count Twelve alleges as the jurisdictional act the mailing of a letter of transmittal and a Bankers stock certificate in the name of Ben and Ann Benson to the United California Bank.

*   *   *

These are counts 75 through 84, and each of them charges one or more of the defendants on trial here with making false statements of material fact or omitting to disclose material facts in documents filed with the Securities and Exchange Commission and, in certain cases, with stock exchanges.

In order to assist in explaining them, I have

split them into two different groups. The first group consists of four counts and relates to allegedly false accountant's certifications rendered on EFCA financial statements for the years 1968, 1969, 1970, and 1971, and included in various registration statements and an annual report on Form 10-K.

Count 75 charges as follows:

On or about April 22, 1969, in the Central District of California, defendants JULIAN S. H. WEINER and MARVIN AL LICHTIG willfully made and caused to be made untrue statements of material fact in a registration statement filed by Equity Funding Corporation of America with the Securities and Exchange Commission pursuant to Title 15, United States Code, Section 77f, the said statements being to the effect that the firm of Wolfson, Weiner, Ratoff and Lapin, certified public accountants, had examined the consolidated statement of financial condition of EFA and its subsidiaries as of December 31, 1968, and the related consolidated statement of earnings and retained earnings and the consolidated statement of additional paid-in capital for the five years then ended, in accordance with generally accepted auditing standards, and that, in the opinion of Wolfson, Weiner, Ratoff and Lapin, the aforesaid financial statement presented fairly the consolidated financial position of EFCA and its subsidiaries as of December 31, 1968, and the consolidated results of operations for the five years then ended in conformity with generally accepted accounting principles applied on a consistent basis.

Count 78 charges defendants Weiner and Block with a similar violation relating to the 1969 consolidated financial statement of EFCA included in the December 9, 1970, EFCA registration statement.

Count 80 again charges defendants Weiner and Block with a similar violation relating to the 1970 consolidated financial statement of EFCA included in the December 7, 1971, EFCA registration statement.

Finally, Count 84 charges defendants Weiner and Block with a similar violation relating to the 1971 consolidated financial statements of EFCA included in the EFCA 10-K report of April 5, 1972.

*　　　*　　　*

The second group of counts relates only to Marvin Lichtig and relates to alleged misrepresentations and failures to disclose done in connection with registration statements, a listing application to the New York Stock Exchange and an annual report on Form 10-K.

Count 76 charges that:

On or about November 4, 1969, in the Central District of California, defendants STANLEY GOLDBLUM and MARVIN AL LICHTIG, in a registration statement (Amendment No. 1) filed with the Securities and Exchange Commission pursuant to Title 15, United States, Code, Section 77f:

1. Willfully made and caused to be made untrue statements of material fact as follows:

a. That on December 31, 1968, there were $34,196,037 in Equity Funding Corporation of America premium loans outstanding;

b. That on December 31, 1968, as set forth in its Consolidated statement of financial condition, EFCA had an asset, Funded Loans and Accounts Receivable of $35,476,037;

c. That on December 31, 1968, as set forth in its consolidated statement of financial condition, EFCA had total assets of $79,005,010;

whereas in truth and in fact, the correct figures for the above, at the times stated were as follows:

a. Premium loans outstanding, not more than approximately $18,000,000;

b. Funded Loans and Accounts Receivable, not more than approximately $18,000,000;

c. Total assets, not more than approximately $62,000,000.

2. Willfully omitted and caused to be omitted statements of material fact required to be stated therein and necessary to make the statements therein not misleading, as follows:

a. That during the calendar year 1968 EFCA incurred liabilities in the form of short-term notes and commercial paper placed through Dishy, Easton & Co. with various lenders in the amount of approximately $4,600,000 (some of which was payable in Swiss francs) which remained outstanding and unpaid on December 31, 1968;

b. That as of June 30, 1969, EFCA had incurred long-term liabilities in the form of Swiss franc notes placed through Dishy, Easton & Co. with Loeb, Rhoades International in the approximate amount of $9,000,000 which were due and payable in Swiss francs in 1972.

Counts 77, 79, 81, 82, and 83 charge defendant Lichtig with similar violations involving similar types of allegedly false statements in various documents.

Count 77 involves the December 9, 1970, EFCA registration statement.

Count 79 involves the December 7, 1971, EFCA registration statement.

Count 81 involves the September 8, 1972, EFCA registration statement.

Count 82 involves EFCA's application for the original listing of its shares on the New York Stock Exchange.

And Count 83 involves the April 5, 1972, EFCA 10-K report.

(The jury was then sent out to deliberate. The court is resumed on May 20, 1975 and the verdicts were returned.)

The Court: I'll ask the clerk to read the verdicts, please.
The Clerk: (Reading)
"UNITED STATES DISTRICT COURT
"CENTRAL DISTRICT OF CALIFORNIA

"UNITED STATES OF AMERICA,
                                      Plaintiff,
            vs.   No. 13390-Criminal
"JULIAN S. H. WEINER,   *V E R D I C T*
                      Defendant.

"We, the jury in the above-entitled cause, find the defendant, *JULIAN S. H. WEINER,*
Guilty as charged in Count 6 of the Indictment;
Guilty as charged in Count 10 of the Indictment;
Guilty as charged in Count 11 of the Indictment;
Guilty as charged in Count 12 of the Indictment;
Guilty as charged in Count 13 of the Indictment;
Guilty as charged in Count 14 of the Indictment;
Guilty as charged in Count 75 of the Indictment;
Guilty as charged in Count 78 of the Indictment;
Guilty as charged in Count 80 of the Indictment;
Guilty as charged in Count 84 of the Indictment.
"Dated May 20, 1975
"At Los Angeles, California

                                      "Charles Flores
                              "Foreman of the Jury."

"UNITED STATES DISTRICT COURT
"CENTRAL DISTRICT OF CALIFORNIA
"UNITED STATES OF AMERICA,
Plaintiff.

vs.

"MARVIN AL LICHTIG,
Defendant.

No. 13390-Criminal
V E R D I C T

"We, the jury in the above-entitled cause, find
the defendant, MARVIN AL LICHTIG,
Guilty as charged in Count 6 of the Indictment;
Guilty as charged in Count 10 of the Indictment;
Guilty as charged in Count 11 of the Indictment;
Guilty as charged in Count 12 of the Indictment;
Guilty as charged in Count 13 of the Indictment;
Guilty as charged in Count 14 of the Indictment;
Guilty as charged in Count 75 of the Indictment;
Guilty as charged in Count 76 of the Indictment;
Guilty as charged in Count 77 of the Indictment;
Guilty as charged in Count 79 of the Indictment;
Guilty as charged in Count 81 of the Indictment;
Guilty as charged in Count 82 of the Indictment;
Guilty as charged in Count 83 of the Indictment.
"Dated May 20, 1975
"At Los Angeles, California

"Charles Flores
"Foreman of the Jury."

"UNITED STATES DISTRICT COURT
"CENTRAL DISTRICT OF CALIFORNIA
"UNITED STATES OF AMERICA,
Plaintiff,

vs.

"SOLOMON BLOCK,
Defendant

No. 13390-Criminal
V E R D I C T

"We, the jury in the above-entitled cause, find
the defendant, SOLOMON BLOCK,
Not Guilty as charged in Count 6 of the
Indictment;
Guilty as charged in Count 10 of the Indictment;
Guilty as charged in Count 11 of the Indictment;
Guilty as charged in Count 12 of the Indictment;
Guilty as charged in Count 13 of the Indictment;
Guilty as charged in Count 14 of the Indictment;
Not Guilty as charged in Count 78 of the
Indictment;
Guilty as charged in Count 80 of the Indictment;
Guilty as charged in Count 84 of the Indictment.
"Dated May 20, 1975
"At Los Angeles, California

"Charles Flores
"Foreman of the Jury."

THE ACCOUNTING PROFESSION EXAMINES ITSELF

In short order, as the magnitude of the Equity Funding swindle became clear, the scandal posed an uncomfortable and inescapable dilemma for the public accounting profession. It became harder and harder to resist the conclusion that Equity Funding must have been an "auditing bust"—an utter failure by the auditors. Yet the obvious question *Where were the auditors?* put the accounting profession in a bind. Public accountants liked to think of themselves as a learned profession, willing and able to hold practitioners to high standards. But the everyday reality was something different. Public accounting was a profession under fire, attacked in the courts, raked over in the press, already on the defensive under criticism more intense than it had ever known before. Confronted with the most stunning fraud in decades, a scandal making headlines across the country, would public accounting cleanse its ranks or close them?

In the years before Equity Funding came to light, there had been no shortage of fraud cases to embarrass the accounting profession. But none of the previous cases had been as pervasive as Equity Funding. In past instances, clever corporate managements had combined dubious accounting practices with outright misrepresentations to construct an exaggerated record of business success. Only in the notorious Salad Oil Swindle, where Tino DeAngelis had forged warehouse receipts backed by empty tanks, had there been a recent instance of enormous amounts of concocted assets. Unlike Equity Funding, however, DeAngelis' company had no auditors, and his swindle centered on the highly professional commodities markets, not the nation's broad securities markets. Thus Equity Funding shaped up as the first instance of complete failure by outside auditors since the McKesson-Robbins case more than three decades before.

Throughout the late 1960s and early 1970s, as lawsuits against accountants (either by regulatory authorities or in the name of aggrieved shareholders) grew into a flood, the profession's official body, the American Institute of Certified Public Accountants, stayed on the sidelines. The Institute insisted that it could not initiate disciplinary steps in such cases until the regulatory authorities or the courts had completed their civil or criminal proceedings. The Institute defended its inaction on grounds of practicality and out of concern for due process for accountants facing accusations. On the one hand, the Institute contended, it couldn't prevent any findings of its ethics proceedings from being obtained and exploited by plaintiffs suing accounting firms. The Institute didn't expect the firms to cooperate in providing ammunition for their adversaries. On the other hand, the Institute was loathe to proceed against its members (even with its limited sanction of expulsion from membership) without their full side of the story. Thus in the face of sharp criticism of its toothlessness, the AICPA nevertheless insisted on waiting out the torturous processes of the American legal system before moving against erring or incompetent auditors. As a practical matter, the large, notorious audit failures dragged on so long in the courts that the Institute rarely took action.

The flood of publicity over

Equity Funding, together with the unprecedented dimensions of the fraud, put enormous pressure on the AICPA to abandon its usual aloofness and begin an immediate inquiry into the auditing at Equity Funding. After a flurry of intramural debate, the Institute moved with surprising dispatch to establish an investigating committee chaired by Marvin Stone, the head of a small Denver firm and a former AICPA president. Another prominent member was Archie E. MacKay, the managing partner of Main, Lafrentz & Co. (perhaps the nation's tenth largest accounting firm) and the man generally credited with inspiring the stiffer accounting rules that burst the profit bubble for the franchise industry in 1971.

The Institute tried to paper over the obvious departure from its ethics policy by charging the Stone committee only with determining whether the Equity Funding disclosures had revealed inadequacies in general accepted auditing standards. By their instructions, the committee members were explicitly *not* to investigate the actual performance of Equity Funding's auditors. Of course, that maneuver proved transparent. If generally accepted auditing standards were *not* at fault—and the Stone committee ultimately concluded they weren't—and the fraud was as pervasive as portrayed, then blame had to fall on the auditors.

With the trustee's report available to it, the Stone committee didn't take long to complete its work. Indeed, it wrapped up its conclusions as the trial of the Wolfson, Weiner auditors was about to start. Then the inevitable debate within the Institute began: How could the Institute publish the committee's report while the Equity Funding auditors were on trial for their professional lives? On the other hand, how could the AICPA continue to avoid saying anything when word was leaking out that the Stone report was ready? The report was withheld until after the verdicts and then published almost immediately. Even that delayed publication wasn't without controversy. Two of the Stone committee's five members objected to releasing the report (but not to its conclusions) before all the civil litigation involving Equity Funding's auditors was settled.

Given its narrow charge, the specificity of "generally accepted auditing standards" (there are ten standards, which are stated in less than 300 words, as compared to "generally accepted *accounting principles*," which have never been set down in one place and which would fill volumes if they were), and the necessary political tightrope it had to walk, the Stone committee cannot be faulted on its product. The message was clear.

Nevertheless, a good deal more remains to be said about the impact of Equity Funding on auditing, if not precisely and narrowly on auditing standards. The committee did not probe some critical questions on basic operations of the accounting profession.

Accountants have been on a merger binge, not unlike that of industry. For various reasons—to gain better national and international coverage, to penetrate individual industries, to cover increasing training and research overhead, and sometimes just to have a bigger, more important firm—many accounting firms have grown through merger. As in industry, a few firms have disdained the merger route, but the phenomenon has been pervasive. Unlike industrial mergers, which have been subject to searching and often unsympathetic scrutiny by the Congress, the Justice Department, the Federal Trade Commission, and hordes of academic economists, few questions, in or out of the profession, have been raised about the effects of accounting firm mergers.

What are the obligations, to the public, of a "big name" accounting firm that acquires a small, less known practice? Can it simply put its imprimatur on the unchanged competence and staff of the acquired firm—as seems to have been the case with Seidman & Seidman in Equity Funding—or is there an obligation to integrate the acquired operation? Are there implicit obligations attached to having and using a national accounting firm name?

Both the Stone committee and the trustee pointed out the difficulty of Haskins & Sells' finding the fraud at EFLIC when it did not have access at the same time to the books of EFC-Cal (which was audited by Wolfson, Weiner). Since then, auditors have instituted stronger requirements for "upstream confirmation," that is, for the auditor of a subsidiary company to check with the auditor of a parent company. But can (or should) different accounting firms, often working thousands of miles apart, audit different portions of one corporation? Testimony in the Peat, Marwick depositions in the Ranger National Life incident (portions not reproduced here) chronicled the problems of coordinating work even between offices of the same firm. When different firms are involved, and many were involved in Equity Funding,

problems of coordination are intensified. Certainly, all of the firms auditing Equity Funding subsidiaries coveted the parent company audit. On the other hand, as soon as Seidman & Seidman acquired Wolfson, Weiner; Peat, Marwick lost the audit of Liberty Savings to Seidman.

It seems fairly clear that had Haskins & Sells audited both EFLIC and EFC-Cal, it would have discovered the fraud. It also seems clear that a good deal of the concealment of the fraud was possible because different elements of Equity Funding had different auditors. Should every corporation have only one auditor and the same auditor for all its significant divisions and subsidiaries?

Even a brief discussion of this possibility would have the small CPAs of the United States up in arms. But it's a valid question and has not been raised.

Most of the Stone committee's report is reproduced here. The omissions are descriptions of the fraud that duplicate material in the trustee's report and other sources. The full AICPA report includes a thorough, accurate description of the fraud.

Report of the Special Committee on Equity Funding

The Adequacy of Auditing Standards and Procedures Currently Applied in the Examination Of Financial Statements

American Institute of Certified Public Accountants

Chapter 1

Introduction

The Equity Funding debacle, like all disasters caused by human actions, offers the promise of useful lessons for the future. Of particular concern to the accounting profession is what may be learned from this debacle about the adequacy of standards governing the work of independent auditors.

The dimensions of the Equity Funding disaster and the general nature of its causes were revealed within a period of a few weeks in the spring of 1973. In March of that year, press reports questioned the integrity of the consolidated financial statements and other records and reports of the apparently successful Equity Funding Corporation of America (EFCA) and its subsidiaries, including Equity Funding Life Insurance Company (EFLIC). Within a month, on April 4, the parent company filed a petition in bankruptcy. It appeared by then that a fraud of substantial proportion had been carried out over several years by certain officers and employees of the Equity Funding companies. The result of the fraud was to present to investors, creditors and regulators a picture of ever-increasing earnings and assets and to stimulate an active market in the securities of the parent corporation. It is now apparent that much of the reported earnings and assets were false. EFCA's publicly held securities, with a previous market value in the hundreds of millions of dollars, are now virtually worthless.

The Equity Funding collapse brought on a host of legal proceedings, many of which are likely to go on for years. In addition to the bankruptcy proceedings, there have been investigations by insurance regulatory agencies of several states, as well as by the Securities and Exchange Commission and other federal agencies, grand jury investi-

5

gations which have resulted in the indictment and in some cases conviction of corporate officers and employees; the indictment of certain of the auditors;* disciplinary proceedings by the New York Stock Exchange; and scores of civil lawsuits.

A number of questions are raised by this disaster. In addition to criminal culpability and civil liability, the questions involve the sufficiency of regulatory procedures affecting publicly owned companies including life insurance companies, and the adequacy of prevailing assumptions about the responsibilities of various kinds of professions and occupations—including accountants, lawyers, actuaries, investment bankers and securities analysts—in relation to enterprises like Equity Funding.

Some of these questions concern standards governing the work of the public accounting profession, for EFCA had published annual consolidated financial statements through December 31, 1971 giving a false and misleading picture of its operations and financial position. These financial statements had carried reports by independent auditors which indicated that the financial statements had been examined in accordance with generally accepted auditing standards and were presented fairly in conformity with generally accepted accounting principles. The examination of the consolidated financial statements which were to be included in the 1972 annual report was substantially complete and printer's proofs were prepared. However, the consolidated financial statements and the auditors' report thereon were never issued.

On May 5, 1973, the Board of Directors of the American Institute of Certified Public Accountants, recognizing the importance of the questions raised with respect to the adequacy of prevailing professional standards, resolved that the president of the Institute should appoint a special committee to study whether auditing standards applicable to the examination of financial statements should be changed in the light of Equity Funding. The Board's resolution was as follows:

WHEREAS, the Institute shares the general public concern about the Equity Funding disaster, which caused enormous losses to investors and creditors apparently by reason of massive and collusive fraud; and

WHEREAS, developments in the Equity Funding matter may suggest that changes in generally accepted auditing standards are called for; and

WHEREAS, identification and implementation of any such changes in

---

* On May 20, 1975 a federal district court jury returned a verdict of guilty in a trial of three of the accountants involved with Equity Funding.

6

generally accepted auditing standards should not await the eventual resolution of litigation or other proceedings concerned with assigning responsibility in respect of Equity Funding.

NOW THEREFORE BE IT RESOLVED, that a special committee be appointed by the president of the Institute to study whether the auditing standards which are currently considered appropriate and sufficient in the examination of financial statements'should be changed in the light of Equity Funding, and report its conclusions to the Board of Directors and the auditing standards executive committee.

The appointment of the special committee to consider the possible larger implications of Equity Funding should not be understood as involving any deviation from the Institute's customary procedure for dealing with possible departures from the requirements of the Code of Professional Ethics. Accordingly, any questions raised by the Equity Funding matter as to adherence to professional standards by members of the Institute will be handled by the division of professional ethics.

This is the report of the special committee appointed pursuant to that resolution.

The Committee's Charge

As the resolution of the Institute's Board makes clear, the committee was not charged with attempting to assess fault or legal responsibility of the accountants or firms involved. Its charge was to consider whether the Equity Funding matter suggested a need for changes in generally accepted auditing standards.

The phrase "generally accepted auditing standards" refers to the ten standards which were formally adopted by the membership of the Institute in 1948 and 1949. These standards—three "General Standards," three "Standards of Field Work," and four "Standards of Reporting"—are explained and interpreted in a substantial body of professional literature of which the most authoritative is a series of pronouncements of the Institute set forth in its Statements on Auditing Standards.

The committee has understood its charge to require appraisal not only of the ten standards, but more particularly of the auditing procedures by means of which auditing standards are implemented. The Institute's Board of Directors has confirmed this understanding.

There were two aspects of this appraisal—one particular and the other general. The first focused on the auditing procedures that would customarily have been applied in the circumstances; the other involved

7

consideration of the general question of the auditor's responsibility to detect fraud.

The specific questions that the committee sought to answer were these:

1. What was the nature of the fraud in Equity Funding and how was it accomplished?

2. Would customary auditing procedures provide a reasonable expectation of detecting such a fraud?

3. Are any changes in customary auditing procedures called for in order to provide such a reasonable expectation?

4. Finally, and more generally, is there a need for change in scope of an auditor's responsibility for the detection of fraud, or for clarification of the auditor's responsibility, for the benefit of the accounting profession and the public at large?

The Conduct of the Committee's Study

To answer these questions, the committee did not consider it necessary to conduct an audit of the financial statements of any of the Equity Funding entities. In any event, to perform an audit for the years in which the fraud occurred would probably have been impractical if not impossible. The auditors appointed by the bankruptcy court completed an audit as of the date of bankruptcy. Their audit report appears in the *Report of the Trustee of Equity Funding Corporation of America* dated February 22, 1974.

The committee also did not determine what procedures actually were followed by the auditors of the Equity Funding entities since determination of fault, if any, was not part of its charge. To fulfill its purposes, the committee needed to gather information only with respect to the nature of the fraud and to relate this information to its understanding of the auditing procedures that would customarily have been applied in the examination of the financial statements of the Equity Funding entities.

The information needed for the study was obtained from the February 22 and October 31, 1974 reports of the Trustee of Equity Funding Corporation of America and through interviews with his executive staff, representatives of the auditing firm engaged by the Trustee, representatives of the California and Illinois Insurance Departments, the conservator for the life insurance subsidiary (EFLIC) and certain

8

of his staff, and some of the Equity Funding personnel who had been retained by the Trustee and the conservator.

The committee's representatives also looked at some of the records of the Equity Funding entities for the purpose of understanding the manner in which certain transactions were recorded on the books of the companies. Access to these records was granted by the Trustee and the conservator.

The committee's conclusions in this report necessarily rest upon the information in the reports of the Trustee and the information gathered in interviews and other investigations. If that information subsequently turns out to be inaccurate, the conclusions could be affected.

The committee generally limited its study to the pertinent Equity Funding entities for the years 1971 and 1972. Although it appears that the fraud began as early as 1964, the committee concluded that for its purposes it would be neither practicable nor necessary to extend its study to years before 1971 or into 1973, for the committee understands that the general pattern of the fraud which had appeared in earlier years or in 1973, could be identified without extending the review beyond these two years.

(Chapters 2 and 3 have been deleted. Editor).

Chapter 4

Conclusions and Recommendations Regarding The Adequacy of Auditing Standards and Procedures Currently Applied in the Examination of Financial Statements

General Conclusion

From its review, the committee has concluded that, except for certain observations relating to confirmation of insurance in force and auditing related party transactions, generally accepted auditing standards are adequate and that no changes are called for in the procedures commonly used by auditors. In reaching this conclusion, the committee is aware that it is possible to hypothesize ways in which virtually any audit procedure may be thwarted. Nevertheless, the committee believes that customary audit procedures properly applied would have provided a reasonable degree of assurance that the existence of fraud at Equity Funding would be detected.

The nature, extent and timing of audit procedures are normally based on a study and evaluation of the system of internal control in existence in the area under examination. While such procedures would not necessarily reveal a fraud, it appears that internal accounting and administrative controls at Equity Funding were so weak as to raise concern about the reliability of the accounting records. The committee believes that in such circumstances customary procedures would be extended because of the internal control weakness, thereby enhancing the likelihood of detecting fraud.

The remainder of this chapter sets forth some of the audit procedures which the committee believes would customarily be applied in the circumstances in testing the validity of certain accounts in which fraudulent entries were made at Equity Funding. Each section heading indicates the areas toward which the selected audit procedures would be primarily directed. However, these audit procedures might have

27

uncovered misstatements in related areas as well. For example, discovery of overstatements in the funded loan account might have led to the discovery of overstatements in the insurance in force, in commission income and in other related accounts. Similarly, discovery of an illogical relationship between commission income and commission expense might have led to discovery of the overstatement of funded loans.

Fictitious Funded Loans Receivable

The committee believes that the following customary audit procedures taken together would provide a reasonable degree of assurance that fictitious funded loans receivable would be detected:

- Prepare under the auditor's control a trial balance of funded loans receivable showing borrowers' names, full account numbers and balances.
- Reconcile the trial balance total with the general ledger control account balance and ascertain the propriety of any reconciling items.
- Review on a test basis the entries recording additions and deductions in the funded loans receivable account and examine documentation supporting the changes.
- Request on a test basis confirmation from borrowers of loan balances and amount of collateral pledged.
- On a test basis, inspect, or request confirmation from custodians of, mutual fund shares pledged as collateral by individual borrowers.

The auditor could carry out the above audit procedures relating to the trial balance and confirmation of funded loans receivable manually or through the use of computer programs designed for that purpose. If a client's computer programs were utilized the auditor would review and test such programs to the extent necessary to satisfy himself that they would produce valid data. To conduct such a review an auditor should have adequate technical training and proficiency in EDP techniques.

Fictitious Commission Income and Expense

The committee believes that the following customary auditing procedures taken together would provide a reasonable degree of assurance that fictitious EFC-Cal commission income and expense would be detected:

28

- Select a sample from the additions to the commission income account and trace the origin of such additions to supporting detail. Recalculate commissions earned on a test basis.

- Select a sample from the additions to the commission expense account and trace the origin of such additions to supporting detail. Recalculate commission expense on a test basis.

- Determine whether a logical relationship exists between insurance commission income and insurance commission expense.

- Test other major sources of commission income by examining supporting documentation or by confirming with the sources of such income.

- Review propriety of consolidation elimination and reclassification entries affecting insurance commission income and expense.

- Test overall reasonableness of insurance commission income by comparing it with first year and renewal premium data.

In the audit of commission income and expense the auditor would be cognizant of the relationship between premium volume and insurance commissions. An awareness of this relationship and more particularly, an awareness of that portion of premium volume attributable to first year sales as distinguished from renewals would permit the auditor to determine the overall reasonableness of recorded insurance commission revenue. Similarly, the overall propriety of recorded insurance commission expense would be established in light of gross premium or commission income and the provisions of agents' commission contracts.

Fictitious Life Insurance Policies

The committee believes that the following customary auditing procedures taken together would provide a reasonable degree of assurance that fictitious life insurance policies included in the inventory of insurance in force would be detected:

- On a test basis trace policies included in the inventory of insurance in force to the related premium collection.

- On a test basis trace premium income to premium collections and the related policies to the inventory of insurance in force.

Since EFLIC received no cash when it wrote new "program" policies, premiums could not be traced to specifically identifiable cash collections within its own records. Premiums on such policies were merely recorded as a charge to EFLIC's intercompany receivable due

29

from EFC-Cal and immediately offset by a credit in the same amount representing the first year commission. Thus, the only independent evidence to support premiums on new "program" business was the note receivable representing a loan made by EFC-Cal to finance the assured's premium.

Similar tests tracing evidence of billing and collection would be applied to renewal premiums. Again, in the case of "program" sales, such premiums were added to income and charged by EFLIC to its intercompany account receivable due from EFC-Cal. While the intercompany account balances were settled periodically, settlements were made on a lump sum basis making it impossible to trace specific premiums to specific cash collections as would customarily be the case.

To perform these audit tests it would be necessary to work with the records of both EFLIC and EFC-Cal, since EFC-Cal maintained the related loan account and billing and commission records in connection with its sales of EFLIC policies. Entries recording premium income and commission expense on EFLIC's books for policies sold by EFC-Cal were based solely on intercompany advices from EFC-Cal. Thus, an auditor could not trace premiums on "program" policies to evidence of billing and collection without gaining access to EFC-Cal's records. Under these circumstances, the auditor of EFLIC would either test the records of EFC-Cal himself or, if the two companies engaged separate auditors, EFLIC's auditor might request and rely upon EFC-Cal's auditor to carry out tests using data supplied by him from EFLIC's inventory of policies in force. In addition, EFC-Cal's commission income and premiums remitted would be compared on a test basis with premium income and commission expense on EFLIC's books to see if they corresponded.

Another auditing procedure, which heretofore has not been considered particularly useful, is verification of the authenticity of a selected number of policies included in the in force inventory by direct confirmation with the policyholders. Such a procedure has not generally been considered necessary because it would be unusual for companies to overstate liabilities. Inflation of the inventory of life insurance in force by a company that follows statutory accounting would result in an overstatement of the liability for future policyholder benefits and a reduction in current earnings. However, when companies report on the basis of generally accepted accounting principles (GAAP) there could be motivation for overstating insurance in force because it could result in an addition to current earnings.

There could be an additional motivation for overstating insurance in force when reinsurance of policies has the effect of materially increasing current earnings, which can occur when a company reports on the

30

basis of either GAAP or statutory accounting. Reinsurance of life insurance policies permits the elimination of the related liability for future policyholder benefits. Under certain circumstances, reinsurance may also result in increasing current earnings to the extent that the proceeds received from reinsurance exceed expenses incurred in connection with the sale and servicing of the reinsured policies.

EFLIC reinsured substantial numbers of both bona fide and fictitious policies. Thus, fictitiously inflating the in force inventory, coupled with the manner in which reinsurance commissions were accounted for, resulted in substantially increasing EFLIC's reported earnings.

The committee believes that when current earnings of a company could be materially increased as a result of either the reinsurance of policies or reporting on the basis of GAAP, there may be occasions when policies should be confirmed with policyholders on a test basis. Nevertheless, the committee cautions against placing too much reliance on such confirmation procedures as a sole means of determining the reasonableness of the in force inventory since such procedures cannot be expected to disclose unrecorded policies.

The committee recommends, therefore, that the Institute's auditing standards executive committee consider whether the Life Insurance Audit Guide requires clarification with regard to the confirmation of policies with policyholders.

Fictitious Securities Transactions

As discussed in Chapter 3, fictitious purchases of investments were recorded in 1971 and 1972 by EFCA and EFLIC to substitute for intercompany account balances between EFCA and EFLIC. The committee believes that the customary audit procedures of inspection of the securities held by the company or confirmation of the securities in safekeeping directly with an independent custodian would provide a reasonable degree of assurance that the non-existence of securities would be revealed.

In connection with the fictitious investments recorded on the books of EFLIC at December 31, 1972, the *Report of the Trustee of Equity Funding Corporation of America* dated October 31, 1974, states that Equity Funding established an office in Chicago using a name very close to that of American National Bank and Trust Co. by leasing space at a different address under the name of "American National Trust." The report states:

> From time to time thereafter, fraud participants sent letters addressed to "American National Bank" at the mail drop address to ac-

31

custom post office employees to delivering mail so addressed to the bogus location.

A print-out of the bogus bond portfolio was prepared on EFCA's System/3 computer, and was given to . . . (the auditors) during the 1972 audit to support purchases of $24 million of the bonds at American National Bank. When the auditors also requested a direct bank confirmation for the bogus bonds, a request for confirmation was prepared, addressed to the fictitious branch office and given to them for mailing. . . . (An officer of EFCA) went to Chicago to receive it at the phony American National Bank branch. Nothing was received for a period of several days, causing great consternation among the conspirators who feared that the post office had delivered the request to the real American National Bank and Trust Co. However, they later learned that . . . (the auditors) simply forgot to mail the confirmation request. . . . When the auditors' confirmation finally arrived at the mail drop . . . (an officer of EFCA) apparently signed and returned it to them in Los Angeles. In this manner, the conspirators concealed the $24 million imbalance in the intercompany account on EFLIC's books at year-end 1972.

While this points up the need for auditors to ascertain that valid addresses are used, such a step is already a customary and integral part of confirmation procedures.

An auditor customarily compares recorded security transactions with supporting broker or bank advices. However, this procedure probably would have been ineffective because certain advices had been forged.

Other Fictitious Receivables and Fraudulently Inflated Assets

With respect to the receivables resulting from the sale of the casualty insurance agency operation, the committee believes that the following customary audit procedures taken together would raise serious questions as to whether the receivables were valid:

- Analyze the accounts and review supporting data including contracts or agreements.
- Examine recent financial statements and credit ratings of the debtors to establish the financial standing of debtors.
- Confirm unpaid balances directly with the debtors.

Although the above auditing procedures would customarily be applied to the Estudios and Grandson receivables, the committee is of the opinion that these procedures might have been ineffective in detecting the fraudulent nature of these accounts since the Trustee has determined that both companies were secretly controlled by EFCA. These audit procedures could have been circumvented through management collusion.

As to the investment in the commercial paper of Apatex, the committee is of the opinion that customary auditing procedures (described in the section Fictitious Securities Transactions) might not have disclosed that the asset was fictitious. This opinion is based on the following:

1. Forged purchase advices were available for inspection.

2. The commercial paper was supposedly held by Bishops Bank, an EFCA subsidiary. Confirmation from the bank that it was holding the paper would not have furnished adequate audit evidence because the bank was not an independent custodian.

3. The bank made a market in this commercial paper and may have had such securities on hand for sale. Accordingly, inspection of $2 million of Apatex commercial paper would have given no assurance that the paper inspected was the property of EFC-Cal.

Circumstances such as those which were present regarding the Estudios, Grandson and Apatex accounts highlight the fact that transactions between related parties pose serious auditing problems. The committee did not attempt to reach any conclusions regarding the problems inherent in auditing such transactions since the auditing standards executive committee of the AICPA is currently studying the need for additional auditing procedures in connection with related party transactions.

With respect to the $5.9 million receivable from insurance companies and from agents, the committee believes that the following customary auditing procedures taken together would provide a reasonable degree of assurance that the highly questionable nature of the accounts would be disclosed.

As to the approximately $4 million receivable from insurance companies:

- Analyze the account balance (which would have shown that it had remained unchanged for several years).

- Review commission collections early in the subsequent year which were applicable to the year-end balance under audit.

33

As to the approximately $1.9 million receivable from agents representing unreconciled differences between the control account total and total of the subsidiary records:

- Review the company's method of clearing unreconciled differences.
- Inquire as to why the difference had not been written off.

With respect to the inflated investment in Bishop's Bank, the committee is of the opinion that customary auditing procedures would have included a review of the net change in the "goodwill" account which was recorded on the books of EFCA. Such a review would provide a reasonable degree of assurance that the inflated account would be discovered.

In regard to the capitalized mineral exploration costs, the committee believes that an attempt to review data supporting the journal entries which gave rise to deferral of such costs would provide reasonable assurance that the impropriety of the asset would be discovered.

Use of the Computer

In the opinion of the committee, a knowledge of computer audit techniques was not essential to the detection of the Equity Funding fraud. Manual application of customary auditing procedures would have provided a reasonable degree of assurance that the fraud would be uncovered.

The committee also believes that the fraud did not contain any elements that involved new or unique computer applications. Thus, no recommendations are made for any new auditing standards or procedures in regard to computer maintained financial records.

34

Chapter 5

Responsibility of Auditors for Detection of Fraud

The extensive fraud at Equity Funding raises fundamental conceptual and practical questions about the responsibility of auditors for detection of fraud, and about the understanding of that responsibility by both the accounting profession and the public. The committee believes it should address these questions even though it has concluded that no significant changes in generally accepted auditing standards and procedures are necessary in the light of Equity Funding.

The understanding of the public accounting profession as to its responsibility for detection of fraud is set forth in Statement on Auditing Standards No. 1, in sections 110.05, .06, .07 and .08, which are reproduced in the Appendix. The propositions contained in that Statement relate to the ten generally accepted auditing standards, which govern the auditor's work in examining financial statements. One of these standards requires that the auditor make a proper study and evaluation of internal control as a basis for reliance thereon and for the determination of the extent of the tests to which auditing procedures are to be restricted. Thus, in the presence of weakness in internal control, the auditor recognizes the possibility that fraud could go undetected; and, correspondingly, modification of the nature, extent and timing of audit tests may be considered necessary.

The ten standards also require adequate technical training and proficiency as an auditor, independence in mental attitude, exercise of due professional care, adequate planning and supervision, and sufficient competent evidential matter to support the auditor's opinion on the financial statements being examined. The auditor's report explicitly states whether his examination has met these standards.

In meeting these standards, the auditor's attitude is one of awareness of the possibility of fraud. Many customary auditing procedures, though not specifically aimed at fraud detection, are nonetheless designed to test the reliability of the books and records and may raise questions as to the possibility of fraud. If the auditor suspects that there is a lack of honesty affecting the records or financial statements, he should modify the nature, extent and timing of his tests so as to either confirm or dispel his suspicion.

Although an auditor's unqualified opinion provides a degree of assurance that there is no material fraud, the committee believes that there is a risk that the opinion may be misunderstood as providing a higher degree of assurance as to the absence of fraud than can reasonably be expected. If such misunderstanding is to be avoided, it is important that the inescapable limitations on an audit be understood.

SAS No. 1, section 110.06, states that the auditor cannot give assurance that all types of fraud have been detected even when the most extensive audit has been conducted. Three examples are given: forgery, collusion and unrecorded transactions.

Forgery may be employed as to signatures and other signs of authenticity, or to entire documents. Throughout history skillful forgers have eluded detection even by experts; and auditors cannot reasonably be expected to be handwriting or documentary experts.

Collusion—as between client personnel and outsiders, or among management or employees of the client—may result in the presentation to the auditor of falsified confirmations or other documents that appear genuine. If the auditor has no reason to suspect the genuineness of the documents, it would be reasonable for him to rely on them. In a scheme to conceal fraud, of course, there is likely to be a combination of forgery and collusion.

Finally, auditing techniques cannot provide assurance that there are no unrecorded transactions. For example, a payable may be concealed, and little short of requesting confirmation from every possible creditor would provide assurance of its discovery.

In addition to the foregoing limitations which are largely insurmountable, there are practical and economic limitations on the degree of assurance that auditors can reasonably be expected to provide. An ordinary audit is not an examination of every transaction and of every document relating to every transaction; rather, an audit involves a testing of transactions and of the related underlying records and other documents. The nature, extent and timing of the testing depend upon a

36

number of factors, including the auditor's study and evaluation of the client's internal control, the results of particular tests, the importance of particular items being tested, and whether grounds for suspicion of fraud are discovered in the course of the audit. In the usual case, to substitute for such an examination one covering every transaction and record of the client would multiply the amount of work involved to an impracticable degree.

"Detailed" audits, which may be undertaken for special purposes, offer a greater likelihood of detecting fraud because they ordinarily involve examination of larger numbers of individual items and transactions than the ordinary audit. Even in detailed audits, however, some types of fraud may escape detection (e.g., unrecorded transactions, forgery, or collusion) because there is necessarily a point where the auditor's inquiry stops.

In every audit, the auditor is expected to be aware of the possibility of fraud. Nonetheless, there must come a point where, unless he has reason for suspicion, the auditor accepts the truth of representations made to him and the genuineness of documents which he inspects. Examples of representations which would normally be accepted (in the absence of specific reasons for suspicion) even though they might be deliberately false would be representations by management as to the completeness of a set of board or executive committee minutes; or by the client's counsel as to the absence of pending material litigation; or by a debtor of the client as to the correctness of an account receivable; or by a bank or depository as to the status of the client's accounts with it.

Yet there will almost always be some further step that could be taken to corroborate the accuracy of the representation made to the auditor. For example, a debtor's response to a request for confirmation of an account receivable could be checked by inspection of the debtor's records reflecting the corresponding account payable, or by a certificate from the debtor's auditor. If the representation is one of counsel, the auditor could ask to inspect the pleadings in the case, he could examine the court records, or he could require an opinion of his own counsel with respect to the opinion of the client's counsel, and so on. Each such incremental step would add a degree of confidence, and yet in few cases would it produce absolute certainty.

Similarly, there is a point where, again assuming that he has no reason for suspicion, the auditor accepts the genuineness of documents: as, for example, the genuineness of securities held by the client and inspected by the auditor, even though these might be skillfully counterfeited; or of contracts or signatures on confirmations, although these might be forged; or of underlying internal documents, although the availability of the client's own forms often makes these relatively easy to falsify. As to any such matter, there is ordinarily some further step that could be taken to test the authenticity of a document on which reliance is placed: the authority of a debtor's officer or employee to sign a confirmation could be authenticated; the genuineness of that person's signature could be verified; the authority of the authenticating officer could itself be authenticated, and the genuineness of that signature checked, and so on. Again each additional step would produce another degree of confidence, still without achieving complete certainty.

Absolute certainty is no more an attainable goal of auditing than it is of any other professional endeavor. What is sought is a reasonable degree of assurance; and what is applied to achieve such reasonable assurance is and must be a professional judgment as to how far inquiry should go. The necessity for such a judgment reflects the fact that there is no ultimate stopping place: each new level of test offers yet another choice between reliance or still a further test. It reflects the fact that each incremental step would increase the work involved and therefore the cost and duration of the audit, without promising ultimate certainty.

The question may be raised whether, even if in ordinary circumstances audits cannot reasonably be expected to detect all material fraud, the expectation should not be different when, as in Equity Funding, the fraud is a "massive" one. In other words, it might be suggested that, assuming the term "massive" could be given a concrete definition, auditing standards should be such that an auditor's opinion would invariably constitute a reasonable assurance that no "massive" fraud existed such as in Equity Funding. The committee does not believe that such a suggestion is sound.

On analysis, three fairly distinct meanings might be assigned to the term "massive": referring to size—the numerical magnitude of the falsified figures or of the losses incurred by investors and others as a result of the fraud; referring to the extent of the collusion—the number of persons involved in the fraudulent scheme and the elaborateness of that scheme; and referring to the number of accounts affected. There is, of course, some connection between these several dimensions of the term, since it is often the case that the larger dollar amounts of falsification, the more accounts will be tainted and the more elaborate will be the precautions necessary to avoid detection of the falsification.

In any of these senses, the more massive a fraud, the greater will be the likelihood of its detection by customary audit tests. The larger the number of accounts and records affected by the falsification, the larger will be the number of potential audit trails leading to its discovery. The

38

larger the dollar amount of falsification resulting from the fraud, the more likely it will be that the fraud will continue and enlarge from year to year; and the longer the fraud continues, the greater will be the chances of its coming to light in one way or another. Moreover, the more extensive the collusion, the more numerous will be the persons who may intentionally or inadvertently betray their guilty knowledge or behave in a manner that will arouse suspicion.

On the other hand, the more skillful the collusion, the less likely will be the discovery of the fraud—regardless of its massiveness in the sense of size or numbers of accounts affected. Fraudulent devices such as forgery and the failure to record transactions are virtually impossible to detect by ordinary auditing, and as to any given auditing procedure, techniques can be devised that will offer reasonable promise of circumventing the procedure in question. Thus, there remains the possibility that even a massive fraud can escape detection by an audit conducted in accordance with generally accepted auditing standards.

It may fairly be said that the more massive the fraud the more likely it is to be detected in a conventional audit; nonetheless there is no definable degree of massiveness as to which such an audit can invariably be relied upon for such detection. Nor, in the committee's view, is there any practicable means of altering auditing standards or procedures so as to provide such an absolute assurance with respect to any set degree of massiveness.

In sum, the committee reaffirms the soundness of the accounting profession's understanding with respect to the role of audits in the detection of fraud. A change in this basic understanding to make the auditor's opinion into more of a guarantee of the absence of fraud would represent a major change in the conception and performance of audits and would vastly increase their expense—yet still not furnish a complete guarantee. To ask that a professional opinion be made into an absolute assurance would, moreover, be to seek a degree of certainty which is seldom to be found in any other area of commercial life—or, for that matter, in any area of our lives, private or public. However, even though such absolute assurance is not feasible, the application of generally accepted auditing standards will often result in the discovery of material frauds. Audits also can be expected to deter frauds which might otherwise occur.

Having said all this, the committee is still concerned that there may be a divergence in the understanding of the public and of the accounting profession with respect to the auditor's responsibility for detection of fraud. Although the committee believes that all of the propositions contained in SAS No. 1, sections 110.05, .06, .07 and .08, are sound, it also concludes that the way they are cast, with its greater emphasis on the limitations rather than on the positive aspects of the matter, may contribute to the risk of disparity in understanding, between the public at large and the public accounting profession, as to what an auditor's responsibility is with respect to the detection of fraud.

On one hand, there seems to be a tendency to view auditors' reports as if they were warranties—absolute assurances against fraud or error—and to ignore the practical limitations on auditors' work, which SAS No. 1 emphasizes. On the other hand, those limitations, even though well understood by the profession, may not be expressed in a persuasive way. The committee believes that a more detailed statement of both the auditor's responsibilities and the limitations of those responsibilities might well be helpful in reducing such misunderstanding. It therefore recommends that the auditing standards executive committee consider restating those sections of SAS No. 1 which relate to the auditor's responsibility for detection of fraud.

In this respect, it seems clear that the auditor has an obligation to discover material frauds that are discoverable through application of customary auditing procedures applied in accordance with generally accepted auditing standards. The auditing profession should, on an ongoing basis, continue to improve the efficiency of customary audit procedures to the end that probability of discovery of material frauds continues to increase within the limits of practicability.

**Respectfully Submitted by the
Special Committee on Equity Funding**

Marvin L. Stone, *Chairman*
J. T. Arenberg, Jr.
Leo E. Burger
Robert C. Holsen
A. E. MacKay

AICPA Staff
Thomas R. Hanley

February 1975

40

Dissent to Publication at This Time

Messrs. Arenberg and Holsen dissent to the publication of this Report prior to the termination of significant litigation involving Equity Funding because (a) the rights of certain litigants may be unfairly affected by the premature publication of this Report, (b) new information that may be brought out during the course of the litigation could, as indicated on page 9 of the Report, affect the committee's conclusions, so that publication would turn out to have been premature, and (c) the absence of recommendations for changes in auditing procedures may lead some readers of the Report to believe that the audits were deficient even though the committee, in keeping with its charge, made no attempt to assess fault. In addition, they believe that publication of the Report at this time may establish an unwarranted and potentially dangerous precedent, particularly when, as in this instance, there has been no discussion of the Report with the auditors involved.

HOW NOT TO BUY AN ACCOUNTING FIRM

On September 1, 1976, the SEC issued its Accounting Series Release No. 196, "In the Matter of Seidman & Seidman et al.," an examination of the Wolfson, Weiner audit practices and, in particular, of the acquisition of Wolfson, Weiner by the Seidman firm.

The following excerpts from ASR No. 196 cover the portions related to Equity Funding—the SEC also took Seidman to task on several other audits.

Unfortunately, while the SEC roundly condemns the Seidman firm's lack of care in the acquisition of Wolfson, Weiner and notes the continued activity on the EFCA audit of the former Wolfson, Weiner auditors, the Commission is silent on the frequently made accusation that this arrangement was specifically agreed to in the merger. Interestingly, the Commission, when discussing the audit of Investors Planning Corp., fails to note that Equity Funding acquired IPC only after the SEC gave permission for it to do so, and after the SEC had turned down other potential buyers.

UNITED STATES OF AMERICA
Before the
SECURITIES AND EXCHANGE COMMISSION

SECURITIES EXCHANGE ACT OF 1934
Release No.12752 /September 1, 1976

ACCOUNTING SERIES
Release No. 196 /September 1, 1976

ADMINISTRATIVE PROCEEDING File No. 3-5072

In the Matter of	:	OPINION AND ORDER
	:	PURSUANT TO RULE 2(e)
SEIDMAN & SEIDMAN et al.	:	OF THE COMMISSION's
	:	RULES OF PRACTICE

This Opinion and Order under Rule 2(e)(1) 1/ of the
Commission's Rules of Practice [17 C.F.R. 201.2(e)(1)]
arises out of: (1) the conduct of Seidman & Seidman
and certain of its partners and employees in connection
with its combination of practices in February, 1972 with the
Los Angeles, California office of Wolfson, Weiner, Ratoff
& Lapin ("Wolfson/Weiner") and of the audits of certain
financial statements of three former Wolfson/Weiner clients--
Equity Funding Corporation of America ("Equity"), Omni-Rx
Health Systems ("Omni-Rx") and SaCom, and (2) certain of the
audits of financial statements of Cenco, Incorporated
("Cenco").

1/ Rule 2(e)(1) provides as follows:

The Commission may deny temporarily or permanently, the
privilege of appearing or practicing before it in any
way to any person who is found by the Commission after
notice of and the opportunity for hearing in the matter
(i) not to possess the requisite qualifications to
represent others, or, (ii) to be lacking in character
or integrity or to have engaged in unethical or improper
professional conduct, or (iii) to have willfully violated,
or willfully aided and abetted the violation of any
provision of the Federal securities laws [15 U.S.C.
77a to 80b-20], or the rules and regulations thereunder.

- 2 -   34-12752

Seidman & Seidman is a partnership engaged in the practice
of public accounting. It has more than 150 partners located
in 43 offices throughout the United States and is affiliated
with a number of accounting firms outside the United States.
Since its creation in 1910, the firm has performed a variety
of auditing, tax, advisory and related services in the
United States and abroad.

Seidman & Seidman has submitted an offer of settlement,
described in detail below, which we have considered and
determined to accept. As contemplated by the settlement
offer, Seidman & Seidman has waived institution of formal
administrative proceedings under Rule 2(e) and, without
admitting or denying any of the statements or conclusions
set forth herein, has consented to the issuance of this
Opinion and Order. The facts developed in the staff
investigations and the related accounting and auditing
issues are set forth in some detail below.

SUMMARY

The matters giving rise to these proceedings are the
result of two unrelated areas of inquiry conducted by the
Commission staff. These matters involved fraudulent conduct
by the client companies in which Seidman & Seidman was deceived.
Nevertheless, we have concluded that Seidman & Seidman did
not fulfill its responsibilities in the manner required by
the standards of the profession.

Three of the audit engagements which are the subject of
this Opinion and Order concern clients obtained by Seidman &
Seidman through its February 1972 combination of practices with
the Los Angeles, California office of Wolfson/Weiner. As a
result of the staff's investigation we have found that the
audit practices employed by Wolfson/Weiner's Los Angeles
office were far below professional standards and that employees
of that office engaged in acts and practices in flagrant
violation of rules of the Commission and standards of the
accounting profession relating to independence.

Seidman & Seidman failed to undertake a reasonable investigation prior to the combination of the firms and failed to
properly review practices and professional qualifications of
staff members of the Wolfson/Weiner office or to adequately
inquire into factors bearing on their independence from
clients. After the combination, Seidman & Seidman failed
to take reasonable steps to ensure the maintenance of

- 3 -   34-12752

professional audit review practices and independence in
connection with former Wolfson/Weiner clients.

In Equity 2/ certain former Wolfson/Weiner and management
personnel were criminally convicted following disclosure of
a massive financial fraud. 3/ Over approximately ten
years, Equity falsified its financial statements by
reporting bogus assets and earnings in the tens of millions
of dollars. Approximately one month after consummation
of the Wolfson/Weiner combination, Seidman & Seidman issued
an unqualified opinion on the December 31, 1971 Equity
financial statements although no pre-combination Seidman and
Seidman personnel had worked on or reviewed the audit and
Seidman & Seidman was aware that Wolfson/Weiner partners
generally did not review audit engagements.

In Omni-Rx 4/, Seidman & Seidman audited financial statements for inclusion in a registration statement for a public
offering and financial statements for a subsequent reporting
period which were included in an Annual Report on Form 10-K.
Seidman & Seidman learned after the offering that a substantial
amount of the offering proceeds had been used to pay debts of
persons in management who were in effective control of Omni-Rx
and that statements by Omni-Rx in a report filed with the
Commission concerning use of proceeds were false. Seidman &
Seidman subsequently issued an opinion on Omni-Rx's financial

----

2/ In April 1973, the Commission filed a complaint in the United
    States District Court for the Central District of California
    seeking injunctive and other relief against Equity and others,
    not including Seidman & Seidman. See Litigation Release
    No. 5849/April 16, 1973.

3/ Julian S.H. Weiner and Solomon Block, both formerly
    associated with the Wolfson/Weiner firm, were convicted in
    the United States District Court for the Central District
    of California of certain criminal violations of the federal
    securities laws. Under the provisions of Rule 2(e)(2)
    of the Commission's Rules of Practice, their right to
    practice before the Commission was automatically suspended
    following that conviction.

4/ The Commission has filed a complaint in the United States
    District Court for the District of Columbia seeking
    injunctive relief against Omni-Rx and others,not including
    Seidman & Seidman. See Litigation Release No. 7540
    September 1, 1976.

- 4 -   34-12752

statements for the year in which these events occurred which
omitted to disclose these facts. In addition, Seidman & Seidman
issued an opinion on the financial statements included in the
registration statement which financial statements failed to
reflect necessary provisions for losses on accounts receivable
due from affiliates and failed to disclose the adverse financial
condition of the affiliates of Omni-Rx.

In SaCom 5/, Seidman & Seidman audited financial statements included in a registration statement, and financial
statements for a subsequent reporting period included in
an Annual Report on Form 10-K. In these audits the firm
accepted management decisions to capitalize material
amounts of costs and to record, without necessary loss
allowances, the full amounts of claims for certain
government contract work without substantial evidential
support for such accounting treatment.

The second, and unrelated area of inquiry is the Cenco
case. 6/ In that case, the staff investigation indicates
that certain members of the former management group and
others engaged in a calculated scheme to falsify Cenco's
financial statements. This was accomplished in large part by
inflation of the quantities and cost of items of inventory.
We have concluded that Seidman & Seidman failed to conduct the
examinations in question in accordance with generally accepted
auditing standards, including ignoring or failing to adequately
pursue significant facts which came to its attention. In
our view the examinations were not properly planned and
staffed and the audit work performed provided an insufficient
basis to support opinions that the financial statements
were fairly presented.

The audits of financial statements of Equity, Omni-Rx,
SaCom and Cenco, the particulars of which are detailed
below, involve serious deficiencies in audit performance,
review, supervision and, except with respect to Cenco,

5/ The Commission has filed a complaint in the United States
District Court for the District of Columbia seeking
injunctive relief against SaCom and others, not including
Seidman & Seidman. See Litigation Release No. 7539
September 1, 1976.

6/ The Commission has filed a complaint in the United States
District Court for the Northern District of Illinois
seeking injunctive relief against certain members of the
former management of Cenco and others, not including
Seidman & Seidman. See Litigation Release No. 7538
September 1, 1976.

independence. The financial statements of these issuers
were not prepared in conformity with generally accepted
accounting principles and the audits were not conducted
in accordance with generally accepted auditing standards
as was represented by Seidman & Seidman in its reports.
In several instances Seidman & Seidman failed to obtain
sufficient competent evidential matter to afford a reasonable basis for its opinions, permitted the examination of
critical audit areas to be performed by persons having
inadequate training or proficiency in audit work, and
placed unwarranted reliance upon management representations.

A firm engaged in practice before the Commission and
persons who undertake responsible positions in such firms must
take appropriate measures to insure the maintenance of professional standards and independence in the conduct, review
and supervision of audit work on financial statements to be
filed with the Commission. Investors and other users of
financial statements properly rely upon reports of auditors
for protection and have a right to assume that such reports
are based upon examinations conducted in accordance with
high professional standards by independent auditors. Under
the circumstances of these cases, we find that Seidman &
Seidman's conduct represented a breach of its ethical and
professional responsibilities in practicing before the
Commission.

COMBINATION OF PRACTICES

Seidman & Seidman was founded in 1910 by M. L. Seidman with a single office in New York, New York. By 1968, the firm had developed into a diverse, nationwide practice. At that time the firm had ten general partners (six Seidman family members and four unrelated persons). In 1968 Seidman & Seidman reorganized into six geographic regions, each under the supervision of a regional partner, and entered upon a program of rapid expansion through combinations of practices with other smaller firms. Since 1968 the number of Seidman & Seidman offices has increased from 24 to 43. It is indicative of the pace of expansion that during the nine years from 1960 to 1969 the firm engaged in only three combinations while in the five years from 1969 to 1973 there were 26 such combinations.

The Wolfson/Weiner firm was founded in about 1957 in Los Angeles by Julian S. H. Weiner and Phillip J. Wolfson. Ten years later this firm and certain other firms scattered throughout the country entered into a loosely affiliated national organization. In 1971, Wolfson/Weiner had 18 partners and about 200 employees in six offices across the United States. Each office was substantially independent of the others. In the Los Angeles office one of the two partners acted principally as the administrative partner while the other was primarily engaged in practice development and in seeking financing and similar activities on behalf of clients of Wolfson/Weiner.

Although Equity was Wolfson/Weiner's major client, a substantial portion of annual revenues resulted from audit work by Wolfson/Weiner for companies in the process of

going public through registered public offerings or offerings
under Regulation A. Wolfson/Weiner had a reputation in
the Los Angeles area for its ability to groom companies
for public offerings and assist them in obtaining financing
and underwriting arrangements. The Wolfson/Weiner clientele
thus consisted largely of unseasoned companies, some of
which were apparently formed for the purpose of going public.
The officers of these companies had little if any knowledge
or experience in the reporting requirements of the Commission,
and the companies frequently had accounting systems unsuited
to such public reporting requirements. Many were undergoing
audits for the first time. Such a practice and clientele
required a high degree of skill and judgment in auditing
which Wolfson/Weiner lacked.

        The staff's investigation indicates that Wolfson/Weiner's
Los Angeles office did not meet the professional standards
necessary for investor protection in many of its client
audit engagements. While on occasion the two partners were
engaged in critical decision making on audit engagements,
they were not familiar with the details of audits and generally
did not review workpapers. In addition many members of Wolfson/
Weiner's audit staff failed to meet the standards of the profession with respect to qualifications and competence. Audit
managers, some of whom were not certified public accountants,
were permitted to sign the firm's name to audit reports.
The Wolfson/Weiner workpapers examined by the staff in its
investigation were replete with audit conclusions which
were not supported by either the audit procedures or the
audit findings, open points left unanswered and statements
by the field auditors disputing conclusions on material
matters reached by the partners or managers of the engagements.
In addition, numerous and gross departures by Wolfson/Weiner
partners and staff from the independence standards of the
profession and requirements of the Commission were found.

        After initial contact by Wolfson/Weiner, discussions
occurred in 1970 concerning a possible combination of the
two firms but Seidman & Seidman rejected the Wolfson/Weiner
proposal. Wolfson/Weiner reopened the discussions in 1971.
Several meetings occurred in late 1971 and early 1972 between
Wolfson/Weiner partners and certain members of the Seidman &
Seidman Policy Group. Seidman & Seidman declined a combination
with the entire Wolfson/Weiner firm and reached an agreement

- 19 -   34-12752

to combine with only its successful Los Angeles practice. 21/
A formal agreement between the parties was completed
on February 18, 1972 and was made retroactive to February 1,
1972.   The separate offices were physically combined during
the Summer of 1972.

     It was the policy of Seidman & Seidman that the regional
partner supervise the pre-merger investigation and that the
results of the investigation together with his recommendation
be presented for the consideration and vote of the Policy
Group of Seidman & Seidman. 22/   Seidman & Seidman had, at the
time, established procedures for the investigation and
evaluation of combination of practice candidates.   These
procedures were set forth in two outlines included in a
merger kit which consisted substantially of information
about Seidman & Seidman. While the merger kit did not specify
the manner in which such reviews were to be conducted it
required that investigations be conducted into, among other
things, the audit practices and procedures and qualifications
of personnel of the firm to be acquired.

     The Commission believes that the pre-combination examination
procedures used by Seidman & Seidman were inadequate. For
example, the Seidman & Seidman procedures contemplated some
investigation of the audit procedures of the combination candidate,
but did not specify the scope of this investigation or the
manner in which it was to be conducted. In this instance,
Seidman & Seidman performed a cursory review for one day of
two of Wolfson/Weiner's audit clients and one non-audit client.
Further, Seidman & Seidman erred in unduly relying upon oral

21/   In April of 1972, Seidman & Seidman, in a separate trans-
      action, combined practices with the Ratoff & Lapin firm
      in White Plains, New York, which had been a part of the
      Wolfson/Weiner affiliated group.

22/   The western regional partner of Seidman & Seidman at the
      time was Robert Spencer. As such, he supervised the pre-
      combination investigation of the Los Angeles office of
      the Wolfson/Weiner firm. In October 1973, he became a
      senior partner of the firm and since then has not been
      involved in the investigation of possible combination of
      practice candidates for Seidman & Seidman. He has assured
      the Commission that he will not be involved in such
      activities in the future. The Commission accepts his
      assurance and directs him to comply therewith.

representations by the partners of Wolfson/Weiner with respect to the nature and quality of its practice.

Moreover, an inadequate investigation was made of the qualifications of the Wolfson/Weiner staff. During its investigation Seidman & Seidman did learn of the lack of participation of the two Wolfson/Weiner partners in the conduct and review of audit engagements as well as of certain concerns as to the qualifications of one senior member of the firm's staff.

Despite these matters the Policy Group approved the combination of practices on the recommendation of the regional partner. The vote of the Policy Group on the combination was taken by telephone and mail instead of at a regularly scheduled meeting as was the general practice.

After the combination and until mid 1973, one of the Wolfson/Weiner partners was assigned the responsibility for the audit engagements of former Wolfson/Weiner clients. This partner continued his former practice of rarely participating in review of audit engagements, a fact known to Seidman & Seidman. The deficiencies in the audit practice of Wolfson/Weiner as discussed above also continued. Over a period of time after the combination of practices, Seidman & Seidman became increasingly aware of material deficiencies in the work product and qualifications of members of the former Wolfson/Weiner staff and failed to adequately supervise the conduct of the continuing audit engagements.

The Commission has become increasingly concerned that the trend in the accounting profession toward growth accomplished through combinations may sometimes weaken professional standards in audit engagements. In situations such as these, the Commission believes that a rigorous examination of the procedures and previous audit work as well as the independence of a candidate are required. Such examinations, while not a perfect safeguard against false statements made by principals of a combination candidate, should be sufficient in scope to permit the acquiring firm to know with a reasonable degree of confidence the quality of the practice it proposes to acquire. A combination of practices should be fully discussed and analyzed by the decision making authorities of the acquiring firm.

- 21 -   34-12752

Furthermore, the Commission believes that accounting firms should be hesitant to rush into combinations of practice. In this instance, there appears to have been a desire by Wolfson/ Weiner, pressed by Equity's management, to conclude the combination so that the 1971 year-end Equity financial statements could carry the name of Seidman & Seidman. The desire to obtain the public relations benefits of financial statements audited by a major accounting firm is not a reasonable excuse for shortening the deliberative process before effecting a combination.

Seidman & Seidman's investigation of Wolfson/Weiner revealed that the two Wolfson/Weiner partners, while actively involved in client relations and some aspects of audit work, did not customarily involve themselves in the review aspects of audits. The involvement of partners in the review of audits is, in the Commission's view, a necessary element of sound auditing practice. Where no partner of a combina- tion candidate regularly performs review functions, it is incumbent upon the acquiring firm to investigate closely the manner in which review functions are performed within the combination candidate. The Commission is not satisfied with the examination by Seidman & Seidman of Wolfson/Weiner in this regard.

Post-combination procedures for assimilation of combined practices are no less important than appropriate and adequate pre-combination examination standards and procedures. Firms which choose to expand through combinations with other practitioners have an obligation to maintain and enforce a high level of professionalism throughout the enlarged practice.

INDEPENDENCE 23/

Various partners and employees in the Seidman & Seidman Los Angeles Office who had previously been employed by Wolfson/ Weiner had direct and indirect financial interests in clients

---

23/ Rule 2.01 of Regulation S-X, promulgated by the Commission, provides in part:

(b) The Commission will not recognize any certified public accountant or public accountant as independent who is not in fact independent. For example, an accountant will be considered not independent with respect to any person or any of its parents, its subsidiaries, or other affiliates (1) in which, during the period of his pro- fessional engagement to examine the financial statements

Footnote continued on next page.

and also engaged in various promotional and financial activities
on behalf of those clients. For those reasons and others specified
below, we have found that Seidman & Seidman was not independent
with respect to its audit of certain financial statements of
of Equity, Omni-Rx, SaCom and certain other clients served by
the Los Angeles Office of that firm. 24/ In two instances, audit
fees were "adjusted" for the sole purpose of reducing related
offering costs shown in a registration statement. In at
least one instance, a finder's fee was paid to secure an
issuer as a client.

It is also the Commission's view that the firm's independence
was compromised in certain instances by the facts and circumstances
of the engagement itself. An accounting firm cannot be considered
independent when the judgment of the auditors is subordinated
to the views of the client, or where the auditors consciously
acquiesce in the concealment of material information. Similarly,
a firm cannot be viewed as independent where it does not take
action with respect to serious past deficiencies arising out
of intentional misconduct by the client.

The staff found evidence of a lack of independence with
respect to other issuers. The two partners entering Seidman &

Footnote continued from preceding page.

being reported on or at the date of his report he or
his firm or a member thereof had, or was committed to
acquire, any direct financial interest or any material
indirect financial interest or (2) with which, during
the period of his professional engagement to examine
the financial statements being reported on, he or
his firm or a member thereof was connected as a
promoter, underwriter, voting trustee, director, officer,
or employee, except that a firm will not be deemed not
independent in regard to a particular person if a
former officer or employee of such person is employed
by the firm and such individual has completely dissociated
himself from the person and its affiliates and does not
participate in auditing financial statements of the
person or its affiliates covering any period of his
employment by the person. For the purpose of Rule 2.01
the term "member" means all partners in the firm and all
professional employees participating in the audit or
located in an office of the firm participating in a
significant portion of the audit.

24/ The independence issues with respect to Omni-Rx and SaCom
    are discussed below in the sections relating to those
    companies.

- 23 -   34-12752

Seidman as a result of the combination of practices were instrumental in the founding of a number of their audit clients.
These partners, as well as former Wolfson/Weiner employees,
held securities of several publicly held client companies prior
to the combination of practices. 25/

The former Wolfson/Weiner partner assigned as audit
partner to each of that firm's former clients frequently engaged
in promotional activity and attempts to secure financing on
behalf of those clients. 26/ These activities included several
instances where he solicited underwriters to join underwriting
syndicates and made calls on banks on behalf of the client.
He also proposed acquisitions to the issuers and made representations to prospective investors and lenders concerning
the managements and future prospects of these issuers, and
otherwise acted as their agents. All of these activities
are inconsistent with the concept of independence.

EQUITY FUNDING CORPORATION OF AMERICA 27/

Equity began inauspiciously in the early 1960's when
it pioneered the "equity funding" concept, involving the sale
of mutual fund shares which were then pledged by the investor
to secure a loan which financed life insurance premiums.
By recording fictitious assets and earnings, Equity showed

25/ In some cases the two partners held such securities
     indirectly in the name of a corporation. The partners and
     employees continued to hold client securities in certain
     instances following the combination of practices. In certain
     instances, independence questionnaires were given to Seidman &
     Seidman which did not disclose such holdings.

26/ The Commission does not suggest that independence is
     impaired when an auditor participates with his client
     in meetings with underwriters and lenders for the
     purpose of assisting the client in explaining his
     financial data. When he represents the client in
     financing negotiations, however, he is assuming a
     management role.

27/ Equity recently emerged from Chapter X bankruptcy and
     has been renamed Orion Corporation.

- 24 -   34-12752

tremendous growth over a short period of time. Following its
first public offering of common stock in November 1964, Equity
became listed on the American Stock Exchange in 1966 and the
Pacific and New York exchanges in late 1970. The company was
constantly in registration from 1965 through its collapse in
1973, during which time it made numerous acquisitions (often
by issuing common stock) and numerous public offerings.

By the time the massive fraud was disclosed, Equity had
in excess of $120 million (net of deferred taxes) in fictitious
or fraudulently inflated assets on its books. In contrast
to the millions of dollars of reported earnings over the years,
Equity appears never to have earned more than a nominal profit
in its entire corporate life. It was in fact struggling to
remain viable at the very time Seidman & Seidman succeeded to
the audit engagement in 1972. 28/

Seidman & Seidman issued an unqualified opinion on the
December 31, 1971 Equity financial statements although the
audit work was performed by Wolfson/Weiner personnel. The
Commission's investigation has indicated that the audit of
Equity's 1971 financial statements (as well as examinations in
prior years) were conducted in a grossly deficient manner. The
1971 working papers, as in the case of working papers for every
year dating back to 1964, failed to reflect sufficient competent
evidential matter to support the unqualified opinions given, and
in fact clearly evidenced the deficient performance of the
examination.

When Seidman & Seidman combined practices with Wolfson/Weiner
in February of 1972, the 1971 audit of Equity was substantially
complete. Although nearly all the personnel conducting the 1971
audit were persons originally associated with the Wolfson/Weiner
firm, Seidman & Seidman, which was aware that prior audits
had not been reviewed by Wolfson/Weiner partners, made no
review of its own. Seidman & Seidman incorrectly assumed,
on the basis of Wolfson/Weiner's representations, that the

28/   For information concerning the fraud and the manner in which
      it was perpetrated see: "Report(s) of the Trustee of Equity
      Funding Corporation", Robert M. Loeffler, Trustee. (October 31,
      1974 and February 22, 1974).

- 25 -   34-12752

1971 Equity audit had been conducted properly, and allowed
its name to appear on the 1971 Equity financial statements.

The staff's investigation has indicated many serious audit
deficiencies in the 1971 engagement, as described in part below.
Among the deficiencies was the virtual absence of review of audit
work by competent senior level personnel, although this deficiency
was concealed from Seidman & Seidman. Nevertheless, the Commission
is of the view that Seidman & Seidman should have reviewed the
1971 Equity workpapers before lending the Seidman & Seidman name
to the audit report, rather than relying upon the representation
of Wolfson/Weiner personnel that the audit had been conducted
properly.

Funded Receivables

Historically, the largest single asset on Equity's consolidated balance sheet was the "funded receivables" account.
These receivables were generated when a program participant
pledged mutual fund shares and borrowed money from Equity to
finance life insurance premiums. Most of these receivables were
carried on the books of one of Equity's wholly owned subsidiaries,
Equity Funding Corporation -- California ("EFC-Cal"). The mutual
fund shares were sold through another subsidiary, Equity Funding
Securities Corporation ("EFSC"). Although EFC-Cal marketed the
related life insurance policies, the insurance in most instances
was issued by Equity Funding Life Insurance Company ("EFLIC"),
a subsidiary of Equity which was not audited by Wolfson/Weiner.

By December 31, 1971, EFC-Cal had recorded approximately
$34 million of fictitious funded receivables (and related
collateral). The only substantive auditing procedure used in
verifying the existence and valuation of this asset was a wholly
inadequate attempt to confirm selected balances with program
participants. This began with a computer prepared list provided
by the client of customer accounts from which the first two
digits of the five digit account number had been dropped. This
device allowed Equity employees to "account" for the approximate
general ledger balance by the simple expedient of having legitimate accounts appear two or three times on the list. 29/ No

---

29/ The auditors were told that the computer "wasn't programmed"
    to print all five digits. The Wolfson/Weiner staff was not
    proficient in the area of electronic data processing and the
    client's explanation was accepted.

conscientious attempt was made by the Wolfson/Weiner auditors to
verify the accuracy of the listing by testing it to the underlying accounting records or otherwise. In fact, documentation
for the fictitious funded receivables was created only if and
when requested by the auditors. 30/ The auditors then permitted
Equity employees to prepare confirmations and supply the missing
two digits for the selected accounts to be confirmed. When dupli-
cates appeared in the sample, Equity employees supplied two
fictitious digits and the names and addresses of confederates.
The client's work was neither supervised nor tested by the
auditors.

Client Contractual Receivables

In early 1969, Equity acquired Investors Planning Corporation ("IPC"), a mutual fund sales operation whose sales were
largely in the form of so-called contractual plans. These
plans established a continuing obligation on the part of the
seller to charge decreasing sales commissions after the first
year of the agreement. The purchaser had no continuing obligations or duties, but did have an incentive to continue to
purchase mutual fund shares over the life of the agreement
because of the favorable commission rate in the later years
of the contract, called a "trail commission".

Equity paid approximately $12 million for IPC of which
about $5 million reflected the fair value of assets acquired
and $7 million was attributed to "goodwill". The goodwill
in effect reflected what Equity was willing to pay in order
to acquire the approximately 100 mutual fund salesmen who
worked for IPC and the right to receive trail commissions
from previously sold contractual plans.

Near the end of 1969, Equity decided to take into current
income all the revenue that would ever be received from trail
commissions on existing purchase plans. This recognition of
income was effected by booking "receivables" which were grouped
with the Funded Loans Receivable in the consolidated financial
statements.

Over $17 million of these "receivables" were included in
the December 31, 1969 balance sheet. No disclosure was made of
their inclusion in the Funded Loan Receivable balance. Recording
the sale of the commission as an asset duplicated assets already
on the books, since the value of the trail commissions had

30/   Internal control at Equity was so poor that documentation
      even for legitimate receivables was often missing.

- 27 -   34-12752

originally been recognized as goodwill at the date of purchase.
In addition, the initial recording of these spurious assets was
made for an amount far in excess of the value of the commissions,
where the right to collect depended on the entirely voluntary
continued participation by customers in the plans.

In 1970 the trail commissions were "sold" to a non-existent
company, Compania de Estudios y Asuntos ("Estudios"), for $13.5
million, but the bogus receivables continued to be carried in the
the "Funded Loan Receivable" account. The $2 million "down
payment" for the sale was provided by Equity itself. The 1970
Wolfson/Weiner workpapers show the "receivable" as $14.5 million
but there is no indication that a copy of the contract of
sale to Estudios or other supporting documentation was obtained.
Further, no effort was made to determine the nature of the
Estudios company or its financial condition, nor was any attempt
made to confirm the existence of the contractual "receivables"
with the individual plan participants.

The 1971 audit workpapers reflect the Estudios receivable
at $13.5 million. As in the prior year, there was no apparent
attempt to confirm the supposed obligation of Estudios nor to
confirm the contractual receivables with the individual plan
investors.

Establissement Grandson

In 1970, Equity recorded a fictitious receivable from
Establissement Grandson ("Grandson"), a company secretly controlled by Equity. This "receivable" was inappropriately used
to offset a previously undisclosed liability of about $9
million. 31/ The receivable was documented by two spurious
notes which were due February 10 and February 14, 1972 and
which were shown to the Wolfson/Weiner auditors. Although
confirmations were mailed during the 1970 audit, they were
intercepted by Equity personnel and fictitious responses were
returned. During the 1971 audit, it appears that no attempt

31/   The liability (a loan from an international brokerage firm)
       had originally been intentionally mis-recorded as a credit to
       the funded receivables account, but was later properly recorded
       when the lender noted its absence from financial statements.

- 28 -   34-12752

was made to confirm the two notes; nor was any investigation
made of payments on the notes, despite the fact that both
supposedly matured before the financial statements were
issued.

Agent Receivables

Receivables from agents (on the books of EPC-Cal) consisted
of advances made to sales agents and items that had been paid
on their behalf. By the end of 1969, EFC-Cal had lost control
of the detail of the amounts making up the balances; where the
company did have detail, a large percentage was uncollectible.
When agents were terminated, the amounts due from them were not
deleted from the receivable account. By the end of 1971 the amount
of valid receivables from agents was approximately $1.2 million
but the amount shown on the books was approximately $3.4 million.
Throughout the years, it appears that no auditor ever asked
for supporting documentation for this asset account, nor did the
auditors ever confirm with outside sources the existence of the
balances.

Exploration Costs

In September 1970, Equity used a journal entry to decrease
the Grandson receivable and recorded "Exploration Costs" (supposedly intangible drilling costs) in the amount of $1,750,000.
This totally fictitious asset was put on Equity's books
because management did not want the oil and gas subsidiary
to know about it. No documentation for the entry was ever
prepared.

A 1970 workpaper schedule shows the item, but there is no
indication of any work performed by the Wolfson/Weiner auditors
regarding the source of the item, the details behind it, any
examination of supporting documents, or any other substantive
audit work. During 1971, additions, some of which were fictitious,
were made to the account. Again a workpaper schedule shows the
item and the additions, but again no audit work was performed.

Insurance Agency Profits

An Equity subsidiary, Equity Casualty Insurance Agency,
("ECIA") sold casualty insurance and had shown only minimal profits through 1970. In 1971 the company's future profits for the
period January 1, 1972 through December 31, 1980, were "sold"
to a non-affiliated insurance company. Consideration for the

- 29 -   34-12752

sale consisted of a note in the amount of $2.5 million, $800,000
of which was included in income for 1971. The remaining credit
of $1.7 million was used to reduce a fictitious accounts receiv-
able and an improper suspense asset account on the books
of Equity itself.

The written agreement, entered into as of December 31, 1971,
provided that the note was to be paid in equal annual installments of $367,556 through March 31, 1981, at which time all
interest and principal then unpaid would become due and payable.
Each year as an installment payment came due there was to
be credited against the installment the greater of (1) ECIA's
net income or (2) $365,000. Thus, if net income was zero,
$365,000 of the then current installment payment would be
forgiven and the installment would be only $2,556. The maximum
installment payment was therefore $2,556 and the minimum was
zero, giving the note a miniscule current value. The 1971
workpapers contain a journal entry with respect to this transaction, but no audit work appears to have been performed.

Commissions Receivable

The books of EFC-Cal for the year ended December 31, 1971
contained an account called "Commissions Receivable" in the
amount of $2.9 million which dated back to the year 1968.
Although the account was carried as a current asset on the
balance sheet, there had been no collection since 1968. The
account was in fact, occasionally used to record non-existent
assets as an alternative to the constant fraudulent inflation
of Funded Loans Receivable. There was no audit evidence whatsoever reflected in the 1971 audit workpapers.

Commercial Paper

Equity transferred cash to EFLIC in 1971 because of
problems EFLIC had in covering its own non-existent assets. 32/
Instead of recording a receivable from EFLIC, Equity recorded
an investment in non-existent commercial paper. Over $19 million
of bogus commercial paper was on the books at December 31, 1971.
Equity had created documentation for the alleged investments,
but the auditors never asked to see it.

The workpapers for the 1971 audit show a listing of commercial paper investments supposedly held by Equity in the amount
of $28,115,000. There was no indication in the workpapers

32/   Principally non-existent life insurance policies which had
      been reinsured with unaffiliated insurers.

of any maturity date for most of the commercial paper, and
the auditors made no attempt to confirm it with any custodian.
Most of the supposed "redemptions" were not traced to cash
receipts or otherwise verified.

In December 1971, Equity recorded an "investment" in the
amount of $2,000,000 supposedly in the commercial paper of a
company called Apatex. The paper was purportedly due to mature
on April 17, 1972, and was carried on the books and records of
Equity as a part of approximately $3,700,000 in other securities
and investments.

The 1971 audit workpapers show no indication that the
auditors verified the existence of these investments by observation or confirmation.

The Wolfson/Weiner audit work discussed above is so
obviously deficient that elaboration seems superfluous. With
respect to Seidman & Seidman's conduct, it should be noted that
a comparison of the recorded assets to the workpapers makes
the total inadequacy of the audit evidence conspicuously clear.
Yet Seidman & Seidman substituted its imprimatur for that of
the Wolfson/Weiner firm on Equity's 1971 financial statements,
without any review of the Wolfson/Weiner audit workpapers.

THE FINANCIAL HISTORY OF EQUITY FUNDING: THERE WERE CLUES

The fascination of Equity Funding is the number of disquieting questions it raises about the American financial system. "Full disclosure" is the cornerstone of our method for keeping financial markets functioning efficiently. It is still possible for a company to avoid much disclosure by issuing condensed financial statements in abbreviated annual reports. If the company does not need to go frequently to public markets for additional capital, it may be public but still rather secretive.

Equity Funding did not try such tactics. Its annual and even quarterly reports provided far more data than were required at the time, even to the extent of giving product line information in greater detail than is called for today. EFCA went repeatedly to the market, issuing an unbroken stream of massive prospectuses. Of course, some of this profuse financial information seems to have lacked careful auditing. Nevertheless, considering the magnitude of the fraud, either Equity Funding did some spectacular doctoring of the information, or too many people were asleep at the switch. Either way, the magical powers of "full disclosure" seem to be subject to question.

Even simple financial analysis would have produced some disquieting, if not conclusive

questioning about EFCA. For example, if the 1970 interim reports, originally issued for three-, six-, and nine-month periods, were merely arrayed with the 1970 annual report, to provide figures for each of the four quarters of the year, the results strongly suggest, as was testified at the trial of the auditors, that the books were held open at year end to create revenues but not expenses. Table 1 shows the reported quarterly profits on the four major products: securities (mutual funds), insurance, natural resources, and real estate. The table was prepared simply by subtracting three-month sales figures from six-month figures, six-month from nine-month, nine-month figures from those in the annual report, and doing the same for expenses.

The four product lines showed a profit of $11.1 million in the fourth quarter, about *double the $5.8 million average for the preceding three quarters.* One would expect a substantial jump in the figures for natural resources at year end, since these were tax shelter investments, but there is no Christmas season in mutual funds or individual life insurance.

The probability that the fourth quarter 1970 books were held open to record additional revenues is even more clearly

TABLE 1 EQUITY FUNDING QUARTERLY PROFITS FOR 1970–1971 (in millions)

	1970				1971	
	1st	*2nd*	*3rd*	*4th*	*1st*	*2nd*
Securities	$2.8	$1.9	$1.9	$4.0	$2.9	$2.3
Insurance	2.9	2.1	2.5	4.0	3.1	2.7
Natural Resources	.2	.2	.2	2.3	.7	.3
Real Estate	.2	1.2	1.3	.8	.8	.9
	$6.1	$5.4	$5.9	$11.1	$7.5	$6.2

shown in the relationship between securities sales commissions revenues and the cost of commission expense. In the second quarter, for example, revenues from securities sales commissions were $3,184,000 with expenses of $1,229,000. In the magical fourth quarter, securities revenues jumped 40 percent to $5,275,000. On the other hand, we are supposed to believe—and apparently most people did—that expenses to produce these commissions actually dropped slightly to $1,211,000. Equity Funding certainly did have a remarkable sales force. This demonstration is intended as an illustration, not as a final indication of all such instances in the reported financial results of Equity Funding. We hope the reader will find more.

Within obvious space limits, we have included as great a variety of published financial information as possible. In addition, a listing of significant prospectuses and other materials is provided at the end of this section.

The materials in this section are arranged chronologically. All have been photoreproduced from the originals, to preserve the original pagination and even some errors. The source of the materials, if not apparent, is indicated. The original financial statements for some years are omitted, and are found only as comparative figures in the statements of the following year. In such instances, there appear to have been no significant reclassifications or restatements between the years. That is, the comparative figures are those originally reported.

Financial Statements, Prospectuses, Interim and Annual Reports

TABLE OF CONTENTS

PROSPECTUS

100,000 Shares
EQUITY FUNDING CORPORATION OF AMERICA
Common Stock
($.30 Par Value)

THESE SECURITIES HAVE NOT BEEN APPROVED OR DISAPPROVED BY THE
SECURITIES AND EXCHANGE COMMISSION NOR HAS THE COMMISSION
PASSED UPON THE ACCURACY OR ADEQUACY OF THIS PROSPECTUS.
ANY REPRESENTATION TO THE CONTRARY IS A CRIMINAL OFFENSE.

	Price to Public	Underwriting Discounts and Commissions (1)	Proceeds to Company (2)
Per Share	$6.00	$.54	$5.46
Total	$600,000	$54,000	$546,000

(1) The Company will issue to the Representative of the Underwriters and to Theodore Goodman, who furnished financial advisory services to the Company, equally, a total of 17,500 non-transferable Common Stock Purchase Warrants ("Warrants"), at an aggregate price of $1,750, in cash, exercisable commencing on December 22, 1965 at $7.20 per share until December 22, 1967, and at $7.80 per share until December 22, 1969, the expiration date. In addition, the Representative and Mr. Goodman have purchased, in equal parts, a total of 10,000 shares of Common Stock from the Company's principal stockholders and executive officers at a price of $.60 per share. The Representative and certain of the Underwriters hereof will acquire additional shares of Common Stock at varying prices which are not expected to exceed approximately $3.00 per share, as more fully described under "Certain Transactions" herein. Such Underwriters, including the Representative, and Mr. Goodman may be deemed "underwriters" under the Securities Act of 1933 with respect to any resale of the aforesaid shares and/or shares issuable upon the exercise of Warrants any may realize a profit on the sale of such securities in addition to the underwriting discounts specified above. None of such shares, however, are being offered at this time. See "Certain Transactions" and "Underwriting".

    The Representative has, for a period of five years, been accorded (a) a right of first refusal on any public or private financing program for the Company and/or its principal stockholders and (b) the right to designate a member of the Board of Directors of the Company. It is contemplated that Nelson Loud, a partner of the Representative, will be elected to the Board as the designee of the Underwriters. Mr. Goodman, who will receive a finder's fee of $5,000, payable by the Representative, also is expected to be elected to the Board of Directors of the Company.

(2) Before deducting expenses payable by the Company estimated at $34,000, including a maximum of $3,000 which the Company has agreed to pay to the Underwriters toward their expenses in connection with the qualification of this offering under certain state securities laws.

There has heretofore been no trading market for the Company's common stock.

These shares are offered by the Underwriters named herein subject to prior sale, when, as and if delivered to and accepted by such Underwriters and subject to approval of certain legal matters by Gibson, Dunn & Crutcher, counsel for the Underwriters and by Glaser & Glaser and Freedman, Levy, Kroll & Simonds, counsel for the Company.

NEW YORK SECURITIES CO.

The date of this Prospectus is December 14, 1964

Between June 1962 and late 1963, the Company was in the process of complying with certain administrative and regulatory requirements applicable to the public offering of its Programs which resulted in a curtailment of its selling activities during that period. The Company's operations in 1962 also were adversely affected by the marked decline in the market value of securities which occurred in May of that year. After compliance with applicable Federal and state requirements, the Programs were offered publicly commencing in late October, 1963, with a resulting increase in the sales volume of life insurance and mutual fund shares. The increase in earnings for the nine-month period ended September 30, 1964, as compared to the same period in 1963, is attributed by the Company to such increased sales.

HISTORY AND BUSINESS

The Company was essentially inactive until March 1961, when it issued 633,334 shares of common stock in equal parts to Stanley Goldblum, Michael R. Riordan, Eugene R. Cuthbertson and Raymond J. Platt, who may be considered the Company's founders. Such shares were issued in exchange for all of the then outstanding common stock of three corporations, two of which are incorporated in California and New York, respectively, under the same name, Equity Funding Corporation, and the other in California as Equity Securities Corporation. The latter has been engaged in the sale of mutual fund shares since 1957. The others have operated as general life insurance agents of various insurance companies since January 1960.

Messrs. Goldblum, Riordan and Cuthbertson are directors as well as the principal executive officers of the Company. Until August 1962, Mr. Platt was a director and a vice-president of the Company, but is no longer connected with it except as a stockholder. The aggregate book value of the stock of the above subsidiaries at the time it was transferred to the Company by such persons was $190,000 and their total cash investment therein was $101,666.

Substantially all of the Company's income is derived from commissions earned on the sale of life insurance, discounts on the sale of mutual fund shares and interest charged on loans to finance life insurance premiums. The percentage of the Company's total gross income attributable to each of such sources for the years ended December 31, 1960 through 1963, and for the nine month periods ended September 30, 1963 and 1964, is as follows:

| | Year Ended December 31: | | | | Nine Months Ended | |
	1960	1961	1962	1963	Sept. 30, 1963	Sept. 30, 1964
Life Insurance Commissions.............	46%	73%	65%	59%	59%	60%
Mutual Fund Discounts.................	41%	18%	22%	16%	16%	16%
Interest on Life Insurance Premium Loans..	3%	6%	12%	23%	22%	19%

The following table indicates the percentage of gross life insurance and mutual fund commission income, combined, which was represented by the sale of coordinated acquisition plans, including the Programs, and by the sale of life insurance and mutual funds independent of such plans, for the years ended December 31, 1960 through 1963, and for the nine month periods ended September 30, 1963 and 1964:

| | Year Ended December 31: | | | | Nine Months Ended | |
	1960	1961	1962	1963	Sept. 30, 1963	Sept. 30, 1964
Coordinated Acquisition Plan Sales.....	92.6%	82.7%	77.9%	44.4%	43.9%	42.3%
Non-Plan Sales	7.4%	17.3%	22.1%	55.6%	56.1%	57.7%
	100%	100%	100%	100%	100%	100%

7

PROSPECTUS

70,148 Shares

EQUITY FUNDING CORPORATION OF AMERICA
Common Stock

($.30 Par Value)

The shares offered hereby are outstanding shares to be sold to the Underwriters by certain stockholders (see "Selling Stockholders"). The Company will receive no part of the proceeds of the sale. Between December 15, 1964, the date of the Company's first public offering, and May 10, 1965, the bid price of the Company's common stock in the over-the-counter market, as reported by the National Quotation Bureau, Inc., ranged from a high of $9¾ to a low of $7¼ per share. On May 10, 1965, the high bid and low asked prices were $9⅝ and $9¾, respectively.

THESE SECURITIES HAVE NOT BEEN APPROVED OR DISAPPROVED BY THE SECURITIES AND EXCHANGE COMMISSION NOR HAS THE COMMISSION PASSED UPON THE ACCURACY OR ADEQUACY OF THIS PROSPECTUS. ANY REPRESENTATION TO THE CONTRARY IS A CRIMINAL OFFENSE.

	Price to Public	Underwriting Discounts and Commissions[1]	Proceeds to Selling Stockholders[2]
Per Share	$9.25	$.70	$8.55
Total	$648,869.00	$49,103.60	$599,765.40

(1) Theodore Goodman, a director of the Company, will receive a finder's fee, payable by the Representative of the Underwriters, equal to 25% of the net underwriting commissions received by the Representative.

(2) Before deducting expenses payable by the Selling Stockholders estimated at $25,000.

In addition to the 70,148 shares offered hereby, the principal stockholders and executive officers of the Company have given the Underwriters the right to purchase from them, equally an aggregate of up to 10,000 shares, at the same net price per share, solely for the purpose of covering over-allotments, if any, in the sale of the 70,148 shares (see "Underwriting").

The shares are offered by the several Underwriters named herein subject to prior sale, when, as and if delivered to and accepted by such Underwriters and subject to approval of certain legal matters by counsel. It is expected that delivery of certificates for such shares will be made on or about May 19, 1965.

NEW YORK SECURITIES CO.

The date of this Prospectus is May 12, 1965

FROM PROSPECTUS DATED
MAY 12, 1965

CONSOLIDATED STATEMENT OF EARNINGS
AND RETAINED EARNINGS

The following Consolidated Statement of Earnings and Retained Earnings has been compiled as explained in Note 1 to Financial Statements. The statements for the five years ended December 31, 1964, has been examined by Wolfson, Weiner & Company, independent certified public accountants, whose opinion appears elsewhere in this Prospectus. This statement should be read in conjunction with the related financial statements and notes thereto included elsewhere in this Prospectus.

	Year Ended December 31,				
	1960 Audited	1961 Audited	1962 Audited	1963 Audited	1964 Audited
INCOME:					
Mutual Fund commissions	$167,002.00	$ 325,093.00	$ 412,291.31	$ 212,270.41	$ 494,155.63
Life Insurance commissions	189,014.00	1,292,766.00	1,192,993.67	787,422.71	1,911,302.67
Interest income	12,901.00	109,774.51	226,382.29	300,418.05	448,681.00
Casualty Insurance commissions	–0–	–0–	–0–	–0–	13,247.19
Securities trading income	40,300.00	38,314.00	4,593.24	24,740.97	250.00
Leasing commission	–0–	–0–	–0–	–0–	1,563.00
TOTAL INCOME	409,217.00	1,765,947.51	1,836,260.51	1,324,852.14	2,869,199.49
EXPENSES:					
Commissions on Mutual Funds	71,943.93	203,018.10	262,757.83	89,661.03	223,195.24
Commissions on Life Insurance	93,359.27	741,295.70	775,117.03	296,386.55	756,392.90
Interest on insurance premium financing loans	6,400.14	59,320.43	169,542.84	251,456.27	328,899.75
Selling, general and administrative (Note 14)	256,679.93	560,696.75	708,884.62	681,440.97	944,304.99
TOTAL EXPENSES	431,383.27	1,564,330.98	1,916,302.32	1,318,944.82	2,252,792.88
EARNINGS (LOSS) BEFORE CAPITAL GAIN AND INCOME TAXES	(22,166.27)	201,616.53	(80,041.81)	5,907.32	616,406.61
CAPITAL GAIN ON SALE OF SECURITIES	–0–	–0–	84,784.00	64,904.00	3,915.05
EARNINGS (LOSS) BEFORE FEDERAL TAXES ON INCOME	(22,166.27)	201,616.53	4,742.19	70,811.32	620,321.66
FEDERAL TAXES ON INCOME (Note 8)	660.00	76,986.24	23,185.19	18,053.25	230,854.72
Less: Operating loss carryback tax credit	–0–	–0–	42,763.68	–0–	–0–
NET TAX PROVISION	660.00	76,986.24	(19,578.49)	18,053.25	230,854.72
NET EARNINGS (LOSS)	(22,826.27)	124,630.29	24,320.68	52,758.07	389,466.94
RETAINED EARNINGS (DEFICIT) BEGINNING OF PERIOD	471.11	(22,355.16)	102,275.13	126,595.81	179,353.88
RETAINED EARNINGS (DEFICIT) END OF PERIOD	($ 22,355.16)	$ 102,275.13	$ 126,595.81	$ 179,353.88	$ 568,820.82
EARNINGS (LOSS) PER SHARE*	($.04)	$.18	$.03	$.07	$.52

* Earnings per share have been computed on the basis of $.30 par value common stock. Earnings per share for the years 1960 thru 1963 were computed on the following number of outstanding shares: 1960 — 633,334 shares, 1961 — 709,400 shares, 1962 — 718,309 shares, and 1963 — 751,678 shares. Earnings per share for the year 1964 were computed on the basis of the average number of shares outstanding in the amount of 753,084 shares.

Under the Company's method of operation, one of its subsidiaries purchases Custodial Notes on a limited interim basis pending their resale in larger aggregate amounts to institutional lenders, who are expected to provide the bulk of the funds to be used by the Company in financing the Programs. Custodial Notes purchased by this subsidiary have been, and it is anticipated that they will be, resold to institutional lenders prior to their maturity. All of the Company's presently outstanding Custodial Notes bear interest at the rate of 5¾% per annum. At this time, $350,000 of such Notes (88% of the total amount outstanding) are held by State Farm Life Insurance Company.

Coordinated Acquisition Plans Sold Prior to October 21, 1963

The coordinated acquisition plans sold by the Company before October 21, 1963, are substantially the same in principle as the Programs. Investors who have initiated such plans, however, assign their mutual fund shares to a subsidiary of the Company with power to hypothecate such shares to secure loans for paying insurance premiums and interest. The shares are pledged with banks as collateral for loans for the aforesaid purpose. Such loans are primarily on a demand or short-term basis, and the arrangement may be terminated at any time by the subsidiary or the investor. The lender may require the assignment of additional shares or repayment of the loan if the value of the collateral declines to a point where the lender feels insecure. If repayment is demanded but not made, the shares may be sold to satisfy the indebtedness, and any excess of proceeds would be remitted to the investor. There are no specific requirements as to termination or minimum collateral values as in the case of the Programs which provide for more formalized overall procedures.

During 1964, the average rate of interest charged the Company on such borrowings was approximately 5½% per annum while the rate charged to investors by the Company was 6%.

Coordinated Acquisition Plan Sales and Terminations

The following table sets forth pertinent statistical information for the periods indicated concerning the sale of all coordinated acquisition plans, including the Programs, by the Company and by the independent insurance agencies which effect sales for the Company:

| | Years Ended December 31, | | | | | |
	1960	1961	1962	1963	1964	Total
Plans Sold						
Number of Plans Initiated	510	2,309	2,180	371	682	6,052
Amount of Premiums Financed	$ 299,877	$ 1,114,396	$ 833,434	$ 134,263	$ 398,780	$ 2,780,750
Face Amount of Life Insurance Policies Sold	$9,578,455	$49,413,836	$43,651,120	$7,243,282	$20,022,835	$129,909,528
Premium Loans Outstanding at End of Period(1)	$ 288,973	$ 1,490,483	$ 3,337,271	$4,912,340	$ 6,913,699	——
Plans Terminated						
Termination of Plans Initiated During Period Indicated, as of December 31, 1964(2)	209	806	292	27	None	1,334
Amount of Annual Premiums Involved in Terminations	$ 108,353	$ 328,217	$ 99,061	$ 14,660	None	$ 350,291
Face Amount of Life Insurance Involved in Terminations(3)	$3,525,779	$13,635,388	$ 4,778,871	$ 499,177	None	$ 22,436,615

(1) Including interest.

(2) Terminations generally result because of reasons which are personal to the investor. As previously noted, no forced liquidations have taken place to date. There is no assurance, of course, that this will be the case in the future.

(3) "Terminations" refer only to the financing arrangement and not necessarily to a termination of the related life insurance policy.

11

The following table reflects sales of life insurance by or through the Company, by quarters, for the year ended December 31, 1960 through March 31, 1965:

Quarter Ended	Face Amount of Life Insurance Sold(1)	Face Amount of Cancellations(2)	Amount of Premium Actually Paid	First Year Gross Commissions	Gross Renewal Commissions(3)	Total Gross Commissions	Commission Expense
1960							
March 31	$ 1,143,589	$ 290,770	$ 24,049	$ 21,666	$ 981	$ 22,647	$ 11,302
June 30	2,388,635	613,612	50,183	44,607	1,064	45,671	22,739
September 30	2,856,088	614,452	62,243	57,104	1,589	58,693	29,806
December 31	3,077,254	800,808	63,731	59,796	2,207	62,003	29,512
1961							
March 31	9,383,534	2,371,632	220,841	204,499	2,987	207,486	118,786
June 30	12,696,717	3,304,707	298,676	279,561	7,579	287,140	164,215
September 30	15,941,630	3,882,993	375,716	344,156	16,861	361,017	207,043
December 31	18,938,519	4,492,755	445,822	417,290	19,833	437,123	251,252
1962							
March 31	18,456,891	1,850,803	434,382	406,582	19,228	425,810	274,647
June 30	14,043,124	1,559,951	329,110	311,009	28,460	339,469	220,315
September 30	11,629,662	1,344,055	273,125	258,377	23,290	281,667	183,365
December 31	5,065,937	823,123	118,668	111,074	34,974	146,048	96,790
1963							
March 31	9,828,515	999,057	246,082	231,564	56,239	287,803	108,358
June 30	5,033,348	307,819	126,244	117,534	68,200	185,734	69,650
September 30	5,512,422	143,305	137,845	126,680	41,885	168,565	62,802
December 31	4,489,102	125,426	111,697	104,884	40,437	145,321	55,577
1964							
March 31	12,431,374	621,107	298,186	291,030	61,429	352,459	147,426
June 30	13,765,452	——	316,487	310,281	94,212	404,493	122,468
September 30	14,475,290	——	341,753	334,999	96,401	431,398	172,439
December 31	29,020,505	——	686,525	624,818	98,135	722,953	314,060
1965							
March 31	30,326,428	——	691,639	631,265	99,268	730,533	317,680

(1) Indicates face amount of life insurance paid for during period indicated.

(2) Indicates cumulative face amount of policies terminated from period indicated through March 31, 1965.

(3) As security for the payment of the 6% Promissory Note issued by the Company to the partnership mentioned in the text, above, the Company assigned, as of June 24, 1964, to such partnership, all of its right to receive renewal commissions on policies previously sold through it, or through two of its officers and directors who act as general agents on behalf of the Company in certain states which only permit individuals to act as general agents. The loan agreement with the partnership provides for certain "events of default" upon the occurrence of which, the partnership shall have the right to demand direct payment to it of the aforesaid renewal commissions until the Company's "notes" are fully paid, with interest. The following are the principal events of default included in such agreement: (i) failure to pay any installment of interest or principal when due; (ii) failure to meet certain production requirements with respect to the sale of insurance; (iii) certain events of bankruptcy, insolvency or reorganization; and, (iv) termination by Pennsylvania Life of any of the general agency agreements with the Company or with certain of its officers and directors (see above) because of Pennsylvania Life's determination that it is not feasible or practicable for it to qualify or comply with Federal or state laws applicable to the coordinated sale of mutual funds shares and life insurance. In case an event of default shall have occurred, the unpaid principal and accrued interest thereon shall immediately become due and payable, except that if the event of default is that described in "(iv)", above, then the unpaid principal amount of the outstanding notes and interest accrued thereon shall be payable 18 months after the occurrence of such event of default.

14

Mutual Fund Sales

The Company has non-exclusive selling agreements with the principal underwriters of 76 mutual funds. The greatest part of its sales, however, are of shares of the various Keystone Custodian Funds, five of whose funds are offered in the Programs. The Company's maximum commission, before deduction of salesmen's commissions (see below) on sales of Keystone Custodian Funds is 6% of the offering price of the shares. With respect to the sale of shares in other mutual funds, such maximum commission is 8% of the offering price of the shares of those funds. The Company does not participate in commissions earned on mutual fund sales effected in Programs sold through the affiliated mutual fund distributors of the independent insurance agencies. All of the mutual fund shares sold by the Company are of the so-called "open-end" type which permit investors to redeem their shares at any time at net asset value. The Company does not itself redeem such shares nor does it earn any commissions or fees for any services it may render its clients in connection with such redemptions.

The following table sets forth pertinent information concerning the sale of mutual fund shares by the Company, by quarters, for the year ended December 31, 1960 through March 31, 1965:

Quarter Ended	Amount of Mutual Fund Shares Sold[1]	Gross Commissions	Commission Expense
1960			
March 31	$ 585,472	$ 35,714	$ 15,321
June 30	523,323	31,661	13,646
September 30	882,638	53,135	22,848
December 31	797,468	46,492	20,129
1961			
March 31	1,017,416	59,848	35,917
June 30	1,110,235	64,926	40,940
September 30	1,630,611	95,637	63,982
December 31	1,789,015	104,682	62,179
1962			
March 31	2,251,921	132,155	84,091
June 30	2,782,338	163,187	110,723
September 30	1,177,931	69,168	42,283
December 31	817,055	47,781	25,661
1963			
March 31	825,981	48,303	20,236
June 30	904,915	52,919	20,456
September 30	937,316	54,654	24,675
December 31	969,413	56,394	24,294
1964			
March 31	981,668	58,906	29,613
June 30	1,558,884	104,698	40,764
September 30	2,464,388	136,517	59,327
December 31	3,337,607	194,035	93,491
1965			
March 31	3,892,651	234,345	115,565

(1) The amounts shown include the applicable sales charge and are based on the total amount of shares sold during the period indicated on which a dealer's discount (commission) was allowed the Company. As no sales charge is applicable on capital gains distributions taken in shares pursuant to automatic reinvestment plans, the amount of such distributions is not included in the table.

15

APPENDIX B
CONSOLIDATED FINANCIAL STATEMENTS

Equity Funding Corporation of America
Consolidated Statement of Earnings and Retained Earnings
For the Year Ended December 31, 1964

	YEAR ENDED DECEMBER 31,	
	1964	1963
INCOME:		
Mutual Fund commissions	$ 494,155.63	$ 212,270.41
Life Insurance commissions	1,911,302.67	787,422.71
Interest income	448,681.00	300,418.05
Casualty Insurance commissions	13,247.19	
Securities trading income	250.00	24,740.97
Leasing commissions	1,563.00	
TOTAL INCOME	$2,869,199.49	1,324,852.14
EXPENSES:		
Commissions on Mutual Funds	223,195.24	89,661.03
Commissions on Life Insurance	756,392.90	296,386.55
Interest on insurance premium financing loans	328,899.75	251,456.27
Selling, general and administrative (Note 14)	944,304.99	681,440.97
TOTAL EXPENSES	2,252,792.88	1,318,944.82
EARNINGS BEFORE CAPITAL GAIN AND INCOME TAXES	616,406.61	5,907.32
CAPITAL GAIN ON SALE OF SECURITIES	3,915.05	64,904.00
EARNINGS BEFORE FEDERAL TAXES ON INCOME	620,321.66	70,811.32
FEDERAL TAXES ON INCOME (NOTE 8)	230,854.72	18,053.25
NET EARNINGS	389,466.94	52,758.07
RETAINED EARNINGS BEGINNING OF PERIOD	179,353.88	126,595.81
RETAINED EARNINGS END OF PERIOD	$ 568,820.82	$ 179,353.88

The accompanying notes are an integral part of this statement.

The financial statements as at and for the year ended December 31, 1963, are shown for comparative purposes only. Reference should be made to the previously issued Annual Report for the Accountant's Report and notes pertaining to those financial statements.

Equity Funding Corporation of America
Consolidated Statement of Financial Condition (Note 1)
December 31, 1964

Assets

CURRENT ASSETS:	DECEMBER 31, 1964		DECEMBER 31, 1963	
Cash		$ 520,230.61		$ 74,640.30
Accounts receivable		298,432.48		28,579.13
Notes receivable		39,886.72		41,587.32
Commissions receivable		563,219.24		216,692.51
Advances to salesmen, employees and officers (Note 2)		52,273.22		28,678.18
Securities at cost (Note 3)		19,361.15		16,480.00
Prepaid expenses		50,129.85		49,386.89
TOTAL CURRENT ASSETS ..		1,543,533.27		456,044.33
FIXED ASSETS AT COST (NOTE 4):				
Furniture, fixtures and equipment	$ 59,617.61		$ 43,197.12	
Less allowance for depreciation.	25,602.79	34,014.82	21,495.54	21,701.58
OTHER ASSETS:				
Cash value—officers' life insurance	227.00			
Loans receivable from clients for premium loans (Note 5)	6,682,075.61		4,912,339.54	
Collateral notes receivable (Note 15)	231,623.21			
Cost of renewal commissions acquired (Note 6)	$279,688.48		$267,188.48	
Less amortization to date	102,518.51	177,169.97	72,831.14	194,357.34
Deposits		33,392.86		24,559.39
Goodwill		12,000.00		12,000.00
Deferred Charges (Note 7):				
Organization expenses, net of amortization	3,943.59		8,153.60	
Cost of opening and developing new offices, net of amortization	429,328.98		351,640.26	
Registration costs, net of amortization	225,806.67	659,079.24	7,795,567.89	264,281.48	624,075.34	5,767,331.61
TOTAL ASSETS		$9,373,115.98		$6,245,077.52

The accompanying notes are an integral part of this statement.

The financial statements as at and for the year ended December 31, 1963, are shown for comparative purposes only. Reference should be made to the previously issued Annual Report for the Accountant's Report and notes pertaining to those financial statements.

Liabilities

		DECEMBER 31, 1964		DECEMBER 31, 1963	
CURRENT LIABILITIES:					
Accounts payable			$ 684,106.51		$ 91,679.13
Notes payable to banks—current portion (Note 9)			120,000.00		60,000.00
Notes payable, others—current portion (Note 10)			94,003.63		380.04
Accrued expenses:					
Commissions		$ 1,574.02		$ 3,625.29	
Taxes (other than federal taxes on income)		11,211.32		9,271.33	
Interest and sundry expenses		10,295.69	23,081.03	3,675.02	16,571.64
Federal taxes on income, estimated (Note 8)			308,673.15		77,734.72
TOTAL CURRENT LIABILITIES ...			1,229,864.32		246,365.53
LONG TERM DEBT:					
Notes payable to banks (Note 9)	$210,000.00				
Less current portion	120,000.00	90,000.00			
Notes payable to others (Note 10)	305,068.20			300,000.00	
Less current portion	94,003.63	211,064.57	301,064.57		300,000.00
OTHER LIABILITIES:					
Notes payable on clients premium loans (Note 5)		5,975,584.54		4,912,339.54	
Custodial collateral notes payable (Note 15)		209,000.00	6,184,584.54	———	4,912,339.54
STOCKHOLDERS' EQUITY:					
Common stock—authorized 4,000,000 shares (Note 1)					
Issued 1,565,494 shares, par value $.15 per share				234,824.10	
Issued 882,769 shares, par value $.30 per share		264,830.70			
Common stock purchase warrants (Note 11)		1,750.00			
Stock options (Note 11)				250.00	
Additional paid in capital		894,875.03		440,618.47	
Retained earnings		568,820.82		179,353.88	
		1,730,276.55		855,046.45	
Less treasury stock (Note 12)					
62,183 shares, par value $.15 per share ..				68,674.00	786,372.45
32,425 shares, par value $.30 per share ..		72,674.00	1,657,602.55		
COMMITMENTS AND CONTINGENT LIABILITIES (NOTE 13):					
TOTAL LIABILITIES AND STOCKHOLDERS' EQUITY			$9,373.115.98		$6,245,077.52

Equity Funding Corporation of America
Notes to Consolidated Financial Statements
December 31, 1964

NOTE 1. PRINCIPLE OF CONSOLIDATION AND SUBSE-
QUENT EVENTS CONCERNING CAPITAL STOCK:

The Company, acting primarily as a holding Company of its wholly
owned subsidiaries, was incorporated in Delaware on September 2,
1960 under the name of Tongor Corporation of America. Its present
name was adopted on January 19, 1961.

Equity Securities Corporation, which handles the mutual fund
aspect of the Company's overall program, was incorporated in California on January 31, 1957 under the name of Investors Investment
Corporation. It adopted the name of Gordon C. McCormick, Inc., on
April 11, 1960. Its present name was adopted on July 20, 1961.

Equity Funding Corporation (California) handles the insurance
aspect of the Company's overall program on the West Coast. It was
incorporated in California under the name of Tongor Corporation
on June 12, 1959. It began conducting business in January 1960 and
adopted its present name on April 7, 1960.

Equity Funding Corporation (New York) handles the insurance
aspect of the Company's overall program on the East Coast. It was
incorporated in New York on August 25, 1960.

Equity Casualty Insurance Agency, which functions as a casualty
insurance broker, was incorporated in California on May 26, 1961
under the name of Equity Funding Casualty Corporation. It adopted
its present name on September 6, 1961. Operations of this Corporation, discontinued as of December 31, 1962, was reinstated as of
September 23, 1963.

Equity Funding Service Corporation was incorporated in Delaware
on August 31, 1961. It was formed to handle the loan aspect of the
Company's overall program, and was activated as of April 15, 1964.

North American Equity Corporation was incorporated on December 11, 1961 in Delaware. This Corporation handles the mutual fund
aspect of the Company's overall program in the state of Colorado.

First Equity Funding Corporation was incorporated in Delaware
on December 18, 1961. This Corporation handles the loan aspect of
the Company's collateralized loans.

Equity Funding Corporation of Arizona was incorporated in
Arizona on December 31, 1963. This Corporation handles the life
insurance aspect of the Company's overall program in Arizona.

Equity Funding Corporation of Maryland was incorporated in
Maryland on July 18, 1963. This Corporation functions as a life
insurance agency in the State of Maryland.

Equity Leasing Corporation, which functions as an equipment
leasing broker, was incorporated in California on September 22, 1964.

Inasmuch as the above corporations were under common control
for the periods audited, the consolidation is considered to represent a
pooling of interests. All intercompany accounts, transactions and
profits of the above corporations have been eliminated from the consolidated financial statements.

The Company had issued stock purchase options in two series to
certain key employees, district and division managers, agents and
associated general agents of the Company. As of December 31, 1964,
there were 7,000 Series A options outstanding entitling optionees to
purchase the Company's $.30 par value stock at a price of $13.00
per share.

Post Audit Note: In regard to the Series A options, as of March 8,
1965, none of the options were exercised and under the terms of the
option agreement all the options have expired as of January 31, 1965.

The Company intends, from time to time in the future, to grant
options on shares of its common stock to certain personnel, including
officers other than Messrs. Goldblum, Riordan and Cuthbertson,
under terms and conditions approved by stockholders on September
1, 1964 and for this purpose has reserved an aggregate of 45,000
shares of common stock.

Production Option Plan: Under this plan, 25,000 shares have been
reserved for the benefit of eligible sales representatives or division
managers. Options granted may be exercised only from June 30, 1966
through June 30, 1968. The options are conditioned upon the optionee
maintaining a continuous relationship with the Company until the
date of exercise and no option may be exercised unless a registration
statement covering the underlying shares is then effective under the
Securities Act of 1933. To the extent that shares are available under
this plan, options will be exercisable in whole or in part by the
optionee within the above period, at the rate of four shares of common stock for each $100 of commissions, bonuses or overrides earned
by the optionee as of December 31, 1965. The purchase price is:
(i) $6.50 per share if the right to exercise the option is earned prior
to April 1, 1965, (ii) the market value per optioned share on April
1, 1965, if the right to exercise is earned from April 1, 1965, to
October 1, 1965, and (iii) market value per share on October 1,
1965, if the right to exercise is earned from October 1, 1965, through
December 31, 1965. ("Market value" is the mean average between
the bid and asked price for the preceding 10 business days.) Options
may be exercised by the optionee's legatees or representatives for a
period of six months after the death of the optionee to the extent
exercisable at the time of death.

Incentive Stock Options: An additional 20,000 shares of common stock have been reserved for incentive stock options to be granted to eligible sales representatives, employees and division managers. Options granted will have a term of four years and will be exercisable from time to time as to not less than 100 shares commencing after the expiration of two years from the date of grant. The purchase price per share is the greater of $6.50 or the market value (as defined above), of the common stock on the date of grant. The options will be conditioned upon the optionee maintaining a continuous relationship with Company until the date of exercise and, in no event, may an option be exercised unless a registration statement covering the underlying shares is then effective under the Securities Act of 1933. In the event the optionee shall cease to be a representative of the Company prior to the expiration of the option, his option shall terminate except that (i) options may be exercised for a period of three months after termination of employment, but not more than four years after the date of grant, and (ii) options may be exercised by the optionee's representatives or legatees within six months of the death of the optionee if death occurs while the optionee is an employee of the Company or within three months after termination of employment to the extent exercisable at the time of death.

Outstanding Options: As of December 31, 1964 there are outstanding options on 9,916 shares of the Company's common stock granted to the optionees under the Production Option Plan.

The Articles of Incorporation of the Company were amended on September 1, 1964 to increase the par value of the Company's common stock from $.15 per share to $.30 per share. On December 22, 1964, a public stock offering of 100,000 shares of the common stock of Equity Funding Corporation of America was made. Pursuant to the amendment and the public stock offering, as of December 31, 1964, there were 882,769 shares of common stock issued having a par value of $.30 per share.

NOTE 2. ADVANCES TO OFFICERS:

As of December 31, 1964 advances made to officers were as follows:

Stanley Goldblum	$ 3,597.33
Eugene R. Cuthbertson	8,912.56
Michael R. Riordan	8,196.22
TOTAL	$20,706.11

NOTE 3. SECURITIES, AT COST:

As of December 31, 1964 the Company owned the following securities:

(a) 1,750 shares of common stock of Equity Funding Corporation of America at a total investment of $15,368.75.

(b) 180 shares of Keystone Mutual Funds, series S3, at a total investment of $1,987.20.

(c) 180 shares of Keystone Mutual Funds, series K2, at a total investment of $2,005.20.

NOTE 4. FIXED ASSETS, AT COST:

It is the policy of the Company to provide for depreciation of office furniture, automobile, fixtures and equipment on a "straight-line" basis predicated on the estimated useful lives of the individual items in the various classes of assets. The principal estimated useful lives in computing depreciation are as follows:

Office furniture and fixtures	10 years
Office equipment	5 years
Leasehold improvements	3 years
Automobile	5 years

NOTE 5. CLIENTS' PREMIUM LOANS AND ASSIGNED COLLATERAL:

Under the method of operation followed prior to October 21, 1963, as contrasted to the Programs described in the Prospectus, clients who coordinate their investment and insurance program assign their purchased mutual fund shares to Equity Funding Corporation with power to hypothecate their shares only to secure loans for paying their insurance premiums and loan interest. These shares are pledged by Equity Funding Corporation to the lending institutions as collateral for the loans made for the aforesaid purpose.

The premium payment loans are primarily on demand or short term basis and either Equity Funding Corporation or the client may terminate the loan or loan program at any time. The lender may require the assignment of additional collateral or repayment of the loan balance if the value of the collateral should decline to an aggregate value at which the lender feels itself insecure. Where repayment is demanded and not received, the lender may sell the collateral and any proceeds in excess of the outstanding obligation will be remitted to the customer.

The loans receivable from clients for premium loans reported under "Other Assets" are offset, in part, by the contra notes payable on premium loans reported under "Other Liabilities." The difference, in the amount of $706,491.07, is held by Equity Funding Corporation of America. The collateral assigned by clients as security for the notes payable on premium loans reported under "Other Liabilities" amounted to $9,896,289.00.

NOTE 6. COST OF RENEWAL COMMISSIONS ACQUIRED:

The Company capitalized the cost of purchasing and acquiring complete right, title and interest to certain of its renewal commissions belonging to the Company as of December 31, 1961. These renewal commissions will be received over a period of nine years and the cost thereof is being amortized over the said nine year period. The cost shown is related to only a portion of the renewal commissions belonging to the Company as of December 31, 1961. This figure is not intended to reflect the actual value of the renewal commissions.

The Company has also capitalized $12,500.00, the cost of purchasing and acquiring complete right, title and interest to all renewal commissions belonging to two independent insurance agencies acquired in the latter part of 1964. The renewal commissions may be received over a period of nine years and the cost thereof will be amortized over a period of five years beginning in 1965.

NOTE 7. DEFERRED CHARGES:

The Company has capitalized organization expense, the cost of opening and developing new offices and registration costs. Costs incurred prior to 1961 are being amortized on an annual basis over a five year period. Costs incurred after December 31, 1960, are being amortized on an annual basis over a three year period commencing in the year after completion of the specific office or project. Costs incurred prior to December 31, 1963, in connection with the registration of the Company's Programs, are being amortized over a three year period commencing January 1, 1964.

The amounts deferred and amortized with respect to the costs of opening and developing new offices and registration costs are as follows:

	OPENING BALANCE	DEFERRED DURING PERIOD	AMORTIZED DURING PERIOD	CLOSING BALANCE
Balance January 1, 1961...	$ — 0 —			
Transactions in 1961:				
Costs of opening and developing new offices.................	$ — 0 —	$ 27,545.75	$ — 0 —	$ 27,545.75
Registration costs	$ — 0 —	11,085.54	— 0 —	11,085.54
	$ — 0 —	$ 38,631.29	$ — 0 —	
Balance December 31, 1961				$ 38,631.29
Transactions in 1962:				
Costs of opening and developing new offices.................	$ 27,545.75	$224,228.37	$ 9,181.92	$242,592.20
Registration costs......................................	11,085.54	100,349.77	— 0 —	111,435.31
	$ 38,631.29	$324,578.14	$ 9,181.92	
Balance December 31, 1962				$354,027.51
Transactions in 1963:				
Costs of opening and developing new offices.................	$242,592.20	$196,472.76	$ 87,424.70	$351,640.26
Registration costs......................................	111,435.31	152,846.17	— 0 —	264,281.48
	$354,027.51	$349,318.93	$ 87,424.70	
Balance December 31, 1963				$615,921.74
Transactions in 1964:				
Costs of opening and developing new offices.................	$351,640.26	$227,104.35	$149,415.63	$429,328.98
Registration costs......................................	264,281.48	49,619.01	88,093.82	225,806.67*
	$15,921.74	$276,723.36	$237,509.45	
Balance December 31, 1964				$655,135.65

*Registration costs for the common stock rescission offer in the amount of $26,815.00 and the registration costs for the public stock offering in the amount of $35,171.84 have been charged to additional paid-in capital (capital surplus) and not included herein.

The amortization charge as reflected in the Company's consolidated financial statements, as contained in the above analysis, have been deducted for federal income tax purposes.

NOTE 8. FEDERAL TAXES ON INCOME:

The provision and the liability for federal income taxes has been computed on the accrual basis. However, certain of the Company's subsidiaries report on the cash basis for income tax purposes. Inasmuch as there is a question as to whether these companies may report on the cash basis, the deferred income tax liability has been reported as a current liability of the Company.

The current year's provision and the liability for federal income taxes have been reduced by the current year's investment credit in the amount of $15,946.41, and the tax effect as the result of net operating loss carryover in certain subsidiaries in the amount of $2,642.72. The provision has also been reduced by the prior year's investment credit in the amount $147.44.

The federal income tax returns of the Company have not been examined by the Internal Revenue Services.

NOTE 9. NOTES PAYABLE TO BANKS:

The Company is indebted on an unsecured note payable to the American City Bank of Los Angeles, California in the amount of $210,000.00 bearing interest at the rate of 6% per annum. This note is payable at the rate of $10,000.00 per month plus interest and is personally guaranteed by the principal officers. This note supersedes and consolidates all prior loans with the American City Bank.

NOTE 10. NOTES PAYABLE, OTHERS:

The Company is indebted to the International Business Machine Company on an installment note having a remaining balance of $152.04. The Company is indebted to the Fidelity Bank on an install-

ment note payable at the rate of $182.08 per month having a remaining balance in the amount of $4,916.16.

The Company is indebted on notes payable to a partnership controlled by certain officers and directors of Pennsylvania Life Insurance Company in the amount of $300,000.00, bearing interest at the rate of 6% per annum and is secured by the assignment of the Company's rights to insurance renewal commissions. The notes are to be repaid by the Company on the following basis:

For the period January 1, 1965 to January 31, 1965, interest only.

For the period February 1, 1965 to January 31, 1966, $8,333.33 per month plus interest.

For the period February 1, 1966 to January 31, 1967, $12,500.00 per month plus interest.

For the period February 1, 1967 to January 31, 1968, $4,166.67 per month plus interest.

The loan was arranged by Pennsylvania Life Insurance Company in connection with a general agency agreement executed between the Company and Pennsylvania Life Insurance Company. The loan agreement provides in effect that if the Company breaches certain terms of the agency agreement the payee of the notes may declare the unpaid principal and any unpaid interest immediately due and payable.

NOTE 11. COMMON STOCK PURCHASE WARRANTS:

The Company has issued to New York Securities Company and to Theodore Goodman, equally, a total of 17,500 non-transferable common stock purchase warrants, at an aggregate price of $1,750.00 in cash, exercisable commencing on December 22, 1965 at $7.20 per share until December 22, 1967, and at $7.80 per share until December 22, 1969, the expiration date.

A stock option given to Mr. Alfred Strelsin to purchase 8,333 shares of the Company's $.30 par value common stock lapsed as of November 12, 1964. The $250.00 the Company received for this option has been transferred to additional paid-in capital.

NOTE 12. TREASURY STOCK:

On January 7, 1963, the Company purchased 2,925 shares of its $.30 par value common stock from Bernard Mazel, a former employee of the Company, whose employment was terminated on December 1, 1962. The purchase price paid by the Company was $11,100.00.

On May 10, 1963, the Company purchased from Raymond J. Platt, a former officer and director of the Company, 27,500 shares of its $.30 par value common stock for a total purchase price of $51,074.00.

On June 28, 1963, the Company purchased from Milton Polland, President of Union Trust Life Insurance Company, 667 shares of its common stock for a total purchase price of $6,500.00. This purchase was made in connection with the termination of the Company's General Agent Agreement with Union Trust Life Insurance Company.

On July 1, 1964, the Company purchased from A. Arthur Sherman, a former officer of the Company, 1,333 shares of $.30 par value stock for a total price of $4,000.00. Total shares held in treasury as of December 31, 1964 amounted to 32,425 shares of $.30 par value stock.

NOTE 13. COMMITMENTS AND CONTINGENT LIABILITIES:

(a) The Company leases offices and equipment at monthly rentals totalling $20,411.19. The leases involved expire in the years 1965 to 1970 except one lease on the home office in Los Angeles involving the sum of $5,470.20 per month expiring in the year 1974.

In regard to the lease on the home office, the Company had an option to cancel as of October 31, 1969 as long as notice to exercise the option was given to the lessor during the month of November, 1968 together with payment of $12,860.10 for the privelege of cancelling the lease. The Company has relinquished its right to cancel the aforsaid lease and will receive as consideration for the relinquishment of this right a $4,500.00 credit from the Kreedman Management and Realty Corp., the lessor, to be applied against the leasehold improvement cost of approximately $8,000.00 contemplated in expanding the total rental facilities of the home office in Los Angeles.

(b) The Company had sold certain of its $.10 and $.15 par value common stock without a California permit. Under the California Corporate Securities Law, the Company might have incurred a contingent liability in the maximum amount of $792,932. As a result of the aforesaid, the Company made an "Offer of Rescission," on terms and conditions satisfactory to the Commissioner of Corporations of California, to all holders of outstanding stock of the Company previously issued without a permit. Of the total number of holders of stock subject to the "Rescission Offer," only five individuals owning, collectively, 11,000 shares of the Company's $.10 par value stock

requested a rescission of their stock purchase. The sum of $29,815.85 was paid to them according to the terms and conditions of the "Rescission Offer." It is the opinion of the Company's counsel that there is, as of December 31, 1964, no material liability to the stockholders who had acquired their shares of the Company's common stock without a California permit.

(c) The Company has, pursuant to an agreement dated November 24, 1964, indemnified Gordon C. and Toni McCormick from certain liabilities that the McCormick's may have to Eugene Roemer arising out of a $50,000 note given by Mr. McCormick to Mr. Roemer. The liability of the McCormicks on such note was the subject of litigation to which the Company was made· a party, but which was dismissed with prejudice on November 30, 1964. The maximum contingent liability of the Company under such indemnification would be $50,000 plus legal fees and interest.

(d) The Company is proceeding to effect, through New York Securities Co., the private placement of approximately $1,000,000 of debt securities to bear interest at the rate of not more than 6% per annum. If such securities are so placed, they will contain a limited privilege of conversion into common stock of the Company, at a price not less than $6.00 per share, restrictions on the payment of dividends and other customary terms and conditions. If such securities are sold, it is expected that a placement fee, plus expenses, will be paid, equally, to New York Securities Co. and Theodore Goodman.

NOTE 14. SUPPLEMENTARY PROFIT AND LOSS INFORMATION:

The following amounts were charged to Selling, General and Administrative expenses:

Maintenance and Repairs	$ 7,723.86
Depreciation of Furniture and Fixtures	$ 6,344.14
Taxes other than federal income taxes:	
Payroll	$ 21,151.70
Personal Property and Licenses	3,747.17
Franchise	2,975.00
	$ 27,873.87
Rents	$144,204.11

NOTE 15: CLIENTS' COLLATERAL NOTES AND COMPANY'S CUSTODIAL COLLATERAL NOTES:

As of December 31, 1964 the Company had received collateral notes in connection with the financing of clients' premiums under the Company's "Programs for the Acquisition of Mutual Fund Shares and Life Insurance" in the amount of $231,623.21. These notes are secured by Keystone mutual funds shares having a value of $494,746.73 and were issued under a custodial collateral note agreement executed between the Company and the New England Merchants National Bank of Boston.

The Company has issued custodial collateral notes to the Pennsylvania Life Company in the amount of $59,000.00 and to the State Farm Life Insurance Company in the amount of $150,000.00. Equity Funding Service Corporation, a fully owned subsidiary, is holding the balance of $22,623.21.

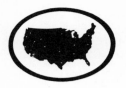

EQUITY FUNDING CORPORATION OF AMERICA
CONSOLIDATED STATEMENT OF EARNINGS AND RETAINED EARNINGS

	FOR THE YEAR ENDED	
	DECEMBER 31, 1966 (AUDITED)	DECEMBER 31, 1965 (AUDITED)
INCOME:		
Mutual Fund Commissions	$1,641,687	$1,139,552
Life Insurance Commissions	4,733,985	3,475,214
Interest income	907,403	662,913
Other income	203,737	85,669
TOTAL INCOME	7,486,812	5,363,348
EXPENSES:		
Commissions on Mutual Funds	828,381	561,913
Commissions on Life Insurance	2,032,337	1,494,342
Interest on insurance premium financing loans	598,818	455,652
Selling, general and administrative (Note 13)	1,849,813	1,433,790
TOTAL EXPENSES	5,309,349	3,945,697
EARNINGS BEFORE MINORITY INTEREST	2,177,463	1,417,651
MINORITY INTEREST (Note 1)	1,936	—
EARNINGS BEFORE FEDERAL TAXES ON INCOME ..	2,179,399	1,417,651
FEDERAL TAXES ON INCOME (Note 7):		
Current portions	26,787	389,996
Deferred portion	975,257	231,711
NET TAX PROVISION	1,002,044	621,707
NET EARNINGS	1,177,355	795,944
RETAINED EARNINGS — BEGINNING OF PERIOD	1,364,765	568,821
RETAINED EARNINGS — END OF PERIOD	$2,542,120	$1,364,765
EARNINGS PER SHARE*	$1.35	$.94

*Earnings per share for the years 1965 and 1966 were computed on the following average number of outstanding shares: 1965 — 850,344 shares and 1966 — 868,769 shares.

The accompanying notes are an integral part of the financial statements.

The financial statements as at and for the year ended December 31, 1965 are shown for comparative purposes only. Reference should be made to the previously issued Annual Report for the Accountants' Report and notes pertaining to those financial statements.

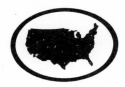

EQUITY FUNDING CORPORATION OF AMERICA

CONSOLIDATED STATEMENT OF FINANCIAL CONDITION (Note 1)

ASSETS

	DECEMBER 31, 1966 (AUDITED)			DECEMBER 31, 1965 (AUDITED)		
CURRENT ASSETS:						
Cash		$ 216,702			$ 2,797,142	
Accounts receivable		521,470			895,116	
Notes receivable		52,113			29,998	
Commissions receivable		1,025,403			1,131,512	
Advances to salesmen and employees		116,819			47,805	
Securities, at cost (Note 2)		19,522			7,992	
Prepaid expenses		82,131			53,433	
TOTAL CURRENT ASSETS		2,034,160			4,962,998	
FIXED ASSETS, AT COST (Note 3):						
Building and leasehold interest	$ 413,092			$ — 0 —		
Furniture, fixtures and equipment	102,650			88,023		
	515,742			88,023		
Less allowance for depreciation	54,330	461,412		35,226	52,797	
OTHER ASSETS:						
Investment in securities, at cost (Note 2)		380,740			275,000	
Loans receivable from clients for premium loans (Note 4)		13,776,971			9,210,597	
Collateral notes receivables (Note 10)		2,700,898			1,162,113	
Deposits		49,476			34,000	
Goodwill		12,000			12,000	
Cost of renewal commissions acquired, net of amortization (Note 5)		114,920			144,983	
Deferred charges (Note 6):						
Organization expense, net of amortization ..	$ 1,928			$ 2,086		
Cost of opening and developing new offices, net of amortization	391,435			319,908		
Registration costs, net of amortization	40,124			121,173		
Acquisition and development costs, net of amortization	11,475			18,992		
Financing costs, net of amortization	192,414	637,376	17,672,381	212,175	674,334	11,513,027
TOTAL ASSETS			$20,167,953			$16,528,822

The accompanying notes are an integral part of the financial statements.

The financial statements as at and for the year ended December 31, 1965 are shown for comparative purposes only. Reference should be made to the previously issued Annual Report for the Accountants' Report and notes pertaining to those financial statements.

LIABILITIES

	DECEMBER 31, 1966 (AUDITED)		DECEMBER 31, 1965 (AUDITED)	
CURRENT LIABILITIES:				
Accounts payable		$ 598,214		$ 1,427,877
Notes payable to bank (Note 8)		500,000		206,250
Notes payable to others — current portion		58,334		148,018
Accrued expenses:				
Commissions	$ 3,223		$ 3,524	
Taxes (other than federal taxes on income) ...	12,342		10,392	
Interest and sundry expenses	80,692	96,257	74,517	88,433
Federal taxes on income, estimated current portion (Note 7)		26,787		922,051
TOTAL CURRENT LIABILITIES		1,279,592		2,792,629
OTHER LIABILITIES:				
Notes payable on clients premium loans (Note 4).	7,439,599		7,079,599	
Custodial Collateral Notes payable (Note 10)....	2,625,000		1,140,000	
Federal taxes on income, deferred portion (Note 7)	1,883,640	11,948,239	— 0 —	8,219,599
LONG TERM DEBT (Note 9):				
Notes payable to others	$62,500		$211,065	
Less current portion	58,334	4,166	148,018	63,047
5¾% Subordinated Promissory Note, Series A...		400,000		400,000
5¾% Subordinated Convertible Promissory Note, Series B		600,000		600,000
5½% Capital Subordinated Notes, ... due December 1, 1980		2,000,000 3,004,166		2,000,000 3,063,047
MINORITY STOCKHOLDERS' INTEREST (Note 1) ..		(686)		— 0 —
STOCKHOLDERS' EQUITY:				
Preferred Stock—Authorized 15,000 shares. par value $100 per share, none issued (Note 1)		— 0 —		— 0 —
Common Stock—Authorized 4,000,000 shares.				
Issued 882,769 shares par value $.30 per share ..			264,831	
Issued 913,406 shares par value $.30 per share..		274,022		
Common stock purchase warrants (Note 11)		625		1,750
Addtional paid in capital		1,192,549		894,875
Retained earnings		2,542,120		1,364,765
		4,009,316		2,526,221
Less treasury stock 32,425 shares, par value $.30 per share, at cost		72,674 3,936,642		72,674 2,453,547
COMMITMENTS AND CONTINGENT LIABILITIES (Note 12)				
TOTAL LIABILITIES AND STOCKHOLDERS' EQUITY		$20,167,953		$16,528,822

The accompanying notes are an integral part of the financial statements.

The financial statements as at and for the year ended December 31, 1965 are shown for comparative purposes only. Reference should be made to the previously issued Annual Report for the Accountants' Report and notes pertaining to those financial statements.

EQUITY FUNDING CORPORATION OF AMERICA
NOTES TO CONSOLIDATED FINANCIAL STATEMENT, DECEMBER 31, 1966

NOTE 1. PRINCIPLE OF CONSOLIDATION AND SUBSEQUENT EVENTS CONCERNING CAPITAL STOCK:

The Company consists of the parent corporation, sixteen wholly-owned subsidiaries and one subsidiary, EFC Management Corporation, in which New York Securities Co. holds a 5% minority interest.

Inasmuch as all of the corporations were under common control for the periods audited, the consolidation is considered to represent a pooling of interests. All intercompany accounts, transactions and profits have been eliminated from the consolidated financial statements.

The Articles of Incorporation of the Company were amended in September 1965 to authorize 15,000 shares of preferred stock $100 par value per share. As of December 31, 1966 none of the preferred stock was issued.

The Company has a Production Option Plan pursuant to which 22,975 shares have been reserved for options granted to eligible sales representatives or division managers. Such options are exercisable during a two-year period ending on June 30, 1968, at the rate of four shares of common stock for each $100 of commissions, bonuses or overrides earned by the optionee as of December 31, 1965. The purchase price per share is $6.50 as to 16,220 shares and $8.125 as to 6,755 shares.

An additional 60,000 shares of common stock have been reserved for Incentive Stock Options granted or to be granted to eligible sales representatives, division managers and employees, other than the Company's two principal executive officers. Such options have a term of four years and are exercisable from time to time in units of not less than 100 shares commencing after the expiration of two years from the date of grant. The purchase price per share is the greater of $6.50, as to 20,000 of the shares reserved, and $10, as to 40,000 of the shares reserved, or the market value, as defined, of the common stock on the date of grant.

The Company has issued stock purchase options to certain employees, district and division managers, agents and associated general agents of the Company. The following shares are subject to options granted under the Production Option Plan and Incentive Stock Options as at March 1, 1967:

	Date of Grant	Number of Shares	Option Price Per Share	Market at Date of Grant High Bid	Market at Date of Grant Low Ask
Production Options:	3/31/65	5,416	$ 6.50	$ 7.75	$ 7.875
	7/28/65	2,661	$ 8.125	$ 7.25	$ 7.375
Incentive Options:	4/15/65	16,408	$ 8.01	$ 9.375	$ 9.50
	1/12/66	26,942	$10.875	$14,625	$14.75
	1/6/67	4,000	$11.50*		
	2/15/67	2.500	$21.875*		

*Option price indicated is equal to the closing price on American Stock Exchange on date of grant.

In addition to its Production Option Plan, and options granted, or to be granted, as Incentive Stock Options, the Board of Directors has adopted, subject to stockholder approval, a qualified Option Plan pursuant to which 22,500 shares of the Company's common stock are reserved for options granted or to be granted to certain key employees of the Company. Such options are intended to qualify as "qualified stock options" as defined in Section 422 of the Internal Revenue Code of 1954, as amended. The options will be exercisable in whole or in part between June 1, 1967 and May 31, 1970, at a price equal to the fair market value of the common stock on the date of grant. If employed until May 1, 1967, the option may be exercised within three months after any subsequent termination of employment of the optionee. In the event of the optionee's death, his option may be exercised by the optionee's estate to the extent not theretofore exercised, until May 31, 1971. As of March 1, 1967 options as to 17,500 shares, exercisable at $10.00 per share, and options as to 1,250 shares, exercisable at $11.375 per share, were outstanding. On March 1, 1967 the Company's common stock closed at $26.00 per share on the American Stock Exchange.

NOTE 2. SECURITIES, AT COST:

As of December 31, 1966, two subsidiaries of the Company owned 1564 shares of common stock of Equity Funding Corporation of America at a total investment of $19,522 (market value $17,790).

On such date, the Company owned the following securities, included under other assets in the Consolidated Statement of Financial Condition:

(a) 50,000 shares of common stock of Congressional Life Insurance Company at a total investment of $275,000 (market value $300,000). These securities are held by the United California Bank as collateral. Refer to Note 8.

(b) 9,200 shares of Equity Growth Fund of America, Inc. at a total investment of $100,740 (market value $107,640).

(c) 740 shares of Kennesaw Life and Accident Insurance Company at a total investment of $5,000 (market value $2,220).

NOTE 3. FIXED ASSETS, AT COST:

It is the policy of the Company to provide for depreciation on a "straight-line" basis predicated on the estimated useful lives of the individual items on the various classes of assets. The principal estimated useful lives in computing depreciation are as follows:

Office furniture and fixtures ....10 years
Office equipment ....5 years
Leasehold improvements ....3 years
Automobile ....5 years
Building ....20 years

The leasehold interest continues until December 31, 2049 and amortization is on a "straight-line" basis.

NOTE 4. CLIENTS' PREMIUM LOANS AND ASSIGNED COLLATERAL:

Under the method of operation followed prior to October 21, 1963, as contrasted to the Programs described in this Prospectus, clients who co-

ordinate their investment and insurance program assign their purchased mutual fund shares to Equity Funding Corporation with power to hypothecate their shares only to secure loans for paying their insurance premiums and loan interest. These shares are pledged by Equity Funding Corporation to the lending institutions as collateral for the loans made for the aforesaid purpose.

The premium payment loans are primarily on demand or short term basis and either Equity Funding Corporation or the client may terminate the loan or loan program at any time. The lender may require the assignment of additional collateral or repayment of the loan balance if the value of the collateral should decline to an aggregate value at which the lender feels itself insecure. Where repayment is demanded and not received, the lender may sell the collateral, and any proceeds in excess of the outstanding obligation is remitted to the client.

The loans receivable from clients for premium loans reported under "Other Assets" are offset, in part, by the contra notes payable on premium loans reported under "Other Liabilities." The difference, in the amount of $6,337,372 is held by Equity Funding Corporation of America. The collateral assigned by clients as security for the notes payable on premium loans reported under "Other Liabilities" and the portion held by Equity Funding Corporation of America amounted to $22,875,652.

NOTE 5. COST OF RENEWAL COMMISSIONS ACQUIRED:

The Company capitalized the cost of purchasing and acquiring complete right, title and interest to certain of its renewal commissions. Costs incurred prior to 1964 are being amortized on an annual basis over a nine-year period. Costs incurred after December 31, 1963 are being amortized on an annual basis over a five-year period. This figure is not intended to reflect the actual value of the renewal commissions.

NOTE 6. DEFERRED CHARGES:

The Company has capitalized organization expense, the cost of opening and developing new offices, registration costs, financing costs and acquisition and development costs. Costs incurred prior to 1961 being amortized on an annual basis over a five year period. The cost of opening and developing new offices incurred after December 31, 1960 are being amortized on an annual basis over a three year period. Registration costs are being amortized over a three year period. Financing costs are being amortized over the life of the respective loans. Acquisition and development costs are being amortized over a three year period.

The amounts deferred and amortized with respect to the costs of opening and developing new offices and registration costs are as follows:

	Opening Balance	Deferred During Period	Amortized During Period	Closing Balance
Balance January, 1961	— 0 —			
Transactions in 1961:				
Cost of opening and developing new offices ..	— 0 —	27,546	— 0 —	27,546
Registration costs	— 0 —	11,085	— 0 —	11,085
	— 0 —	38,631	— 0 —	
Balance December 31, 1961				38,631
Transactions in 1962:				
Cost of opening and developing new offices ..	27,546	224,228	9,182	242,592
Registration costs	11,085	100,350	— 0 —	111,435
	38,631	324,578	9,182	
Balance December 31, 1962				354,027
Transactions in 1963:				
Cost of opening and developing new offices ..	242,592	196,473	87,425	351,640
Registration costs	111,435	152,846	—0—	264,281
	354,027	349,319	87,425	
Balance December 31, 1963				615,921
Transactions in 1964:				
Cost of opening and developing new offices ..	351,640	227,104	149,415	429,329
Registration costs	264,281	49,619	88,094	225,806
	615,921	276,723	237,509	
Balance December 31, 1964				655,135
Transactions in 1965:				
Cost of opening and developing new offices ..	429,329	115,199	224,620	319,908
Registration costs	225,806	— 0 —	104,633	121,173
	655,135	115,199	329,253	
Balance December 31, 1965				441,081
Transactions in 1966:				
Cost of opening and developing new offices ..	319.908	276,821	105,294	391,435
Registration costs	121,173	25,501	106,550	40,124
	441,081	302,322	311,844	
Balance December 31, 1966				431,559

The amortization charge as reflected in the Company's consolidated financial statements, as contained in the above analysis, has been deducted for federal income tax purposes.

NOTE 7. FEDERAL TAXES ON INCOME:

The provision and the liability for federal income taxes have been computed on the accrual basis. The Company reports on the cash basis for income tax purposes and has reported the current portion of the income tax liability under "Current Liabilities" in the "Consolidated Statement of Financial Condition." The deferred portion of the income tax liability has been reported under "Other Liabilities," instead of under "Current Liabilities" as in prior years.

In the past, the Company has reported the deferred income tax liability under "Current Liabilities," pending a review by the Internal Revenue Service through the process of an income tax examination, as to whether the Company may report on a cash basis. Such a review has not as yet been made.

Since the Company believes that it may properly report on the cash basis, the deferred income tax liability has been reported under "Other Liabilities."

NOTE 8. NOTES PAYABLE TO BANK:

The Company is indebted to the United California Bank of Los Angeles, California in the amount of $500,000 on two notes as follows:
(1) A demand note in the amount of $250,000 bearing interest at the rate of 5¾% per annum. This note is secured by 50,000 shares of Congressional Life Insurance Company common stock.
(2) An unsecured note dated December 12, 1966 in the amount of $250,000 due in 91 days and bearing interest at the rate of 6¾% per annum. This note was paid in full on March 13, 1967.

NOTE 9. LONG TERM DEBT:

The Company is indebted on notes payable to a partnership controlled by certain officers and directors of Pennsylvania Life Insurance Company in the amount of $62,500, bearing interest at the rate of 6% per annum and is secured by the assignment of the Company's rights to insurance renewal commissions. The notes are to be repaid by the Company on the following basis:

For the month of January, 1967, $12,500 plus interest.

For the period February 1, 1967 to January 31, 1968, $4,167 per month plus interest.

The Company is indebted on two unsecured subordinated notes payable to the Paul Revere Life Insurance Company in the amount of $1,000,000, bearing interest at the rate of 5¾% per annum with interest payable semi annually commencing August 1, 1965. These notes are to be repaid by the Company on the following basis:

The Series A Note is in the amount of $400,000. Payments of $130,000 are due on February 1, 1968 and 1969 and the balance of $140,000 is due on February 1, 1970.

The Series B Note in the amount of $600,000 is convertible into the common stock of the Company at any time up to February 1975, limited to the amount of indebtedness at the time of conversion. The conversion price shall be $7.14 per share subject to adjustments on the payment of dividends and other customary terms and conditions. Five payments of $120,000 each are due February 1, 1971 through 1975.

On December 29, 1965, the Company issued $2,000,000 of 5½% Capital Subordinated Notes due December 1, 1980. The Notes are subject to optional redemption at fixed percentages of the principal amount during the period December 1, 1966 to December 1, 1980. The Notes are also subject to redemption in part on December 1, 1969, and on each December 1 thereafter to and including December 1, 1979, through the operation of a Sinking Fund.

Each Capital Subordinated Note is accompanied by a non-detachable Warrant for the purchase of common stock, $.30 par value, of the Company at the rate of 40 shares of common stock for each $1,000 principal amount of Capital Subordinated Notes and unless previously exercised expires at the close of business on December 1, 1975. The applicable Warrant prices are as follows:

If Exercised on or Prior to December 1,	Price per share
1968	$12
1971	14
1975	16

Long term debt maturing during each of the five years subsequent to 1966, is as follows:

1967	$ 58,333
1968	134,167
1969	130,000
1970	140,000
1971	120,000

NOTE 10. CLIENTS' COLLATERAL NOTES AND COMPANY'S CUSTODIAL COLLATERAL NOTES:

As of December 31, 1966, the Company had received collateral notes in connection with the financing of clients' premiums under the Company's "Programs for the Acquisition of Mutual Fund Shares and Life Insurance" in the amount of $2,700,898. These notes are secured by Keystone Mutual Fund Shares having a value of $5,863,265 and were issued under a Custodial Collateral Note Agreement executed between the Company and the New England Merchants National Bank of Boston.

The Company has issued Custodial Collateral Notes to the Pennsylvania Life Company in the amount of $375,000 and to the State Farm Insurance Company in the amount of $2,250,000. Equity Funding Service Corporation, a wholly owned subsidiary, is holding the balance of $75,898.

NOTE 11. COMMON STOCK PURCHASE WARRANTS:

As of December 31, 1966, Theodore Goodman holds stock purchase warrants with respect to 6250 shares at a price of $625.

NOTE 12. COMMITMENTS AND CONTINGENT LIABILITIES:

The Company leases offices and equipment at monthly rentals totalling $41,501. The leases involved expire in the years 1967 to 1975.

NOTE 13. SUPPLEMENTARY PROFIT AND LOSS INFORMATION:

The following amounts were charged to Selling, General and Administrative expenses:

	Year Ended December 31, 1966
Maintenance and repairs	$ 19,245
Depreciation of furniture and fixtures	$ 13,971
Taxes other than federal income taxes:	
Payroll	$ 47,848
Personal property and licenses	25,776
Franchise	9,979
	$ 83,603
Rents	$225,486

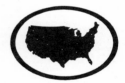

EQUITY FUNDING CORPORATION OF AMERICA

CONSOLIDATED STATEMENT OF EARNINGS AND RETAINED EARNINGS

The following Consolidated Statement of Earnings and Retained Earnings has been compiled as explained in Note 1 to the Financial Statements of Equity Funding. The statements for the five years ended December 31, 1967, have been examined by Wolfson, Weiner, Ratoff & Lapin, independent certified public accountants, whose opinion appears elsewhere in this Offering Circular. With respect to the unaudited periods, Equity Funding believes that all adjustments (which consist of normal recurring accruals) necessary for a fair statement of the results of operations for such periods have been made. This statement should be read in conjunction with the related financial statements and notes thereto included elsewhere in this Offering Circular.

	Year Ended December 31,					Nine Months Ended	
	1963	1964	1965	1966	1967	September 30, 1967 unaudited	September 30, 1968 unaudited
INCOME:							
Life Insurance commissions	$ 787,423	$1,911,303	$3,475,214	$4,733,985	$ 6,930,950	$4,474,746	$ 7,373,679
Mutual Fund commissions	212,270	494,156	1,139,552	1,641,687	2,043,964	1,283,575	2,899,417
Interest income	300,418	448,681	662,913	907,403	1,304,793	864,864	1,300,564
Other income	24,741	15,060	85,669	203,737	899,236	419,203	1,617,800
Total Income	1,324,852	2,869,200	5,363,348	7,486,812	11,178,943	7,042,388	13,191,461
EXPENSES:							
Commissions on Life Insurance	296,387	756,393	1,494,342	2,032,337	2,803,444	1,820,260	2,881,167
Commissions on Mutual Funds	89,661	223,195	561,913	828,381	1,006,705	633,412	1,236,930
Interest on insurance premium financing loans	251,456	328,900	455,652	598,818	714,304	470,992	631,073
Selling, general and administrative (Note 13)	681,441	944,305	1,433,790	1,849,813	3,217,416	1,471,655	2,634,216
Total Expenses	1,318,945	2,252,793	3,945,697	5,309,349	7,741,869	4,396,319	7,383,386
EARNINGS BEFORE CAPITAL GAINS	5,907	616,407	1,417,651	2,177,463	3,437,074	2,646,069	5,808,075
Capital gain on sale of securities	64,904	3,915	—	—	—	—	—
EARNINGS BEFORE MINORITY INTEREST	70,811	620,322	1,417,651	2,177,463	3,437,074	2,646,069	5,808,075
Minority interest	—	—	—	1,936	—	—	—
EARNINGS FROM OPERATIONS	70,811	620,322	1,417,651	2,179,399	3,437,074	2,646,069	5.808,075
EARNINGS FROM UNCONSOLIDATED SUBSIDIARIES:							
Earnings (loss) excluding non-recurring reinsurance agreements	—	—	—	—	148,667	—	146,213
Earnings from non-recurring reinsurance agreements	—	—	—	—	600,000	—	632,000
Total earnings from unconsolidated subsidiaries	—	—	—	—	748,667	—	778,213
EARNINGS BEFORE FEDERAL TAXES ON INCOME	70,811	620,322	1,417,651	2,179,399	4,185,741	2,646,069	6,586,288
Federal taxes on income (Note 7):							
Current portion	64	8,326	389,996	26,787	31,236	15,192	501,363
Deferred portion	17.989	222.528	231,711	975,257	1,624,125	1,184,673	2.565,968
Total tax provision	18,053	230,854	621,707	1,002.044	1,655,361	1,199,865	3.067,331
NET EARNINGS	52,758	389,468	795,944	1,177,355	2,530,380	1,446,204	3,518,957
RETAINED EARNINGS—BEGINNING OF YEAR	126,595	179,353	568,821	1,364,765	2,542,120	2,542,120	3,601,189
Less: Stock dividend paid	—	—	—	—	(1,469,376)	(1,478,273)	(2,008,732)
Adjustment for minority interest	—	—	—	—	(1,935)	—	—
RETAINED EARNINGS—END OF YEAR*	$ 179.353	$ 568.821	$1,364,765	$2.542,120	$ 3,601.189	$2,510,051	$ 5,111,414
EARNINGS PER SHARE:							
Before non-recurring reinsurance agreements	$.02	$.16	$.29	$.42	$.59	$.43	$.71
From non-recurring reinsurance agreements	—	—	—	—	$.16	—	$.16
Total earnings per share**	$.02	$.16	$.29	$.42	$.75	$.43	$.87
PRO FORMA EARNINGS PER SHARE***				$.35	$.62	$.38	$.80

* See Note 14 to the Financial Statements of Equity Funding with respect to dividend restrictions applicable to retained earnings as of December 31, 1967 and September 30, 1968.

** Earnings per share have been computed on the basis of $0.30 par value common stock. Earnings per share for the year 1963 were computed on 2,438,818 outstanding shares. Earnings per share for the years 1964 thru 1967 were computed on the following average number of outstanding shares: 1964—2,443,380 shares, 1965—2,758,942 shares, 1966—2,818,718 shares, and 1967—3,371,670 shares. Earnings per share for the nine-months ended September 30, 1967 were computed on 3,360,986 average number of outstanding shares and the earnings for the nine-months ended September 30, 1968 were computed on 4,054,842 average number of outstanding shares. (The foregoing number of shares are as adjusted for the five percent stock dividend paid on April 15, 1967, the three-for-two stock split effected December 6, 1967, the three percent stock dividend paid on March 14, 1968 and the two-for-one stock split effected November 1, 1968.)

*** 1966—The pro forma earnings per share for 1966 were computed on the basis of an average of 2,818,718 outstanding shares and on the assumption that (a) Equity Funding's 5¾% Subordinated Convertible Promissory Note, Series B, outstanding at December 31, 1966 was converted and 272,646 additional shares of Common Stock were issued, eliminating the related interest on such Note, less applicable income tax of $16,560, and that (b) all of Equity Funding's Common Stock Purchase Warrants and stock options outstanding on December 31, 1966 were exercised (reduced by the equivalent number of shares which could be purchased with the proceeds at an assumed market price of approximately $10⅜ per share) and that 372.976 shares of Common Stock were issued.

1967—The pro forma earnings per share for 1967 were computed on the basis of an average of 3,371,670 outstanding shares and on the assumption that (a) Equity Funding's Convertible Subordinated Debentures, Convertible Subordinated Junior Notes and Convertible Subordinated Junior Capital Notes outstanding at December 31, 1967 were converted and 748,156 additional shares of Common Stock were issued, eliminating the related interest on such securities, less applicable income tax of $115,071, and that (b) all of Equity Funding's Common Stock Purchase Warrants and stock options outstanding on December 31, 1967 were exercised (reduced by the equivalent number of shares which could be purchased with the proceeds at an assumed market price of approximately $17½ per share) and that 187,376 shares of Common Stock were issued.

Nine months ended September 30, 1967 and September 30, 1968—The pro forma earnings per share were computed on the basis of an average number of shares outstanding in the amount of 3,360,986 and 4,054,842 respectively and on the assumption that (a) all of Equity Funding's Common Stock Purchase Warrants and stock options outstanding on September 30, 1967 and 1968 were exercised (reduced by the equivalent number of shares which could be purchased with the proceeds at an assumed market price of approximately $10⅜ and $43⅝ per share respectively), and that (b) Equity Funding's Convertible Debentures outstanding at September 30, 1967 and 1968 were converted, eliminating the related interest on such securities, less applicable income tax resulting in total shares of 3,897,796 and 4,707,002 and earnings of $1,517,466 and $3,781,457, respectively.

The annual interest to be paid by Equity Capital on the Debentures offered hereby initially will be approximately $1,312,500.

BUSINESS OF EQUITY FUNDING

General

The greatest part of Equity Funding's income is derived from commissions earned on the sale of life insurance and mutual fund shares. Sales are effected primarily through Equity Funding's own sales organization consisting of approximately 2,500 salesmen, who are licensed as insurance and/or securities salesmen and are employed on a commission basis. Equity Funding's 106 sales offices, 36 of which were opened in 1968, are located in Alabama, Arizona, Arkansas, California, Colorado, Florida, Georgia, Hawaii, Illinois, Indiana, Kentucky, Louisiana, Michigan, Minnesota, Mississippi, Missouri, New Jersey, New Mexico, New York, Ohio, Oregon, Pennsylvania, Tennessee, Texas, Utah, Washington, District of Columbia and Okinawa. Up to 25 more new sales offices are planned for opening during 1969, depending upon the availability of managerial personnel.

The percentage of Equity Funding's total gross income attributable to the above sources for the years ended December 31, 1963 through 1967, and for the nine-month period ended September 30, 1968, is as follows:

	Year Ended December 31,					Nine Months Ended September 30, 1968
	1963	1964	1965	1966	1967	
Life insurance commissions	59%	67%	66%	63%	62%	56%
Mutual fund commissions	16%	17%	21%	22%	18%	22%

The dollar amount of commissions earned by Equity Funding in connection with the sale of life insurance and mutual fund shares for the years ended December 31, 1963 through 1967, and for the nine-month period ended September 30, 1968, is as follows:

	Year Ended December 31,					Nine Months Ended September 30, 1968
	1963	1964	1965	1966	1967	
Gross life insurance commissions	$787,422	$1,911,303	$3,475,214	$4,733,985	$6,930,950	$7,373,679
Less: Commissions to salesmen	296,387	756,393	1,494,342	2,032,337	2,803,444	2,881,167
Net commissions	$491,035	$1,154,910	$1,980,872	$2,701,648	$4,127,506	$4,492,512
Gross mutual fund commissions	$212,270	$ 494,156	$1,139,552	$1,641,687	$2,043,964	$2,899,417
Less: Commissions to salesmen	89,661	223,195	561,913	828,381	1,006,705	1,236,930
Net commissions	$122,609	$ 270,961	$ 577,639	$ 813,306	$1,037,259	$1,662,487

Coordinated Acquisition Plans

The following table indicates the percentage of aggregate gross insurance and mutual fund commission income represented by the sale of coordinated acquisition plans and by the sale of insurance and mutual fund shares independent of the plans for the years ended December 31, 1963 through 1967, and for the nine-month period ended September 30, 1968:

	Year Ended December 31,					Nine Months Ended September 30, 1968
	1963	1964	1965	1966	1967	
Coordinated acquisition plan sales	44.4%	42.8%	43.7%	46.9%	44.6%	40.5%
Non-plan sales	55.6%	57.2%	56.3%	53.1%	55.4%	59.5%

15

Coordinated Acquisition Plan Sales and Terminations

The table below sets forth statistical information for the periods indicated concerning the sale of all coordinated acquisition plans by Equity Funding and by certain independent insurance agencies. No representation is made that sales of the proposed modified programs described below will be effected at the rate shown below for "Programs" sold during the periods covered.

	Year Ended December 31.				
"Programs" Sold	1963	1964	1965	1966	1967
Number of "Programs" Sold (1)	371	682	1,525	2,763	3,912
Amount of Premiums Financed	$ 134,263	$ 398,780	$ 799,293	$ 1,489,033	$ 2,071,778
Face Amount of Life Insurance Policies Sold	$7,243,282	$20,022,835	$45,073,171	$83,176,572	$116,262,182
Premium Loans Outstanding at End of Period(2)	$4,912,340	$ 6,913,998	$10,372,709	$16,477,869	$ 25,094,811
Amount of Mutual Funds Purchased in Financing of Premiums(3)	$2,048,917	$ 5,771,765	$ 9,641,715	$11,007,640	$ 13,687,157
"Programs" Terminated					
Termination of "Programs" Sold During Period Indicated, as of December 31, 1967(4)	96	111	159	147	None
Amount of Annual Premiums Involved in Terminations	$ 32,229	$ 67,545	$ 83,862	$ 81,794	None
Face Amount of Life Insurance Involved in Terminations(5)	$1,174,540	$ 3,365,838	$ 4,723,217	$ 4,499,021	None

(1) The number of programs sold by Equity Funding alone, exclusive of programs sold through independent insurance agencies, and the percentage of total program sales represented by such Equity Funding sales, in each of the periods shown in the table, is as follows: 1963—77 (21%); 1964—676 (99%); 1965—1,499 (98%); 1966—2,733 (99%) and, 1967—3,912 (100%). The information shown in the table also includes programs involving fire and casualty insurance, except that the amount of the coverage included in such insurance in programs sold and terminated is not reflected because of the complex variety of fire and casualty protection provided under those policies.

(2) Including interest.

(3) Represents amount of mutual fund shares sold in programs sold by Equity Funding alone. It is not practicable under Equity Funding's method of accounting to determine the amount of shares sold by mutual fund distributors affiliated with independent insurance agencies.

(4) Terminations generally result because of reasons which are personal to the investor. Only two forced liquidations have taken place to date. Of course, no representations can be made as to the extent of any future forced liquidations.

(5) "Terminations" refer only to the financing arrangement and not necessarily to a termination of the related life insurance policy.

For the nine months ended September 30, 1968, Equity Funding sold 6,646 Programs, under which $3,500,178 of insurance premiums were financed, $191,436,263 face amount of life insurance policies were issued and $23,267,565 of mutual fund shares were purchased. At the end of such period, $33,540,512 of insurance premium loans were outstanding.

The average face amount of the life insurance policies sold in all coordinated acquisition plans is approximately $24,000. The average amount of the first year loan made to participants is approximately $510.

The sale and continuation of Equity Funding's Programs and the continuation of substantially similar plans sold by Equity Funding prior to October 1963 (the "old Plans") are dependent upon Equity Funding's ability to obtain funds for financing insurance premiums. Equity Funding obtains funds for this purpose from institutional lenders, including banks, from the public sale of its debt securities and

16

through cash generated in its own operations. At September 30, 1968, $8,360,000 of bank loans effected by Equity Funding were utilized in the financing of old Plans, $2,530,000 of loans effected by Equity Funding with certain insurance companies, including $170,000 of loans from Presidential, were used in connection with the financing of the Programs, and approximately $22,600,000 of Equity Funding's internally generated funds and proceeds of debt underwritings were used in the financing of old Plans and Programs. See Equity Funding's Financial Statements herein.

On December 10, 1968, the United States Federal Reserve Board ("Board") announced proposals to broaden the coverage of its margin regulations so that they would apply to loans made under plans for the acquisition of mutual fund shares and insurance such as the Programs. If such proposals are adopted, Programs offered or sold after April 30, 1969, would be subject to the Board's margin requirements. Equity Funding understands that the margin requirements will not apply to subsequent borrowings made to complete, in accordance with their original terms, Programs and old Plans sold prior to the effective date of such proposals.

Under the Board's current margin requirements, the maximum loan value of mutual fund shares pledged in a Program would be 20% of their net asset value. However, under the Programs now offered by Equity Funding the initial borrowing on pledged mutual fund shares may be as high as 43%, and, thereafter, annual borrowings may be as high as 65%, of the value of the pledged shares. Equity Funding has implemented plans to offer a modified coordinated mutual fund share and life insurance acquisition program designed to meet existing margin requirements. It is anticipated that the modified programs, which in principle will be the same as the Programs now being offered, will, in general, require proportionately higher investments in mutual fund shares and the application of cash values to reduce the amount of premium financed through Equity Funding. The offering of such modified programs is subject to compliance with various governmental regulations and no representation can, of course, be made as to when, or as to the actual form in which, they will be available.

Equity Funding has also considered other alternative practicable procedures which it could adopt to comply with the Board's existing margin requirements. Adoption of any of such procedures, including the modified program described above, may involve temporary delays or interruptions in the sale of coordinated acquisition programs which could have a temporary adverse effect on Equity Funding's operations. Equity Funding believes, however, that these revisions would not, under present margin requirements, have a long-range adverse effect on its operations, although there can, of course, be no assurance that this will be the case.

A material deterioration in stock market conditions could adversely affect Equity Funding's business.

Life Insurance Sales

In addition to the insurance business it conducts through Presidential which is described under "Life Insurance Company Operations", below, Equity Funding also is a general agent for Pennsylvania Life Insurance Company ("Penn Life") and Congressional Life Insurance Company ("Congressional") in three States in which Presidential is not qualified to do business. Equity Funding owns approximately 5% of Congressional's outstanding capital stock. Prior to the acquisition of Presidential, the greater part of Equity Funding's life insurance sales was in policies issued by Penn Life. During 1968, substantially all of Equity Funding's life insurance business was applied for through Presidential.

The insurance policies sold by Equity Funding are whole life and term. Premium income is primarily represented by the sale of whole life insurance policies. Term policies do not, at this time, account for a substantial part of such income. The amount of the annual premium due on any insurance contract varies with the size and type of the policy, the age of the insured and the extent of any supplemental benefits desired.

The following table reflects pertinent information with respect to life insurance sales by or through Equity Funding for the years ended December 31, 1963 through 1967:

Year	Premiums in Force Beginning of Year	Premiums Billed During Year	Premiums Lapsed During Year	Premiums Paid and in Force at End of Year	Gross Com- missions	Com- mission Expense	Net Com- mission Income
1963	$ 2,155,285	$ 2,777,153	$ 202,187	$ 2,574,966	$ 787,423	$ 296,387	$ 491,035
1964	2,574,966	4,217,917	246,186	3,971,731	1,911,303	756,393	1,154,910
1965	3,971,731	7,187,678	394,035	6,793,643	3,475,214	1,494,342	1,980,872
1966	6,793,643	11,273,921	741,934	10,531,987	4,733,985	2,032,337	2,701,648
1967	10,531,987	16,954,305	1,191,260	15,763,045	6,930,950	2,803,444	4,127,506

Mutual Fund Sales

Although Equity Funding has selling agreements with the distributors of a large number of mutual funds, the greater part of its mutual fund sales is in shares of Equity Growth Fund, which is described below, and in shares of the various Keystone Custodian Funds, five of which are offered in the Programs. Currently, about 32% of Equity Funding's total mutual fund sales are in shares of Equity Growth Fund and about 21% of such sales are in shares of the various Keystone Custodian Funds. During 1967, shares of Equity Growth Fund and of the various Keystone Custodian Funds accounted for about 28% and 25%, respectively, of Equity Funding's total mutual fund sales. Equity Funding's maximum commission, before deduction of salesmen's commissions, on sales of Keystone Custodian Funds is 6% of the offering price of the shares. One of Equity Funding's subsidiaries also acts as a wholesale representative of Axe Securities Corporation in the sale of shares of Axe-Houghton Stock Fund Inc. (the "Axe Fund") for which it receives an amount equal to five-sixths of the sales charge (after deduction of the applicable dealers' discount) and bears certain costs relating to the sale of such shares. Equity Funding intends to concentrate its mutual fund sales in shares of Equity Growth Fund, Republic and such other mutual funds as it may in the future manage and serve as principal distributor.

The following table sets forth pertinent information concerning the sale of mutual fund shares by Equity Funding for the years ended December 31, 1963 through 1967, and for the nine months ended September 30, 1968:

Year	Amount of Mutual Fund Shares Sold*	Gross Commissions	Commission Expense	Net Commissions
1963	$ 3,637,625	$ 212,270	$ 89,661	$ 122,609
1964	$ 8,342,547	$ 494,156	$ 223,195	$ 270,961
1965	$19,673,058	$1,139,552	$ 561,913	$ 577,639
1966	$29,865,320	$1,641,687	$ 828,381	$ 813,306
1967	$36,235,687	$2,043,964	$1,006,705	$1,037,259
Nine-months ended September 30, 1968	$43,411,112	$2,614,532	$1,194,680	$1,419,852

* The amounts shown include the applicable sales charge and are based on the total amount of shares sold during the period indicated on which a dealer's discount (commission) was allowed Equity Funding. As no sales charge is applicable on capital gains distributions taken in shares pursuant to automatic reinvestment plans, the amount of such distributions is not included in the table.

Mutual Fund Management and Distribution

Equity Growth Fund

Equity Growth Fund was incorporated in March 1966 and commenced the sale of its shares of common stock as an open-end investment company in August 1966. Its total net assets at December 31, 1968 amounted to $42,466,669. Investments of Equity Growth Fund are managed by EFC Management Corporation ("EFC Management"), a subsidiary of Equity Funding. For services and

18

duct an overseas banking business, principally involving the financing of commercial transactions in which Equity Funding, its subsidiaries, or affiliates may participate. It may also serve as a derivative source of foreign capital which may be loaned to Equity Funding to finance its Programs or to meet its other working capital requirements. There is, of course, no assurance that this transaction will be consummated.

Oil and Gas Exploration

In November 1968, Equity Funding agreed to purchase, on behalf of International, all the outstanding capital stock of Traserco, Inc. ("Traserco Delaware"), a Delaware corporation, from unaffiliated persons for 3,500 shares of Equity Funding's Common Stock. Traserco Delaware is the owner of all of the outstanding stock of Traserco C.A. ("Traserco Panama"), a Panamanian corporation, which is the owner of an undivided 23.75% interest in various petroleum concessions previously granted by the Government of Ecuador and now owned by a consortium of which Traserco Panama is a member. The concessions cover approximately 3,500,000 acres off the coast of Ecuador. The consortium has engaged an operating company to conduct off-shore oil and gas exploration in the area covered by the concessions. Upon the consummation of the transaction, which is subject to various conditions including the consent of the Government of Ecuador and the members of the consortium, Traserco Panama will be merged into Traserco Delaware, which will change its name to Traserco C.A. As part of the transaction, Equity Funding also has agreed to pay $97,750 to the sellers as reimbursement for certain advances previously made by them in payment of the balance of the purchase price of Traserco Panama's concession interest.

Equitex Petroleum Corporation, a California corporation, was formed by Equity Funding in September 1968, to enter into oil and gas exploration ventures overseas, primarily Africa and the Middle East. It has not yet entered into any concession agreements.

At this time, the concession interest of Traserco Panama, and any concession interests developed by Equitex, may only be regarded as having speculative value.

IPC TRANSACTIONS

Equity Funding entered into an agreement on October 31, 1968, for the purchase of substantially all of the assets of IPC at a price of $6.8 million, plus the net book value of the specific assets to be transferred as of the closing date, which is to take place not later than April 15, 1969. The purchase price, which is expected to total not more than approximately $9.3 million, is to be paid 81% in cash and the balance in shares of Equity Funding's Common Stock, valued at its average closing price on the American Stock Exchange for the five business days preceding the closing. Such shares will be distributed by IPC to its stockholders other than I.O.S., Ltd. (S.A.) ("IOS"), a Panama corporation, which owns 81% of IPC's outstanding capital stock. Of the total purchase price, $2.5 million will be held in escrow for a one-year period, subject to reduction in certain events.

The assets of IPC to be acquired by Equity Funding include all of the assets, properties, business and goodwill of IPC related to the operations of IPC in the United States. Assets related to the overseas operations of IPC, encompassing all operations of IPC not carried on in any State of the United States, are not being acquired by Equity Funding. The proposed transaction is subject to various conditions, including the approval of certain matters by stockholders of IPC and of Fund of America, and there is, therefore, no assurance that it will be consummated.

In addition to the approval of the sale by IPC's stockholders, the purchase agreement requires that a new management agreement and a new underwriting agreement between Equity Funding or a subsidiary thereof be approved by the shareholders of Fund of America. The new agreements are to be identical in all material respects with the existing agreements.

Pursuant to an order dated May 23, 1967, under which the United States Securities and Exchange Commission ("SEC") accepted an offer of settlement of an administrative proceeding brought against IOS by the SEC (although not in connection with IOS's interest in IPC), IOS is required to dispose of its interest in IPC's United States operations, subject to the SEC's consent. Equity Funding is informed that the SEC has advised IOS that it has approved the proposed sale to Equity Funding.

Assuming that the proposed acquisition is consummated, Equity Funding plans to form a new Delaware corporation to be known as IPC Management Corporation ("New IPC"). New IPC will act as investment adviser and principal distributor for Fund of America, and as sponsor for the four contractual plans presently sponsored by IPC.

Business of IPC to Be Acquired

Sales of Securities

IPC sponsors and sells plans for the accumulation of shares of four mutual funds and also sells mutual fund securities directly. Its principal offices are located in New York City. IPC has 29 branch offices in 21 states and the District of Columbia, and expects to have not less than approximately 150 full-time and 1800 part-time sales representatives at the close of the acquisition by Equity Funding. IPC sponsors and distributes plans for the accumulation of the shares of Fund of America, Axe-Houghton Fund B., Inc., Axe Science Corporation and National Investors Corporation, all of which are registered investment companies under the United States Investment Company Act of 1940, as are the plans themselves. IPC offers plans in 20 states and in the District of Columbia.

As the sponsor of the plans, IPC receives creation and sales charges applicable to the plans. These charges compensate IPC for its services and costs in creating the plans and arranging for their administration; for making the mutual fund shares available at net asset value; and for all related selling expenses and commissions. The creation and sales charges range from 8.5% to 1% of the payments made depending upon the plan purchased. IPC also receives fees for certain administrative and investor services which the custodians of all four plans have delegated to IPC.

IPC offers and sells shares of Fund of America, as principal distributor, in 18 states and the District of Columbia. Fund of America shares are sold at net asset value plus a sales charge which ranges from 8.5% on purchases of less than $25,000 to 1% on purchases of $500,000 or more. A major portion of the sales charge is paid as commissions to sales representatives and regional divisional managers. IPC retains approximately 30% of the sales charge. Under its distributorship agreement, IPC bears the expenses of federal and state registrations, sales promotion, prospectuses, sales literature, and proxy material and reports to shareholders used in connection with the continuous offering. During its last fiscal year, IPC also sold, as a dealer, shares of approximately 144 mutual funds.

Investment Management

Fund of America Management Corporation ("Management Corporation"), which is wholly-owned by IPC, now serves as investment adviser to Fund of America, pursuant to a management agreement under which Management Corporation assists in the administration of the fund, supervises and manages its investment portfolio, and directs the purchase and sale of investment securities subject to the supervision and control of the fund's Board of Directors. Management Corporation furnishes to the fund complete office facilities, internal accounting and auditing, personnel, telephone and other mechanical services. Officers, directors or employees of Management Corporation, who may be officers, directors or employees of Fund of America, serve without additional compensation from the fund.

For these services the fund pays Management Corporation a monthly fee of 1/24 of 1% of the net asset value of the fund on the last business day of each month, which amounts to ½ of 1% on an annual basis. To the extent that the fund's annual operating expenses, including the fee of Management Corporation, but excluding interest and taxes, exceed 1% of the fund's average net assets, such excess is

EQUITY FUNDING CORPORATION OF AMERICA

CONSOLIDATED STATEMENT OF FINANCIAL CONDITION (NOTE 1)

ASSETS

	December 31, 1967 Audited		September 30, 1968 Unaudited	
CURRENT ASSETS:				
Cash		$ 1,155,074		$ 3,463,831
Accounts receivable		2,803,408		3,511,365
Notes receivable		45,650		67,117
Commissions receivable		870,861		1,866,004
Advances to salesmen and employees		106,963		148,278
Securities, at cost (Note 2)		402,693		3,596,384
Prepaid and sundry expenses		132,016		109,989
Total Current Assets		5,516,665		12,762,968
PROPERTY AND EQUIPMENT (Note 3):				
Building and leasehold interest	$ 492,538		$ 525,944	
Furniture, fixtures and equipment	163,832		259,644	
	656,370		785,588	
Accumulated depreciation and amortization	84,759	571,611	121,196	664,392
OTHER ASSETS:				
Investment in securities, at cost (Note 2)	380,817		544,627	
Loans receivable from clients for premium loans (Note 4)	19,512,475		23,006,473	
Collateral notes receivable (Note 5)	5,582,336		10,534,039	
Deposits	59,574		71,598	
Goodwill	12,000		12,000	
Cost of renewal commissions acquired, net of amortization (Note 6)	218,368		182,842	
Deferred charges, net of amortization (Note 7):				
Organization expense	$ 1,388		$ 8,891	
Cost of opening and developing new offices	956,792		1,438,214	
Registration costs	15,084		7,478	
Acquisition and development costs	3,958		—	
Financing costs	469,268	1,446,490	515,962	1,970,545
Investment in unconsolidated subsidiaries (Note 8):				
Equity in unconsolidated subsidiaries	5,454,847		6,232,700	
Excess of cost over related net assets of unconsolidated subsidiaries	4,994,980	10,449,467	4,994,980	11,227,680
Covenant not to compete	30,000		30,000	
Excess of cost over net book value on date of acquisition of consolidated subsidiaries (Note 1)	—	37,691,527	1,039,629	48,619,433
		$43,779,803		$62,046,793

38

EQUITY FUNDING CORPORATION OF AMERICA

CONSOLIDATED STATEMENT OF FINANCIAL CONDITION (NOTE 1)

LIABILITIES

	December 31, 1967 Audited		September 30, 1968 Unaudited	
CURRENT LIABILITIES:				
Accounts payable		$ 2,658,160		$ 1,813,212
Notes payable—current portion (Note 10)		1,028,179		555,780
Commissions payable		7,792		40,665
Taxes (other than federal taxes on income)		32,166		38,287
Accrued interest and sundry expenses		205,396		569,398
Federal taxes on income, estimated current portion (Note 9)		31,236		568,163
Total Current Liabilities		3,962,929		3,585,505
OTHER LIABILITIES:				
Notes payable on clients premium loans (Note 4)	$ 8,443,194		$ 8,360,000	
Custodial collateral notes payable (Note 5)	2,775,000		2,530,000	
Federal taxes on income, deferred portion (Note 9)	3,511,197	14,729,391	6,091,622	16,981,622
LONG TERM DEBT (Note 10):				
Notes payable to banks	2,500,732		—	
Notes payable to others	753,685		777,561	
	3,254,417		777,561	
Less current portion	1,028,179		555,780	
	2,226,238		221,781	
5½% convertible subordinated debentures due 1982	5,906,000		—	
5¾% convertible subordinated junior notes due 1972	1,600,000		—	
5½% capital subordinated notes due 1980	1,940,000		1,896,500	
5½% convertible subordinated junior capital notes due 1972	1,976,800		—	
5¼% convertible subordinated debentures due 1983	—	13,649,038	15,000,000	17,118,281
STOCKHOLDERS' EQUITY:				
Preferred stock—authorized 15,000 shares, par value $100 per share, none issued (Note 1)	—			
Authorized 1,000,000 shares, no par value, none issued (Note 1)			—	
Common stock — authorized 4,000,000 shares at December 31, 1967 and 8,000,000 shares at September 30, 1968 par value $.30 per share, issued 1,848,589 shares and 2,334,319 shares respectively	554,577		700,296	
Common stock purchase warrants (Note 11)	625		625	
Additional paid-in capital	7,354,728		18,621,724	
Retained earnings	3,601,189		5,111,414	
	11,511,119		24,434,059	
Less treasury stock 32,425 shares, par value $.30 per share, at cost	72,674	11,438,445	72,674	24,361,385
COMMITMENTS AND CONTINGENT LIABILITIES (Note 12)				
		$43,779,803		$62,046,793

39

NOTES TO CONSOLIDATED FINANCIAL STATEMENTS—(Continued)

The leasehold interest continues until December 31, 2049 and amortization is on a "straight-line" basis.

Expenditures for additions, major renewals and improvements are capitalized, and expenditures for maintenance and repairs are charged to income as incurred. Upon sale or retirement of items of equipment and improvements, the cost and related accumulated depreciation are eliminated from the accounts and the resulting gain or loss, if any, is reflected in income. Equipment becoming obsolete or unusable is written down to salvage value.

Note 4. Clients' Premium Loans and Assigned Collateral:

Under the method of operation followed prior to October 21, 1963, as contrasted to the Programs described in this Prospectus, clients who coordinate their investment and insurance program assign their purchased mutual fund shares to a subsidiary with power to hypothecate their shares only to secure loans for paying their insurance premiums and loan interest. These shares are pledged by the subsidiary to the lending institutions as collateral for the loans made for the aforesaid purposes.

The premium payment loans are primarily on a demand or short-term basis, and either the subsidiary or the client may terminate the loan or loan program at any time. The lender may require the assignment of additional collateral or repayment of the loan balance if the value of the collateral should decline to an aggregate value at which the lender feels insecure. Where repayment is demanded and not received, the lender may sell the collateral, and any proceeds in excess of the outstanding obligation is remitted to the client.

The loans receivable from clients for premium loans reported under "Other Assets" are offset, in part, by the contra notes payable on premium loans reported under "Other Liabilities." The difference in the amount of $11,069,281 is held by Equity Funding. The collateral assigned by clients as security for the loans receivable on premium loans reported under "Other Assets" amounted to $32,398,513.

Note to Unaudited September 30, 1968 Consolidated Financial Statements:

As of September 30, 1968 the difference between the loans receivable from clients and the notes payable on premium loans, in the amount of $14,646,473 was held by Equity Funding. The collateral assigned by clients as security amounted to $39,571,134.

Note 5. Clients' Collateral Notes and Company's Custodial Collateral Notes:

As of December 31, 1967, Equity Funding had received collateral notes in connection with the financing of clients' premiums under Equity Funding's "Programs for the Acquisition of Mutual Fund Shares and Life Insurance" in the amount of $5,582,336. These notes are secured by mutual fund shares having a value of $12,113,669 and were issued under a Custodial Collateral Note Agreement executed between Equity Funding and the New England Merchants National Bank of Boston.

Equity Funding has issued Custodial Collateral Notes to the Pennsylvania Life Company in the amount of $325,000, to the State Farm Insurance Company in the amount of $2,250,000 and to The Presidential Life Insurance Company of America, a wholly-owned subsidiary, in the amount of $200,000. Equity Funding Service Corporation, a wholly owned subsidiary, is holding the balance of $3,099,836.

Note to Unaudited September 30, 1968 Consolidated Financial Statements:

As of September 30, 1968 Equity Funding had received collateral notes in the amount of $10,534,039. These notes are secured by mutual fund shares having a value of $21,436,769. Equity Funding has issued custodial collateral notes to the State Farm Life Insurance Company, the Pennsylvania Life Company and the Presidential Life Insurance Company, in the amount of $2,250,000, $110,000 and $170,000 respectively. Equity Funding Service Corporation is holding the balance of $8,004,039.

Note 6. Cost of Renewal Commissions Acquired:

Equity Funding capitalized the cost of purchasing and acquiring complete right, title and interest to certain of its renewal commissions. Costs incurred prior to 1964 are being amortized on an annual basis over a nine-year period. Costs incurred after December 31, 1963 are being amortized on an annual basis over a five-year period. This figure is not intended to reflect the actual value of the renewal commissions.

Note 7. Deferred Charges:

Equity Funding has capitalized organization expenses, the cost of opening and developing new offices, registration costs, financing costs and acquisition and development costs. The costs of opening and developing new offices incurred after December 31, 1960 are being amortized on an annual basis over a three year period. Registration costs are being amortized over a three year period. Financing costs are being amortized over the life of the respective loans. Acquisition and development costs are being amortized over a three year period.

CONSOLIDATED STATEMENT OF EARNINGS

(UNAUDITED)

	Nine Months Ended Sept. 30, 1968		Nine Months Ended Sept. 30, 1967	
INCOME				
Mutual Fund Commissions...	$2,899,418		$1,283,575	
Life Insurance Commissions..	7,373,679		4,474,746	
Interest Income	1,300,564		864,864	
Other Income	1,617,800		419,203	
TOTAL INCOME		$13,191,461		$7,042,388
EXPENSES				
Commissions on Mutual Funds	1,236,930		633,412	
Commissions on Life Insurance	2,881,167		1,820,260	
Interest on Insurance Premium Financing Loans	631,073		470,992	
Selling General and Administrative	2,634,216		1,471,654	
TOTAL EXPENSES		7,383,386		4,396,318
Net Earnings from Operations		5,808,075		2,646,070
Net Earnings from Unconsolidated Subsidiaries		778,214		
EARNINGS BEFORE FEDERAL TAXES ON INCOME		6,586,289		2,646,070
FEDERAL TAXES ON INCOME				
Current Portion	501,363		15,192	
Deferred Portion	2,565,968		1,184,674	
Net Tax Provision		3,067,331		1,199,866
NET EARNINGS		$ 3,518,958		$1,446,204
EARNINGS PER SHARE		$ 1.74		$ .87
AVERAGE NUMBER OF SHARES OUTSTANDING .		2,027,434		1,669,616
Proforma Earnings Per Share.		$ 1.61		$ .69

CONSOLIDATED STATEMENT OF FINANCIAL CONDITION

September 30, 1968

(UNAUDITED)

ASSETS

CURRENT ASSETS

Cash	$ 2,463,831
Certificates of Deposit	1,000,000
Accounts Receivable	3,511,365
Investment Securities	3,596,384
Notes Receivable	67,117
Commissions Receivable	1,866,004
Advances to Salesmen and Employees	148,277
Prepaid and Sundry Expenses	109,990
	12,762,968
PROPERTY AND EQUIPMENT (Schedule "A")	664,392
OTHER ASSETS (Schedule "B")	48,652,281
TOTAL ASSETS	$62,079,641

LIABILITIES AND STOCKHOLDERS' EQUITY

CURRENT LIABILITIES

Accounts Payable	$ 1,813,212
Notes Payable—Current Portion	555,780
Commissions Payable	40,665
Taxes (Other Than Federal Taxes on Income)	38,287
Accrued Interest and Sundry Expenses	569,397
Federal Taxes on Income, Estimated Current Portion	568,163
	3,585,504
OTHER LIABILITIES (Schedule "C")	16,981,622
LONG TERM DEBT (Schedule "D")	17,118,281
STOCKHOLDERS' EQUITY (Schedule "E")	24,394,234
Total Liabilities and Stockholders' Equity	$62,079,641

SUPPORTING SCHEDULES TO THE CONSOLIDATED STATEMENT OF FINANCIAL CONDITION

September 30, 1968

(UNAUDITED)

PROPERTY AND EQUIPMENT
AT COST (SCHEDULE "A")

Building and Leasehold Interest	....	$ 525,944
Furniture, Fixtures, Equipment	....	259,644
		785,588
Accumulated Depreciation and Amortization	....	121,196
		$ 664,392

OTHER ASSETS (SCHEDULE "B")

Investments in Securities at Cost	....	$ 544,627
Loans Receivable from Clients for Premium Loans	....	23,006,473
Collateral Notes Receivable	....	10,534,039
Deposits	....	71,298
Goodwill	....	12,300
Cost of Renewal Commissions, Net of Amortization	....	182,842
Deferred Charges, Net of Amortization		
Organization Expense	....	8,891
Cost of Opening and Developing New Offices	....	1,438,214
Registration Costs	....	7,478
Financing Costs	....	515,962
Investment in Unconsolidated Subsidiaries		
Equity in Unconsolidated Subsidiaries	....	6,232,700
Excess of Cost Over Related Net Assets of		
Unconsolidated Subsidiaries	....	6,067,457
Covenant Not to Compete	....	30,000
		$48,652,281

SUPPORTING SCHEDULES TO THE CONSOLIDATED STATEMENT OF FINANCIAL CONDITION

September 30, 1968
(UNAUDITED)

OTHER LIABILITIES (SCHEDULE "C")

Notes payable on clients' premium loans	$ 8,360,000
Custodial Collateral Notes Payable	2,530,000
Federal Taxes on Income, Deferred Portion	6,091,622
	$16,981,622

LONG TERM DEBT (SCHEDULE "D")

Notes Payable to Banks	$ 25,000
Notes Payable Others	752,561
	777,561
Less Current Portion	555,780
	221,781
5¼% Convertible Subordinated Debentures due May 1, 1983	15,000,000
5½% Capital Subordinated Notes due December 1, 1980	1,896,500
	$17,118,281

STOCKHOLDERS' EQUITY (SCHEDULE "E")

Preferred Stock Authorized 15,000 Shares Par value $100.00 per Share None Issued	
Common Stock Authorized 8,000,000 Shares Par Value $.30	
Issued 2,334,319 Shares	$ 700,296
Common Stock Purchase Warrants	625
Additional Paid-In Capital	18,601,724
Retained Earnings	5,164,263
	24,466,908
Less Treasury Stock 32,425 Shares, Par Value $.30 per Share at Cost	72,674
	$24,394,234

PROSPECTUS

Equity Funding Corporation of America

404,925 Shares of Common Stock

This Prospectus covers shares of Common Stock, par value $.30 per share (the "Common Stock") of Equity Funding Corporation of America (the "Company") which are issuable upon conversion of 5¼% Guaranteed (Subordinated) Debentures due 1989 (the "Debentures") heretofore issued and sold by Equity Funding Capital Corporation N.V. ("Equity Capital"), a subsidiary of the Company. The Indenture pursuant to which the Debentures were issued provides for conversion on or after November 1, 1969 (unless redeemed prior to conversion), until maturity of the Debentures, at the rate of 15.87 shares of Common Stock for each $1,000 principal amount of Debentures (equivalent to a conversion price of $63.00 per share), subject to adjustment in certain events. As a result of a 2% Common Stock dividend paid by the Company in April 1969, the adjusted conversion rate as of the date hereof is 16.197 shares of Common Stock for each $1,000 principal amount of Debentures (equivalent to a conversion price of $61.74 per share).

The Common Stock is listed on the American Stock Exchange. See "Price Range of Common Stock" herein with respect to the market prices for the Company's Common Stock during recent periods. On November 10, 1969, the closing price of the Common Stock on the American Stock Exchange was $68.25 per share.

THESE SECURITIES HAVE NOT BEEN APPROVED OR DISAPPROVED BY THE SECURITIES AND EXCHANGE COMMISSION NOR HAS THE COMMISSION PASSED UPON THE ACCURACY OR ADEQUACY OF THIS PROSPECTUS. ANY REPRESENTATION TO THE CONTRARY IS A CRIMINAL OFFENSE.

The date of this Prospectus is November 14, 1969

EQUITY FUNDING CORPORATION OF AMERICA
CONSOLIDATED STATEMENT OF EARNINGS
AND RETAINED EARNINGS

The following consolidated statement of earnings and retained earnings has been compiled as explained in Note 1 to the Company's Financial Statements. The statements for the five years ended December 31, 1968, have been examined by Wolfson, Weiner, Ratoff & Lapin, independent certified public accountants, whose opinion appears elsewhere in this Prospectus. With respect to the unaudited periods, the Company believes that all adjustments (which consist only of normal recurring accruals) necessary for a fair statement of the results of operations for such periods have been made. This statement should be read in conjunction with the related financial statements and notes thereto included elsewhere in this Prospectus. (See Note C, below, as to pro forma results of the proposed acquisition of Liberty for the periods indicated.)

	Year Ended December 31,					Six Months Ended June 30,	
	1964 Audited	1965 Audited	1966 Audited	1967 Audited	1968 Audited	1968 Unaudited	1969 Unaudited
							(Note B)
INCOME:							
Life Insurance commissions	$1,911,303	$3,475,214	$4,733,985	$ 6,930,950	$ 9,511,866	$5,346,226	$ 6,244,662
Mutual Fund commissions	494,156	1,139,552	1,641,687	2,043,964	5,001,777	1,835,337	10,995,834
Interest income	448,681	662,913	907,403	1,304,793	1,759,106	966,553	1,261,159
Other income	15,060	85,669	203,737	899,236	2,906,368	849,825	2,842,178
Total Income	2,869,200	5,363,348	7,486,812	11,178,943	19,179,117	8,997,941	21,343,833
EXPENSES:							
Commissions on Life Insurance	756,393	1,494,342	2,032,337	2,803,444	3,330,661	2,319,105	2,461,858
Commissions on Mutual Funds	223,195	561,913	828,381	1,006,705	2,061,166	856,394	4,746,742
Interest on insurance premium financing loans	328,900	455,652	598,818	714,304	931,454	455,563	616,815
Selling, general and administrative (Note 13)	944,305	1,433,790	1,849,813	3,217,416	3,835,531	1,785,533	8,592,127
Total Expenses	2,252,793	3,945,697	5,309,349	7,741,869	10,158,812	5,416,595	16,417,542
EARNINGS BEFORE CAPITAL GAINS	616,407	1,417,651	2,177,463	3,437,074	9,020,305	3,581,346	4,926,291
Capital gain on sale of securities	3,915	—	—	—	—	—	—
EARNINGS BEFORE MINORITY INTEREST	620,322	1,417,651	2,177,463	3,437,074	9,020,305	3,581,346	4,926,291
Minority interest	—	—	1,936	—	—	—	—
EARNINGS FROM OPERATIONS	620,322	1,417,651	2,179,399	3,437,074	9,020,305	3,581,346	4,926,291
Earnings from unconsolidated subsidiaries, net of extraordinary items (Note A)	—	—	—	698,667	757,537	334,552	1,480,576
EARNINGS BEFORE FEDERAL AND STATE TAXES ON INCOME	620,322	1,417,651	2,179,399	4,135,741	9,777,842	3,915,898	6,406,867
Federal and State taxes on income (Note 9):							
Current portion	8,326	389,996	26,787	31,236	546,333	19,492	353,582
Deferred portion	222,528	231,711	975,257	1,624,125	3,546,704	1,858,965	2,003,629
Total tax provision	230,854	621,707	1,002,044	1,655,361	4,093,037	1,878,457	2,357,211
NET EARNINGS BEFORE EXTRAORDINARY ITEMS	389,468	795,944	1,177,355	2,480,380	5,684,805	2,037,441	4,049,656
Extraordinary items, net of applicable Federal and State taxes (Notes 2 and 8)	—	—	—	50,000	2,141,052	52,000	634,796
NET EARNINGS	389,468	795,944	1,177,355	2,530,380	7,825,857	2,089,441	4,684,452
RETAINED EARNINGS—BEGINNING OF YEAR	179,353	568,821	1,364,765	2,542,120	3,610,189	3,601,189	9,436,810
Less: Stock dividends paid	—	—	—	(1,469,376)	(2,008,732)	(1,992,115)	(5,908,564)
Adjustment for minority interest	—	—	—	(1,935)	—	—	—
RETAINED EARNINGS—END OF PERIOD*	$ 568,821	$1,364,765	$2,542,120	$ 3,601,189	$ 9,418,314	$3,698,515	$ 8,212,698
EARNINGS PER COMMON SHARE—ASSUMING NO DILUTION:							
Before extraordinary items (Note A)	$.16	$.28	$.41	$.72	$1.35	$.51	$.81
Extraordinary items	—	—	—	.02	.52	.01	.13
Total earnings per common share— assuming no dilution**	$.16	$.28	$.41	$.74	$1.87	$.52	$.94
EARNINGS PER COMMON SHARE—ASSUMING FULL DILUTION:							
Before extraordinary items (Note A)			$.34	$.56	$1.10	$.44	$.72
Extraordinary items			—	.04	.48	.03	.16
Total earnings per common share— assuming full dilution***			$.34	$.60	$1.58	$.47	$.88
COMMON STOCK DISTRIBUTIONS:							
Dividends				5%	3%	3%	2%
Splits				3-for-2	2-for-1	—	—

9

EQUITY FUNDING CORPORATION OF AMERICA
PRO FORMA STATEMENT OF FINANCIAL CONDITION

The following pro forma statement of financial condition of the Company at December 31, 1968 gives effect to the acquisition of the United States assets of IPC, the acquisition of Ankony Angus and the proposed acquisition of Liberty. This statement should be read in conjunction with financial statements and related notes of the Company, IPC, Ankony Angus and Liberty included elsewhere herein. The Company's statement of financial condition at June 30, 1969, includes IPC and Ankony Angus. The pro forma statement at June 30, 1969 gives effect to the proposed acquisition of Liberty.

Columns 2–8 are headed **December 31, 1968**; columns 9–11 are headed **June 30, 1969**.

ASSETS	Company (Audited)	IPC (Audited)	Ankony Angus (Unaudited)	Adjustments	Pro Forma Combined (Unaudited)	Liberty Adjustments	Pro Forma Combined (Unaudited)	Company (Unaudited)	Liberty Adjustments	Pro Forma Combined (Unaudited)
Current assets	$18,707,571	$6,927,181	$947,100	($6,264,866)	$20,316,986		$20,316,986	$45,630,204		$45,630,204
Property and equipment, at cost	671,330	320,586	3,526,634		4,518,550		4,518,550	10,951,494		10,951,494
Excess of cost over net book value on date of acquisition of consolidated subsidiaries:	1,039,628				1,039,628		1,039,628			
IPC				6,922,300(2)	6,922,300		6,922,300			
Ankony Angus				2,500,000(4)	2,500,000		2,500,000			
Excess of cost over related net assets of unconsolidated subsidiaries	4,994,980				4,994,980	$2,628,161(5)	7,623,141	7,719,222	$2,628,161(5)	10,347,383(6)
Equity in unconsolidated subsidiaries	10,174,823				10,174,823	3,671,839(5)	13,846,662	12,903,156	3,671,839(5)	16,574,995
Other assets	43,416,678	416,535	8,037,730		51,870,943		51,870,943	56,349,104		56,349,104
Investment—IPC				{ 10,234,403 (1); (10,234,403)(2) }						
Investment—Ankony Angus				{ 13,000,000 (3); (13,000,000)(4) }						
	$79,005,010	$7,664,302	$12,511,464	$3,157,434	$102,338,210	$6,300,000	$108,638,210	$133,553,180	$6,300,000	$139,853,180

LIABILITIES	Company (Audited)	IPC (Audited)	Ankony Angus (Unaudited)	Adjustments	Pro Forma Combined (Unaudited)	Liberty Adjustments	Pro Forma Combined (Unaudited)	Company (Unaudited)	Liberty Adjustments	Pro Forma Combined (Unaudited)
Current liabilities	$9,295,423	$4,352,199	$889,940		$14,537,562		$14,537,562	$20,167,457		$20,167,457
Other liabilities	23,970,378		1,121,524		25,091,902		25,091,902	29,740,570		29,740,570
Long-term debt	16,927,215			{ $6,500,000(3); 2,025,000(1) }	25,452,215		25,452,215	29,305,787		29,305,787
Capital stock	1,389,004			{ 27,326(3); 8,049(1) }	1,424,379	$29,097(5)	1,453,476	1,625,787	$29,097(5)	1,654,884
Warrants	625				625		625	625		625
Additional capital	18,076,725			{ 6,472,674(3); 1,936,488(1) }	26,485,887	6,270,903(5)	32,756,790	44,571,930	6,270,903(5)	50,842,833
Retained earnings	9,418,314				9,418,314		9,418,314	8,213,698		8,213,698
Treasury stock	(72,674)				(72,674)		(72,674)	(72,674)		(72,674)
Excess of assets over liabilities:										
IPC		3,312,103		(3,312,103)(2)						
Ankony Angus			10,500,000	(10,500,000)(4)						
Liberty										
	$79,005,010	$7,664,302	$12,511,464	$3,157,434	$102,338,210	$6,300,000	$108,638,210	$133,553,180	$6,300,000	$139,853,180

The following transactions are reflected in the pro forma adjustments:

(1) The purchase by the Company of the United States operations of IPC and the related indebtedness incurred, the common stock issued for such purchase and the cash paid for such purchase.

(2) Elimination on consolidation of the excess of assets over liabilities of IPC. The assumed total cost of the assets of IPC purchased is $6,922,300 greater than the net equity of IPC at December 31, 1968, which amount has been added to "excess of cost over net book value on date of acquisition of consolidated subsidiaries" on consolidation.

(3) The purchase of Ankony Angus and the related indebtedness incurred and the common stock issued for such purchase.

(4) Elimination on consolidation of the excess of assets over liabilities of Ankony Angus. The assumed total cost of the assets of Ankony Angus at December 31, 1968, which amount has been added to "excess of cost over net book value on date of acquisition of consolidated subsidiaries" on consolidation.

(5) The proposed acquisition of Liberty in exchange for 90,322 shares of the Company's common stock having a total value equal to approximately $6,300,000.

(6) The Company does not intend to amortize these amounts since it believes that there has been no diminution in value.

(7) Pro forma income statements have not been included in the Prospectus since IPC and Ankony Angus are included in the consolidated financial statements of the Company from January 1, 1969, and the combined results of operations of the Company and Liberty on a pooling of interests basis for the five years and six months ended June 30, 1969 are set forth in Note C to the Company's Consolidated Statement of Earnings and Retained Earnings.

20

INSURANCE OPERATIONS

Presidential

In October 1967, the Company acquired all of the outstanding stock of Presidential and Presidential Life Insurance Agency, Inc. ("Presidential Agency") from unaffiliated sellers. The consideration paid by the Company consisted of $1,099,000 in cash, a $500,000, 5½% promissory note which has been paid, 82,447 shares of the Company's Common Stock and $2,002,300 principal amount of its 5½% Convertible Subordinated Junior Capital Notes, which have been converted into Common Stock of the Company.

Presidential was incorporated in June 1959 and is authorized under Illinois law to write life and accident and health insurance. It is presently qualified to write life and accident and health insurance in the District of Columbia and in all states except Connecticut, New Jersey, New York, North Carolina and West Virginia. Of the life insurance presently in force, approximately 29% was written in California and approximately 16% was written in Illinois. Presidential Agency is a general agent of Presidential.

The insurance sold by Presidential includes individual whole life and endowment, term, group, mortgage and accident and health insurance. Premium rates are believed by the Company to be generally competitive with similar types of insurance written by other companies. At this time, the policies being written by Presidential are non-participating.

The following table shows, for the five years ended December 31, 1968, Presidential's life insurance in force, new insurance written, premium income and admitted assets:

	1964	1965	1966	1967	1968
Admitted Assets	$ 2,602,244	$ 2,145,822	$ 2,838,466	$ 2,678,780	$ 8,208,779
Capital Stock and Surplus	2,131,305	1,393,272	1,471,162	2,122,466	6,335,118
Ratio of Capital Stock and Surplus to Total Liabilities	452.5%	185.1%	107.6%	381.5%	338.1%
Life Insurance in Force:					
Whole Life and Endowment	5,937,602	27,877,227	48,234,308	77,373,441	105,395,534
Term and Other Policies	27,881,149	41,625,068	31,850,927	15,091,049	59,958,011
Total Individual	33,818,751	69,502,295	80,085,235	92,464,490	165,353,545
Group	7,709,750	20,770,300	28,680,900	16,763,250	22,172,780
Total Life Insurance in Force*	$41,528,501	$90,272,595	$108,766,135	$109,227,740	$187,526,325
Life Insurance—Direct New Business:					
Whole Life and Endowment	$ 2,041,432	$22,243,908	$ 29,825,339	$ 49,401,253	53,601,191
Term and Other Policies	10,152,662	17,385,002	1,186,771	2,748,616	45,334,633
Total Individual	12,194,094	39,628,910	31,012,110	52,149,869	98,935,824
Group	6,711,500	12,063,000	—	—	180,000
Total Direct New Business	18,905,594	51,691,910	31,012,110	52,149,869	99,115,824
Individual Assumed Reinsurance Paid For	—	—	—	—	—
Group Assumed Reinsurance Paid For	—	2,592,800	—	—	—
Total Life Insurance Paid For	$18,905,594	$54,284,710	$ 31,012,110	$ 52,149,869	99,115,824
Premium Income:					
Individual Life	$ 152,831	$ 851,245	$ 1,400,780	$ 673,704	698,205
Group	42,768	72,683	150,422	150,689	81,874
Individual A & H	—	1,829	34,398	29,100	1,566,036
Total Premium Income	$ 195,599	$ 925,757	$ 1,585,600	$ 853,493	2,346,115
***Includes Ceded Reinsurance and Assumed Reinsurance as follows:**					
Ceded Reinsurance:					
Individual	$28,027,154	$46,455,442	$ 44,849,650	$ 85,759,115	143,900,711
Group	1,999,250	1,842,000	2,045,250	—	1,897,250
Total Ceded Reinsurance	$30,026,404	$48,297,442	$ 46,894,900	$ 85,759,115	145,797,961
Assumed Reinsurance:					
Individual	—	—	—	—	—
Group	—	2,592,800	10,288,400	13,830,120	15,971,030
Total Assumed Reinsurance	—	$ 2,592,800	$ 10,288,400	$ 13,830,120	15,971,030

EQUITY FUNDING CORPORATION OF AMERICA

CONSOLIDATED STATEMENT OF FINANCIAL CONDITION (NOTE 1)

ASSETS

	December 31, 1968 Audited		June 30, 1969 Unaudited	
CURRENT ASSETS:				
Cash		$ 2,814,974		$ 6,632,924
Accounts receivable		6,066,422		10,065,205
Notes receivable		96,384		2,323,804
Commissions receivable		2,813,193		2,846,909
Inventory—Livestock		—		2,100,970
Advances to salesmen and employees		279,160		467,576
Securities, at cost (Note 2)		6,626,276		20,544,112
Prepaid and sundry expenses		11,162		648,704
Total Current Assets		18,707,571		45,630,204
PROPERTY AND EQUIPMENT, AT COST (Note 3):				
Real Estate and leasehold interest	$ 541,508		$ 4,300,796	
Furniture, fixtures and equipment	263,774		736,707	
Livestock—Breeding herd	—		6,808,550	
	805,282		11,846,053	
Accumulated depreciation and amortization	133,952	671,330	894,559	10,951,494
OTHER ASSETS:				
Investments, at cost (Note 2)	3,731,703		4,341,288	
Funded loans and accounts receivable (Note 4)	35,476,037		35,720,927	
Loans receivable from officers and directors (Note 4)	835,000		835,000	
Deposits and sundry assets	112,503		821,951	
Cost of renewal commissions acquired, net of amortization (Note 5)	158,453		131,118	
Deferred charges, net of amortization (Note 6):				
Organization expense $ 1,002			$ 2,250	
Cost of opening and developing new offices 2,249,572			2,098,526	
Registration costs 6,584			1,350	
Acquisition and development costs 202,667			429,294	
Financing costs 619,157	3,078,982		776,651	3,308,071
Investment in unconsolidated subsidiaries (Note 7):				
Equity in unconsolidated subsidiaries 10,174,823			12,902,156	
Excess of cost over related net assets of unconsolidated subsidiaries 4,994,980	15,169,803		7,719,222	20,621,378
Covenant not to compete	24,000		21,000	
Excess of cost over net book value on date of acquisition of consolidated subsidiaries (Note 8)	1,039,628	59,626,109	11,169,749	76,970,482
		$79,005,010		$133,552,180

See accompanying notes.

56

EQUITY FUNDING CORPORATION OF AMERICA

CONSOLIDATED STATEMENT OF FINANCIAL CONDITION (NOTE 1)

LIABILITIES

	December 31, 1968 Audited		June 30, 1969 Unaudited	
CURRENT LIABILITIES:				
Accounts payable	$ 4,626,545		$ 5,587,744	
Notes payable (Note 10)..................	507,500		8,019,988	
Other payables (Note 10).................	—		3,000,000	
Current portion of long-term debt (Note 10)..	2,043,280		431,501	
Commissions payable	94,354		281,456	
Taxes (other than federal taxes on income)....	58,345		98,384	
Accrued interest and sundry expenses........	271,440		707,963	
Federal and State taxes on income, estimated current portion (Note 9)...............	1,693,959		2,040,421	
Total Current Liabilities........		9,295,423		20,167,457
OTHER LIABILITIES:				
Notes payable on funded loans and accounts receivable (Note 4)	$15,564,629		$18,956,159	
Other payables (Note 10).................	—		2,500,000	
Federal and State taxes on income, deferred portion (Note 9).......................	8,405,749		10,654,402	
Deferred income	—	23,970,378	130,009	32,240,570
LONG-TERM DEBT (Note 10):				
Notes payable to banks....................	2,020,000		—	
Notes payable to others....................	242,995		2,237,288	
	2,262,995		2,237,288	
Less current portion.............	2,043,280		431,501	
	219,715		1,805,787	
5¼% convertible subordinated debentures due 1983	14,866,000			
5½% capital subordinated notes due 1980....	1,841,500			
5¼% guaranteed (subordinated) debentures due 1989	—	16,927,215	25,000,000	26,805,787
STOCKHOLDERS' EQUITY:				
Preferred stock—authorized 1,000,000 shares, no par value, none issued (Note 1)........	—		—	
Common stock—authorized 8,000,000 shares, par value $.30 per share, issued 4,630,012 shares and 5,419,290 shares respectively....	1,389,004		1,625,787	
Common stock purchase warrants (Note 11)...	625		625	
Additional paid-in capital..................	18,076,725		44,571,930	
Retained earnings [includes undistributed earnings from unconsolidated subsidiaries of $1,687,502 and $3,620,693 respectively (see Note 14)]	9,418,314		8,212,698	
	28,884,668		54,411,040	
Less treasury stock 32,425 shares, par value $.30 per share, at cost	72,674	28,811,994	72,674	54,338,366
COMMITMENTS AND CONTINGENT LIABILITIES (Note 12)				
		$79,005,010		$133,552,180

See accompanying notes.

Equity Funding Corporation of America & Subsidiaries
Consolidated Statement of Additional Paid-in Capital

20

	Year Ended December 31	
	1968	1967
Balance, beginning of year	$ 7,354,728	$1,192,549
Net proceeds in excess of par from:		
Sale of stock	8,597,692	4,529,804
Stock dividend	1,991,757	1,455,601
Stock split	132,548	176,774
	10,721,997	6,162,179
	$18,076,725	$7,354,728

from the 1968
Annual Report of
Equity Funding

Equity Funding Corporation of America & Subsidiaries
Notes To Consolidated Financial Statements   December 31, 1968

NOTE 1. PRINCIPLE OF CONSOLIDATION AND SUBSEQUENT EVENTS CONCERNING CAPITAL STOCK:

The accounts of the Company and all of its subsidiaries (excluding the savings and loan, life insurance and Bermuda subsidiaries), after elimination of inter-company items, have been consolidated. The investments in The Presidential Life Insurance Company of America and Crown Savings and Loan Association are recorded at cost plus equity in undistributed earnings since acquisition. The investment in Electronics International Management, Limited, a Bermuda corporation, is recorded at cost.

On February 14, 1968, the Board of Directors declared a 3% stock dividend payable March 14, 1968 to holders of common stock of record at March 1, 1968.

The Articles of Incorporation of the Company were amended on April 22, 1968 to authorize 1,000,000 shares of preferred stock without par value and to increase the authorized common stock to 8,000,000 shares.

On September 6, 1968, the Board of Directors declared a two-for-one stock split payable November 1, 1968 to holders of common stock of record at October 1, 1968.

On March 3, 1969, the Board of Directors declared a 2% stock dividend payable April 30, 1969 to holders of common stock of record at March 20, 1969. This transaction has been reflected only in the pro forma earnings per share computation in the Consolidated Statement of Earnings and Retained Earnings.

The Company has issued stock purchase options to certain employees, district and division managers, agents and associated general agents. Information as of December 31, 1968 with respect to options granted under the plans is as follows (adjusted for 3% stock dividend and two-for-one stock split):

Date of Grant	Number of Shares	Option Per Share	Option Total	Market Value At Date of Grant Per Share	Market Value At Date of Grant Total
Production Options:					
1968	100,000	$26.12-$43.12	$2,827,900	$26.12-$43.12	$2,827,900
Incentive Options:					
1965	2,154	$2.47	$5,320	$2.89	$6,225
1966	13,870	$3.35	$46,464	$4.47	$61,999
1967	17,907	$3.54-$9.94	$91,824	$3.54-$10.56	$93,069
1968	45,000	$26.12-$48.25	$1,268,674	$26.12-$48.25	$1,268,674
Qualified Options:					
1966	26,368	$3.08	$81,213	$3.08	$81,213
1967	67,903	$17.07	$1,159,100	$17.07	$1,159,100
1968	64,332	$19.66-$56.00	$2,611,311	$19.66-$56.00	$2,611,311
	337,534		$8,091,806		$8,109,491

NOTE 2: SECURITIES, AT COST:

On December 31, 1968, the Company owned the following investments included under the caption "Current Assets" in the Consolidated Statement of Financial Condition:

(a) Utility and school bonds of various districts of Mexico, maturing at various dates up to January 29, 1969, at a total investment of $75,369 (market value—no material difference).

21

(b) The Company has a net investment of $6,550,907 in various listed securities that it intends to hold for a short-term period (market value—no material difference).

On December 31, 1968 the Company also owned the following securities and notes included under "Other Assets" in the Consolidated Statement of Financial Condition:

(a) 50,000 shares of common stock of Congressional Life Insurance Company at a total investment of $275,000 (market value $387,500).

(b) Five Mississippi Improvement Bonds due in 1979 bearing interest at the rate of 3¾% per year at a total investment of $5,077 (market value $4,800).

(c) 274,800 shares of common stock of Whittington Oil Co., Inc. subject to an investment letter, for a total investment of $2,984,126 (market value, less estimated discount factor attributable to investment letter feature, $5,015,100). 150,000 shares were received as compensation as a result of the Company's participation with Whittington Oil in an oil exploration program in 1968. The compensation in the amount of $1,923,900 (net of applicable income taxes of $2,458,960) is included under the caption "Special items" in the Consolidated Statement of Earnings and Retained Earnings. A portion of the 150,000 shares was transferred to an unconsolidated subsidiary.

(d) 26,068 shares of the Enterprise Fund at a total investment of $250,000 (market value $309,949).

(e) The Company owns several notes at a total investment of $217,500. These notes are secured, bear interest at rates between 7%-8%, and are payable over five years.

NOTE 3. FUNDED LOANS AND ACCOUNTS RECEIVABLE:

Under the method of operations of the Company, this represents, in the aggregate, the amount that clients owe as a result of the various "funding programs" offered by the Company, together with loans and/or receivables where "funding programs" have terminated and where the respective shares have not been liquidated as of December 31, 1968.

The Funded Loans And Accounts Receivable are offset, in part, by the contra Notes Payable on Funded Loans and Accounts Receivable. The difference in the amount of $20,746,408 is held by Equity Funding Corporation of America or one of its subsidiaries.

The collateral assigned by clients as security for the notes payable held by the various lending institutions amounted to $43,503,138.

NOTE 4. INVESTMENT IN UNCONSOLIDATED SUBSIDIARIES:

The amount by which the Company's investment in The Presidential Life Insurance Company of America and Crown Savings and Loan Association exceeds the net book value of such businesses has been allocated to excess of cost over net assets at dates of acquisition, and the Company does not intend to amortize these amounts since it believes that there has been no diminution in value.

The investment in Electronics International Management, Limited, a Bermuda corporation, is reflected at cost.

NOTE 5. PROPERTY AND EQUIPMENT, AT COST:

It is the policy of the Company to provide for depreciation on a "straight-line" basis predicated on the estimated useful lives of the individual items on the various classes of assets. The principal estimated useful lives in computing depreciation are as follows:

Office furniture and fixtures	10 years
Office equipment	5 years
Leasehold improvements	3 years
Automobile	5 years
Building	20 years

The Company has a leasehold interest that continues until December 31, 2049 and amortization is on a "straight-line" basis.

Expenditures for additions, major renewals and betterments are capitalized and expenditures for maintenance and repairs are charged to income as incurred. Upon sale or retirement of items of equipment and improvements the cost and related accumulated depreciation are eliminated from the accounts and the resulting gain or loss, if any, is reflected in income. Equipment becoming obsolete or unusable is written down to salvage value.

NOTE 6. COST OF RENEWAL COMMISSIONS ACQUIRED:

The Company capitalized the cost of purchasing and acquiring complete right, title and interest to certain of its renewal commissions. Costs incurred prior to 1964 are being amortized on an annual basis over a nine-year period. Costs incurred after December 31, 1963 are being amortized on an annual basis over a five-year period. This figure is not intended to reflect the actual value of the renewal commissions.

22

NOTE 7. DEFERRED CHARGES:

The Company has capitalized certain expenditures as follows:

Item	Amortization Period
Organization expense	5 Years
Cost of opening and developing new offices	3 Years
Registration costs	3 Years
Financing costs	Life of loan
Acquisition and development costs	3 Years

The amortization charge as reflected in the Company's Consolidated Financial Statements, as contained in the above analysis, has been deducted for Federal income tax purposes.

NOTE 8. EXCESS OF COST OVER NET BOOK VALUE ON DATE OF ACQUISITION OF CONSOLIDATED SUBSIDIARIES:

During 1968 the Company acquired RMF Corporation (formerly known as Salik Management Corporation) and effectively acquired Palm Escrow Co. and Presidential Life Insurance Agency, Inc. The amount paid for these companies was $1,523,767. The amount by which the Company's investment exceeds the net book value of the respective companies is reflected in this account. The investments in the subsidiaries is recorded at cost and is eliminated in the Consolidated Financial Statements.

NOTE 9. FEDERAL AND STATE TAXES ON INCOME:

The provision and the liability for Federal and State income taxes have been computed on the accrual basis. The Company reports on the cash basis for income tax purposes and has reported the current portion of the tax liability under "Current Liabilities" in the Consolidated Statement of Financial Condition. The deferred portion of the income tax liability has been separately stated. The provision for State income taxes has been reflected in the Consolidated Statement of Earnings and Retained Earnings for 1968.

Federal income tax returns of the Company and subsidiaries are being examined through 1967. Currently, no determination has been made. The Company believes there will be no material effect on the earnings of the Company as reported through 1967.

NOTE 10. LONG-TERM LIABILITIES AND DEBENTURES:

Long-term debt at December 31, 1968 is as follows:

The Company is indebted to the United California Bank on an unsecured 7½% promissory note, due February 22, 1969	$ 2,000,000
A subsidiary of the Company is indebted to the City National Bank on an unsecured 7% promissory note, due May 15, 1969 . .	20,000
The Company is indebted to the Wallace Moir Co. on a real estate loan bearing interest at the rate of 7% per annum and providing for monthly payments of $1,940 including principal and interest. This loan is secured by the building owned by the Company	242,995
The Company is indebted to the Searsfund & Co. on a 7¾% note, due February 27, 1969	500,000
A subsidiary is indebted on a non-interest bearing note, due and payable April 1, 1969	7,500
	$ 2,770,495
Less current portion	2,550,780
	$ 219,715

On December 29, 1965, the Company issued $2,000,000 of 5½% Capital Subordinated Notes due December 1, 1980. The Notes are subject to optional redemption at fixed percentages of the principal amount during the period December 1, 1966 to December 1, 1980. The Notes are also subject to redemption in part on December 1, 1969 and on each December 1 thereafter to and including December 1, 1979 through the operation of a sinking fund. Each Note is accompanied by a non-detachable Warrant for the purchase of the Company's common stock at the rate of 129.78 shares of common stock for each $1,000 principal amount of Notes and unless previously exercised expires at the close of business on December 1, 1975. The applicable Warrant prices if exercised on or prior to December 1, 1971—$4.32, 1975—$4.94 per share   1,841,500

23

On May 1, 1968 the Company issued $15,000,000 of 5¼% Convertible Subordinated Debentures due May 1, 1983. The Debentures are subject to optional redemption at fixed percentages of the principal amount during the period May 1, 1969 to maturity. The Debentures are also subject to redemption in part on May 1, 1977 and on each May 1 thereafter to and including May 1, 1982 through the operation of a sinking fund. The Debentures are convertible into common stock of the Company at $30.50 a share through May 1, 1973. $33.00 a share through May 1, 1978 and $36.00 a share through May 1, 1983 14,866,000

Total Long-Term Liabilities And Debentures $16,927,215

Long-term debt maturing during each of the five years subsequent to 1968 is as follows:

1969	$2,550,780
1970	23,280
1971	47,780
1972	143,280
1973	163,280

POST-AUDIT NOTE:

As of January 22, 1969, Equity Funding Capital Corporation N.V., a wholly owned subsidiary of Equity Funding Corporation of America, issued $25,000,000 of 5¼% Guaranteed (Subordinated) Debentures due 1989. These debentures are convertible on and after November 1, 1969 at $63 per share into common stock of, and guaranteed as to payment of principal, interest and sinking fund, by Equity Funding Corporation of America. These debentures were not offered in the United States of America, its territories or possessions or to nationals or residents thereof.

NOTE 11. COMMON STOCK PURCHASE WARRANTS:

On December 31, 1968, Theodore Goodman held stock purchase warrants with respect to 20,278 shares which he acquired at a cost of $625.

NOTE 12. COMMITMENTS AND CONTINGENT LIABILITIES:

The Company leases offices and equipment at monthly rentals totalling approximately $79,472, plus property taxes and insurance in some instances. The leases involved expire in the years 1969 to 1975.

On November 13, 1968, the Company signed a lease with Century City, Inc. for location of its home office. The lease shall commence on October 1, 1969 and will end on September 30, 1979. The monthly rental will be approximately $32,500. The Company intends to sublease the premises it now occupies.

On October 31, 1968, the Company entered into an agreement to acquire certain of the assets, properties, business and goodwill of Investors Planning Corporation of America for approximately $10,000,000 (subject to adjustment on date of closing) payable in cash of approximately $6,100,000, a note for $2,000,000 and the balance of approximately $1,900,000 in common stock of the Company. It is contemplated by the Company that the closing will occur in April, 1969.

On October 31, 1968, the Company entered into an agreement to acquire approximately 80% of the outstanding stock of Pension Life Insurance Company of America for $2,000,000 (subject to adjustment on date of closing) payable with a promissory note, without interest, due within one year from the date of closing. It is contemplated by the Company that the closing will occur in April, 1969.

In the opinion of general counsel, lawsuits filed against the Company are without merit or, in any event, will not result in a material adverse effect on the operations or property of the Company.

NOTE 13: SUPPLEMENTARY PROFIT AND LOSS INFORMATION:

The following amounts were charged to Selling, General and Administrative expenses:

	1968	1967
Maintenance and repairs	$ 26,844	$ 24,211
Depreciation of furniture and fixtures	$ 22,860	$ 16,338
Taxes other than income taxes:		
Payroll	$ 62,535	$ 53,467
Personal property and licenses	33,874	31,685
Franchise	20,586	13,645
	$116,995	$98,797
Rents	$375,298	$317,519

Equity Funding Corporation of America and Subsidiaries

QUARTERLY
REPORT

Consolidated Statement of Earnings (Unaudited)

	For the Three Months Ended	
	March 31, 1969	March 31, 1968
Income:		
Mutual Fund Commissions	$5,404,851	$ 872,482
Life Insurance Commissions	3,076,094	2,338,679
Interest income	593,182	477,465
Other income	1,934,578	336,938
Total Income	$11,008,705	$4,025,564
Expenses:		
Commissions on Mutual Funds	2,330,326	423,558
Commissions on Life Insurance	1,140,801	925,472
Interest on insurance premium financing loans	277,668	225,136
Selling, general and administrative	4,740,117	871,297
Total Expenses	8,488,912	2,445,463
Earnings from Operations	2,519,793	1,580,101
Earnings from Unconsolidated Subsidiaries	798,527	158,809
Earnings Before Federal and State Taxes on Income	3,318,320	1,738,910
Federal and State Taxes on Income:		
Current portion	222,676	15,744
Deferred portion	1,069,123 1,291,799	729,243 744,987
Net Earnings Before Special Item	2,026,521	993,923
Special Item, Less Applicable Federal and State Taxes of $293,704	229,796	—0—
Net Earnings	$ 2,256,317	$ 993,923
Earnings per Share:		
Earnings before special item	$.41	$.25
Special item	.05	—
Total Earnings	$.46	$.25
Pro Forma Earnings per Share:		
Earnings before special item	$.37	$.20
Special item	.04	—
Total Pro Forma Earnings	$.41	$.20

QUARTERLY
REPORT

Equity Funding Corporation of America and Subsidiaries

Consolidated Statement of Earnings (Unaudited)

	Six Months Ended	
	June 30, 1969	June 30, 1968
Income:		
Mutual Fund Commissions $10,995,834		$1,835,337
Life Insurance Commissions 6,244,662		5,346,226
Interest income 1,261,159		966,553
Other income 2,842,178		849,825
Total Income	$21,343,833	$8,997,941
Expenses:		
Commissions on Mutual Funds 4,746,742		856,394
Commissions on Life Insurance 2,461,858		2,319,105
Interest on insurance premium financing loans 616,815		455,563
Selling, general and administrative 8,592,127		1,785,533
Total Expenses	$16,417,542	$5,416,595
Earnings from Operations	4,926,291	3,581,346
Earnings from Unconsolidated Subsidiaries	1,886,576	386,552
Earnings before Federal and State Taxes on income	6,812,867	3,967,898
Federal and State Taxes on Income:		
Current portion 353,582	19,492	
Deferred portion 2,003,629 2,357,211	1,858,965 1,878,457	
Net Earnings before Special Item	$ 4,455,656	$2,089,441
Special Item, Less Applicable Federal and State Taxes	229,796	—
Net Earnings	$ 4,685,452	$2,089,441
Earnings per Share:		
Earnings before special item	$ .89	$ .52
Special item	.05	—
Total Earnings per Share	$ .94	$ .52
Pro Forma Earnings per Share:		
Earnings before special item	$ .84	$ .47
Special item	.04	—
Total Pro Forma Earnings per Share	$ .88	$ .47

QUARTERLY
REPORT

Equity Funding Corporation of America and Subsidiaries

Consolidated Statement of Earnings (Unaudited)

	For the Nine Months Ended			
	September 30, 1969		September 30, 1968	
Income:				
Mutual Fund Commissions	$14,849,739		$2,899,418	
Life Insurance Commissions	10,025,287		7,373,679	
Interest income	1,889,901		1,300,564	
Other operating income	3,829,923		1,617,800	
Total Income		$30,594,850		$13,191,461
Expenses:				
Commissions on Mutual Funds	5,434,671		1,236,930	
Commissions on Life Insurance	3,050,517		2,881,167	
Interest on insurance premium financing loans	967,628		631,073	
Selling, general and administrative	12,608,677		2,634,216	
Total Expenses		22,061,493		7,383,386
Earnings from Operations		8,533,357		5,808,075
Earnings from Unconsolidated Subsidiaries, Net of Extraordinary Items		1,723,266		684,214
Earnings before Federal and State Taxes on Income		10,256,623		6,492,289
Federal and State Taxes on Income:				
Current Portion	397,876		501,363	
Deferred Portion	3,375,124	3,773,000	2,565,968	3,067,331
Net Earnings before Extraordinary Items		6,483,623		3,424,958
Extraordinary Items, Less Applicable Federal and State Taxes		779,796		94,000
Net Earnings		$ 7,263,419		$ 3,518,958
Earnings per Share Assuming No Dilution:				
Before Extraordinary Items		$1.29		$ .83
Extraordinary Items		.16		.02
Earnings Per Share—No Dilution		$1.45		$ .85
Earnings per Common Share Assuming Full Dilution:				
Before Extraordinary Items		$1.23		$ .77
Extraordinary Items		.14		.02
Earnings Per Share—Full Dilution		$1.37		$ .79

2

PROSPECTUS

Equity Funding Corporation of America

$20,000,000

9½% Debentures Due 1990

with

Warrants to Purchase 500,000 Shares of Common Stock

The Debentures and Warrants are being offered in Units each consisting of a $1,000 Debenture and Warrants to purchase 25 shares of Common Stock.

The Debentures will be fully registered as to both interest and principal. Interest is payable on June 1 and December 1 of each year beginning June 1, 1971. Subsequent to December 1, 1975, the Debentures are redeemable at the option of the Company at prices set forth herein, except that prior to December 1, 1980 no redemptions may be made from or in anticipation of monies borrowed at an interest cost to the Company of less than 9½% per annum. The Debentures are also redeemable through operation of a sinking fund beginning in 1976.

The Warrants are exercisable at $25¼ per share, payable in cash, subject to adjustment upon the occurrence of certain events, and will expire on December 1, 1975. The Warrants will not be exercisable until 90 days from the date of this Prospectus, nor will the Debentures and Warrants be separately transferable until such date or such earlier date as shall be determined by the Representative of the Underwriters.

On December 8, 1970, the closing price of the Company's Common Stock on the New York Stock Exchange was $24⅛. There is presently no market for the Debentures or the Warrants, which will be traded in the over-the-counter market. Application has been made for the listing of the Debentures on the New York Stock Exchange. The Company intends to make application to list the Warrants on the American Stock Exchange.

THESE SECURITIES HAVE NOT BEEN APPROVED OR DISAPPROVED BY THE SECURITIES AND EXCHANGE COMMISSION NOR HAS THE COMMISSION PASSED UPON THE ACCURACY OR ADEQUACY OF THIS PROSPECTUS. ANY REPRESENTATION TO THE CONTRARY IS A CRIMINAL OFFENSE.

	Price to Public(1)	Underwriting Discounts and Commissions(2)	Proceeds to Company(3)
Per Unit	$1,000	$27.50	$972.50
Total	$20,000,000	$550,000	$19,450,000

(1) Plus accrued interest from December 1, 1970.

(2) The Estate of Theodore Goodman is to receive from the Representative of the Underwriters 25% of its net underwriting commissions and representative's fee pursuant to a previous agreement between the Representative and Theodore Goodman.

(3) Before deducting expenses payable by the Company estimated at $255,000. The Company has agreed to indemnify the Underwriters against certain civil liabilities, including liabilities under the Securities Act of 1933.

(4) The Company has granted to the Underwriters a right to purchase up to an additional $2,000,000 principal amount of Debentures with Warrants to purchase up to an additional 50,000 shares of Common Stock at the price to the public less underwriting discounts and commissions shown in the table, solely for the purpose of covering over-allotments, if any. If all of such additional $2,000,000 principal amount of Debentures with Warrants to purchase 50,000 shares of Common Stock are purchased by the Underwriters, the "Total" figures under "Price to Public", "Underwriting Discounts and Commissions" and "Proceeds to Company" will be $22,000,000, $605,000 and $21,395,000, respectively. See "Underwriting".

The Units are offered, subject to prior sale, cancellation, withdrawal or modification of the offer, when, as and if issued and delivered by the Company, and subject to approval of certain legal matters by counsel. See "Underwriting". In addition, Units are being offered to certain institutions for delivery on January 7, 1971 pursuant to Delayed Delivery Contracts as set forth under "Delayed Delivery Arrangements" herein.

NEW YORK SECURITIES CO.

Incorporated

The date of this Prospectus is December 9, 1970

EQUITY FUNDING CORPORATION OF AMERICA AND SUBSIDIARIES
CONSOLIDATED STATEMENT OF EARNINGS AND RETAINED EARNINGS

The following consolidated statement of earnings and retained earnings has been compiled as explained in Note 1 to the Company's financial statements. The statements for the five years ended December 31, 1969, have been examined by Wolfson, Weiner, Ratoff & Lapin, independent certified public accountants, whose opinion appears elsewhere in the Prospectus. With respect to the unaudited periods, the Company believes that all adjustments (which consist only of normal recurring accruals) necessary for a fair statement of the results of operations for such periods have been made. This statement should be read in conjunction with the related financial statements and notes thereto included elsewhere in this Prospectus. (See Note C, below, as to pro forma results of the proposed acquisition of Liberty.)

	Year Ended December 31,					Six Months Ended June 30,	
	1965 (Audited)	1966 (Audited)	1967 (Audited)	1968 (Audited)	1969 (Audited)	1969 (Unaudited)	1970 (Unaudited)
INCOME:							
Insurance sales commissions	$3,475,214	$4,733,985	$ 6,930,950	$10,464,355	$15,247,569	$ 6,244,662	$ 7,602,173
Securities sales commissions	1,139,552	1,641,687	2,043,964	5,001,777	19,954,887	10,995,834	7,741,436
Real estate operations	—	—	—	6,789	981,822	788,185	3,989,189
Natural resources operations	—	—	—	83,531	3,502,519	1,651,641	1,040,354
Investment management income	—	—	—	1,425,291	2,556,459	824,024	844,935
Interest income	662,913	907,403	1,304,793	1,759,106	2,918,399	1,405,226	2,482,351
Other income	85,669	203,737	899,236	438,268	409,988	366,513	83,569
Total income	5,363,348	7,486,812	11,178,943	19,179,117	45,571,643	22,276,085	23,784,007
EXPENSES:							
Commissions on insurance	1,494,342	2,032,337	2,803,444	3,330,661	5,284,437	2,461,858	2,654,887
Commissions on securities	561,913	828,381	1,006,705	2,061,166	7,880,604	4,746,742	3,031,267
Real estate operations	—	—	—	37,229	750,000	615,867	2,608,998
Natural resources operations	—	—	—	58,859	2,312,650	1,070,894	557,825
Interest and amortization of debt expense	527,386	790,968	1,144,414	1,272,000	4,049,984	1,647,105	3,281,523
Selling, general and administrative (Note 13)	1,362,056	1,657,663	2,787,306	3,398,897	12,703,690	6,816,449	8,155,974
Total expenses	3,945,697	5,309,349	7,741,869	10,158,812	32,981,365	17,358,915	20,290,474
EARNINGS BEFORE MINORITY INTEREST	1,417,651	2,177,463	3,437,074	9,020,305	12,590,278	4,917,170	3,493,533
Minority interest	—	1,936	—	—	—	—	—
EARNINGS FROM CONSOLIDATED OPERATIONS BEFORE INCOME TAXES	1,417,651	2,179,399	3,437,074	9,020,305	12,590,278	4,917,170	3,493,533
FEDERAL AND STATE TAXES ON INCOME (Note 9):							
Current portion	389,996	26,787	31,236	546,333	284,707	350,982	67,300
Deferred portion	231,711	975,257	1,624,125	3,546,704	5,194,593	2,003,629	1,306,800
Total tax provision	621,707	1,002,044	1,655,361	4,093,037	5,479,300	2,354,611	1,374,100
EARNINGS FROM CONSOLIDATED OPERATIONS	795,944	1,177,355	1,781,713	4,927,268	7,110,978	2,562,559	2,119,433
Earnings from unconsolidated subsidiaries, net of taxes and extraordinary items* (Notes A and B)	—	—	698,667	757,537	3,094,648	1,481,576	3,297,940
NET EARNINGS BEFORE EXTRAORDINARY ITEMS	795,944	1,177,355	2,480,380	5,684,805	10,205,626	4,044,135	5,417,373
Extraordinary items, net of applicable Federal and State taxes (Note 1 and Note B)	—	—	50,000	2,141,052	706,006	634,796	—
NET EARNINGS	795,944	1,177,355	2,530,380	7,825,857	10,911,632	4,678,931	5,417,373
RETAINED EARNINGS — BEGINNING OF PERIOD	568,821	1,364,765	2,542,120	3,601,189	9,418,314	9,418,314	14,421,382
Add: Retained earnings resulting from Diversified Land Company pooling (Note 1)	—	—	—	—	—	1,414,826	1,635,191
Less: Dividends paid	—	—	(1,469,376)	(2,008,732)	(5,908,564)	(4,380,318)	(6,283,984)
Adjustment for minority interest	—	—	(1,935)	—	—	—	—
RETAINED EARNINGS — END OF PERIOD	$1,364,765	$2,542,120	$ 3,601,189	$ 9,418,314	$14,421,382	$11,131,753	$15,189,962
EARNINGS PER COMMON SHARE — ASSUMING NO DILUTION							
Before extraordinary items (Note A)	$ .28	$ .40	$ .71	$1.33	$1.95	$ .79	$ .97
Extraordinary items	—	—	.01	.50	.14	.12	—
Total earnings per common share — assuming no dilution**	$ .28	$ .40	$ .72	$1.83	$2.09	$ .91	$ .97
EARNINGS PER COMMON SHARE — ASSUMING FULL DILUTION:							
Before extraordinary items		$ .33	$ .58	$1.14	$1.90	$ .73	$ .94
Extraordinary items		—	.01	.41	.13	.11	—
Total earnings per common share — assuming full dilution***		$ .33	$ .59	$1.55	$2.03	$ .84	$ .94
COMMON STOCK DISTRIBUTIONS:							
Stock dividends			5%	3%	2%	2%	2%
Cash dividends							$ .10
Stock splits			3-for-2	2-for-1	—	—	—

(See accompanying notes next page. Numerical note references are to notes to the Company's financial statements.)

6

NOTES:

* For all periods included in the above statements, net earnings from unconsolidated subsidiaries do not include gains (losses) sustained by the life insurance subsidiary from the sale of securities since the insurance company reports its income on the statutory method of accounting whereby capital gains and losses and certain other items are not included in determining net income. In 1968 and 1969, securities losses were sustained by the insurance subsidiary in the amount of ($6,905) and ($631,750) respectively. There were no gains (losses) from the sale of securities in the other periods. The effect of these losses is to decrease extraordinary earnings per share, assuming no dilution, in the amount of none and 13¢ for 1968 and 1969 respectively. On a fully diluted basis, the decrease for extraordinary earnings per share would be none and 11¢ respectively.

The Company was listed on the New York Stock Exchange on October 19, 1970, and pursuant to its regulations, the method of accounting of its unconsolidated life insurance subsidiary will be changed from statutory accounting practices to generally accepted accounting principles. This change will be implemented in the financial statements commencing with the annual report for December 31, 1970 and where prior statements are included for comparison purposes, they will be restated as necessary.

** Earnings per common share—assuming no dilution have been computed on the basis of $.30 par value stock, and on the following average number of outstanding shares: 1965—2,870,402 shares, 1966—2,932,594 shares, 1967—3,507,885 shares, 1968—4,269,341 shares, 1969—5,232,321 shares, for the six months ended June 30, 1969—5,149,124 shares, and for the six months ended June 30, 1970—5,605,798 shares.

*** Earnings per common share—assuming full dilution shown were computed on the basis of the average number of shares outstanding, 1966—2,932,594 shares, 1967—3,507,885 shares, 1968—4,269,341 shares, 1969—5,232,321 shares, June 30, 1969—5,149,124 shares, and June 30, 1970—5,605,798 shares respectively and on the assumption that the Company's convertible promissory notes and debentures where applicable, were converted, eliminating the related interest on the notes and debentures less applicable income tax (resulting in fully diluted earnings of $1,195,295, $2,655,040, $8,098,723, $11,003,250, $4,918,987 and $5,799,624 respectively), and that all of the Company's warrants and stock options were in fact exercised, resulting in the total number of fully diluted shares as follows: 1966—3,604,297 shares, 1967—4,481,213 shares, 1968—5,239,214 shares, 1969—5,407,280 shares, June 30, 1969—5,836,272 shares, and June 30, 1970—6,165,513 shares. The above fully diluted shares have been reduced by the equivalent number of shares which could be purchased with the proceeds that the Company would receive were the common stock purchase warrants and stock options exercised.

The foregoing number of average and fully diluted shares are as adjusted for all stock dividends and stock splits through December 31, 1969 and the two percent stock dividend paid April 24, 1970.

Note A. Earnings from unconsolidated subsidiaries include $660,000, $535,782, $2,342,777, $954,076 and $2,940,000 or $.19, $.13, $.45, $.19 and $.52 per common share—assuming no dilution, for the years 1967, 1968 and 1969, and for the six months ended June 30, 1969 and 1970, respectively, attributable to coinsurance transactions of Equity Funding Life Insurance Company (formerly "The Presidential Life Insurance Company of America"). To the extent that these coinsurance earnings were realized during the periods indicated, earnings from the policies coinsured will not be available in future periods.

A portion of the earnings from unconsolidated subsidiaries attributable to Crown Savings and Loan Association includes earnings allocated to general reserves on the books of Crown in the amounts of $83,254, $130,000 and none for the years ended December 31, 1967, 1968 and 1969, respectively, and none for the six months ended June 30, 1969 and 1970.

Note B. Earnings from unconsolidated subsidiaries net of taxes as reported by Equity Funding Corporation of America consist of the following:

	1967	1968	1969	Six Months Ended June 30, 1969	Six Months Ended June 30, 1970
Equity Funding Life Insurance Company (formerly the Presidential Life Insurance Company of America):					
Ordinary	$623,733	$338,367	$2,448,876	$1,149,641	$3,000,361
Extraordinary Item	50,000	136,000	480,000	405,000	—
	$673,733(1)	$474,367	$2,928,876	$1,554,641	$3,000,361
Crown Savings and Loan Association:					
Ordinary	$ 74,934	$419,170	$ 468,401	$ 200,953	$ 177,045
Extraordinary Item	—	45,298	—	—	—
	$ 74,934(2)	$464,468	$ 468,401	$ 200,953	$ 177,045
Bishops Bank and Trust Company Limited:					
Ordinary	$ —	$ —	$ 177,371	$ 130,982	$ 120,534
Extraordinary Item	—	—	—	—	—
	$ —	$ —	$ 177,371	$ 130,982	$ 120,534
Total					
Ordinary	$698,667	$757,537	$3,094,648	$1,481,576	$3,297,940
Extraordinary Item	$ 50,000	$181,298	$ 480,000	$ 405,000	$ —

	1967 Earnings Prior to Acquisition	1967 Earnings as Reported by Parent	1967 Earnings as Reported by Unconsolidated Subsidiary
(1) Equity Funding Life Insurance Company (formerly The Presidential Life Insurance Company of America).......	($534,946)	$673,733	$138,787
(2) Crown Savings and Loan Association..................	$ 77,153	$ 74,934	$152,087

Note C. The following summary combines the results of operations of the Company and Liberty for the periods shown, assuming a pooling of interests. The pro forma earnings per share computations give effect to the proposed issuance of 65,050 shares of the Company's preferred stock as if such shares had been converted into 185,856 shares of the Company's common stock.

	Year Ended December 31,					Six Months Ended June 30,	
	1965 (Unaudited)	1966 (Unaudited)	1967 (Unaudited)	1968 (Unaudited)	1969 (Unaudited)	1969 (Unaudited)	1970 (Unaudited)
Pro Forma Net Earnings..	$1,597,103	$1,221,631	$2,202,713	$7,905,793	$11,282,156	$4,856,474	$5,441,777
Pro Forma Earnings Per Common Share—assuming no dilution	$ .52	$ .39	$ .60	$1.77	$2.08	$ .91	$ .94
Pro Forma Earnings Per Common Share—assuming full dilution		$ .33	$ .50	$1.51	$2.03	$ .85	$ .92

The annual interest to be paid on the Debentures offered hereby (excluding interest with respect to Debentures reserved for over-allotments) will initially be $1,900,000.

Of the $2,141,052 shown in the consolidated statement of earnings and retained earnings as an extraordinary item in 1968, $1,482,087 is attributable to net compensation received in the form of securities by the Company as a result of its distribution of interests in an oil and gas exploration program conducted in that year. See "Oil and Gas Exploration" under the heading "Description of Business—Natural Resources Operations" in this connection. The Company has written down, as of October 31, 1970, its investment in such securities by $2,944,571 to a book value based on the market price of the securities on that date. During October 1970, the Company also realized a gain of $900,000 upon the repurchase, at a discount, of certain promissory notes, as described following the table under "Capitalization." Such transactions resulted in an extraordinary loss of $897,571 after applicable taxes as reflected in the following summary of the results of the Company's operations for the four months ended October 31, 1969 and 1970, and for the ten months then ended. The figures shown in the summary are unaudited and all adjustments, consisting only of normal recurring accruals and the write-down described above, necessary for a fair presentation of the results of operations shown have been made. (The earnings per common share have been adjusted to give effect to the applicable stock dividends described under "Dividends".)

	Ten Months Ended October 31,		Four Months Ended October 31,	
	1969	1970	1969	1970
Total income	$36,393,421	$39,044,495	$14,117,336	$15,260,488
Net earnings before extraordinary items	$ 7,626,946	$ 9,578,162	$ 3,582,811	$ 4,102,089
Extraordinary items, net of applicable Federal and State taxes	709,796	(897,571)	75,000	(897,571)
Net earnings	$ 8,336,742	$ 8,680,591	$ 3,657,811	$ 3,204,518
Earnings per common share—assuming no dilution:				
Before extraordinary items	$1.48	$1.69	$.69	$.72
Extraordinary items	.14	(.16)	.02	(.16)
Total earnings per common share—assuming no dilution	$1.62	$1.53	$.71	$.58

8

EQUITY FUNDING LIFE INSURANCE COMPANY
(Formerly The Presidential Life Insurance Company of America)
STATEMENT OF OPERATIONS

The following statement of operations for the two full years ended December ? , 1969 has been examined by Haskins & Sells, independent certified public accountants; the opinion of said firm, which as referred to therein is based, as to policy reserves on the opinion of independent consulting actuaries, and, as to amounts applicable to certain accident and health business on the report of other independent accountants, appears elsewhere in this Prospectus. The statement for the three years ended December 31, 1967 has been examined by Arthur Young & Company, independent certified public accountants, as set forth in their report included elsewhere in this Prospectus. The statement for the six month periods ended June 30, 1969 and 1970 is unaudited; however, in the opinion of Equity Life, such unaudited statement includes all adjustments (which consisted only of normal recurring accruals) necessary for a fair presentation of the results of operations for such interim periods. The operating results for interim periods are not necessarily indicative of the results for an entire year. This statement should be read in conjunction with its notes and the other Equity Life financial statements and the notes thereto, together with the above-mentioned opinions and reports, included elsewhere in this Prospectus.

	Year Ended December 31,					Six Months Ended June 30,	
	1965	1966	1967(a)	1968(b)	1969(b)	1969(b) (Unaudited)	1970(b) (Unaudited)
Premiums and other considerations (net of reinsurance):							
Life	$1,000,944	$1,557,559	$ 811,719	$ 780,079	$3,130,791	$1,015,280	$3,931,844
Accident and health	5,501	34,398	42,352	1,566,036	2,100,502	3,221,095	85,078
Considerations for supplementary contracts without life contingencies	—	—	—	—	144,052	—	—
Total	1,006,445	1,591,957	854,071	2,346,115	5,375,345	4,236,375	4,016,922
Investment income:							
Interest on bonds	75,533	90,660	99,885	74,475	75,405	43,622	19,797
Interest on policy loans	7,528	9,622	11,260	734	1,965	1,010	842
Interest on certificates of deposit	4,514	9,974	—	8,410	248,221	101,468	73,894
Interest on mortgage loan	—	—	—	—	18,548	—	27,794
Interest on collateral loans and unsecured notes receivable from parent company and its affiliates	—	—	—	55,342	28,750	—	218,700
Other	4,073	2,096	4,314	—	—	—	—
Total investment income	91,648	112,352	115,459	138,961	372,889	146,100	341,027
Investment expense	(3)	180	1,727	647	2,541	224	620
Net investment income	91,651	112,172	113,732	138,314	370,348	145,876	340,407
Other income:							
Coinsurance considerations (Note 4)	—	—	—	535,782	2,342,777	954,076	2,940,000
Service fees from parent company	—	—	—	205,651	89,820	24,661	66,000
Total	—	—	—	741,433	2,432,597	978,737	3,006,000
Total income	1,098,096	1,704,129	967,803	3,225,862	8,178,290	5,360,988	7,363,329
Policy benefits and reserves:							
Death and other benefits under life policies	150,421	316,924	264,494	179,030	90,606	73,469	131,868
Benefits under accident and health policies	997	14,157	14,793	101,929	383,704	429,619	2,685
Increase (decrease) in aggregate life reserves (Note 1)	207,032	463,940	(702,490)	98,185	(289,014)	(290,555)	190,738
Increase (decrease) in aggregate accident and health reserves	—	—	—	613,992	(574,580)	868,769	(7,305)
Increase (decrease) in reserves for supplementary contracts without life contingencies	—	—	—	—	140,652	—	(4,800)
Total	358,450	795,021	(423,203)	993,136	(248,632)	1,081,302	313,186
Remainder	739,646	909,108	1,391,006	2,232,726	8,426,922	4,279,686	7,050,143
Operating expenses:							
Commissions(c)	392,208	602,447	453,302	836,608	3,936,984	2,210,677	2,410,683
Salaries and other general expenses	993,993	1,114,135	761,979	867,722	925,795	390,036	643,688
Taxes, licenses and fees	43,222	57,752	61,726	86,554	164,636	102,941	102,770
Increase (decrease) in loading on deferred and uncollected premiums	105,374	21,349	(25,007)	(32,525)	120,631	21,391	(7,359)
Total	1,534,797	1,795,683	1,252,000	1,758,359	5,148,046	2,725,045	3,149,782
	(795,151)	(886,575)	139,006	474,367	3,278,876	1,554,641	3,900,361
Dividends to life policyholders	—	770	219	—	—	—	—
Gain (loss) from operations before Federal income taxes and extraordinary credit	(795,151)	(887,345)	138,787	474,367	3,278,876	1,554,641	3,900,361
Provision for Federal income taxes (Notes 1 and 6)	—	—	50,000	136,000	830,000	405,000	900,000
Gain (loss) from operations before extraordinary credit	(795,151)	(887,345)	88,787	338,367	2,448,876	1,149,641	3,000,361
Credit resulting from tax loss carryover (Note 6)	—	—	50,000	136,000	480,000	405,000	—
Net gain (loss) from operations (Notes 1, 4 and 5)	$ (795,151)	$ (887,345)	$ 138,787	$ 474,367	$2,928,876	$1,554,641	$3,000,361

(See accompanying notes next page)

9

NOTES:

(a) In December 1967, the Company entered into an agreement with respect to the reinsurance of a block of business for a consideration of $600,000. As a result of this agreement, the provision in 1967 for aggregate life reserves was reduced approximately $1,142,000, premium income was decreased approximately $542,000 and net gain from operations was increased approximately $600,000. Another reinsurance agreement was modified during 1967 to retroactively reinsure an additional block of business. The principal effect of this agreement was to reduce premium income for the year approximately $570,000 ($173,000 applicable to prior years) and to reduce expenses and provision for aggregate life reserves approximately $630,000 ($158,000 applicable to prior years). The net effect was to increase 1967 net gain from operations approximately $60,000 of which a portion (not material) was attributable to the prior two years. The approximate effect on 1967 results of operations of the two foregoing agreements was to decrease premium income by $1,112,000 and to increase net income by $660,000. See "Reinsurance" under the caption "Description of Business — Insurance Operations" elsewhere in this Prospectus for additional information.

(b) Net gain from operations for 1968 includes approximately $1,035,000 of which $882,000 is applicable to certain coinsurance transactions (including a nonrecurring expense allowance of $250,000 and reserve assumptions of $96,000) and $153,000 relates to an accident and health business agreement.

Net gain from operations for 1969 includes approximately $2,209,000 consisting of $2,343,000 applicable to certain coinsurance transactions less $134,000 relating to an accident and health business agreement.

Net gain from operations for the six month periods ended June 30, 1969 and 1970 includes $954,000 and $2,940,000, respectively, applicable to certain coinsurance transactions.

Substantially all of the Company's accident and health business was 100% coinsured as of July 1, 1969.

For additional information, see Notes 4 and 5 to the Equity Life financial statements and "Ceded Reinsurance" and "Certain Factors Affecting Operations" under the caption "Description of Business — Insurance Operations" appearing elsewhere in this Prospectus.

(c) Commissions paid to subsidiaries of the Company's parent were approximately $896,000, $3,046,000, $1,197,000, and $2,529,000 during the years ended December 31, 1968 and 1969, and the six months ended June 30, 1969 and 1970, respectively.

(d) Numerical note references are to notes to the Equity Life financial statements.

As of June 30, 1970, approximately 27,500 Programs were being maintained. During the first six months of 1970, 5,018 Programs were sold and 1,512 Programs were terminated. From the introduction of the Programs in 1960 through September 30, 1970, a total of 117 have been terminated as the result of forced liquidations, including 115 Programs which were so terminated during the first nine months of 1970. The average face amount of the life insurance policies sold in all Programs is approximately $31,307. The average amount of the first year loan made to participants is approximately $608.

At this time, all of the states in which Programs are being offered have so-called "anti-combination" or "anti-inducement" statutes. In some states in which the Company does not do business, these statutes have been interpreted to prohibit the sale of the Programs. In the Company's opinion, however, its inability to sell in those jurisdictions will not materially affect its business.

Other Marketing Activities

The Company recently commenced the sale of parcels of unimproved land located primarily in California. Currently, it is also engaged in the public sale, through a subsidiary, of units of interest in a limited partnership formed to acquire and operate certain apartment buildings located in California. See "Real Estate, Banking and Finance Operations", below, in this connection. The Company recently began to market publicly interests in a cattle breeding limited partnership. The general partner of each of such limited partnerships is a subsidiary of the Company. In this connection, The National Association of Securities Dealers, Inc. currently has under consideration certain proposed rules which would regulate, and possibly prohibit, the distribution of limited partnership interests through dealers which are affiliated with the general partner of such partnerships. Whether, or the extent to which, the adoption of such rules would have a materially adverse effect on the Company cannot now be determined.

INSURANCE OPERATIONS

Equity Life

In October 1967, the Company acquired all of the outstanding stock of Equity Life (formerly "The Presidential Life Insurance Company of America") and Presidential Life Insurance Agency, Inc. from unaffiliated sellers. The consideration paid by the Company consisted of $1,099,000 in cash, a $500,000, 5½% promissory note which has been paid, 164,894 shares of the Company's Common Stock and $2,002,300 principal amount of its 5½% Convertible Subordinated Junior Capital Notes, which have been converted into 66,660 shares of Common Stock of the Company.

Equity Life was incorporated in June 1959 and is authorized under Illinois law to write life and accident and health insurance. It is presently qualified to write life and accident and health insurance in the District of Columbia and in all states except Connecticut, New Jersey, New York, North Carolina and West Virginia. Of the life insurance presently in force, approximately 36% was written in California and approximately 17% was written in Illinois.

The insurance sold by Equity Life includes individual whole life and endowment, term, group, mortgage and accident and health insurance. Premium rates are believed by the Company to be generally competitive with similar types of insurance written by other companies. The policies being written by Equity Life are non-participating.

The following table shows, for the five years ended December 31, 1969, Equity Life's admitted assets, capital stock and surplus, premium income and certain information relating to its life insurance in force:

	1965	1966	1967	1968	1969
Admitted Assets	$ 2,145,823	$ 2,838,466	$ 2,678,780	$ 8,208,779	$ 10,686,567
Capital Stock and Surplus	$ 1,316,896	$ 1,471,162	$ 2,122,466	$ 6,335,118	$ 8,939,837
Ratio of Capital Stock and Surplus to Total Liabilities	158.9%	107.6%	381.5%	338.1%	511.8%
Premiums and other considerations (net of ceded reinsurance):					
Individual Life	$ 931,933	$ 1,407,137	$ 674,282	$ 698,205	$ 3,108,693
Group	72,683	150,422	150,689	81,874	22,098
Individual A & H	1,829	34,398	29,100	1,566,036	2,100,502
Considerations for supplementary contracts without life contingencies	—	—	—	—	144,052
Total Premium Income	$ 1,006,445	$ 1,591,957	$ 854,071	$ 2,346,115	$ 5,375,345

Life Insurance:	1965	1966	1967	1968	1969
In Force Beginning of Year—					
Whole Life and Endowment........	$ 5,937,602	$ 27,877,227	$ 48,234,308	$ 77,373,441	$105,395,534
Term and Other Policies...........	27,881,149	41,625,068	31,850,927	15,091,049	59,958,011
Group	7,709,750	20,770,300	28,680,900	16,763,250	22,172,780
Total in Force Beginning of Year....	41,528,501	90,272,595	108,766,135	109,227,740	187,526,325
Paid-for New Business—					
Direct:					
Whole Life and Endowment......	22,532,375	29,875,339	51,352,220	53,648,605	161,888,562
Term and Other Policies.........	18,132,554	1,186,771	2,773,016	45,434,633	188,516,000
Group	12,063,000	8,303,100	96,500	5,657,817	36,691,982
Total Direct New Business.......	52,727,929	39,365,210	54,221,736	104,741,055	387,096,544
Reinsurance Assumed:					
Whole Life and Endowment......	—	—	—	—	6,197,000
Term and Other Policies.........	—	—	—	—	—
Group	2,592,800	—	—	—	—
Total Reinsurance Assumed	2,592,800	—	—	—	6,197,000
Total Paid-for New Business	55,320,729	39,365,210	54,221,736	104,741,055	393,293,544
Terminations—					
Whole Life and Endowment........	592,750	9,518,258	22,213,087	25,626,512	49,381,034
Term and Other Policies...........	4,388,635	10,960,912	19,532,894	567,671	18,845,958
Group	1,595,250	392,500	12,014,150	248,287	6,263,162
Total Terminations	6,576,635	20,871,670	53,760,131	26,442,470	74,490,154
In Force End of Year—					
Whole Life and Endowment........	27,877,227	48,234,308	77,373,441	105,395,534	224,100,062
Term and Other Policies...........	41,625,068	31,850,927	15,091,049	59,958,011	229,628,053
Group	20,770,300	28,680,900	16,763,250	22,172,780	52,601,600
Total in Force End of Year........	90,272,595	108,766,135	109,227,740	187,526,325	506,329,715
Reinsurance Ceded—					
Individual	46,455,442	44,849,650	85,759,115	143,900,711	432,037,339
Group	1,842,000	2,045,250	—	1,897,250	20,091,118
Total Reinsurance Ceded	48,297,442	46,894,900	85,759,115	145,797,961	452,128,457
Net in Force End of Year—					
After Reinsurance Ceded	$ 41,975,153	$ 61,871,235	$ 23,468,625	$ 41,728,364	$ 54,201,258

The following tabulation sets forth certain mortality and general expense information pertaining to life insurance operations for the five years ended December 31, 1969:

TOTAL LIFE INSURANCE	1965	1966	1967	1968	1969
Expected mortality	$167,714	$283,403	$303,504	$223,374	$670,352
Actual mortality	$121,627	$249,698	$735,924	$298,296	$466,649
Ratio — Actual to Expected mortality	73.8%	88.1%	242.5%	133.5%	69.6%
Ratio of general insurance expenses to premiums and other considerations	98.8%	70.0%	89.2%	37.0%	17.2%

The following tabulation shows the termination ratios of direct individual life policies including reinsurance for the years 1965 through 1969:

	Individual Life
1965................................	6.8%
1966................................	15.3%
1967................................	29.1%
1968................................	13.6%
1969................................	6.9%

19

These ratios are calculated by dividing the amounts of insurance lapsed, surrendered, expired or matured by the sum of the insurance in force at the beginning of the year and the new business written during the year.

The following table shows the cash and invested assets of Equity Life at December 31, 1968 and 1969.

	1968		1969	
	Admitted Asset Value	Percent of Total	Admitted Asset Value	Percent of Total
Cash and Certificates of Deposit ...	$3,905,895	51%	$6,414,026	69%
Bonds:				
Governments	1,228,902	16	286,445	3
Public Utilities	203,522	3	203,461	2
Industrial and Miscellaneous	243,738	3	294,907	3
Total Bonds	1,676,162	22	784,813	8
Common Stocks	2,021,566	27	1,250,000	14
Mortgage Loan	—	—	819,340	9
Policy Loans	17,707	—	25,874	—
Total	$7,621,330	100%	$9,294,053	100%

The following tabulation shows, for the years 1965 through 1969, Equity Life's cash and invested assets as of the end of each period, net investment income and net investment yield on average cash and invested assets:

	Cash and Invested Assets	Net Investment Income	Net Investment Yield
1965	$2,018,265	$ 91,651	4.05%
1966	2,487,193	112,172	5.05%
1967	2,427,222	113,732	4.68%
1968	7,621,330	138,314	2.77%
1969	9,294,053	370,348	4.44%

Sales. Since July 1968, all of Equity Life's life insurance policies have been sold through the Company's own sales force. Prior thereto, Equity Life's policies were sold through general agents, independent agents, salaried representatives and brokers. However, all of such marketing arrangements have been terminated. See Note 5 to Equity Life's Financial Statements with respect to accident and health insurance policies sold in recent periods.

Ceded Reinsurance. In January 1968, Equity Life entered into a coinsurance agreement with an unaffiliated insurance company requiring the cession of an aggregate of $250,000,000 face amount of life insurance sold to customers of the Company over a three year period ending December 31, 1970. Under the terms of the agreement, Equity Life is entitled to receive certain credits toward the amount of insurance it is required to cede for insurance sold by Equity Life in excess of specified yearly requirements and for certain other insurance policies issued to customers of the Company. The agreement will terminate upon the ceding of $250,000,000 of insurance, including the above-described credits, but if such amount is not reached by the end of 1970, the agreement will continue in force until that amount is realized. As of September 30, 1970, Equity Life had been credited with approximately $230,000,000 face amount of life insurance under the agreement.

In March 1969, Equity Life entered into a coinsurance agreement with an unaffiliated insurance company under which Equity Life coinsured approximately $99,000,000 face amount of life insurance sold to customers of the Company from March 31, 1968 to March 31, 1969 which were in effect on June 30, 1969 for a total consideration of approximately $1,099,000. In addition to the consideration received, Equity Life will retain as an expense allowance a portion of all renewal premiums attributable to the policies and riders coinsured under the agreement, and have the right to recapture the business coinsured at any time after 1979.

In October 1969 Equity Life entered into a coinsurance agreement with an unaffiliated insurance company under which such company has agreed to coinsure up to one billion dollars face amount of life insurance sold to customers of the Company from July 1, 1969 through December 31, 1973. During 1969, Equity Life ceded approximately $140,000,000 face amount of life insurance and received a total consideration of approximately $1,300,000. For the six months ended June 30, 1970, Equity Life ceded approximately $276,000,000 face amount of life insurance and received a total consideration of approximately $2,900,000. The maximum amount of first year reinsurance premiums which may be ceded under this agreement is approximately $15,000,000. Equity Life also will retain, as an expense allowance, a portion of all renewal premiums attributable to policies and riders under the agreement, will have the right, after the eighth policy year, to recapture annually a portion of the amounts reinsured on any policy. The reinsurance agreement may be terminated by either party thereto as to further reinsurance and is subject to certain persistency requirements.

Certain Factors Affecting Operations. Under state laws and regulations governing accounting procedures for life insurance companies, costs incurred in putting a new insurance policy in force are required to be charged in full against current income. These costs typically include medical and investigation expenses, sales commissions, reserve requirements and other overhead and special items which, in the aggregate, are normally greater than the amount of the first year's premium. Thus, in the case of a new, expanding life insurance company, where the amount of new insurance written is high in relation to the amount of insurance already in force, losses are normally reported during the early years. In subsequent years, the annual costs of maintaining a policy in force are lower since charges such as medical and investigation expenses are eliminated and commissions are considerably reduced. The lapse of policies prior to the recovery of first year costs will have an adverse effect on earnings. Policies remaining in force, however, represent continuing value to a life insurance company. To the extent that new insurance policies are reinsured, Equity Life will reduce its first year costs and increase its current income. The profits shown in Equity Life's operations since 1967 are attributable to reinsurance agreements. In this connection, Equity Life intends to continue for the foreseeable future to cede significant blocks of insurance from time to time as it has in the past, in the ordinary course of its operations, under reinsurance or coinsurance agreements with non-affiliated companies. The extent to which this will affect future earnings or losses of Equity Life cannot, of course, be ascertained at this time, since this depends on mortality, persistency, conversions and other policy changes. See Note 4 to Equity Life's Financial Statements in this connection. As a general practice Equity Life retains a small portion of the face amount of life insurance written. Equity Life will not receive renewal premium income on the ceded portion of its policies; however, it will receive an allowance for servicing such policies.

Regulation. As an insurance company, Equity Life is subject to regulation and supervision in each of the states in which it does business. Although different in each state, such regulations generally establish supervisory agencies with broad administrative powers over the granting of licenses to transact business, licensing of agents, approval of policy forms, reserve requirements, the form and content of financial statements and the character of investments. Equity Life must file annual reports with state agencies and is subject to examination by them at any time.

Reserves. Under Illinois law, Equity Life is required to provide reserves to meet its policy obligations. These reserves are carried as liabilities and, together with net premiums received and interest compounded annually at certain assumed rates, are calculated to be sufficient to meet policy obligations as

21

EQUITY FUNDING CORPORATION OF AMERICA AND SUBSIDIARIES

CONSOLIDATED STATEMENT OF FINANCIAL CONDITION (Note 1)

ASSETS

	December 31, 1969 (Audited)		June 30,1970 (Unaudited)	
CURRENT ASSETS:				
Cash and short term investments.............		$ 12,424,731		$ 9,582,306
Securities, at cost (Note 2).................		19,966,061		10,329,989
Contracts, notes and loans receivable..........		8,202,587		9,936,470
Accounts receivable		4,758,610		4,987,492
Commissions receivable		2,704,308		2,668,266
Advances to salesmen and employees..........		948,659		1,283,391
Inventories of cattle and real estate, at cost		—		10,709,872
Prepaid expenses and other current assets......		747,556		1,148,783
Total current assets		49,752,512		50,646,569
PROPERTY AND EQUIPMENT, AT COST (Notes 3 and 8):				
Real estate and leasehold improvements.......	$ 5,123,979		$ 7,585,853	
Furniture, fixtures and equipment............	1,555,384		2,167,244	
Livestock—Breeding herd	4,435,339		5,055,139	
	11,114,702		14,808,236	
Accumulated depreciation and amortization	817,944	10,296,758	1,160,620	13,647,616
OTHER ASSETS:				
Investments, at cost (Note 2)...............		527,830		4,394,283
Funded loans and accounts receivable (Note 4)		51,188,119		57,978,277
Contracts and notes receivable..............		—		5,183,942
Loans receivable—unconsolidated subsidiaries..		—		2,000,000
Loans receivable—officer		—		134,448
Deposits and sundry assets.................		2,346,659		2,579,620
Cost of renewal commissions acquired, net of amortization (Note 5)...................		329,082		267,502
Deferred charges, net of amortization (Note 6):				
Organization expense	$ 17,593		$ 21,876	
Cost of opening and development of new offices	4,181,515		3,317,662	
Registration costs	68,556		179,175	
Acquisition and development costs..........	365,109		621,069	
Financing and other costs................	1,068,262		1,263,148	
Development and exploration costs— natural resources	883,226	6,584,261	—	5,402,930
Investment in unconsolidated subsidiaries (Notes 1 and 7):				
Equity in unconsolidated subsidiaries........	16,691,382		22,022,109	
Excess of cost over related net assets of un- consolidated subsidiaries	7,719,222	24,410,604	7,719,222	29,741,331
Excess of cost over net book value on date of acquisition of consolidated subsidiaries (Note 1)		15,237,190	100,623,745	15,237,190	122,919,523
			$160,673,015		$187,213,708

The accompanying notes are an integral part of the financial statements.

EQUITY FUNDING CORPORATION OF AMERICA AND SUBSIDIARIES

CONSOLIDATED STATEMENT OF FINANCIAL CONDITION (Note 1)

LIABILITIES AND STOCKHOLDERS' EQUITY

	December 31, 1969 (Audited)		June 30, 1970 (Unaudited)	
CURRENT LIABILITIES:				
Accounts payable		$ 4,656,060		$ 1,445,099
Notes and loans payable—unconsolidated subsidiaries		—		5,958,977
Notes and loans payable (Note 8)		4,997,488		6,612,492
Other payables (Note 8)		3,000,000		1,250,000
Current portion of long-term debt (Note 8) ...		1,906,281		934,922
Commissions payable		4,738,342		5,015,583
Taxes (other than Federal and State taxes on income)		101,844		61,083
Accrued interest and sundry expenses........		1,592,093		947,526
Federal and State taxes on income, current portion (Note 9)		284,707		352,007
Total current liabilities		21,276,815		22,577,689
OTHER LIABILITIES:				
Notes payable on funded loans and accounts receivable (Note 4)	$21,703,968		$16,912,327	
Other payables (Note 8)	2,500,000		1,250,000	
Federal and State taxes on income, deferred portion (Note 9)	15,484,149	39,688,117	18,108,789	36,271,116
LONG-TERM DEBT (Note 8):				
Notes payable—secured	2,730,812		12,084,028	
Notes payable—other	2,687,944		13,917,611	
	5,418,756		26,001,639	
Less current portion	1,906,281		934,922	
	3,512,475		25,066,717	
5¼% Guaranteed (subordinated) debentures due 1989	23,872,000		23,872,000	
7½% Guaranteed (subordinated) notes due 1974	10,000,000	37,384,475	10,000,000	58,938,717
COMMITMENTS AND CONTINGENT LIABILITIES (Note 10)		—		—
STOCKHOLDERS' EQUITY:				
Preferred stock—authorized 1,000,000 shares, no par value, issued none and 20,000 shares respectively (Note 11)		—		2,000,000
Common stock—authorized 20,000,000 shares, par value $.30, issued 5,552,458 shares and 5,761,210 shares respectively		1,665,737		1,728,363
Additional paid-in capital		46,269,236		50,521,992
Retained earnings [Includes undistributed earnings from unconsolidated subsidiaries of $5,262,150 and $8,560,090, respectively (Note 12).]		14,421,382		15,189,962
		62,356,355		69,440,317
Less treasury stock, 14,611 shares and 6,303 shares respectively, at cost.......		32,747 62,323,608		14,131 69,426,186
		$160,673,015		$187,213,708

The accompanying notes are an integral part of the financial statements.

EQUITY FUNDING CORPORATION OF AMERICA AND SUBSIDIARIES

NOTES TO CONSOLIDATED FINANCIAL STATEMENTS
December 31, 1969

Note 1. Principle of Consolidation and Other Matters:

The consolidated financial statements include the accounts of the Company and subsidiaries after elimination of inter-company accounts, except for the following which are stated at cost plus equity in undistributed earnings and advances where applicable since acquisition:

    (a) Equity Funding Life Insurance Company (formerly "The Presidential Life Insurance Company of America")

    (b) Crown Savings and Loan Association

    (c) Bishops Bank and Trust Company Limited, a Bahama Islands Corporation.

On April 30, 1969 the Company paid a 2% stock dividend declared by the Board of Directors on March 3, 1969.

The Articles of Incorporation of the Company were amended on August 7, 1969 to increase the authorized common stock to 20,000,000 shares.

During the current period the Company purchased certain assets and assumed certain liabilities of Ankony Angus, Investors Planning Corporation of America, and Affiliated Insurance Agency, Inc. and acquired 78.7% of the outstanding stock of Pension Life Insurance Company of America. The total consideration paid for these acquisitions was $25,554,403. Pension Life Insurance Company was subsequently sold in the current period by the Company. The gain on this transaction of $229,796, net of Federal and State income taxes of $293,704, has been shown as an extraordinary item in the consolidated statement of earnings and retained earnings. In addition, included in extraordinary items is $480,000 which represents the tax benefit from the operating loss carry-forward of the insurance subsidiary, and sundry adjustments aggregating $3,790.

During the year the Company acquired 97.3% of the outstanding capital stock of Bishops Bank and Trust Company Limited for approximately $5,180,000.

The amount by which the Company's investment in consolidated and unconsolidated subsidiaries exceeds the net book value on date of acquisition has not been amortized in the current period since the Company believes that there has been no diminution in value.

On March 4, 1970 the Board of Directors declared a $.10 cash dividend and a 2% stock dividend payable April 24, 1970 to holders of record on March 20, 1970.

The Company has issued stock purchase options to certain employees, district and division managers, agents and associated general agents of the Company. Information as of December 31, 1969 with respect to options granted under the plans is as follows (adjusted for all stock dividends and stock splits through December 31, 1969):

	Production Options	Production Options	Incentive Options	Incentive Options
Option price per share (range)	$54.00–$72.375	$25.61–$42.28	$3.286	$ 6.61
Year of grant	1969	1968	1965	1966
Number of shares subject to options outstanding at 12/31/69	84,678	79,258	1,986	2,964
Market value at date of grant:				
Per share (range)	$54.00–$72.375	$25.61–$42.28	$3.286	$ 6.61
Total	$5,438,235	$2,186,929	$6,526	$19,592

	Production Options	Production Options	Incentive Options	Incentive Options
Number of shares subject to options exercisable during 1969	None	11,500	3,687	10,161
Market value at date options became exercisable:				
Per share (range)	Not Applicable	$49.625–$80.75	$10.23	$20.15
Total	Not Applicable	$807,070	$37,718	$204,744
Number of shares subject to options exercised during 1969	None	8,900	1,701	7,197
Market value at date options were exercised:				
Per share (range)	Not Applicable	$55.00 –$71.125	$51.00–$73.00	$51.00–$68.50
Total	Not Applicable	$523,814	$113,899	$443,250

EQUITY FUNDING CORPORATION OF AMERICA AND SUBSIDIARIES

NOTES TO CONSOLIDATED FINANCIAL STATEMENTS (CONTINUED)

	Incentive Options	Incentive Options	Incentive Options	Qualified Options	Qualified Options
Option price per share (range)..	$9.74	$25.61–$62.01	$54.04–$63.25	$16.74–$56.96	$49.02–$80.00
Year of grant...............	1967	1968	1969	1967	1968
Number of shares subject to options outstanding at 12/31/69	1,576	46,971	45,173	59,511	125,745
Market value at date of grant:					
Per share (range).........	$9.74	$25.61–$62.01	$54.04–$63.25	$16.74–$56.96	$49.02–$80.00
Total	$15,350	$1,476,944	$2,579,846	$1,270,541	$7,043,382
Number of shares subject to options exercisable during 1969	20,633	None	None	61,978	46,014
Market value at date options became exercisable:					
Per share (range)........	$49.625–$80.75	Not Applicable	Not Applicable	$19.00	$49.02–$80.00
Total	$1,241,694	Not Applicable	Not Applicable	$1,177,582	$7,037,186
Number of shares subject to options exercised during 1969	19,057	None	None	2,467	2,101
Market value at date options were exercised:					
Per share (range)	$49.625–$73.00	Not Applicable	Not Applicable	$55.00–$72.625	$59.75–$70.50
Total	$1,123,253	Not Applicable	Not Applicable	$ 147,287	$ 142,441

Options granted under any of the Company's Production or Incentive Stock Option Plans will not be "qualified stock options" within the meaning of the Internal Revenue Code of 1954 (the "Code"). Accordingly, when exercised, these options will result in taxable income to the optionee in an amount equal to the difference, if any, between the option price and the fair market value of the Company's Common Stock on the exercise date. Upon any such exercise, the Company will be entitled to a corresponding federal income tax deduction in an amount equal to the income, if any, so taxed to the optionee.

Options granted under any of the Company's Qualified Stock Option Plans are designed to be "qualified stock options" under Section 422 of the Code. Accordingly, under the applicable provisions of the Code, an employee will not realize any taxable income upon either the receipt or the exercise of an option granted under one of the Qualified Option Plans. If the stock issued pursuant to the option is held for at least three years, the difference between the amount realized by the employee upon its subsequent disposition and the amount which he paid for the stock will be taxed as a long-term capital gain or loss. In such cases the Company will not be entitled to any deduction for federal income tax purposes in connection with either the grant of an option or the issuance of stock when an option is exercised.

Notes to Unaudited June 30, 1970 Consolidated Financial Statements:

During the current period the Company acquired all of the outstanding capital stock of Diversified Land Company. The acquisition was treated as a pooling of interests. As a result of the pooling, retained earnings of Diversified in the amount of $1,635,191 was added to the retained earnings of the Company. The Company's earnings for six months ended June 30, 1969 and 1970, only, have been adjusted to reflect the earnings of the Company and Diversified on a pooling of interests basis.

56

EQUITY FUNDING CORPORATION OF AMERICA AND SUBSIDIARIES

NOTES TO CONSOLIDATED FINANCIAL STATEMENTS (CONTINUED)

Information as of June 30, 1970 with respect to options granted under the Company's various plans is as follows (adjusted for all stock dividends and stock splits through June 30, 1970):

Year (or Period) of Grant	No. of Shares	Option Price or Range		Market Value at Date of Grant	
		Per Share Range	Total	Per Share Range	Total
Year ended December 31, 1967:					
Incentive Options	1,607	$ 9.55	$ 15,347	$ 9.55	$ 15,347
Qualified Options	20,405	$16.41	$ 334,846	$16.41	$ 334,846
Year ended December 31, 1968:					
Incentive Options	39,520	$25.11–$60.79	$ 1,249,169	$25.11–$60.79	$ 1,249,169
Qualified Options	65,154	$16.41–$53.82	$ 2,875,042	$16.41–$53.82	$ 2,875,042
Production Options	81,155	$25.11–$41.45	$ 2,192,510	$25.11- $41.45	$ 2,192,510
Year ended December 31, 1969:					
Incentive Options	41,544	$52.98–$62.01	$ 2,334,580	$52.98–$62.01	$ 2,334,580
Qualified Options	75,151	$48.06–$78.43	$ 4,250,092	$48.06–$78.34	$ 4,250,092
Production Options	87,789	$52.98–$69.57	$ 5,510,321	$52.98–$69.57	$ 5,510,321
Six months ended June 30, 1970:					
Incentive Options	1,844	$18.44–$62.01	$ 63,958	$18.44–$62.01	$ 63,958
Qualified Options	33,394	$15.00–$52.94	$ 1,154,465	$15.00–$52.94	$ 1,154,465
Production Options	13,493	$52.38	$ 706,763	$52.38	$ 706,763
			$20,687,093		$20,687,093

The Company is presently in the process of acquiring the remaining 2.7% of outstanding capital stock of Bishops Bank and Trust Company, Limited.

Note 2. Securities, at Cost:

On December 31, 1969 the Company owned the following investments included under the caption "Current Assets" in the Consolidated Statement of Financial Condition:

a) Utility and school bonds of various districts of Mexico, maturing at various dates up to August 31, 1970 at a total investment of $2,359,575 (market value—no material difference)

b) The Company has a net investment of $17,606,486 in various listed securities that it intends to hold for a short term period (market value—no material difference).

On December 31, 1969, the Company also owned investments aggregating $467,830 in various limited partnerships engaged in cattle breeding, and sundry investments totalling $60,000, included as investments under "Other Assets" in the Consolidated Statement of Financial Condition.

Note to Unaudited June 30, 1970 Consolidated Financial Statements:

On June 30, 1970, the Company owned the following securities and investments included in the Consolidated Statement of Financial Condition:

a) "Securities, at Cost" include investments of $10,329,989 in various listed securities that the Company intends to hold for a short term period. As of June 30, 1970, the market value was approximately $7,093,000. No reserves for market decline have been provided since the Company believes that such decline is of a temporary nature. (As of September 30, 1970, the market value of the securities held on June 30, 1970, was approximately $8,665,000.)

EQUITY FUNDING CORPORATION OF AMERICA AND SUBSIDIARIES

NOTES TO CONSOLIDATED FINANCIAL STATEMENTS (CONTINUED)

b) The investments under "Other Assets" include various securities, at cost, and undistributed income in two limited partnerships totalling $326,872. The balance of $4,067,411 represents common stock of Whittington Oil Co., Inc. for which the Company paid $726,000 in cash. A portion of the Whittington common stock in the amount of $3,376,360 was received as compensation as a result of the Company's participation with Whittington Oil in an oil exploration program in 1968. This amount, net of applicable taxes of $1,894,273, was included as extraordinary income in the Company's 1968 financial statements. As of June 30, 1970, the market value was approximately $635,000. (As of September 30, 1970, the market value was approximately $736,000.) See page 31 of this Prospectus under the caption "Oil and Gas Exploration" for additional information.

Note 3. Property and Equipment, at Cost:

It is the policy of the Company to provide for depreciation primarily on a "straight-line" basis predicted on the estimated useful lives of the individual items on the various classes of assets. The principal estimated useful lives in computing depreciation are as follows:

Breeding herd	3 to 8 years
Building and improvements	20 to 25 years
Leasehold improvements	3 to 10 years
Office furniture, fixtures and equipment	5 to 10 years

Expenditures for additions, major renewals and betterments are capitalized and expenditures for maintenance and repairs are charged to income as incurred. Upon sale or retirement of items of equipment and improvements the cost and related accumulated depreciation are eliminated from the accounts and the resulting gain or loss, if any, is reflected in income. Equipment becoming obsolete or unusable is written down to salvage value.

Note to Unaudited June 30, 1970 Consolidated Financial Statements:

During the current period the Company reclassified accumulated costs of exploration and development of natural resources from "Deferred Charges" to "Property and Equipment". The Company intends to amortize these costs on the "unit of production" method.

Note 4. Funded Loans and Accounts Receivable:

Under the Company's method of operations, this represents, in the aggregate, the amount that clients owe as a result of the various "Equity Funding Programs" offered by the Company, and net contracts receivable together with loan and/or receivables where "Equity Funding Programs" have terminated and where the respective shares have not been liquidated as of December 31, 1969.

The Funded Loans and Accounts Receivable are offset, in part, by the contra Notes Payable on Funded Loans and Accounts Receivable. The difference in the amount of $29,484,151 is held by Equity Funding Corporation of America and its subsidiaries.

Of the total issued collateral assigned by clients as security to the Company, $47,441,885 is used to secure notes payable in the amount of $21,703,968 held by various lending institutions.

Note to Unaudited June 30, 1970 Consolidated Financial Statements:

On June 30, 1970 the difference between Funded Loans and Accounts Receivable and the Notes Payable on Funded Loans and Accounts Receivable, in the amount of $41,065,950, was held by Equity Funding Corporation of America and its subsidiaries. Of the total issued collateral assigned by clients as security to the Company, $33,642,001 is used to secure notes payable in the amount of $16,912,327 held by various lending institutions.

Note 5. Cost of Renewal Commissions Acquired:

The Company capitalized the cost of purchasing and acquiring complete right, title and interest to certain of its renewal commissions. Costs incurred prior to 1964 are being amortized on an annual basis over a nine year period. Costs incurred after December 31, 1963 are being amortized on an annual basis over a five-year period. This figure is not intended to reflect the actual value of the renewal commissions.

EQUITY FUNDING CORPORATION OF AMERICA AND SUBSIDIARIES

NOTES TO CONSOLIDATED FINANCIAL STATEMENTS (CONTINUED)

Note 6. Deferred Charges:

The Company has capitalized certain expenditures as follows:

Item	Amortization Period
Acquisition and development costs..........................	3 years
Cost of opening and developing new offices....................	3 years
Covenant not to compete................................	5 years
Exploration and development of natural resources.............	Unit of production
Financing costs	Life of loan
Organization expense	5 years
Registration costs	3 years

The amounts deferred and amortized with respect to the costs of opening and developing new offices and registration costs are as follows:

	Opening Balance	Deferred During Period	Amortized During Period	Closing Balance
Balance, January 1, 1961.................				
Transactions 1961 through 1968:				
Cost of opening and developing new offices	$ —	$3,916,864	$1,667,292	$2,249,572
Registration costs	—	339,401	332,818	6,583
	$ —	$4,256,265	$2,000,110	
Balance, December 31, 1968...............				$2,256,155
Transactions in 1969:				
Cost of opening and developing new offices	$2,249,572	$2,953,278	$1,021,335	$4,181,515
Registration costs	6,583	73,937	11,964	68,556
	$2,256,155	$3,027,215	$1,033,299	
Balance, December 31, 1969..............				$4,250,071
Transactions January 1, 1970 to June 30, 1970 (unaudited):				
Cost of opening and developing new offices	$4,181,515	$ 129,930	$ 993,783	$3,317,662
Registration costs	68,556	129,081	18,462	179,175
	$4,250,071	$ 259,011	$1,012,245	
Balance, June 30, 1970 (unaudited).........				$3,496,837

The amortization charge as reflected in the Company's consolidated financial statements, as contained in the analysis, has been deducted for Federal and State income tax purposes.

Note 7. Investment in Unconsolidated Subsidiaries:

The amount by which the Company's investment in Equity Funding Life Insurance Company (formerly "The Presidential Life Insurance Company of America"), Crown Savings and Loan Association and Bishops Bank and Trust Company, Limited exceeds the net book value of such business has been allocated to excess of cost over net assets at dates of acquisition. The Company did not amortize these amounts since it believes that there has been no diminution in value.

EQUITY FUNDING CORPORATION OF AMERICA AND SUBSIDIARIES

NOTES TO CONSOLIDATED FINANCIAL STATEMENTS (CONTINUED)

An unconsolidated subsidiary holds loans receivable of $835,000 from officers and directors representing loans made in connection with a public offering of limited partnership interest in Equity Resources Limited Partnership 1968. Such notes bear interest at 7½% per annum, mature in 1973, and are secured, in the aggregate, by 26,365 shares of the Company's common stock.

Note 8. Notes Payable and Long-Term Debt:

Long-term debt at December 31, 1969 is as follows:

	Current Notes Payable	Current Other Payables	Other Payables	Long-Term Debt Current Portion	Long-Term Debt Deferred Portion
A subsidiary of the Company is indebted on notes secured by trust deeds on land and buildings in process of construction:					
8½% note due January, 1971					$ 750,000
9½% note due January, 1971					400,000
9¾% note due August, 1970				$1,500,000	
Various notes on land due between 1970 and 1972				21,108	59,704

On January 22, 1969, Equity Funding Capital Corporation N.V., a wholly owned subsidiary of Equity Funding Corporation of America issued $25,000,000 of 5¼% guaranteed (subordinated) debentures due 1989. The debentures are subject to optional redemption of fixed percentages of the principal amount during the period February 1, 1972 to maturity. The debentures are also subject to redemption in part on February 1, 1980 and on each February 1 thereafter to and including February 1, 1988 through the operation of a sinking fund as follows:

Year	Percentage of Aggregate Principal Amount of Debentures Outstanding on November 20, 1979
1981	10%
1982	10%
1983	10%
1984	10%
1985	10%
1986	10%
1987	10%
1988	10%

The debentures are convertible into common stock of Equity Funding Corporation of America at $61.74 per share on and after November 1, 1969. Balance of unconverted debentures at December 31, 1969   23,872,000

60

EQUITY FUNDING CORPORATION OF AMERICA AND SUBSIDIARIES

NOTES TO CONSOLIDATED FINANCIAL STATEMENTS (CONTINUED)

	Current Notes Payable	Current Other Payables	Other Payables	Long-Term Debt Current Portion	Long-Term Debt Deferred Portion
During the year Equity Funding Capital Corporation N.V., issued 7½% guaranteed (subordinated) notes due 1974, with detachable warrants which entitle the holder thereof to purchase 100,000 shares of common stock of the Company at $74.625 per share commencing after November 1, 1970. The notes may be applied at face value in payment of the exercise price of the warrants					10,000,000
A subsidiary of the Company is indebted to several individuals on unsecured loans ..				385,173	2,302,771
The Company is indebted to various individuals in the amount of $6,500,000 in connection with Ankony Angus acquisition as follows: (1) $1,000,000 note bearing interest at 7% per annum, due January 2, 1970 (paid at maturity) included in notes payable under current liabilities, and (2) $3,000,000, $1,250,000 and $1,250,000 due on April 15, 1970, 1971 and 1972 respectively, subject to certain earnings requirements. The latter amounts may be adjusted downward if such requirements are not met. Accordingly, the investment account for Ankony Angus would also be reduced	$1,000,000	$3,000,000	$2,500,000		
The Company is indebted to I.O.S. Ltd. (S.A.) on two unsecured non-interest bearing notes due April 1, 1970. These notes were issued in connection with the acquisition of the assets of Investors Planning Corporation and the majority of common stock of Pension Life Insurance Company	3,954,988				
Post Audit Note: The Company is contesting this liability to the extent of approximately $2,600,000.					
One of the Company's subsidiaries, Palm Escrow, is indebted to City National Bank on an unsecured 7¼% note due February 1970	42,500				
TOTALS	$4,997,488	$3,000,000	$2,500,000	$1,906,281	$37,384,475

Long-term debt maturing during each of the five years subsequent to December 31, 1969 is as follows:

1970	$ 1,906,281
1971	$ 1,632,211
1972	$ 294,253
1973	$ 107,656
1974	$10,100,810

61

EQUITY FUNDING CORPORATION OF AMERICA AND SUBSIDIARIES

NOTES TO CONSOLIDATED FINANCIAL STATEMENTS (CONTINUED)

Notes to Unaudited June 30, 1970 Consolidated Financial Statements:

Long-term debt at June 30, 1970 is as follows:

	Current Notes Payable	Current Other Payables	Other Payables	Long-Term Debt Current Portion	Long-Term Debt Deferred Portion
Subsidiaries of the Company are indebted on various Notes secured by trust deeds on land and buildings in process of construction, interest rates from 5% to 13%, payable at various dates				$934,922	$ 6,512,712
A subsidiary is indebted on a 10¼% loan due in March 1971, secured by collateral of $5,775,000 assigned by clients as security for funded loans and accounts receivable...................					4,636,394(A)
5¼% guaranteed (subordinated) debentures due 1989					23,872,000
7½% guaranteed (subordinated) notes due 1974.					10,000,000
The Company is indebted on various unsecured loans:					
10% note due December 1970............					4,621,221(A)
9½% note due February 1972............					4,535,195
8⅞% note due February 1972............					4,533,195
The Company is indebted on various unsecured loans, and loans secured by trust deeds on property and equipment......................	$4,587,492				228,000
The Company is indebted to I. O. S. Ltd. on unsecured non-interest bearing notes due April 1, 1970. These notes were issued in connection with the acquisition of Investors Planning Corporation and the majority of common stock of Pension Life Insurance Company. The Company is contesting this liability....................	2,025,000				
The Company is indebted to various individuals in the amount of $2,500,000 in connection with Ankony Angus acquisition as follows: $1,250,000 and $1,250,000, due on April 15, 1971 and 1972 respectively, subject to certain earnings requirements		$1,250,000	$1,250,000		
Totals	$6,612,492	$1,250,000	$1,250,000	$934,922	$58,938,717

Long-term debt maturing during each of the twelve month periods subsequent to June 30, 1970 is as follows:

1971....................	$ 934,922
1972....................	$20,215,078
1973....................	$ 473,631
1974....................	$ 504,034
1975....................	$10,768,566

(A) The Company is presently negotiating to renew these loans; accordingly, they are classified as deferred. These notes will be maturing during the twelve month period ended June 30, 1972.

Note 9. Federal and State Taxes on Income:

The provision and the liability for Federal and State income taxes have been computed on the accrual basis. The Company reports on the cash basis for income tax purposes and has reported the current portion of the tax liability under "Current Liabilities" in the Consolidated Statement of Financial Condition. The deferred portion of the income tax liability has been separately stated.

Federal income tax returns of the Company and subsidiaries are being examined through 1968. Currently, no determination has been made. The Company believes there will be no material effect on the earnings of the Company as reported through 1968.

EQUITY FUNDING CORPORATION OF AMERICA AND SUBSIDIARIES

NOTES TO CONSOLIDATED FINANCIAL STATEMENTS (CONTINUED)

Note 10. Commitments and Contingent Liabilities:

The Company leases offices and equipment at monthly rentals totalling approximately $162,000, plus property taxes and insurance in some instances. The leases involved expire in the years 1970 through 1980.

The Company has been advised by counsel that the lawsuits filed against the Company are without merit or, in any event, will not result in a material adverse effect on the operations or property of the Company.

Notes to Unaudited June 30, 1970 Consolidated Financial Statements:

The Company is guarantor on a loan of 8,600,000 Swiss francs ($1,998,977) made to an unconsolidated subsidiary (see page 4 of this Prospectus for additional guarantees).

In July 1970 the Company entered into a Merger Agreement to acquire the outstanding guaranteed stock of Liberty Savings and Loan Association, in exchange for preferred stock having a value of approximately $6,505,000. The acquisition is conditioned, among other things, upon approval of the various regulatory agencies involved.

Note 11. Preferred Stock:

During the current period, the Board of Directors authorized the issuance of 20,000 shares of Series A Preferred Stock, stated value $100 per share, with liquidating value of $100 per share; the shares are to pay a semi-annual dividend at the rate of 4¼% of stated value per annum, are entitled to voting rights, and are convertible into common stock, no later than five years from date of issue, at the rate of one common share for each $45 of stated value of the preferred shares. The preferred shares are redeemable in whole or in part by the Company at any time after June 30, 1972. The preferred shareholders may require the Company to redeem up to a maximum of 50% of the preferred shares at any time after two years from date of issue. As of June 30, 1970, 20,000 shares of preferred stock were issued and outstanding.

Note 12. Dividend Restrictions and Other Matters Concerning Potential Earnings:

As of December 31, 1969 there was available for the payment of cash dividends out of the consolidated retained earnings the amount of $11,222,243. Consolidated retained earnings attributable to the Company's life insurance subsidiary in the amount of $3,666,189 are unavailable for the payment of cash dividends due to such subsidiary's surplus deficit at the date of its acquisition by the Company.

Note to Unaudited June 30, 1970 Consolidated Financial Statement:

As of June 30, 1970 there was available for payment of cash dividends out of the consolidated retained earnings the amount of $11,582,473. Consolidated retained earnings attributable to the Company's life insurance subsidiary in the amount of $3,666,189 are unavailable for the payment of cash dividends due to such subsidiary's surplus deficit at the date of its acquisition by the Company.

Subsequent Events:

Equity Funding Life Insurance Company (Formerly The Presidential Life Insurance Company of America) during November 15, 1970, declared a cash dividend of $1,100,000 payable on December 20, 1970 to its parent, Equity Funding Corporation of America.

Note 13. Supplementary Profit and Loss Information:

The following amounts were charged to Selling, General and Administrative Expenses:

	Year Ended December 31,					Six Months Ended June 30,	
	1965	1966	1967	1968	1969	1969	1970
Maintenance and repairs	$ 14,459	$ 19,245	$ 24,211	$ 26,844	$ 101,840	$ 66,331	$ 56,986
Depreciation of property and equipment	$ 9,623	$ 19,104	$ 30,429	$ 49,552	$ 590,326	$ 46,544	$405,277
Taxes other than Federal income taxes:							
Payroll	$ 32,413	$ 47,848	$ 53,467	$ 62,535	$ 275,333	$172,857	$215,274
Property and licenses	11,308	25,776	31,685	33,874	236,118	160,448	52,358
Franchise	10,811	9,979	13,645	20,586	27,993	259,403	37,048
	$ 54,532	$ 83,603	$ 98,797	$116,995	$ 539,444	$592,708	$304,680
Rents	$197,957	$225,486	$317,519	$375,298	$1,386,738	$868,959	$991,703

CONSOLIDATED STATEMENT OF EARNINGS AND RETAINED EARNINGS

INCOME THREE MONTHS ENDED MARCH 31	1970	1969
Securities sales commissions	$ 4,557,253	$ 5,404,851
Insurance sales commissions	4,528,639	3,076,094
Natural resources operations	630,651	1,204,600
Real estate operations	1,357,400	--
Investment management income	370,309	425,213
Interest income	1,049,342	593,182
Other income	31,627	304,765
Total Income	12,525,221	11,008,705

EXPENSES

Commissions on securities	1,802,016	2,330,326
Commissions on insurance	1,600,173	1,140,801
Natural resources operations	378,266	795,224
Real estate operations	1,226,200	—
Interest and amortization of debt expense	1,476,133	706,031
Selling, general and administrative	3,628,468	3,188,554
Depreciation and amortization	495,960	327,976
Total Expenses	10,607,216	8,488,912
Earnings From Operations	1,918,005	2,519,793
Earnings From Unconsolidated Subsidiaries, Net of Extraordinary Items:		
Life insurance subsidiary, net of applicable taxes of $420,000 and $165,000 respectively	1,250,011	489,641
Bank and savings and loan subsidiaries, net of applicable taxes of $121,645 and $61,449 respectively	254,127	143,886
Earnings Before Federal and State Taxes on Income	3,422,143	3,153,320
Federal and State Taxes on Income:		
Current portion	32,217	222,676
Deferred portion	753,935	1,069,123
Total Tax Provision	786,152	1,291,799
Net Earnings Before Extraordinary Items	2,635,991	1,861,521
Extraordinary Items, Less Applicable Federal and State Taxes of $293,704	—	394,796
Net Earnings	2,635,991	2,256,317
Retained Earnings—January 1, 1970	14,421,382	9,418,314
Adjustments for Dividends	(6,283,984)	(5,495,103)
Retained Earnings—March 31, 1970	$10,773,389	$ 6,179,528

CONSOLIDATED STATEMENT OF EARNINGS AND RETAINED EARNINGS

INCOME SIX MONTHS ENDED JUNE 30	1970	1969
Insurance sales commissions	$ 7,602,173	$ 6,244,662
Securities sales commissions	7,741,436	10,995,834
Real estate operations	3,989,189	788,185
Natural resources operations	1,040,354	1,651,641
Investment management income	844,935	824,024
Interest income	2,482,351	1,405,226
Other income	83,569	366,513
Total Income	23,784,007	22,276,085

EXPENSES

	1970	1969
Commissions on insurance	2,654,887	2,461,858
Commissions on securities	3,031,267	4,746,742
Real estate operations	2,608,998	615,867
Natural resources operations	557,825	1,070,894
Interest and amortization of debt expense	3,281,523	1,647,105
Selling, general and administrative	6,576,710	6,151,336
Depreciation and amortization	1,579,264	665,113
Total Expenses	20,290,474	17,358,915
Earnings from consolidated operations before income taxes	3,493,533	4,917,170
Federal and State Taxes on Income:		
Current portion	67,300	350,982
Deferred portion	1,306,800	2,003,629
Total Tax Provision	1,374,100	2,354,611
Earnings from Consolidated Operations	2,119,433	2,562,559
Earnings from Unconsolidated Subsidiaries, Net of Extraordinary Items:		
Life insurance subsidiary, net of applicable taxes of $1,000,000 and $405,000 respectively	3,000,361	1,149,641
Bank and savings and loan subsidiaries, net of applicable taxes of $167,000 and $149,000 respectively	356,279	331,935
Net Earnings Before Extraordinary Items	5,476,073	4,044,135
Extraordinary Items, Less Applicable Federal and State Taxes of $293,704	—	634,796
Net Earnings	5,476,073	4,678,931
Retained Earnings—January 1	14,421,382	9,418,314
Adjustments for Stock Dividends and Acquisitions	(4,648,793)	(4,380,318)
Retained Earnings—June 30	$15,248,662	$ 9,716,927

CONSOLIDATED STATEMENT OF EARNINGS AND RETAINED EARNINGS

INCOME NINE MONTHS ENDED SEPTEMBER 30

	1970	1969
Insurance sales commissions	$11,605,926	$10,025,287
Securities sales commissions	10,656,467	14,849,739
Real estate operations	5,878,720	1,636,511
Natural resources operations	1,315,702	1,997,076
Investment management income	1,257,671	1,458,020
Interest income	4,024,423	2,118,438
Other income	114,588	374,826
Total Income	34,853,497	32,459,897

EXPENSES

	1970	1969
Commissions on insurance	4,118,948	3,050,517
Commissions on securities	4,129,301	5,434,671
Real estate operations	3,181,299	1,159,250
Natural resources operations	665,201	1,192,919
Interest and amortization of debt expense	5,021,730	2,922,617
Selling, general and administrative	9,663,056	8,884,536
Depreciation and amortization	2,464,441	1,088,442
Total Expenses	29,243,976	23,732,952
Earnings from consolidated operations before income taxes	5,609,521	8,726,945
Federal and State Taxes on Income:		
Current portion	110,700	412,076
Deferred portion	2,077,000	3,430,624
Total Tax Provision	2,187,700	3,842,700
Earnings from Consolidated Operations	3,421,821	4,884,245
Earnings from Unconsolidated Subsidiaries, Net of Extraordinary Items:		
Life insurance subsidiary, net of applicable taxes of $1,467,000 and $480,000 respectively	4,400,891	1,293,784
Bank and savings and loan subsidiaries, net of applicable taxes of $178,000 and $151,200 respectively	668,068	499,482
Net Earnings Before Extraordinary Items	8,490,780	6,677,511
Extraordinary Items, Less Applicable Federal and State Taxes of $293,704	—	709,796
Net Earnings	$ 8,490,780	7,387,307
Retained Earnings—January 1	14,421,382	9,418,314
Adjustments for Stock Dividends & Acquisitions	(4,642,729)	(4,380,318)
Retained Earnings—September 30	$18,269,433	$12,425,303

EQUITY FUNDING CORPORATION OF AMERICA AND SUBSIDIARIES

CONSOLIDATED STATEMENT OF FINANCIAL CONDITION

SEPTEMBER 30, 1970

ASSETS

Current Assets:

Cash and short-term investments	$ 9,420,141
Marketable securities, at cost	11,655,937
Contracts, notes and loans receivable	5,703,108
Accounts and commissions receivable	9,793,636
Inventory—Natural resources and real estate operations, at cost	14,468,926
Prepaid expenses and other current assets	1,624,143
Total Current Assets	52,665,891
Funded Loans and Accounts Receivable	61,574,857
Property and Equipment, at Cost, Net of accumulated depreciation and amortization	14,838,135

Investment in Subsidiaries:

Excess of cost over net book value on date of acquisition of consolidated subsidiaries	16,056,115
Equity in unconsolidated subsidiaries, including excess cost over related net assets of $7,843,373	30,248,688

Investments and Other Assets:

Contracts and notes receivable, due after one year	14,066,113
Investments, at cost	4,467,594
Deferred charges, net of accumulated amortization	5,454,224
Deposits and sundry assets	1,488,184
	$200,859,801

LIABILITIES AND STOCKHOLDERS' EQUITY

Current Liabilities:

Accounts payable and accrued expenses	$ 9,927,531
Notes and loans payable	9,327,382
Current portion of long-term debt	1,140,360
Federal and State income tax payable, current portion	558,843
Other current liabilities	1,250,000
Total Current Liabilities	22,204,116
Notes Payable on Funded Loans and Accounts Receivable	17,695,105
Long-term Debt, less current portion shown above	35,221,760
Other Liabilities	1,250,000
Deferred Federal and State Income Taxes Payable	16,673,910
Subordinated Debt	32,917,000

STOCKHOLDERS' EQUITY

Preferred stock—authorized 1,000,000 shares, $100 stated value, issued 20,000	2,000,000
Common stock—authorized 20,000,000 shares, $.30 par value, issued 5,926,836	1,778,051
Additional paid-in capital	52,864,501
Retained earnings	18,269,433
	74,911,985
Less treasury stock, at cost	14,075
Total Stockholders' Equity	74,897,910
	$200,859,801

PROSPECTUS

December 7, 1971

Equity Funding Corporation of America

$35,000,000 5½% Convertible Subordinated Debentures due 1991

The Debentures will be issued in registered form and are convertible, unless previously redeemed, into the Company's Common Stock at $36¾ per share, subject to adjustment in certain events. Payments under a Sinking Fund commencing on December 1, 1982 are designed to retire 90% of the Debentures prior to maturity (see "Description of Debentures"). The Debentures are also redeemable at the option of the Company at an initial redemption price of 105½% of the principal amount thereof and thereafter at declining redemption prices as set forth herein. On December 6, 1971, the last reported sale price of the Common Stock on the New York Stock Exchange was $32¼ per share.

The Company has applied for listing of the Debentures on the New York Stock Exchange.

THESE SECURITIES HAVE NOT BEEN APPROVED OR DISAPPROVED BY THE SECURITIES AND EXCHANGE COMMISSION NOR HAS THE COMMISSION PASSED UPON THE ACCURACY OR ADEQUACY OF THIS PROSPECTUS. ANY REPRESENTATION TO THE CONTRARY IS A CRIMINAL OFFENSE.

	Price to Public	Underwriting Discount(2)	Proceeds to Company(3)(4)
Per Debenture	100%	1.75%	98.25%
Total	$35,000,000(1)	$612,500	$34,387,500

(1) Plus accrued interest from December 1, 1971 to date of delivery.

(2) The Estate of Theodore Goodman is to receive from New York Securities Co. Incorporated, one of the Representatives of the Underwriters, 25% of its net underwriting commissions and representative's fee pursuant to a previous agreement between New York Securities Co. Incorporated and Mr. Goodman.

(3) The Company has agreed to indemnify the several Underwriters against certain civil liabilities, including liabilities under the Securities Act of 1933.

(4) Before deducting expenses estimated at $365,000 payable by the Company.

(5) The Company has granted to the Underwriters an option to purchase at the Price to Public less Underwriting Discounts up to an additional $3,500,000 principal amount of Debentures to cover over-allotments, if any. To the extent that such option is exercised, the Underwriters will offer such additional Debentures at the Per Debenture Price to Public set forth above, and the Total Price to Public, Underwriting Discount and Proceeds to Company will be increased accordingly. See "Underwriting".

The Debentures are offered subject to prior sale and when, as and if delivered to and accepted by the Underwriters, and subject to approval of certain legal matters by their counsel and by counsel to the Company. Delivery to the Underwriters is expected on or about December 14, 1971.

BACHE & CO.
Incorporated

NEW YORK SECURITIES CO.
Incorporated

EQUITY FUNDING CORPORATION OF AMERICA AND SUBSIDIARIES

CONSOLIDATED STATEMENT OF EARNINGS AND RETAINED EARNINGS

The following Consolidated Statement of Earnings and Retained Earnings has been compiled as explained in Note 1 to the Company's financial statements. The statements for the five years ended December 31, 1970, have been examined by Wolfson, Weiner, Ratoff & Lapin, independent certified public accountants, whose opinion appears elsewhere in the Prospectus. With respect to the unaudited periods, the Company believes that all adjustments (which consist only of normal recurring accruals) necessary for a fair statement of the results of operations for such periods have been made. This statement should be read in conjunction with the related financial statements and Notes thereto included elsewhere in this Prospectus. As to the results of operations of Diversified Land Company, which are included in the Company's Consolidated Statement of Earnings and Retained Earnings, see Note (G) to such statement and "Description of Business—Real Estate".

	Year Ended December 31,					Six Months Ended June 30,	
	1965 (Audited)	1967 (Audited)	1968 (Audited)	1969 (Audited)	1970 (Audited)	1970 (Unaudited)	1971 (Unaudited)
INCOME:							
Insurance sales commissions(A)	$ 4,733,985	$ 6,930,950	$10,464,355	$15,247,569	$17,638,207	$ 7,602,173	$ 8,900,795
Securities sales commissions	1,641,687	2,043,964	5,001,777	19,954,887	15,931,895	7,741,436	8,035,776
Real estate operations	1,657,170	1,143,263	804,822	3,096,165	12,010,129	3,989,189	12,959,721
Natural resources operations	—	—	83,531	3,502,519	7,668,212	1,040,354	3,407,636
Investment management income	—	—	1,425,291	2,556,459	1,741,193	844,935	942,894
Interest income(B)	1,214,551	1,613,857	2,071,745	3,265,821	5,626,377	2,482,351	3,709,378
Other income	203,737	899,236	438,268	409,988	296,861	83,569	255,955
Total income	9,451,130	12,631,270	20,289,789	48,033,408	60,912,874	23,784,007	38,212,155
EXPENSES:							
Commissions on insurance(A)	2,032,337	2,803,444	3,330,661	5,284,437	6,054,342	2,654,887	3,111,429
Commissions on securities	828,381	1,006,705	2,061,166	7,880,604	5,340,826	3,031,267	2,845,462
Real estate operations	1,164,363	1,227,327	843,623	2,147,831	8,488,264	2,608,998	11,250,450
Natural resources operations	—	—	58,859	2,312,650	4,795,101	557,825	2,416,185
Interest and amortization of debt expense(C)	1,026,404	1,413,926	1,529,791	4,297,281	7,501,855	3,281,523	4,428,600
Selling, general and administrative(A)	1,915,868	3,041,572	3,721,634	13,118,662	17,981,120	8,155,974	8,586,862
Total expenses	6,967,353	9,492,974	11,545,734	35,041,465	50,161,508	20,290,474	32,638,988
EARNINGS BEFORE MINORITY INTEREST	2,483,777	3,138,296	8,744,055	12,991,943	10,751,366	3,493,533	5,573,167
Minority interest	1,936	—	—	—	—	—	—
EARNINGS FROM CONSOLIDATED OPERATIONS BEFORE INCOME TAXES	2,485,713	3,138,296	8,744,055	12,991,943	10,751,366	3,493,533	5,573,167

8

FEDERAL AND STATE TAXES ON INCOME (Note 7):							
Current portion	144,987	31,236	452,033	312,800	209,000	67,300	106,000
Deferred portion	975,257	1,540,425	3,546,704	5,347,800	3,756,000	1,306,800	1,842,000
Total tax provision	1,120,244	1,571,661	3,998,737	5,660,600	3,965,000	1,374,100	1,948,000
EARNINGS FROM CONSOLIDATED OPERATIONS	1,365,469	1,566,635	4,745,318	7,331,343	6,786,366	2,119,433	3,625,167
Earnings from unconsolidated subsidiaries, net of taxes and extraordinary items(D)(E)(F)(G)	44,276	371,000	812,030	3,132,711	5,981,954	3,613,303	4,098,904
NET EARNINGS BEFORE EXTRAORDINARY ITEMS	1,409,745	1,937,635	5,557,348	10,464,054	12,768,320	5,732,736	7,724,071
Extraordinary items, net of applicable Federal and State taxes(H)	—	50,000	2,221,453	636,006	(1,021,309)	—	—
NET EARNINGS	1,409,745	1,987,635	7,778,801	11,100,060	11,747,011	5,732,736	7,724,071
DIVIDENDS ON PREFERRED STOCK	—	—	—	—	42,500	—	42,500
NET EARNINGS AVAILABLE FOR COMMON STOCK	1,409,745	1,987,635	7,778,801	11,100,060	11,704,511	5,732,736	7,681,571
RETAINED EARNINGS — BEGINNING OF PERIOD	6,466,424	7,876,169	8,392,493	14,162,562	19,354,058	19,354,058	24,700,486
Less: Dividends paid on common stock	—	(1,469,376)	(2,008,732)	(5,908,564)	(6,358,083)	(6,283,984)	(396,532)
Adjustment for minority interest	—	(1,935)	—	—	—	—	—
RETAINED EARNINGS — END OF PERIOD	$ 7,876,169	$ 8,392,493	$14,162,562	$19,354,058	$24,700,486	$18,802,810	$31,985,525
EARNINGS PER COMMON AND COMMON EQUIVALENT SHARE — ASSUMING NO DILUTION(I):							
Before extraordinary items	$ .44	$ .52	$1.23	$1.91	$2.15	$ .99	$1.21
Extraordinary items	—	.01	.49	.12	(.17)	—	—
Total earnings per common and common equivalent share — assuming no dilution	$ .44	$ .53	$1.72	$2.03	$1.98	$ .99	$1.21
EARNINGS PER COMMON SHARE — ASSUMING FULL DILUTION(J):							
Before extraordinary items	$ .36	$ .43	$1.04	$1.83	$2.08	$ .96	$1.16
Extraordinary items	—	.01	.40	.11	(.16)	—	—
Total earnings per common share — assuming full dilution	$ .36	$ .44	$1.44	$1.94	$1.92	$ .96	$1.16
COMMON STOCK DISTRIBUTIONS:							
Stock dividends	—	5%	3%	2%	2%	2%	—
Cash dividends	—	—	—	—	$ .10	$ .10	$ .10
Stock splits	—	3-for-2	2-for-1	—	—	—	—
RATIO OF EARNINGS TO FIXED CHARGES(K):							
Net earnings before extraordinary items	2.43	2.74	5.42	3.74	2.74	2.80	2.92
Net earnings available for common stock	2.43	2.77	7.54	3.88	2.54	2.80	2.92

(See accompanying notes next page. Numerical note references are to the Company's financial statements.)

NOTES TO CONSOLIDATED STATEMENT OF EARNINGS AND RETAINED EARNINGS

(A) Insurance commission income includes commissions received from the unconsolidated life insurance subsidiary (Equity Funding Life Insurance Company), of $896,000, $3,046,000, $10,125,000, $2,529,000 and $6,065,000 for the years ended December 31, 1968, 1969, 1970 and the six months ended June 30, 1970 and 1971, respectively. The amounts included above representing first-year insurance commission income from the unconsolidated life insurance subsidiary are offset by first-year commission expenses of $546,000, $1,732,000, $4,151,000, $1,514,000, and $2,500,000 and other acquisition costs included in "selling, general and administrative expenses", of $418,000, $1,861,000, $6,246,000, $1,642,000, and $3,973,000. The practice of not deferring the amount of expenses in excess of first-year commission income is acceptable treatment under generally accepted accounting principles.

(B) Interest income includes interest received from an unconsolidated banking subsidiary (Bishops Bank and Trust Company Limited) of $225,115, $715,077, $365,658 and $231,587 for the years ended December 31, 1969 and 1970 and the six months ended June 30, 1970 and 1971, respectively.

(C) Interest and amortization of debt expenses includes interest paid to the unconsolidated banking subsidiary of $644,554, $1,491,270, $771,439 and $262,665 for the years ended December 31, 1969 and 1970 and the six months ended June 30, 1970 and 1971, respectively.

(D) The Company's life insurance subsidiary changed its method of reporting earnings from the "statutory method" to "generally accepted accounting principles". (See Note 1 to the Company's financial statements.)

  Net earnings of the unconsolidated life insurance subsidiary before extraordinary earnings under the statutory method were $338,367, $2,448,876, $2,438,989, $3,000,361 and $1,987,578 for the years ended December 31, 1968, 1969 and 1970 and for the six months ended June 30, 1970 and 1971, respectively as compared to $384,325, $2,116,415, $5,094,646, $3,291,320 and $3,479,646 under generally accepted accounting principles for the same periods. In addition, under generally accepted accounting principles, there were extraordinary earnings of $145,000 (originally $136,000) for 1968 and $410,000 (originally $480,000) for 1969. The net effect of the change for 1968 was an increase in ordinary earnings of $45,958 and an increase in extraordinary earnings of $9,000; for 1969 the net effect was a decrease in ordinary earnings of $332,461 and a decrease in extraordinary earnings of $70,000; for 1970 the net effect was an increase in ordinary earnings of $2,655,657; and for the six months ended June 30, 1970 and 1971 the net effect was an increase in ordinary earnings of $290,959 and $1,492,068 respectively. The financial statements for 1968 through June 30, 1971 only have been restated.

(E) Earnings from unconsolidated subsidiaries include $660,000, $535,782, $2,342,777, $4,374,200, $2,940,000 and $3,246,010 or $.18, $.12, $.43, $.74, $.51 and $.51 per common and common equivalent share—assuming no dilution, for the years 1967, 1968, 1969, 1970 and for the six months ended June 30, 1970 and 1971 respectively, attributable to coinsurance transactions of Equity Funding Life Insurance Company (formerly "The Presidential Life Insurance Company of America"). To the extent that these coinsurance earnings were realized during the periods indicated, earnings from the policies coinsured will not be available unless and until the policies are recaptured.

  A portion of the earnings from unconsolidated subsidiaries attributable to Liberty Savings and Loan Association includes earnings allocated to general reserves on the books of Liberty in the amounts of $224,273, $37,945, ($399,202) and $127,211, for the years 1966, 1967, 1968 and 1969, respectively, and none for 1970 and the six months ended June 30, 1970 and 1971.

(F) Earnings from unconsolidated subsidiaries net of taxes as reported by Equity Funding Corporation of America consist of the following:

	1966 (Audited)	1967 (Audited)	1968 (Audited)	1969 (Audited)	1970 (Audited)	Six Months Ended June 30, 1970 (Unaudited)	1971 (Unaudited)
Equity Funding Life Insurance Company:							
Ordinary	—	$ 623,733	$ 384,325	$2,116,415	$5,094,646	$3,291,320	$3,479,646
Extraordinary item .	—	50,000	145,000	410,000	—	—	—
	— (1)	673,733 (2)	529,325	2,526,415	5,094,646	3,291,320	3,479,646

10

NOTES TO CONSOLIDATED STATEMENT OF EARNINGS
AND RETAINED EARNINGS—(Continued)

	1966 (Audited)	1967 (Audited)	1968 (Audited)	1969 (Audited)	1970 (Audited)	Six Months Ended June 30, 1970 (Unaudited)	Six Months Ended June 30, 1971 (Unaudited)
Liberty Savings and Loan Association:							
Ordinary	$ 44,276	(252,733)	427,705	838,925	522,071	201,449	389,894
Extraordinary item .	—	—	116,699	—	—	—	—
	44,276(1)	(252,733)(2)	544,404	838,925	522,071	201,449	389,894
Bishops Bank and Trust Company Limited:							
Ordinary	—	—	—	177,371	325,837	120,534	216,010
Extraordinary item .	—	—	—	—	—	—	—
	—	—	—	177,371	325,837	120,534	216,010
New Era Development Corp. (51% owned):							
Ordinary	—	—	—	—	41,381	—	18,499
Extraordinary item .	—	—	—	—	—	—	—
	—	—	—	—	41,381	—	18,499
Equity Immobiliare Industriale, S.p.A.:							
Ordinary	—	—	—	—	(1,981)	—	(5,145)
Extraordinary item .	—	—	—	—	—	—	—
	—	—	—	—	(1,981)	—	(5,145)
Total ordinary	$ 44,276	$ 371,000	$ 812,030	$3,132,711	$5,981,954	$3,613,303	$4,098,904
Total extraordinary item.	—	$ 50,000	$ 261,699	$ 410,000			

	Equity Funding Life Insurance Company	Liberty Savings and Loan Association
(1) 1966 earnings:		
As reported by parent...........................	—	$ 44,276
Prior to acquisition	($887,345)	96,685
As reported by subsidiary	($887,345)	$140,961
(2) 1967 earnings:		
As reported by parent...........................	$673,733	($252,733)
Prior to acquisition	(534,946)	77,153
As reported by subsidiary	$138,787	($175,580)

(G) The total income, net earnings and earnings per share attributable to Diversified Land Company and Liberty Savings and Loan Association for the years 1966 through 1970 and for the six months ended June 30, 1970 and 1971 are as follows:

	1966 (Audited)	1967 (Audited)	1968 (Audited)	1969 (Audited)	1970 (Audited)	Six Months Ended June 30, 1970 (Unaudited)	Six Months Ended June 30, 1971 (Unaudited)
Total income:							
Before poolings	$7,486,812	$11,178,943	$19,179,117	$45,571,643	$55,303,028	$21,152,218	$35,827,775
Diversified Land Co.	1,964,318	1,452,327	1,110,672	2,461,765	5,609,846	2,631,789	2,384,380
After poolings	$9,451,130	$12,631,270	$20,289,789	$48,033,408	$60,912,874	$23,784,007	$38,212,155

Liberty Savings and Loan Association is not included in the above reconciliation of total income since only its net income is included as a part of earnings from unconsolidated subsidiaries.

	1966 (Audited)	1967 (Audited)	1968 (Audited)	1969 (Audited)	1970 (Audited)	Six Months Ended June 30, 1970 (Unaudited)	Six Months Ended June 30, 1971 (Unaudited)
Net earnings:							
Before poolings	$1,177,355	$ 2,530,380	$ 7,880,815	$10,509,171	$11,250,036	$ 5,419,463	$ 7,343,835
Diversified Land Co. .	188,114	(215,078)	(181,950)	220,365	465,589	288,869	(9,658)
Liberty Savings and Loan Association ..	44,276	(327,667)	79,936	370,524	31,386	24,404	389,894*
After poolings	$1,409,745	$ 1,987,635	$ 7,778,801	$11,100,060	$11,747,011	$ 5,732,736	$ 7,724,071

* Includes the merged operations of Crown Savings and Loan Association.

11

NOTES TO CONSOLIDATED STATEMENT OF EARNINGS
AND RETAINED EARNINGS—(Continued)

	1966	1967	1968	1969	1970	Six Months Ended June 30, 1970	1971
	(Audited)	(Audited)	(Audited)	(Audited)	(Audited)	(Unaudited)	(Unaudited)
Earnings per common and common equivalent share—assuming no dilution:							
Before pooling—							
Ordinary	$ .40	$ .71	$1.36	$1.89	$2.15	$ .98	$1.20
Extraordinary ...	—	.01	.49	.12	(.17)	—	—
Total	$ .40	$ .72	$1.85	$2.01	$1.98	$ .98	$1.20
Diversified Land Co.	$ .05	$(.08)	$(.07)	$ .02	$ .06	$ .04	$(.02)
Liberty Savings and Loan Association	(.01)	(.11)	(.06)	—	(.06)	(.03)	.03
Total	$ .04	$(.19)	$(.13)	$ .02	$ —	$ .01	$ .01
After poolings—							
Ordinary	$ .44	$ .52	$1.23	$1.91	$2.15	$ .99	$1.21
Extraordinary ..	—	.01	.49	.12	(.17)	—	—
Total	$ .44	$ .53	$1.72	$2.03	$1.98	$ .99	$1.21
Earnings per share—assuming full dilution:							
Before poolings—							
Ordinary	$ .33	$ .58	$1.16	$1.85	$2.11	$ .97	$1.16
Extraordinary ...	—	.01	.40	.11	(.16)	—	—
Total	$ .33	$ .59	$1.56	$1.96	$1.95	$ .97	$1.16
Diversified Land Co. .	$ .04	$(.06)	$(.08)	$(.02)	$ .03	$ .02	$(.03)
Liberty Savings and Loan Association ..	(.01)	(.09)	(.04)	—	(.06)	(.03)	.03
Total	$ .03	$(.15)	$(.12)	$(.02)	$(.03)	$(.01)	
After poolings—							
Ordinary	$ .36	$ .43	$1.04	$1.83	$2.08	$ .96	$1.16
Extraordinary ...	—	.01	.40	.11	(.16)	—	—
Total	$ .36	$ .44	$1.44	$1.94	$1.92	$ .96	$1.16

(H) The extraordinary income shown for 1967 is the result of a credit from a tax loss carryover as reflected in the books of Equity Funding Life Insurance Company. Of the 1968 extraordinary income, $145.000 was due to the tax loss carryover of the insurance company. The remaining portion was made up of the following items: The net gain recognized on Whittington Oil Co., Inc. securities — $1,923,900, the sale of various securities — $35,854, a franchise tax refund — $41,440 and the net gain on the sale of real estate — $75,259. The applicable taxes were $2,458,960, $11,952, $9,800 and $41,400 respectively. In 1969 the insurance company tax loss carryover of $410,000 was credited to extraordinary income. Also included was the net gain of $229,796 from the sale of Pension Life Insurance Co. The related taxes were $293,704. The remaining debit item of $3,790 is due to miscellaneous adjustments. In 1970 the items credited to extraordinary income were the gain realized upon the repurchase, at a discount, of certain promissory notes — $425,196, net of taxes of $474,804 and the effect of Equity Funding Life Insurance Company's change to generally accepted accounting principles in the amount of $67,462. The net reductions to extraordinary income were the write-downs to market value of Whittington Oil Co., Inc. securities — $1,391,133 and the reduction in the investment in a cattle partnership — $122,834. These amounts are net of tax reductions of $1,553,438 and $137,166 respectively.

(I) Earnings per common and common equivalent share — assuming no dilution, has been computed on the basis of the following average number of outstanding common and common equivalent shares: 1966 — 2,992,594 shares and the Series B preferred stock having common stock equivalents of 185,640 shares, 1967 — 3,567,885 shares and the Series B preferred stock having common stock equivalents of 185,640 shares, 1968 — 4,329,341 shares and the Series B preferred stock having common stock equivalents of 185,640 shares, 1969 — 5,292,321 shares and the Series B preferred stock having common stock equivalents of 185,640 shares, 1970 — 5,720,412 shares and the Series B preferred stock having common stock equivalents of 185,640 shares and 6,777 earn-out shares earned in 1970, the six months ended June 30, 1970 — 5,605,798 shares and the Series B preferred stock having common stock equivalents

NOTES TO CONSOLIDATED STATEMENT OF EARNINGS
AND RETAINED EARNINGS—(Continued)

of 185,640 shares, and the six months ended June 30, 1971 — 6,005,734 shares, the Series A and Series B preferred stock having common stock equivalents of 198,815 shares, and options and warrants having common stock equivalents of 195,414 shares.

(J) Earnings per common share — assuming full dilution, were computed on the basis of the average number of outstanding common and common equivalent shares, and on the assumption that the Company's convertible preferred stock, promissory notes and debentures where applicable, were converted, eliminating the related interest on the notes and debentures less applicable income tax (resulting in fully diluted earnings of $1,427,685, $2,112,295, $8,051,667, $11,191,678, $12,418,557, $6,113,900 and $8,047,266 in 1966, 1967, 1968, 1969, 1970, and the six months ended June 30, 1970 and 1971 respectively), and that all of the Company's warrants and stock options were in fact exercised, resulting in the total number of fully diluted shares as follows: 1966 — 3,954,381 shares, 1967 — 4,831,297 shares, 1968 — 5,589,298 shares, 1969 — 5,757,364 shares, 1970 — 6,459,456 shares, six months ended June 30, 1970 — 6,351,153 shares, and the six months ended June 30, 1971 — 6,951,050 shares. The above fully diluted shares have been reduced by the equivalent number of shares which could be purchased with the proceeds that the Company would receive were the common stock purchase warrants and stock options exercised.

The foregoing number of average and fully diluted shares are as adjusted for all stock dividends and stock splits through June 30, 1971.

(K) Ratio of earnings to fixed charges represents the number of times that interest, debt expense, one-third of rentals and preferred dividends were covered by the sum of earnings before income taxes, interest, debt expense and one-third of rentals. Assuming a maximum interest rate of 5¾%, the pro-forma ratio of earnings to fixed charges for the year ended December 31, 1970 and the six months ended June 30, 1971 is as follows:

	Year Ended December 31, 1970	Six Months Ended June 30, 1971
Net earnings before extraordinary items.........	2.69	2.88
Net earnings available for common stock........	2.49	2.88

(L) The following pro forma summary combines the results of operations of the Company and Bankers National Life Insurance Company ("Bankers") for the periods as shown, assuming a pooling of interests. The pro forma earnings per share computation gives effect to the issuance of 1,600,000 shares of the Company's common stock in connection with the acquisition of Bankers.

	Year Ended December 31,					Six Months Ended June 30,	
	1966	1967	1968	1969	1970	1970	1971
	(Unaudited)	(Unaudited)	(Unaudited)	(Unaudited)	(Unaudited)	(Unaudited)	(Unaudited)
Net earnings of EFCA and subsidiaries— Common Stock ...	$ 1,409,745	$ 1,987,635	$ 7,778,801	$11,100,060	$11,704,511	$ 5,732,736	$ 7,681,571
Net Income of Bankers National Life Insurance Company	1,153,859	582,830	1,324,013	1,647,484	1,588,510(1)	523,924(1)	1,120,082
Pro forma Net Earnings	$ 2,563,604	$ 2,570,465	$ 9,102,814	$12,747,544	$13,293,021	$ 6,256,660	$ 8,801,653
Pro forma Earnings Per Common and Common Equivalent share—assuming no dilution....	$ .54	$ .48	$1.49	$1.80	$1.77(1)	$ .85(1)	$1.11
Pro forma Earnings Per Common share—assuming full dilution	$ .46	$ .42	$1.30	$1.75	$1.74(1)	$ .83(1)	$1.07

(1) Includes an extraordinary loss of $219,127 or $.03 per Common share.

The annual interest to be paid on the Debentures offered hereby (excluding interest with respect to Debentures reserved for over-allotments) will initially be $1,925,000.

13

The following summary table shows the results of operations of EFCA, Bankers, and EFCA and Bankers on a pro forma basis, for the three months ended September 30, 1970 and 1971, and for the nine months then ended. The figures shown in this table are unaudited and all adjustments, consisting only of normal recurring accruals, necessary for a fair presentation of the results of operations shown have been made. The earnings per common share have been adjusted to give effect to applicable stock dividends.

	Nine Months Ended September 30,		Three Months Ended September 30,	
	1970	1971	1970	1971
EFCA:				
Total income	$34,853,497	$51,044,685	$11,069,490	$12,832,530
Net earnings	$ 8,727,245	$11,476,852	$ 2,994,509	$ 3,752,781
Earnings per common share and common equivalent share—assuming no dilution.........	$1.49	$1.78	$ .50	$ .57
Earnings per common share—assuming full dilution	$1.44	$1.71	$ .48	$ .55
Bankers:				
Total income	$30,589,156	$28,236,564	$10,656,448	$ 8,753,994
Net income	$ 1,116,790(A)	$ 1,728,550	$ 592,866	$ 608,468
Pro Forma:				
Earnings per common share and common equivalent share—assuming no dilution(B).......	$1.32(A)	$1.64	$ .47	$ .53
Earnings per common share—assuming full dilution(B)......	$1.29(A)	$1.59	$ .46	$ .52

(A) Includes extraordinary loss of $219,127 or $.03 per common share.

(B) Reflects 1,600,000 shares of Common Stock of EFCA issued in connection with the acquisition of Bankers on October 15, 1971.

14

EQUITY FUNDING LIFE INSURANCE COMPANY

STATEMENT OF OPERATIONS

The following statement of operations has been prepared on the basis of generally accepted accounting principles (adjusted basis) with respect to the three years ended December 31, 1970, and the six month periods ended June 30, 1970 and 1971 and on the basis of accounting practices prescribed or authorized by the Insurance Department of the State of Illinois (statutory basis) with respect to the two years ended December 31, 1967. The statement for the three full years ended December 31, 1970, has been examined by Haskins & Sells, independent certified public accountants; the opinion of said firm, which as referred to therein is based, as to policy reserves, net deferred and uncollected life premiums, and accrued costs of recapture of reinsured policies on the opinion of independent consulting actuaries, and as to amounts applicable to certain accident and health business on the report of other independent accountants, appears elsewhere herein. The statement for the two years ended December 31, 1967, has been examined by Arthur Young & Company, independent certified public accountants, as set forth in their report included elsewhere herein. The statement for the six month periods ended June 30, 1970 and 1971, is unaudited; however, in the opinion of Equity Life, such unaudited statement includes all adjustments (which consisted only of normal recurring accruals) necessary for a fair presentation of the results of operations for such interim periods. The operating results for interim periods are not necessarily indicative of the results for an entire year. This statement should be read in conjunction with its notes and the other Equity Life financial statements and the notes thereto, together with the above-mentioned opinions and reports, included elsewhere herein.

	Statutory Basis(a)		Adjusted Basis(c)				
	Year Ended December 31,		Year Ended December 31,			Six Months Ended June 30,	
	1966	1967(b)	1968	1969	1970	1970 (Unaudited)	1971 (Unaudited)
Premiums and other considerations (net of reinsurance ceded):							
Life	$1,557,559	$811,719	$786,079	$3,130,791	$11,010,514	$3,931,844	$6,090,847
Accident and health(e)	34,398	42,352	1,566,036	2,100,502	173,919	85,078	207,694
Considerations for supplementary contracts without life contingencies	—	—	—	144,052	10,166	—	—
Total	1,591,957	854,071	2,346,115	5,375,345	11,194,599	4,016,922	6,298,541
Coinsurance considerations(d)	—	—	535,782	2,342,777	4,374,200	2,940,000	3,246,010
Investment income:							
Interest on bonds	90,660	99,885	74,475	75,405	55,282	19,797	222,269
Interest on policy loans	9,622	11,260	734	1,965	2,253	842	953
Interest on certificates of deposit	9,974	—	8,410	248,221	89,514	73,894	98,308
Interest on mortgage loans	—	—	—	18,548	33,927	27,794	1,208
Interest on collateral loans and unsecured notes receivable from parent company and its affiliates	—	—	55,342	28,750	497,989	218,700	57,233
Other	2,096	4,314	—	—	1,060	—	—
Total investment income	112,352	115,459	138,961	372,889	680,025	341,027	379,971
Investment expense	180	1,727	647	2,541	2,094	620	817
Net investment income	112,172	113,732	138,314	370,348	677,931	340,407	379,154
Other income — Service fees from parent company	—	—	205,651	89,820	100,000	66,000	—
Total income	1,704,129	967,803	3,225,862	8,178,290	16,346,730	7,363,329	9,923,705

16

Policy benefits and reserves:							
Death and other benefits under life policies	316,924	264,494	179,030	90,606	156,660	131,868	166,008
Benefits under accident and health policies(e)	14,157	14,793	101,929	383,704	19,277	2,685	13,092
Increase (decrease) in policy reserves:							
Life	463,940	(702,490)	58,794	(366,181)	3,257,850	287,134	987,866
Accident and health(e)	—	—	613,992	(574,580)	25,754	(4,265)	22,716
Supplementary contracts without life contingencies	—	—	—	118,101	(567)	(1,732)	(8,500)
Total	795,021	(423,203)	953,745	(348,350)	3,458,974	415,690	1,181,182
Remainder	909,108	1,391,006	2,272,117	8,526,640	12,887,756	6,947,639	8,742,523
Operating expenses:							
Life commissions(g) (Note 3)	591,574	453,188	78,997	1,299,836	3,921,254	1,661,442	2,867,385
Accident and health commissions(e)	10,873	114	769,618	2,041,077	112,426	29,669	33,433
Other policy acquisition costs (including recapture costs of $233,167 in 1969, $511,241 in 1970 and $275,013 and $326,812 in the six months ended June 30, 1970 and 1971) (Note 3)	—	—	25,765	859,988	1,115,667	597,252	689,051
Salaries and other general expenses	1,114,135	761,979	804,912	189,537	362,182	201,927	230,911
Taxes, licenses, and fees	57,752	61,726	85,259	148,717	197,663	97,115	154,981
Increase (decrease) in loading on deferred and uncollected premiums	21,349	(25,007)	(28,664)	226,320	362,414	(17,086)	137,116
Total	1,795,683	1,252,000	1,735,887	4,765,475	6,071,606	2,570,319	4,112,877
Dividends to life policyholders							
Income (loss) before loss on sale of investments, etc.	(886,575)	139,006	536,230	3,761,165	6,816,150	4,377,320	4,629,646
Loss on sale of investments	770	219	6,905	631,750	41,504	—	—
Income (loss) before Federal income taxes and extraordinary credit	(887,345)	138,787	529,325	3,129,415	6,774,646	4,377,320	4,629,646
Provision for Federal income taxes(f)	—	50,000	145,000	1,013,000	1,680,000	1,086,000	1,150,000
Income (loss) before extraordinary credit	(887,345)	88,787	384,325	2,116,415	5,094,646	3,291,320	3,479,646
Credit resulting from tax loss carryover(f)	—	50,000	145,000	410,000	—	—	—
Net income (loss)	$(887,345)	$ 138,787	$ 529,325	$ 2,526,415	$ 5,094,646	$ 3,291,320	$ 3,479,646

(See accompanying notes next page)

17

EQUITY FUNDING LIFE INSURANCE COMPANY
NOTES TO STATEMENT OF OPERATIONS

(a) The statement of operations for the two years ended December 31, 1967 has been prepared on the basis of accounting practices prescribed or authorized by the Insurance Department of the State of Illinois (statutory basis), which practices differ in certain respects from generally accepted accounting principles. The more important differences applicable to the aforementioned statement pertain to the accounting for commissions and other acquisition costs applicable to the issuance of new policies which were charged to operations when incurred rather than amortized over the expected policy lives and to policy reserves which were based on statutory requirements. In the opinion of management of Equity Life, the effects of variances from generally accepted accounting principles on the statement of operations for the two years ended December 31, 1967 are not practicably or reasonably determinable.

(b) In December 1967, Equity Life entered into an agreement with respect to the reinsurance of a block of business for a consideration of $600,000. As a result of this agreement, the provision in 1967 for aggregate life reserves was reduced approximately $1,142,000, premium income was decreased approximately $542,000 and income (loss) before Federal income taxes and extraordinary credit was increased approximately $600,000. Another reinsurance agreement was modified during 1967 to retroactively reinsure an additional block of business. The principal effect of this agreement was to reduce premium income for the year approximately $570,000 ($173,000 applicable to prior years) and to reduce expenses and provision for aggregate life reserves approximately $630,000 ($158,000 applicable to prior years). The net effect was to increase 1967 income (loss) before Federal income taxes and extraordinary credit approximately $60,000 of which a portion (not material) was attributable to the prior two years. The approximate effect on 1967 results of operations of the two foregoing agreements was to decrease premium income by $1,112,000 and to increase net income by $660,000.

(c) At December 31, 1970, Equity Life adopted the practice of preparing its financial statements, other than those issued pursuant to requirements of insurance regulatory authorities, in conformity with generally accepted accounting principles, and restated its financial statements for 1968 and 1969 to conform to such practice. See Note 1 to Equity Life's financial statements elsewhere in this Prospectus for additional information. A reconciliation of net gain from operations, determined pursuant to statutory accounting and reporting requirements (which as to 1968 and 1969 also represents amounts previously reported to Equity Life's parent company for inclusion in its financial statements for those years), and net income as reported herein is as follows:

	Year Ended December 31,			Six Months Ended June 30,	
	1968	1969	1970	1970	1971
				(Unaudited)	(Unaudited)
Statutory net gain from operations.......	$474,367	$2,928,876	$2,438,989	$3,000,361	$1,714,487
Add (Deduct):					
Net change in deferred and accrued policy acquisition and recapture costs	179,629	354,143	5,710,678	569,736	3,191,097
Recalculation of policy reserve increase	39,391	99,718	(1,076,371)	(102,504)	(191,170)
Deferred Federal income taxes........		(253,000)	(2,030,000)	(186,000)	(1,150,000)
Net realized loss on sale of investments	(6,905)	(631,750)	(41,504)	—	—
Other	(157,157)	28,428	92,854	9,727	(84,768)
Total	54,958	(402,461)	2,655,657	290,959	1,765,159
Net income reported herein............	$529,325	$2,526,415	$5,094,646	$3,291,320	$3,479,646

(d) During 1968, an aggregate cash consideration of $535,782 was received pursuant to the terms of two coinsurance agreements and policy reserves of about $96,000 were assumed by a coinsurer under one of the agreements. Equity Life discontinued writing business on the coinsured policy forms in 1968. Also a $250,000 expense allowance was received pursuant to the terms of a 1967 coinsurance agreement.

18

EQUITY FUNDING LIFE INSURANCE COMPANY

NOTES TO STATEMENT OF OPERATIONS—(Continued)

During the years 1969 and 1970, the Company entered into significant coinsurance agreements with respect to its new business. The Company's policy has been to reinsure substantial portions of its life business and it intends to continue that policy in the ordinary course of conducting its operations. Under these agreements, the Company retains the first-year premiums on ceded life business and receives considerations from the reinsurers, which, in general, are defined in the agreements as various first year allowances. The Company will not receive renewal premium income on the coinsured portion of its policies; however, it retains all policy fees and the reinsurers will pay the Company commission and expense allowances ranging from approximately 12% to 15% of the renewal premiums. The applicable policy acquisitions and recapture costs have been charged against income. The foregoing coinsurance transactions are summarized as follows:

	Year Ended December 31,		6 Months Ended June 30,	
	1969	1970	1970	1971
			(Unaudited)	(Unaudited)
Premiums retained	$3,023,000	$5,479,000	$3,680,000	$4,058,000
Coinsurance considerations	2,343,000	4,374,000	2,940,000	3,246,000
Policy acquisition and recapture cost	(2,132,000)	(4,298,000)	(2,260,000)	(3,577,000)
Excess of premiums and considerations over acquisition and recapture costs	$3,234,000	$5,555,000	$4,360,000	$3,727,000

For additional information, see Notes 3 and 5 to the Equity Life financial statements and "Ceded Reinsurance" under the caption "Description of Business—Insurance Operations" appearing elsewhere in this Prospectus.

(e) Substantially all of the accident and health business for 1968 and 1969 was produced by a nonrelated company under an agreement which, in general, provided that Equity Life's earnings thereunder would be a specified percentage of net premiums written. As of July 1, 1969, the business covered by the agreement was 100% coinsured and the reinsurer assumed the assets and liabilities related to the business.

Amounts included in the financial statements for 1968 and 1969 regarding this business are based on schedules of accounts which were submitted by the producing company.

(f) The provisions for Federal income taxes consists of the following:

	Year Ended December 31,				Six Months Ended June 30,	
	1967	1968	1969	1970	1970	1971
					(Unaudited)	(Unaudited)
Current (credit)			$ 350,000	$ (350,000)	$ 900,000	
Charge equivalent to tax reduction resulting from utilization of tax operating loss carryforward.......	$50,000	$145,000	410,000			
Deferred			253,000	2,030,000	186,000	$1,150,000
Total	$50,000	$145,000	$1,013,000	$1,680,000	$1,086,000	$1,150,000

Deferred Federal income taxes relate primarily to the excess of deductions for life policy reserves and policy acquisition costs claimed for tax purposes over amounts charged against income for financial accounting purposes. See Note 6 to Equity Life's financial statements elsewhere in this Prospectus for additional information relating to Federal income taxes.

(g) Commissions paid to subsidiaries of Equity Life's parent were approximately $896,000, $3,046,000, $10,125,000, $2,529,000 and $6,065,000 during the years ended December 31, 1968, 1969, 1970 and six months ended June 30, 1970 and 1971, respectively.

(h) Numerical note references are to notes to the Equity Life financial statements.

19

insurance company, the Company has become a general agent of Bankers in Connecticut and New Jersey, and a general agent of Palisades in New York. The Company intends to place all of its life insurance business in Connecticut and New Jersey with Bankers and in New York with Palisades. Equity Life is not now qualified in any of such states.

Under its general agency agreements with Equity Life, Bankers and Palisades and other insurers, the Company is entitled to first year and renewal commissions. The policies sold by the Company primarily are ordinary straight-life insurance policies. Term policies also are offered by the Company, but do not at this time account for a substantial part of premium income. The Company sells fire and casualty and accident and health insurance, but this phase of business has not been significant to date.

The following table reflects pertinent information with respect to the Company's total life insurance sales, including policies written by both affiliated and unaffiliated insurers, for the five years ended December 31, 1970:

Year	Premiums in Force Beginning of Year	Premiums Billed During Year	Premiums Lapsed During Year	Premiums Paid and in Force at End of Year	Gross Commissions	Commission Expense	Net Commission Income
1966	$ 6,793,643	$11,273,921	$ 741,934	$10,531,987	$ 4,733,985	$ 2,032,337	$ 2,701,648
1967	10,531,987	16,954,305	1,191,260	15,763,045	6,930,950	2,803,444	4,127,506
1968	15,763,045	23,673,165	1,622,324	22,050,841	10,464,355	3,330,661	7,133,694
1969	22,050,841	38,320,772	3,057,117	35,263,655	15,247,569	5,284,437	9,963,132
1970	35,263,655	52,918,236	4,636,020	48,282,216	17,638,207	6,054,342	11,583,905

Mutual Fund Sales and Distribution

The Company's subsidiary, Equity Funding Securities Corporation ("Equity Securities"), is a mutual fund dealer and in that connection it has selling agreements with the distributors of a large number of mutual funds; however, about 52% of its current mutual fund sales is in shares of Equity Growth Fund, Equity Progress Fund and Fund of America. All of the mutual fund shares sold by the Company are redeemable at any time at net asset value.

EFC Distributors Corporation ("EFC Distributors"), a subsidiary of the Company, acts as the principal distributor for shares of Equity Growth Fund, Equity Progress Fund and Fund of America under agreements which may be terminated by either of the respective parties thereto, without penalty, upon not more than 60 days' notice. Such agreements must be approved at least annually by the directors of the respective mutual funds, including a majority of the directors who are not "interested persons" within the meaning of the Investment Company Act of 1940, as amended (the "1940 Act").

Shares of Equity Growth Fund, Equity Progress Fund and Fund of America are sold to EFC Distributors at their net asset value, and are offered to the public at net asset value plus a sales charge of 8.75% of the offering price on single purchases of less than $25,000. A 7% discount on such purchases is reallowed dealers, including subsidiaries of the Company, and the balance of the sales charge is retained by EFC Distributors. The amount of the sales charge, including the dealers discount, is reduced in larger transactions. Under each of its distributor agreements, EFC Distributors bears a portion of the expenses of such funds.

EFC Sponsors Corporation ("EFC Sponsors"), a subsidiary of the Company, sells and sponsors contractual plans for the accumulation of shares of Fund of America, Axe Science Corporation and National Investors Corporation. As the sponsor of such plans, EFC Sponsors receives sales commissions applicable to the plan which range from 8.75% to 1% of the total payments made, depending upon the plan purchased. EFC Sponsors also receives fees for certain administrative and investor services which have been delegated to it.

The following table sets forth pertinent information concerning the sale of mutual fund shares by the Company for the five years ended December 31, 1970, and for the six-months ended June 30, 1971:

Year	Mutual Fund Shares and Contractual Plans Sold(1)	Gross Commissions(2)	Commission Expense	Net Commissions
1966	$ 29,865,320	$ 1,641,687	$ 828,381	$ 813,306
1967	36,235,687	2,043,964	1,006,705	1,037,259
1968	64,450,778	5,001,777	2,061,166	2,940,611
1969	202,165,256	19,954,887	7,880,604	12,074,283
1970	125,607,166	12,746,247	4,816,280	7,929,967
Six months ended June 30, 1971	55,320,409	5,377,278	2,040,381	3,336,897

(1) Based on offering price of mutual fund shares and payments under contractual plans, including applicable sales charges. The marked increase in mutual fund and contractual plans sold in 1969 was in large part due to the acquisition as of January 1, 1969, of substantially all of the domestic assets of Investors Planning Corporation of America, which had acted as principal distributor for Fund of America and had sponsored and sold contractual plans. Such plans were not offered by the Company prior thereto. See "Recent Acquisitions".

(2) Includes gross commissions attributable to the sale of contractual plans (including commissions on plans sold in prior years) in 1969 of $6,948,528, in 1970 of $5,490,736 and for the six months ended June 30, 1971 of $2,167,176.

Certain of the Company's subsidiaries are subject to regulation by the Securities and Exchange Commission (the "Commission") under the Securities Exchange Act of 1934 and by state and quasi-governmental agencies. The Commission requires such subsidiaries to report regularly with respect to their capital and other aspects of their business, and to conform to the rules and regulations promulgated under the various securities laws, which change from time to time. As members of the National Association of Securities Dealers, Inc., a registered securities association, such subsidiaries are also subject to the supervision of that organization.

On December 14, 1970, Federal legislation was enacted into law which may result in a lowering in the amount of sales commissions on mutual fund shares. Further, as a result of such law, the Company restructured its front-end sales commission arrangement on contractual plans, effective June 14, 1971, so that not more than 20% of any one year's payments by an investor is deducted for sales commissions and the sales commission deducted from the payments during the first four years of the contractual plan does not exceed an average of 16%. Because the Company realized approximately 50% of the total charges applicable to a plan in the first year under plans sold before June 14, 1971, the new law will significantly affect the amount of the first year commissions received on contractual plan sales. The new law could also adversely affect the Company's operations in other respects, to an extent which is not now ascertainable. In 1969, 1970 and for the six months ended June 30, 1971, the Company's first year commissions on contractual plan sales which would have been affected by following the new front-end sales commission arrangement now in effect amounted to $2,918,000, $1,995,000, $852,000, respectively.

Equity Funding Programs

The following table indicates the percentage of gross insurance and mutual fund commission income represented (i) by the sale of *Equity Funding* Programs and (ii) by the sale of insurance and mutual

29

fund shares independent of the Programs for the five years ended December 31, 1970, and for the six months ended June 30, 1971:

	Year Ended December 31,					Six Months Ended June 30, 1971
	1966	**1967**	**1968**	**1969**	**1970**	
Program sales	47%	45%	52%	35%	44%	54%
Non-Program sales	53%	55%	48%	65%	56%	46%

The Programs enable participants to finance their insurance premiums through loans from the Company which are secured by mutual fund shares purchased by the participant for cash. The Company requires a minimum annual premium of $300 and the investment in shares must equal at least 2.5 times each premium loan. Thus at this time the minimum initial investment in mutual fund shares is $750. It is intended that loans and the refinancing of previous borrowings recur annually for a period of ten years, unless the Program is sooner terminated. A Program may be terminated at any time by a Participant, by the Company on the anniversary date or in the event of a participant's inability to meet minimum collateral requirements of 135% of the amount borrowed. Most policies financed in the Programs are ordinary life policies. Although the Company does not now anticipate any material difficulty in obtaining funds for the financing of insurance premiums, there is, of course, no assurance that this will be the case in the future. See "Financing of *Equity Funding* Programs" in this connection.

Programs offered or sold after August 31, 1969, are subject to regulations of the Federal Reserve Board which limit insurance premiums loans to an amount not in excess of 40% of the value of the mutual fund shares pledged for each borrowing. Under such regulations, the amount which may be loaned in a Program may be reduced, or loans may be precluded, by action of the Board. Program participants, as well as the Company, could be adversely affected by any such action.

The following table sets forth statistical information, for the periods indicated, concerning the sale and termination of Programs:

	Year Ended December 31,				
	1966	**1967**	**1968**	**1969**	**1970**
Programs Sold					
Number of Programs Sold(1)	2,763	3,912	5,783	9,354	11,139
Amount of Premiums Financed in First Year Programs Sold(1) .... $	1,489,033	$ 2,071,778	$ 3,164,048	$ 5,694,476	$ 7,583,097
Amount of Mutual Funds Purchased in Financing of First Year Premiums..... $	11,007,640	$ 13,687,157	$ 19,253,232	$ 35,259,256	$ 36,224,454
Face Amount of Life Insurance Policies Sold .... $	83,176,572	$116,262,182	$172,774,122	$296,587,278	$528,520,008
Premium Loans Outstanding at End of Period(2) .... $	16,477,869	$ 25,094,811	$ 36,311,037	$ 51,188,119	$ 63,324,413
Total Number of Programs in Effect at Year End	8,477	12,020	16,682	23,939	31,892
Programs Terminated					
Termination of Programs Sold During Period Indicated, as of December 31, 1970(3) ..	1,032	1,045	1,078	1,018	71
Amount of Annual Premiums Involved in Terminations(4) .... $	530,611	$ 550,440	$ 594,244	$ 572,838	$ 34,701
Face Amount of Life Insurance Involved in Terminations(4) .... $	31,389,413	$ 31,107,357	$ 32,085,363	$ 32,089,775	$ 2,524,050
Total Number of Programs Terminated During Year	366	369	1,121	2,097	3,186

(1) Includes Programs involving fire and casualty and accident and health insurance, but the sale of Programs with such insurance has not, to date, been significant.

(2) Including interest and renewal premiums financed.

(3) Terminations generally result because of reasons which are personal to the investor. See text below in this connection.

(4) "Terminations" refer only to the financing arrangement and not necessarily to a termination of the related insurance policy.

As of June 30, 1971, approximately 36,251 Programs were being maintained. During the first six months of 1971, 6,636 Programs were sold and 2,277 Programs were terminated. From the introduction of the Programs in 1960 through June 30, 1971, a total of 164 have been terminated as the result of forced liquidations, including 140 Programs which were so terminated during 1970. The average face amount of the life insurance policies sold in all Programs is approximately $49,000. The average amount of the first year loan made to participants is approximately $660.

North American Equity Corporation

North American Equity Corporation ("NAEC"), a subsidiary of the Company, is a member of the Midwest Stock Exchange, Pacific Coast Stock Exchange and the Philadelphia-Baltimore-Washington Stock Exchange. Substantially all of NAEC's business is restricted to the handling of transactions for institutions and others engaged in the securities business.

Commissions earned by NAEC are included in securities sales commissions in the Company's Consolidated Statement of Earnings and Retained Earnings and in the table under "Description of Business" showing income sources. NAEC's total commission income in 1970 and for the six months ended June 30, 1971, amounted to $1,620,504 and $1,700,233. This was derived primarily from direct execution for funds managed by EFC Management (approximately 45%) and the balance was realized in approximately equal parts from direct execution for unaffiliated persons and reciprocal business. As described below, the reciprocal business results in an offset against the management fees payable to the Company by the mutual funds under its management.

Pursuant to the terms of the advisory and management agreements between Equity Growth Fund, Fund of America and Equity Progress Fund, and EFC Management, the management fee otherwise payable by such funds is reduced by 50% of that portion of the "net income after taxes", as defined, of NAEC which is attributable to any "reciprocal business" of NAEC resulting from stock exchange transactions effected for the fund. To date, the amount of the reduction in the management fee paid by the funds has not been material. NAEC may effect transactions for the above funds on the New York or American Stock Exchanges through members of such exchanges who may direct brokerage business originated with their customers to NAEC if such business (referred to as reciprocal business) can be executed on a regional stock exchange of which NAEC is a member.

Other Marketing Activities

In 1970 EFCA formed a limited partnership to engage in the breeding of beef cattle and publicly sold $10,000,000 of limited partnership interests therein. In 1970 and 1971, it also sold $5,237,000 of units of interest in a limited partnership formed to acquire and operate certain apartment buildings located in California. In addition, a real estate limited partnership was formed in 1971 and an aggregate of $6,000,000 of interests therein are currently being offered by the Company. A cattle limited partnership also was formed in 1971 by the Company and it is proposed to publicly offer an aggregate of $5,000,000 of limited partnership interests in the cattle partnership prior to the end of 1971, although there is no assurance that such will be the case. The general partner of each of such limited partnerships is a subsidiary of the Company. In this connection, the Company understands that The National Association of Securities Dealers, Inc. has under consideration certain rules which would regulate the distribution of these types of limited partnership interests. The effect on the Company of the adoption of any such rules cannot now be determined. During 1970, the Company commenced the sale of parcels of unimproved land located primarily in California but it has recently taken steps to terminate this aspect of its business. See "Real Estate", below. In the past, the Company sold interests in oil and gas limited partnerships.

INSURANCE OPERATIONS

Equity Life

Equity Life was incorporated under Illinois law in June 1959 and is authorized to write life and accident and health insurance. It is presently qualified to write life and accident and health insurance in the District of Columbia and in all states except Connecticut, New Jersey and New York. Of the life insurance presently in force, approximately 38% was written in California, 7% was in Illinois and 6% in Florida.

The insurance sold by Equity Life includes individual whole life and endowment, term, group, and accident and health insurance. Premium rates are believed by the Company to be generally competitive with similar types of insurance written by other companies. The policies written by Equity Life are non-participating and are sold through the Company's own sales force.

The following table shows, for the five years ended December 31, 1970, Equity Life's assets, capital stock and surplus, premium income and certain information relating to its life insurance in force:

	1966	1967	1968	1969	1970
Assets	$ 2,838,466	$ 2,678,780	$ 8,540,868	$ 11,312,193	$ 21,033,511
Capital Stock and Surplus	$ 1,471,162	$ 2,122,466	$ 6,431,793	$ 8,958,209	$ 12,952,855
Ratio of Capital Stock and Surplus to Total Liabilities	107.6%	381.5%	305.0%	380.4%	160.3%
Premiums and other considerations (net of ceded reinsurance):					
Individual Life	$ 1,407,137	$ 674,282	$ 698,205	$ 3,108,693	$ 10,930,848
Individual Annuities	—	—	—	—	2,000
Group	150,422	150,689	81,874	22,098	89,678
Individual A & H	34,398	29,100	1,566,036	2,100,502	161,907
Considerations for supplementary contracts without life contingencies	—	—	—	144,052	10,165
Total Premium Income	$ 1,591,957	$ 854,071	$ 2,346,115	$ 5,375,345	$ 11,194,599
Life Insurance:					
In Force Beginning of Year —					
Whole Life and Endowment	$ 27,877,227	$ 48,234,308	$ 77,373,441	$105,395,534	$ 224,100,062
Term and Other Policies	41,625,068	31,850,927	15,091,049	59,958,011	229,628,053
Group	20,770,300	28,680,900	16,763,250	22,172,780	52,601,600
Total in Force Beginning of Year ..	90,272,595	108,766,135	109,227,740	187,526,325	506,329,715
Paid-for New Business —					
Direct:					
Whole Life and Endowment	29,875,339	51,352,220	53,648,605	161,888,562	482,031,529
Term and Other Policies	1,186,771	2,773,016	45,434,633	188,516,000	346,725,934
Group	8,303,100	96,500	5,657,817	36,691,982	5,345,241
Total Direct New Business	39,365,210	54,221,736	104,741,055	387,096,544	834,102,704
Reinsurance Assumed:					
Whole Life and Endowment	—	—	—	6,197,000	6,125,182
Total Reinsurance Assumed	—	—	—	6,197,000	6,125,182
Total Paid-for New Business	39,365,210	54,221,736	104,741,055	393,293,544	840,227,886
Terminations —					
Whole Life and Endowment	9,518,258	22,213,087	25,626,512	49,381,034	59,566,497
Term and Other Policies	10,960,912	19,532,894	567,671	18,845,958	52,475,703
Group	392,500	12,014,150	248,287	6,263,162	257,708
Total Terminations	20,871,670	53,760,131	26,442,470	74,490,154	112,299,908
In Force End of Year —					
Whole Life and Endowment	48,234,308	77,373,441	105,395,534	224,100,062	652,690,276
Term and Other Policies	31,850,927	15,091,049	59,958,011	229,628,053	523,878,284
Group	28,680,900	16,763,250	22,172,780	52,601,600	57,689,133
Total in Force End of Year	108,766,135	109,227,740	187,526,325	506,329,715	1,234,257,693
Reinsurance Ceded —					
Individual	44,849,650	85,759,115	143,900,711	432,037,339	739,095,537
Group	2,045,250	—	1,897,250	20,091,118	16,128,127
Total Reinsurance Ceded	46,894,900	85,759,115	145,797,961	452,128,457	755,223,664
Net in Force End of Year —					
After Reinsurance Ceded	$ 61,871,235	$ 23,468,625	$ 41,728,364	$ 54,201,258	$ 479,034,029

The following tabulation sets forth for the last five calendar years certain mortality and general expense information pertaining to life insurance operations of Equity Life:

	1966	1967	1968	1969	1970
Ratio of voluntary terminations to mean number of individual policies in force	15.3%	29.1%	13.6%	6.9%	5.8%
Ratio — Actual to expected mortality for individual life insurance policies	88.1%	242.5%	133.5%	69.6%	93.2%
Ratio of statutory general insurance expenses to premiums and other considerations	70.0%	89.2%	37.0%	17.2%	14.6%

The average face amount of ordinary life policies (non-group policies) sold in the years 1968, 1969 and 1970 was $18,734, $33,262 and $44,003.

Investments. The following table shows the cash and invested assets of Equity Life at December 31, 1969 and 1970.

	1969		1970	
	Amount	Percent of Total	Amount	Percent of Total
Cash and Certificates of Deposit ..	$ 6,414,027	71%	$ 3,882,622	34%
Bonds:				
Governments	286,445	3	659,186	6
Public Utilities	203,461	2	—	—
Industrial and Miscellaneous ..	294,907	3	5,110,839	45
Total Bonds	784,813	8	5,770,025	51
Common Stock	975,000	12	—	—
Collateral Loan	—	—	1,350,000	12
Mortgage Loans	819,340	9	247,492	2
Policy Loans	25,874	—	60,851	1
Total	$ 9,019,054	100%	$11,310,990	100%

The following tabulation shows, for the years 1966 through 1970, Equity Life's cash and invested assets as of the end of each period, net investment income and net investment yield on average cash and invested assets:

	Cash and Invested Assets	Net Investment Income	Net Investment Yield
1966	$ 2,487,193	$112,172	5.05%
1967	2,427,222	113,732	4.68%
1968	7,638,764	138,314	2.77%
1969	9,019,054	370,348	4.44%
1970	11,310,990	677,931	6.90%

33

Ceded Reinsurance. Equity Life coinsures substantial amounts of its life insurance with various unaffiliated companies. The majority of its life coinsurance are based on the agreements described below. In January 1968, Equity Life entered into a coinsurance agreement requiring the cession of an aggregate of $250,000,000 face-amount of life insurance sold to customers of the Company, less certain credits. The requirements of this agreement were met as of December 31, 1970. In October 1969, Equity Life entered into a coinsurance agreement under which an unaffiliated insurer has agreed to assume up to $1 billion face-amount of life insurance sold from July 1, 1969 through December 31, 1973, for a maximum amount of first-year reinsurance premiums of approximately $14 million. During 1969 Equity Life entered into another coinsurance agreement covering policies issued between March 31, 1968 and June 30, 1969. During 1970, Equity Life entered into two coinsurance agreements with one reinsurer to cede approximately $1,750,000 of premium. This agreement was renewed to cover the period during the first six months of 1971. The requirements of this agreement were met as of September 30, 1971.

The table below shows, for the periods indicated, the approximate face-amount of life insurance ceded and the coinsurance considerations received by Equity Life under all of its coinsurance agreements.

Period	Approximate Face Amount Ceded	Coinsurance Considerations
1968	$ 33,000,000	$ 535,782
1969	239,000,000	2,342,777
1970	435,000,000	4,374,200
First six months of 1971	326,000,000	3,246,010

The effect of ceding insurance is to realize, as current income, coinsurance considerations and to forego the profits or losses in subsequent periods prior to the recapture of the business coinsured. As a general rule, Equity Life retains a small portion of each of the policies reinsured. Under its coinsurance agreements, Equity Life also retains, as an expense allowance, a portion of all renewal premiums attributed to policies and writers coinsured. Under the agreements entered into after 1968, Equity Life has the right to recapture the business coinsured under such agreements during various periods ranging from six to fourteen years from the date of cession. (See Note 5 to Equity Life's Financial Statements in this connection.)

Bankers

Bankers was incorporated in New Jersey in 1927 and is a legal reserve life insurance company. It writes, on both a participating and non-participating basis, individual ordinary life, individual credit life, group credit life, other group life and group accident and health insurance, and it also writes some annuity contracts on a non-participating basis. It is licensed to do business in the District of Columbia, Puerto Rico and all states, except New York. Of the Bankers life insurance in force at June 30, 1971, excluding reinsurance accepted, approximately 18% was written in New Jersey, 10% in Pennsylvania and 7% in California. Palisades was incorporated in New York in 1964, and is licensed only in New York. See Note 3 of Notes to Financial Statements of Bankers for condensed balance sheets and operating statements of Palisades.

The following table sets forth the five years ended December 31, 1970, Bankers' admitted assets and stockholders' equity and the ratio of stockholders' equity to total liabilities and participating policyholders' surplus, all determined on a statutory basis, the amount of premiums and other considerations (net of reinsurance ceded) received during each period, life insurance in force at the beginning and end of each period, and the changes therein during each period.

EQUITY FUNDING CORPORATION OF AMERICA AND SUBSIDIARIES

CONSOLIDATED STATEMENT OF FINANCIAL CONDITION

ASSETS

	December 31, 1970 (Audited)		June 30, 1971 (Unaudited)	
CURRENT ASSETS:				
Cash and short-term investments............		$ 21,742,396		$ 11,443,330
Marketable securities, at cost (which approximates market)		8,584,232		4,759,907
Contracts, notes and loans receivable (Notes 6 and 11)		11,296,792		17,947,117
Accounts receivable		7,043,275		7,226,317
Commissions receivable		3,993,266		4,088,266
Advances to salesmen and employees........		1,515,682		1,265,438
Inventories (Notes 2 and 6)..............		9,087,390		7,595,999
Prepaid expenses and other currents assets....		884,671		1,252,861
Total Current Assets...........		64,147,704		55,579,235
PROPERTY AND EQUIPMENT, AT COST (Notes 4 and 6):				
Real estate and leasehold improvements......	$ 4,753,454		$ 6,188,498	
Furniture, fixtures and equipment...........	3,183,084		3,716,100	
Livestock—breeding herd	3,914,764		2,062,006	
Exploration and development of natural resources	5,807,737		7,557,239	
	17,659,039		19,523,843	
Accumulated depreciation and amortization	1,491,228	16,167,811	1,999,056	17,524,787
OTHER ASSETS:				
Investments at cost.....................	2,127,181		3,761,942	
Funded loans and accounts receivable (Note 3)	63,324,413		76,021,472	
Contracts and notes receivable (Notes 6 and 11)	23,869,857		16,589,840	
Loans receivable—officers	181,435		—	
Discount on debt securities (Note 5)........	3,989,700		3,889,958	
Deferred charges, net of amortization (Note 5):				
Cost of opening and developing new offices..	2,324,920		1,330,549	
Financing and other costs..............	2,017,552		1,910,162	
Organization expense	16,696		18,868	
Registration costs	272,291		239,691	
Costs of renewal commissions acquired.....	211,668		178,097	
Deferred compensation—Employee Stock Bonus Plan	—		1,539,938	
Deposits and sundry assets...............	1,764,052		2,070,346	
Investment in unconsolidated subsidiaries (Note 1):				
Equity in unconsolidated subsidiaries......	28,516,057		33,171,087	
Excess of cost over related net assets of unconsolidated subsidiaries	7,926,276		7,926,276	
Excess of cost over net book value on date of acquisition of consolidated subsidiaries (Note 1)	16,176,565	152,718,663	16,014,000	164,662,226
		$233,034,178		$237,766,248

The accompanying notes are an integral part of the financial statements.

EQUITY FUNDING CORPORATION OF AMERICA AND SUBSIDIARIES

CONSOLIDATED STATEMENT OF FINANCIAL CONDITION

LIABILITIES AND STOCKHOLDERS' EQUITY

	December 31, 1970 (Audited)		June 30, 1971 (Unaudited)	
CURRENT LIABILITIES:				
Accounts payable		$ 7,255,522		$ 4,399,761
Notes and loans payable—unconsolidated subsidiaries		1,998,997		—
Notes and loans payable.		7,220,542		9,260,886
Current portion of long-term debt (Note 6) . . .		2,978,330		11,644,730
Commissions payable		2,664,411		1,657,491
Taxes payable (other than income).		51,857		10,065
Federal and State income taxes payable, current portion (Note 7).		209,000		106,000
Other payables		1,250,000		950,000
Accrued interest and sundry expenses.		2,747,824		2,034,284
TOTAL CURRENT LIABILITIES. . . .		26,376,483		30,063,217
NOTES PAYABLE ON FUNDED LOANS AND ACCOUNTS RECEIVABLE (Note 3).	$ 18,966,246		$ 20,862,189	
LONG-TERM DEBT, LESS CURRENT PORTION SHOWN ABOVE (Note 6).	55,574,603		43,231,382	
OTHER LIABILITIES	1,250,000		—	
DEFERRED INCOME (Note 12)	1,468,300		1,446,821	
DEFERRED FEDERAL AND STATE INCOME TAXES PAYABLE (Note 7).	17,484,948		19,236,000	
SUBORDINATED DEBT (Note 6)	26,187,000	120,931,097	26,187,000	110,963,392
COMMITMENTS AND CONTINGENT LIABILITIES (Note 8)		—		—
STOCKHOLDERS' EQUITY:				
Preferred stock—authorized 1,000,000 shares, no par, $100 stated value, issued and outstanding 84,974 shares and 57,607 shares respectively (Note 9)	8,497,400		5,760,700	
Common stock—authorized 20,000,000 shares, $.30 par value, issued 5,929,315 shares (outstanding 5,924,037 shares) and 6,161,922 shares (outstanding 6,156,644 shares) respectively	1,778,795		1,848,577	
Additional paid-in capital	50,761,751		57,156,671	
Retained earnings (includes undistributed earnings from unconsolidated subsidiaries of $12,886,589 and $17,264,839 respectively) (Note 10)	24,700,486		31,985,525	
	85,738,432		96,751,473	
Less treasury stock, 5.278 shares, at cost.	11,834		11,834	
TOTAL STOCKHOLDERS' EQUITY . . .		85,726,598		96,739,639
		$233,034,178		$237,766,248

The accompanying notes are an integral part of the financial statements.

73

EQUITY FUNDING CORPORATION OF AMERICA AND SUBSIDIARIES

CONSOLIDATED STATEMENT OF SOURCE AND APPLICATION OF FUNDS

	Year Ended December 31,			Six Months Ended June 30,	
	1968	1969	1970	1970	1971
	(Audited)	(Audited)	(Audited)	(Unaudited)	(Unaudited)
Source of Funds:					
Net Earnings	$ 7,778,801	$11,100,060	$11,747,011	$ 5,732,736	$ 7,724,071
Charges (Credits) to Earnings not Affecting Working Capital:					
Depreciation and amortization........	991,379	1,909,165	3,265,501	1,579,264	1,452,746
Equity in undistributed income of unconsolidated subsidiaries	(1,073,729)	(3,542,711)	(4,394,416)	(3,613,303)	(4,098,904)
Deferred Federal income taxes........	4,809,850	5,641,504	2,540,200	1,306,800	1,842,000
Other	—	—	(640,000)	—	256,656
Compensation received in the form of securities	(3,376,360)	—	—	—	—
Funds provided from operations.	9,129,941	15,108,018	12,518,296	5,005,497	7,176,569
Increase in Long-Term Debt..............	13,221,719	34,558,923	40,418,973	18,446,087	—
Proceeds from Exercise of Stock Options and Warrants	199,017	792,097	1,149,065	598,717	221,680
Other, Net	125,344	56,069	—	—	157,976
	22,676,021	50,515,107	54,086,334	24,050,301	7,556,225
Application of Funds:					
Decrease in Long-Term Debt.............	—	—	—	—	14,338,039
Increase in Long-Term Receivables........	5,869,013	11,252,616	30,937,142	15,377,316	3,361,143
Additions to Property and Equipment, Net..	148,912	133,044	7,587,018	4,072,653	900,132
Acquisitions of and Advances to Subsidiaries.	3,661,969	16,796,495	5,576,760	2,032,787	256,126
Increase in Investments and Other Assets...	3,985,624	4,005,960	1,702,086	4,226,043	314,990
Cash Dividends, Common and Preferred Stock	—	—	598,600	556,100	640,998
Other, Net	—	—	279,748	82,763	—
	13,665,518	32,188,115	46,681,354	26,347,662	19,811,428
Increase (decrease) in Working Capital....	$ 9,010,503	$18,326,992	$ 7,404,980	$(2,297,361)	$(12,255,203)

The accompanying notes are an integral part of the financial statements.

EQUITY FUNDING CORPORATION OF AMERICA AND SUBSIDIARIES

CHANGES IN WORKING CAPITAL

	Year Ended December 31,			Six Months Ended June 30,	
	1968 (Audited)	**1969** (Audited)	**1970** (Audited)	**1970** (Unaudited)	**1971** (Unaudited)
Increases in Working Capital:					
Increase in:					
Cash and short-term investments........	$ 1,643,729	$ 9,617,659	$ 9,285,881	$ —	$ —
Marketable securities, at cost...........	6,223,583	13,339,785	—	—	—
Contracts, notes and loans receivable....	580,654	7,139,339	2,259,886	899,564	6,650,325
Accounts and commissions receivable....	5,095,533	—	5,069,506	1,456,432	27,798
Inventories	580,605	718,359	6,709,239	8,331,721	—
Prepaid expenses and other current assets.	210,990	1,309,509	—	—	368,190
Decrease in:					
Accounts payable and accrued expenses..	—	—	—	4,207,620	4,918,013
Current portion of long-term debt........	897,272	—	—	1,435,898	—
Federal and State income taxes payable, current portion	—	1,095,920	398,055	255,048	103,000
Other current liabilities................	—	—	1,750,000	1,750,000	—
	15,232,366	33,220,571	25,472,567	18,336,283	12,067,326
Decreases in Working Capital:					
Increase in:					
Accounts payable and accrued expenses..	2,032,013	6,473,069	1,042,703	—	—
Notes and loans payable..............	2,527,500	2,469,988	4,222,051	7,573,981	41,347
Current portion of long-term debt.......	—	1,553,624	607,510	—	8,666,400
Federal and State income taxes payable, current portion	1,662,350	—	—	—	—
Other current liabilities................	—	3,000,000	—	—	—
Decrease in:					
Cash and short-term investments........	—	—	—	2,874,209	10,299,066
Marketable securities	—	—	11,381,829	9,636,072	3,824,325
Accounts and commissions receivable....	—	1,396,898	—	—	—
Inventories	—	—	—	—	1,491,391
Prepaid expenses and other current assets.	—	—	813,494	549,382	
	6,221,863	14,893,579	18,067,587	20,633,644	24,322,529
Increase (decrease) in working capital.....	$ 9,010,503	$18,326,992	$ 7,404,980	$(2,297,361)	$(12,255,203)

The accompanying notes are an integral part of the financial statements.

Consolidated Statement of Earnings and Retained Earnings

QUARTERLY REPORT

Sales and Revenues

	Three Months Ended March 31	
	1971	1970
Insurance	$ 4,852,749	$ 4,528,639
Securities	4,390,561	4,557,253
Real estate	5,699,899	2,419,618
Natural resources	1,582,467	630,651
Investment management	474,174	370,309
Interest	1,727,652	1,139,948
Other	51,986	31,627
	18,779,488	13,678,045

Cost of Sales and Operating Expenses

Insurance	1,708,260	1,600,173
Securities	1,500,121	1,802,016
Real estate	4,894,120	1,945,010
Natural resources	937,147	378,266
Interest and amortization of debt expense	2,312,142	1,561,268
Selling, general and administrative expenses	4,516,747	4,250,861
	15,868,537	11,537,594
Earnings from Consolidated Operations Before Income Taxes	2,910,951	2,140,451
Federal and State Income Taxes:		
Current portion	61,000	47,817
Deferred portion	961.000	851,735
Total Tax Provision	1,022,000	899,552
Earnings from Consolidated Operations	1,888,951	1,240,899
Earnings from Unconsolidated Operations:		
Life insurance subsidiary, net of applicable income taxes of $560,000 and $513,000 respectively	1,680,121	1,555,659
Bank and savings and loan subsidiaries, net of applicable income taxes of $82,000 and $147,000 respectively	207,794	282,160
Net Earnings from Operations	3,776,866	3,078,718
Retained Earnings—January 1	20,969,154	19,354,058
Adjustments for Dividends and Acquisitions	3,279,087	(6,283,984)
Retained Earnings—March 31	$28,025,107	$16,148,792

Consolidated Statement of Earnings and Retained Earnings

Sales and Revenues

	Six Months Ended June 30	
	1971	1970
Insurance	$ 8,900,795	$ 7,602,173
Securities	8,035,776	7,741,436
Real estate	12,959,721	3,989,189
Natural resources	3,407,636	1,040,354
Investment management	942,894	844,935
Interest	3,709,378	2,482,351
Other	255,955	83,569
	38,212,155	23,784,007

Cost of Sales and Operating Expenses

Insurance	3,111,429	2,654,887
Securities	2,845,462	3,031,267
Real estate	11,250,450	2,608,998
Natural resources	2,416,185	557,825
Interest and amortization of debt expense	4,428,600	3,281,523
Selling, general and administrative expenses	8,586,862	8,155,974
	32,638,988	20,290,474
Earnings from Consolidated Operations Before Income Taxes	5,573,167	3,493,533
Federal and State Income Taxes:		
Current portion	106,000	67,300
Deferred portion	1,842,000	1,306,800
Total Tax Provision	1,948,000	1,374,100
Earnings from Consolidated Operations	3,625,167	2,119,433
Earnings from Unconsolidated Operations:		
Life insurance subsidiary, net of applicable income taxes of $1,150,000 and $1,086,000 respectively	3,479,646	3,291,320
Bank and savings and loan subsidiaries, net of applicable income taxes of $222,039 and $294,306 respectively	619,258	321,983
Net Earnings from Operations	7,724,071	5,732,736
Retained Earnings—January 1	24,700,486	19,354,058
Dividends and Adjustments	(439,032)	(6,283,984)
Retained Earnings — June 30	$31,985,525	$18,802,810

Consolidated Statement of Earnings and Retained Earnings

QUARTERLY REPORT

Sales and Revenues

	Nine Months Ended Sept. 30	
	1971	1970
Insurance	$14,152,455	$11,605,926
Securities	11,084,331	10,656,467
Real estate	13,488,164	5,878,720
Natural resources	4,886,184	1,315,702
Investment management	1,365,396	1,257,671
Interest	5,761,977	4,024,423
Other	306,178	114,588
	51,044,685	34,853,497
Cost of Sales and Operating Expenses:		
Insurance	4,939,007	4,118,948
Securities	3,808,719	4,129,301
Real estate	11,727,533	3,181,299
Natural resources	3,451,288	665,201
Interest and amortization of debt expense	6,742,124	5,021,730
Selling, general and administrative expenses	12,417,239	12,127,497
	43,085,910	29,243,976
Earnings from Consolidated Operations Before Income Taxes	7,958,775	5,609,521
Federal and State Income Taxes:		
Current portion	280,000	110,700
Deferred portion	2,511,000	2,077,000
Total Tax Provision	2,791,000	2,187,700
Earnings from Consolidated Operations	5,167,775	3,421,821
Earnings from Unconsolidated Operations:		
Life insurance subsidiary, net of applicable income taxes of $1,732,000 and $1,496,000 respectively	5,225,130	4,536,217
Bank and savings and loan subsidiaries, net of applicable income taxes of $314,507 and $312,440 respectively	1,083,947	769,207
Net Earnings from Operations	11,476,852	8,727,245
Retained Earnings—January 1	24,700,486	19,354,058
Dividends and Adjustments	(439,034)	(6,277,920)
Retained Earnings—September 30	$35,738,304	$21,803,383

Consolidated Statement of Financial Condition

Assets

	September 30 1971
Current Assets:	
Cash and short-term investments	$ 8,708,714
Marketable securities, at cost	4,784,742
Contracts, notes and loans receivable	15,720,466
Accounts and commissions receivable	13,060,847
Inventory—Natural resources and real estate operations, at cost	9,827,377
Prepaid expenses and other current assets	1,153,673
Total Current Assets	53,255,819
Funded Loans and Accounts Receivable	83,226,684
Property and Equipment, at Cost, Net of accumulated depreciation and amortization of $1,540,322	18,361,547
Investment in Subsidiaries:	
Excess of cost over net book value on date of acquisition of consolidated subsidiaries	16,014,000
Equity in unconsolidated subsidiaries, including excess cost over related net assets of $7,926,275	43,307,536
Investments and Other Assets:	
Contracts and notes receivable, due after one year	18,576,914
Investments, at cost	3,869,324
Discount on debt securities	3,840,086
Deferred charges, net of accumulated amortization of $7,718,703	3,223,148
Deferred compensation—Employee Stock Bonus Plan	1,539,938
Deposits and sundry assets	1,857,233
	$247,072,229

Liabilities

	September 30 1971
Current Liabilities:	
Accounts payable and accrued expenses	$ 8,691,884
Notes and loans payable	11,819,324
Current portion of long-term debt	15,074,823
Federal and State income taxes payable, current portion	280,000
Other current liabilities	950,000
Total Current Liabilities	36,816,031
Notes Payable on Funded Loans and Accounts Receivable	23,945,496
Long-term Debt, less current portion shown above	37,520,060
Deferred Income	2,282,308
Deferred Federal and State Income Taxes Payable	19,869,771
Subordinated Debt	26,187,000

Stockholders' Equity

Preferred stock — authorized 1,000,000 shares, $100 stated value, issued 56,546	5,654,600
Common stock — authorized 20,000,000 shares $.30 par value, issued 6,165,626 shares	1,849,688
Additional paid-in capital	57,220,805
Retained earnings	35,738,304
Less treasury stock, at cost	11,834
Total Stockholders' Equity	100,451,563
	$247,072,229

Equity Funding
Corporation of
America
and Subsidiaries

EQUITY FUNDING CORPORATION OF AMERICA

PROSPECTUS
September 11, 1972

I. **801,871 Shares of Common Stock offered by the Selling Stockholders.**

II. **32,700 Common Stock Purchase Warrants (expiring 1974) and 41,856 Shares of Common Stock issuable thereunder.**

III. **337,902 Shares of Common Stock subject to Stock Option Plans.**

IV. **172,450 Shares of Common Stock subject to Employee Stock Bonus Plan.**

V. **550,000 Shares of Common Stock issuable upon exercise of Warrants (expiring 1975).**

VI. **462,782 Shares of Common Stock issuable upon conversion of 5¼% Guaranteed (Subordinated) Debentures due 1989.**

A description of the offerings covered by this Prospectus begins at Page 62. The Company will not receive any of the proceeds from the sale of shares by the Selling Stockholders, from the sale of any of the 1974 Warrants or from the sale of shares issued thereunder. The Company will receive and add to its working capital, proceeds from the issuance of Common Stock upon any exercise of the 1974 Warrants, upon the exercise of the 1975 Warrants and upon the exercise of options granted under the Stock Option Plans.

As of the date of this Prospectus, the exercise prices of the 1974 Warrants and 1975 Warrants were $58.46 per share and $25.25 per share, respectively; the conversion price of the 5¼% Guaranteed (Subordinated) Debentures was $49.52 per share; and the exercise prices of the options granted pursuant to the Stock Option Plans ranged from $14.75 to $74.51 per share.

The Company's Common Stock is listed on the New York, Pacific Coast and Midwest Stock Exchanges (symbol "EQF"), and the Warrants (1975) for 550,000 shares of Common Stock are listed on the American Stock Exchange. On September 11, 1972, the closing price of the Common Stock on the New York Stock Exchange was $36¼ per share.

A SUMMARY DESCRIPTION OF THE COMPANY BEGINS AT PAGE 3. MORE DETAILED INFORMATION IS SET FORTH IN OTHER SECTIONS OF THE PROSPECTUS BEGINNING AT PAGE 6. SEE TABLE OF CONTENTS AT PAGE 2.

Table of Contents

SUMMARY DESCRIPTION OF THE COMPANY

The following is a summary description of the Company, in non-technical form, condensed from the material contained in this Prospectus. For more detailed information, please refer to the other sections of the Prospectus.

MARKETING — FINANCIAL SERVICES PRODUCTS

The Company is primarily engaged in the marketing of financial services products offered by its subsidiaries or by other companies it manages, insurance operations, and the management of assets derived from its marketing activities and insurance operations. The principal financial products offered by the Company are:

- **Life Insurance** — Approximately $1.7 billion of new life insurance was written by the Company's insurance subsidiaries and sold through its marketing organization during 1971. Those subsidiaries had approximately $4.6 billion of life insurance in force at December 31, 1971.

    During 1971, approximately 55% of the Company's total revenues was realized from insurance sales and operations, including insurance asset management operations, and approximately 67% of the Company's net earnings before taxes and extraordinary items was represented by such sales and operations.

- **Mutual Funds** — Approximately $108 million of mutual fund shares were sold by the Company in 1971, of which about one-half was in mutual funds managed by the Company.

- ***Equity Funding* Programs** — The Company created and offers the *Equity Funding** Programs — an insurance premium funding program — which enables a customer to use mutual fund shares he purchases for cash as collateral for a loan to pay his insurance premiums. The Programs are sold through the Company's marketing organization. They include insurance issued by subsidiaries of the Company, mutual funds managed by the Company and insurance premium financing through loans made by the Company to the customer. During 1971, approximately 53% of the Company's gross life insurance and mutual fund commission income was represented by sales made in the Programs.

- **Limited Partnership Investments** — In 1971, the Company marketed approximately $14,161,000 of interests in real estate and cattle limited partnerships created and managed by the Company.

The Company's marketing organization consists of over 130 sales offices with approximately 4,000 representatives, and over 240 insurance general agents. Sales offices or general agencies are located in 39 states.

ASSET MANAGEMENT

Virtually all of the Company's asset management functions result from its marketing operations. Each of the financial products marketed by the Company — insurance, mutual fund shares and limited partnership investments — is paralleled by asset management operations.

Thus, as part of its insurance operations, at December 31, 1971, the Company's insurance subsidiaries managed assets totaling $176,270,000.

The Company manages three mutual funds for which it acts as principal distributor and a dealer. The total assets of those funds were approximately $221,253,068 at June 30, 1972.

---

*Equity Funding is the trademark of Equity Funding Corporation of America.

3

SUMMARY DESCRIPTION OF THE COMPANY (Continued)

Under each of the cattle and real estate limited partnerships formed by the Company, a subsidiary acts as general partner and manages the assets of the partnership, which at June 30, 1972, had an aggregate book value of approximately $69,000,000.

The Company also owns a savings and loan association, and is engaged (i) in real estate construction and development, (ii) cattle operations, as well as (iii) certain stock exchange brokerage, international investment banking and oil and gas exploration, activities.

RECENT DEVELOPMENTS

Recent developments relating to the Company's business include:

• **Bankers Acquisition** — The acquisition in October 1971 of Bankers National Life Insurance Company, a New Jersey corporation, which had $2.4 billion face amount of life insurance in force at December 31, 1971 and $627 million face amount of new life insurance sales in 1971. As a result of this acquisition, the Company is qualified to market life and accident and health insurance in all 50 states, as well as the District of Columbia and Puerto Rico. The Banker's acquisition has been treated for accounting purposes as a pooling of interests.

• **Northern Acquisition** — The acquisition in June 1972 of a 91.2% interest in Northern Life Insurance Company, a Washington corporation ("Northern"), which had $673 million face amount of life insurance in force at December 31, 1971, and $76.5 million face amount of new life insurance sales in 1971. The acquisition of Northern has been treated for accounting purposes as a purchase as of June 30, 1972.

• **Revolving Credit Agreement** — In June 1972, the Company entered into a Revolving Credit Agreement which provides for a $75 million secured line of credit with four banks through June 1975, subject to various terms and conditions.

SUMMARY DESCRIPTION OF THE COMPANY (Continued)

CONDENSED FINANCIAL AND STATISTICAL INFORMATION

The following table summarizes significant financial information with respect to the consolidated operations of the Company and furnishes certain statistical data with respect to the life insurance operations of its subsidiaries, Equity Funding Life Insurance Company ("Equity Funding Life") and Bankers National Life Insurance Company ("Bankers"), mutual fund assets under the Company's management and *Equity Funding* Program sales.

	1967 (Restated)	1968 (Restated)	1969 (Restated)	1970 (Restated)	1971
	(In thousands except for per share and *Equity Funding* Programs data.)				
Total Revenues	$ 47,684	$ 60,519	$ 95,056	$ 106,413	$ 130,951
Earnings Before					
Extraordinary Items	$ 2,736	$ 7,063	$ 11,891	$ 13,891	$ 19,332
Net Earnings	$ 2,786	$ 9,285	$ 12,527	$ 12,870	$ 18,192
Earnings Per Common and Common Equivalent Share —					
Before Extraordinary Items	$ .52	$ 1.17	$ 1.69	$ 1.86	$ 2.45
Net Earnings	$ .53	$ 1.53	$ 1.79	$ 1.72	$ 2.31
Earnings Per Common Share — Assuming Full Dilution —					
Before Extraordinary Items	$ .46	$ 1.04	$ 1.67	$ 1.84	$ 2.36
Net Earnings	$ .46	$ 1.36	$ 1.75	$ 1.71	$ 2.23
Life Insurance Sold —					
Equity Funding Life	$ 54,222	$ 104,741	$ 393,294	$ 840,228	$1,149,732
Bankers	375,084	431,390	311,739	364,363	630,539
Total	$ 429,306	$ 536,131	$ 705,033	$1,204,591	$1,780,271
Life Insurance In Force At Year End —					
Equity Funding Life	$ 109,228	$ 187,256	$ 506,330	$1,234,258	$2,163,549
Bankers	1,858,304	2,066,691	2,155,107	2,263,254	2,472,440
Total	$1,967,532	$2,254,217	$2,661,437	$3,497,512	$4,635,989
Mutual Fund Assets Under Management At Year End	$ 15,418	$ 75,475	$ 194,862	$ 174,116	$ 210,554
Equity Funding Programs —					
Sold	3,912	5,783	9,354	11,139	13,813
In Effect At Year End	12,020	16,682	23,939	31,892	41,121

See Financial Statements of the Company at pages 11 to 13, the insurance operations tables at pages 31 and 32, mutual fund management information at page 41, and the *Equity Funding* Programs sales tables at page 36. Information concerning the life insurance operations of Northern Life Insurance Company begins at page 51.

THE COMPANY

Equity Funding Corporation of America (the "Company" or "EFCA") is primarily engaged in the marketing of financial services products offered by its subsidiaries or other companies it manages, insurance operations and the management of assets resulting from its marketing activities and insurance operations. The products sold by the Company include life and accident and health insurance, which, together with related insurance operations, accounted for 55% of the Company's total revenues and 67% of its net earnings, before taxes and extraordinary items in 1971, and mutual fund shares and limited partnership investments. EFCA created and is the recognized leader in the sale of insurance premium funding programs — plans for the acquisition of mutual fund shares and insurance, which involve the financing of insurance premiums through loans secured by the investor's mutual fund shares. The programs offered by the Company are known as *Equity Funding* Programs. As a result of the marketing of financial service products offered by subsidiaries and other companies managed by EFCA, the Company also engages in significant asset management operations.

Until 1966, EFCA was engaged almost exclusively in the sale of life insurance policies and mutual fund shares issued by others. Since then, the Company has become directly involved in the insurance and mutual fund businesses through the acquisition of four insurance companies and the formation and acquisition of mutual fund managers and distributors. Within the past several years the Company has substantially increased its sales force as a result of internal growth and acquisitions, has acquired two savings and loan associations and has become involved in real estate and cattle operations and oil and gas ventures, as well as certain stock exchange brokerage activities. See "Certain Recent Acquisitions."

The following table indicates, for the periods shown, the approximate percentages of the Company's total revenues and the percentage of its net earnings before taxes and extraordinary items, which are represented by its significant revenue sources. Insurance operations, except for 1967, are reflected in the table shown on the basis of generally accepted accounting principles.

Revenue Sources	1967	1968	1969	1970	1971
Total Revenues (Including Unconsolidated Subsidiary) (000's)	$ 53,589	$ 66,855	$ 99,586	$114,079	$138,218
Percentage of Total Revenues (Including Unconsolidated Subsidiary):					
Insurance Sales and Operations(1)	80%	77%	61%	59%	55%
Securities Sales(2)	4%	8%	20%	14%	10%
Real Estate Operations	—	—	—	—	14%
Net Earnings Before Taxes and Extraordinary Items (Including Unconsolidated Subsidiary) (000's)	$ 6,292	$ 12,116	$ 19,490	$ 20,544	$ 26,904
Percentage of Net Earnings Before Taxes and Extraordinary Items (Including Unconsolidated Subsidiary) (3):					
Insurance Sales and Operations	92%	63%	54%	63%	67%
Securities Sales(2)	9%	16%	26%	14%	10%
Real Estate Operations	—	—	—	—	3%

(1) Consisting of the following:

	1967	1968	1969	1970	1971
Premiums	55%	52%	40%	43%	40%
Commissions (Unaffiliated Sources)	13%	14%	12%	7%	5%
Interest and Investment Income	12%	11%	9%	9%	10%

(2) Until 1970 virtually all securities sales income was represented by commissions on sales of mutual fund shares or mutual fund contractual plans. During 1970 and 1971, 11% and 8% of total revenues was represented by commissions on mutual funds and mutual fund contractual

plan sales, and the balance of the Company's securities sales revenues was accounted for by regional stock exchange brokerage commissions, the sale of limited partnership interests, and other securities activities.

(3) Selling, general and administrative expense and interest and amortization of debt expense has been allocated to the various sources of income in such amounts as the Company considers appropriate.

The Company has a continuous need for funds to finance its *Equity Funding* Programs and for general corporate purposes. Such funds are realized from cash generated in the Company's operations and the sale of debt securities which in the past have, in some cases, included rights to acquire Common Stock of the Company. The Company may at any time be involved in negotiations with lenders, including banks, or it may be involved in acquisition discussions which also could involve the issuance of its debt or equity securities. See "Capitalization" in this connection. The Company has no current agreements, nor do any agreements in principle exist, for any significant acquisitions. The Company has in the past guaranteed, and expects from time to time in the future to guarantee, debt and other obligations of its subsidiaries and affiliates. A material deterioration in stock market conditions might adversely affect the Company's business.

EFCA was incorporated in Delaware in 1960. Its executive offices are located at 1900 Avenue of the Stars, Los Angeles, California 90067. Its telephone number at that address is 213-553-2100. Unless the context otherwise requires, the term "Company" or "EFCA" as used herein includes the Company's subsidiaries all of which are wholly-owned directly or indirectly, except for Northern Life Insurance Company which is 91.2% owned by the Company.

DIVIDENDS

During the five years ended December 31, 1971, the Company has paid cash or stock dividends and has effected stock splits as indicated in its Consolidated Statement of Earnings. On May 8, 1972, the Company also paid a cash dividend of $.10 per share of Common Stock. The payment of dividends in the future will be in the discretion of the Company's Board of Directors and will depend upon conditions then existing, including the Company's earnings, financial requirements, general business conditions and other factors, and will be subject to the prior dividend rights, if any, of the Company's then outstanding preferred stock and limitations contained in certain of its debt instruments. Under the Revolving Credit Agreement, described under "Capitalization", which imposes the most restrictive of such limitations, if borrowings are outstanding thereunder, the payment of cash dividends in any fiscal year is limited to 25% of the Company's net income for the immediately preceding fiscal year. Borrowings are currently outstanding under the Revolving Credit Agreement. For the balance of 1972, approximately $3,807,000 is available for the payment of cash dividends under the limitations contained in the Revolving Credit Agreement.

PRICE RANGE OF COMMON STOCK

The following tables sets forth the high and low prices for the Company's Common Stock on the American Stock Exchange through October 16, 1970, and on the New York Stock Exchange after that date, for the periods indicated through September 11, 1972. All prices have been adjusted for stock dividends and stock splits.

	1970 Quarters			1971 Quarters				1972 Quarters		
	2nd	3rd	4th	1st	2nd	3rd	4th	1st	2nd	3rd*
High	52½	31	30	43⅜	47	45⅜	43⅝	43	46½	42⅜
Low	12¾	17	21⅝	23⅞	36½	33⅜	27¾	31¾	35¼	33⅞

* Through September 11, 1972

On September 11, 1972, the closing price of the Common Stock on the New York Stock Exchange was $36¼ per share. The Company's Common Stock is also listed on the Pacific Coast and Midwest Stock Exchanges.

7.

CAPITALIZATION

The following table shows the capitalization of the Company and its consolidated subsidiaries at June 30, 1972. No adjustment has been made to give effect to the issuance of Common Stock upon the exercise of outstanding options or warrants, the conversion of any of the 5¼% Guaranteed (Subordinated) Debentures due 1989, or the reduction in the principal amount of such Debentures upon any conversion thereof. There is, of course, no assurance that any options or warrants will, in fact, be exercised or that any conversions will be effected.

	Amount Outstanding	Amount To Be Outstanding
Short-Term Debt:		
Notes Payable to Banks bearing interest ranging from 5¼% to 7%	$10,317,000	$10,317,000
Current Portion of Long-Term Debt:		
7% and 8½% Promissory Notes due 1972	5,168,000	5,168,000
Other	3,449,000	3,449,000
Equity Funding Programs Debt:		
Notes Payable for Insurance Premium Loans(1)	2,713,000	2,713,000
Custodial Collateral Notes(2)	31,306,000	31,306,000
Long-Term Debt:		
Senior Debt—		
5¼% Promissory Notes(3)	41,000,000	41,000,000
9½% Debentures due 1990, $40,000,000 authorized exclusive of bond discount	22,000,000	22,000,000
8⅝% Promissory Note due 1975(4)	5,030,000	5,030,000
7¼% Promissory Notes due 1974 and 1975	6,000,000	6,000,000
Sundry Notes Payable bearing interest ranging from 3½ to 8¾%	20,098,000	20,098,000
Subordinated Debt—		
5¼% Guaranteed (Subordinated) Debentures due 1989	22,917,000	22,917,000
7½% Guaranteed (Subordinated) Notes due 1974	3,270,000	3,270,000
5½% Convertible Subordinated Debentures due 1991	38,500,000	38,500,000
Capital Stock:		
Preferred Stock, no par value, 2,000,000 shares authorized	24,562 Shs.(5)	24,562 Shs.(5)
Common Stock, $.30 par value, 30,000,000 shares authorized(6)	7,860,408 Shs.(7)	7,860,408 Shs.(7)

NOTES TO CAPITALIZATION

(1) Represented by various borrowings bearing interest at an average rate of approximately 6½% per annum. The notes are secured directly or indirectly by mutual fund shares relating to Programs sold prior to October 1963, and, except as to $1,113,000 principal amount of notes maturing on several dates through September 1972, are demand notes. The notes are included in "Notes and Loans Payable: Funded loans and accounts receivable" in the Company's Consolidated Balance Sheet.

(2) Issued in connection with the financing of Programs. The Custodial Collateral Notes mature not later than ten years from the date of their issuance and bear an average interest rate of approximately 5½% per annum. The principal amount of the Custodial Collateral Notes is secured by an equal principal amount of notes receivable from investors participating in the Programs. The notes receivable are collateralized by mutual fund shares purchased by such investors who have no personal liability as to any deficiencies on their notes. EFCA has no liability with respect to $3,306,000 of Custodial Collateral Notes, except as to interest. The Custodial Collateral Notes are included in "Notes and Loans Payable: Funded loans and accounts receivable" in the Company's Consolidated Balance Sheet.

(3) Issued under the Revolving Credit Agreement described below.

(4) Secured by 200,000 shares of Equity Funding Life Common Stock, representing 40% of that subsidiary's outstanding shares.

(5) Series B Convertible Voting Preferred Stock, $100 stated value and convertible into Common Stock of EFCA.

(6) Except where the context otherwise requires, all references in this Prospectus to number of shares of Common Stock have been adjusted to give effect to stock dividends and splits of the Company's Common Stock.

(7) Does not include (i) 63,568 treasury shares, and (ii) a total of 3,274,817 shares reserved as follows: (a) 709,238 shares reserved for stock option plans (the 337,902 shares subject to options are issuable at prices ranging from $14.75 to $74.51, see "The Offerings — Stock Options Plans"), (b) 41,856 shares reserved for Common Stock Purchase Warrants (exercisable at $58.46 per share) originally attached to the 7½% Guaranteed (Subordinated) Notes due 1974, (c) 462,782 shares reserved for conversion of the 5¼% Guaranteed (Subordinated) Debentures due 1989 (convertible at $49.52 per share), (d) 30,900 shares reserved for Common Stock Purchase Warrants (exercisable at $68 per share) granted in connection with the acquisition of Independent Securities Corporation, (e) 550,000 shares reserved for Warrants (exercisable at $25.25 per share) issued with the 9½% Debentures due 1990, (f) 70,471 shares reserved for conversion of the Series B Convertible Preferred Stock (convertible at $35 per share), (g) 343,780 shares reserved for the Company's Employee Stock Bonus Plan, (h) 1,047,620 shares reserved for issuance upon conversion of the 5½% Convertible Subordinated Debentures due 1991 (convertible at $36.75 per share, and (i) 18,170 shares reserved for issuance under the terms of an acquisition agreement.

(8) In addition to consolidated debt of EFCA, (i) at June 30, 1972, Liberty Savings and Loan Association ("Liberty"), an unconsolidated subsidiary of EFCA, had deposits of $94,712,000 and notes payable in installments through 1974 in the total principal amount of $7,445,000, and (ii) the Company has guaranteed payment of certain indebtedness of the cattle partnerships it manages. (See "Business — Asset Management — Limited Partnership Management".)

SCHEDULE OF FIXED PAYMENTS

Fixed payments of the Company and its consolidated subsidiaries on long-term debt, representing principal and interest requirements, rental payments and real and personal property taxes (based on payments made during the year ended December 31, 1971) for each of the five years ending December 31, 1976 are as follows:

	1972	1973	1974	1975	1976
Long-Term Debt: (1)					
Principal	$17,510,000 (2)	$ 4,625,000	$10,444,000	$ 6,649,000	$ 3,885,000
Interest	9,282,000	10,022,000	9,724,000	8,769,000	8,424,000
Rental Payments	3,294,000	3,294,000	3,294,000	3,294,000	3,294,000
Real & Personal Property Taxes	201,000	201,000	201,000	201,000	201,000
	$30,287,000	$18,142,000	$23,663,000	$18,913,000	$15,804,000

(1) Does not include debt secured by notes and mutual fund shares of participants in *Equity Funding* Programs.

(2) Of this amount, $4,992,000 has been paid from the proceeds of a long-term debt obligation. The principal and interest requirements of such obligation are included in the table. Also included in the table are the principal and interest requirements for three unsecured notes totaling $8,000,000 issued in the acquisition of Northern Life Insurance Company and $41,000,000 of notes issued under the Revolving Credit Agreement.

Liberty is not included in the above table. Its fixed payments are as follows:

	1972	1973	1974	1975	1976
Advances From Federal Home Loan Bank:					
Principal	$12,725,000	$ 441,000	$ 1,136,000	$ 441,000	$ 441,000
Interest	698,000	281,000	239,000	165,000	135,000
Rental Payments	180,000	180,000	180,000	180,000	180,000
Real & Personal Property Taxes	33,000	33,000	33,000	33,000	33,000
	$13,634,000	$ 935,000	$ 1,588,000	$ 819,000	$ 789,000

Of the long-term debt due in 1972, $9,907,000 of consolidated debt (exclusive of the $4,992,000 referred to in Note (2) above) has been paid by the Company and $9,502,000 of Liberty's debt has been paid as of June 30, 1972.

REVOLVING CREDIT AGREEMENT

The Company has entered into a Revolving Credit Agreement ("Agreement"), dated as of June 29, 1972, with First National City Bank, Franklin National Bank, The Wells Fargo Bank, National Association and National Bank of North America ("Banks") under which it may effect borrowings not to exceed $75,000,000 at any one time until June 30, 1975. Loans will be evidenced by notes payable by the Company in quarterly installments due between September 30, 1976, and June 30, 1980. Each note shall bear a fluctuating per annum rate of interest of (i) the prime rate of interest charged from time to time by First National City Bank on 90-day loans to June 30, 1973, (ii) ¼% above such prime rate thereafter to June 30, 1975. (iii) thereafter to June 30, 1976, at ½% above the prime rate, and (iv) thereafter until payment in full at 1% above the prime rate. The Company also must pay a commitment fee at the rate of ½% per annum, from the date of the Agreement to June 30, 1975, on the average daily unused portion of the commitment of the Banks.

Borrowings under the Agreement are secured by the pledge of all of the outstanding stock of Bankers National Life Insurance Company, 91.2% of the outstanding stock of Northern Life Insurance Company, and 60% of the outstanding stock of Equity Funding Life Insurance Company, the Company's principal life insurance subsidiaries. Upon the acquisition by the Company of the minority interest in Northern Life Insurance Company and the release of the balance of the outstanding stock of Equity Funding Life Insurance Company, which now secures other indebtedness of the Company, all of such shares must be pledged under the Agreement.

Among other terms of the Agreement, the Company must, so long as any note is outstanding under the Agreement, unless otherwise permitted by any three banks holding 66⅔% or more of the notes: (1) maintain "consolidated tangible net worth" of not less than $150,000,000; (2) prepay notes outstanding under the Agreement in an amount equal to the net cash proceeds received by the Company from (i) any sale or issuance of debt securities, with certain exceptions, or (ii) any sale or other disposition of the Company's assets, other than in the ordinary course of business; and (3) add to the collateral securing the notes any securities received by the Company as a result of any sale referred to in (2) above.

Furthermore, so long as any note is outstanding under the Agreement the Company may not without the consent of three banks holding 66⅔% or more of the notes: (1) incur certain indebtedness and liens; (2) incur consolidated long-term lease obligations in excess of $4,000,000 annually; (3) incur any liability under an obligation of anyone other than a subsidiary of the Company, except by endorsement of negotiatble instruments or in other transactions in the ordinary course of business; (4) effect any merger, consolidation, sale, lease or other transfer of assets, deemed material by the Banks; (5) acquire for cash, the stock, assets or obligations of anyone (except U.S. government obligations), except in the ordinary course of business; (6) make loans or advances to Bishops Bank and Trust Company, a Company subsidiary, in an amount at any one time exceeding $5,000,000 on a consolidated basis; (7) make cash investments which exceed the cumulative amount at any one time outstanding of $12,000,000 in oil and gas exploration or development, $20,000,000 in real property with certain exceptions, $5,000,000 in livestock and breeding herds, and $5,000,000 in any other business other than the marketing of life insurance or mutual fund shares and (8) declare or pay cash dividends during any fiscal year in excess of 25% of the Company's net income for the immediately preceding fiscal year.

Each borrowing under the Agreement is subject to certain conditions as to compliance with representation and warranties and other matters. The Company has effected $41,000,000 of borrowings under the Agreement to date, of which $31,200,000 was used to meet part of the purchase price for the acquisition of Northern Life Insurance Company.

Some of the lending banks under this Agreement are also involved in financing loans in connection with the Company's *Equity Funding* Programs. See "Marketing — Financial Services Products — *Equity Funding* Programs".

EQUITY FUNDING CORPORATION OF AMERICA AND SUBSIDIARIES

Consolidated Statement of Earnings

The following consolidated statement of earnings has been compiled as explained in Note 1 to the Company's consolidated financial statements. The statements for the four years ended December 31, 1970 have been examined by Wolfson, Weiner, Ratoff & Lapin, independent certified public accountants, whose opinion appears elsewhere in this Prospectus. The statement for the year ended December 31, 1971 has been examined by Seidman & Seidman, independent certified public accountants, successors to the practice of Wolfson, Weiner, Ratoff & Lapin, and whose opinion also appears elsewhere in this Prospectus. This statement should be read in conjunction with the related consolidated financial statements and notes thereto included elsewhere in this Prospectus.

				Year Ended December 31,	
	1967	**1968**	**1969**	**1970**	**1971**
	Restated (A)	Restated (A)	Restated (A)	Restated (A)	
REVENUES					
Insurance — premiums and commissions	$36,748,000	$44,179,000	$51,909,000	$ 56,540,000	$ 62,482,000
Securities	2,044,000	5,002,000	19,955,000	16,022,000	14,824,000
Real estate	—	7,000	3,329,000	8,731,000	18,996,000
Natural resources	—	83,000	3,502,000	7,668,000	10,532,000
Investment management	—	1,557,000	2,134,000	1,446,000	1,712,000
Interest and investment income	7,571,000	8,543,000	12,468,000	15,160,000	20,314,000
Other	950,000	720,000	920,000	324,000	1,276,000
Earnings from Liberty Savings and Loan Association (Note 1)	(253,000)	428,000	839,000	522,000	815,000
Statutory earnings from Equity Funding Life Insurance Co.	624,000	—			
Total Revenues	47,684,000	60,519,000	95,056,000	106,413,000	130,951,000
COSTS AND EXPENSES					
Insurance:					
Insurance benefits	14,325,000	15,511,000	17,133,000	16,685,000	16,959,000
Increase in reserves	9,213,000	10,355,000	8,293,000	13,463,000	14,657,000
Commissions	7,287,000	7,653,000	10,636,000	9,065,000	10,260,000
	30,825,000	33,519,000	36,062,000	39,213,000	41,876,000
Securities commissions	1,007,000	2,061,000	7,880,000	5,341,000	5,021,000
Real estate, cost of sales	—	37,000	3,000,000	7,740,000	17,472,000
Natural resources, cost of sales	—	59,000	2,313,000	4,795,000	7,236,000
Interest and amortization of debt expense	1,432,000	1,620,000	4,922,000	6,964,000	9,325,000
Selling, general and administrative expenses	5,661,000	8,888,000	18,531,000	19,006,000	19,907,000
Dividends and income allocable to policyholders	1,920,000	1,897,000	2,251,000	2,874,000	3,478,000
Minority interest	(24,000)	(27,000)	3,000	76,000	—
Total Costs and Expenses	40,821,000	48,054,000	74,962,000	86,009,000	104,315,000
Earnings Before Income Taxes	6,863,000	12,465,000	20,094,000	20,404,000	26,636,000
Income taxes (Note 7)	4,127,000	5,402,000	8,203,000	6,513,000	7,304,000
Earnings before Extraordinary Items	2,736,000	7,063,000	11,891,000	13,891,000	19,332,000
Extraordinary items, less applicable income taxes (B)	50,000	2,222,000	636,000	(1,021,000)	(1,140,000)
Net Earnings	2,786,000	9,285,000	12,527,000	12,870,000	18,192,000
Dividends on Preferred Stock	—	—	—	(43,000)	(21,000)
Net Earnings Available for Common Stock	$ 2,786,000	$ 9,285,000	$12,527,000	$ 12,827,000	$ 18,171,000
Earnings per common and common equivalent share (C):					
Earnings before extraordinary items	$ .52	$1.17	$1.69	$1.86	$2.45
Extraordinary items	.01	.36	.10	(.14)	(.14)
Net Earnings	$ .53	$1.53	$1.79	$1.72	$2.31
Earnings per common share assuming full dilution (C):					
Earnings before extraordinary items	$ .46	$1.04	$1.67	$1.84	$2.36
Extraordinary items	—	.32	.08	(.13)	(.13)
Net Earnings	$ .46	$1.36	$1.75	$1.71	$2.23
COMMON STOCK DISTRIBUTIONS:					
Stock dividends	5%	3%	2%	2%	—
Cash dividends	—	—	—	$ .10	$ .10
Stock splits	3 for 2	2 for 1	—	—	—

See accompanying notes following this page. Numerical note references are to notes to the Company's consolidated financial statements.

(A) The amounts by which revenues, net earnings and earnings per share have been restated to give effect to the acquisitions of Bankers National Life Insurance Co. and Liberty Savings and Loan Association, accounted for as poolings of interests, are as follows:

| | Year Ended December 31, | | | |
	1967	1968	1969	1970
Revenues:				
Before poolings	$11,878,000	$21,922,000	$51,204,000	$ 61,476,000
Bankers	36,134,000	38,588,000	43,481,000	44,906,000
Liberty	(328,000)	9,000	371,000	31,000
Restated	$47,684,000	$60,519,000	$95,056,000	$106,413,000
Net earnings:				
Before poolings	$ 2,531,000	$ 7,881,000	$10,509,000	$ 11,250,000
Bankers	583,000	1,324,000	1,647,000	1,589,000
Liberty	(328,000)	80,000	371,000	31,000
Restated	$ 2,786,000	$ 9,285,000	$12,527,000	$ 12,870,000
Earnings per common and common equivalent share:				
Before extraordinary items:				
Before poolings	$ .71	$1.34	$1.89	$2.16
Bankers and Liberty	(.19)	(.17)	(.20)	(.30)
Restated	$ .52	$1.17	$1.69	$1.86
Net earnings:				
Before poolings	$ .72	$1.85	$2.01	$1.98
Bankers and Liberty	(.19)	(.32)	(.22)	(.26)
Restated	$ .53	$1.53	$1.79	$1.72
Earnings per common share assuming full dilution:				
Before extraordinary items:				
Before poolings	$ .58	$1.15	$1.84	$2.11
Bankers and Liberty	(.12)	(.11)	(.17)	(.27)
Restated	$ .46	$1.04	$1.67	$1.84
Net earnings:				
Before poolings	$ .59	$1.56	$1.96	$1.94
Bankers and Liberty	(.13)	(.20)	(.21)	(.23)
Restated	$ .46	$1.36	$1.75	$1.71

The results of operations shown in the Consolidated Statement of Operations have also been restated to give effect to the rescission of the Company's Diversified Land Company acquisition. See Note 1 to the Company's Consolidated Financial Statements.

(B) The extraordinary income shown for 1967, $50,000, is the result of a credit from a tax loss carryover as reflected in the books of Equity Funding Life Insurance Company. Of the 1968 extraordinary income, $145,000 was due to the tax loss carryover of the insurance company. The remaining portion was made up of the following items: The net gain recognized on Whittington Oil Co., Inc. securities — $1,924,000, the sale of various securities — $36,000, a franchise tax refund — $42,000 and the net gain on the sale of real estate — $75,000. The applicable taxes were $2,459,000, $12,000, $10,000 and $42,000 respectively. In 1969 the insurance company tax loss carryover of $410,000 was credited to extraordinary income. Also included was the net gain of $230,000 from the sale of Pension Life Insurance Co. The related taxes were

$294,000. The remaining debit item of $4,000 is due to miscellaneous adjustments. In 1970 the items credited to extraordinary income were the gain realized upon the repurchase, at a discount, of certain promissory notes — $425,000, net of taxes of $475,000 and the effect of Equity Funding Life Insurance Company's change to generally accepted accounting principles in the amount of $68,000. The net reductions to extraordinary income were the write-downs to market value of Whittington Oil Co., Inc. securities — $1,391,000 and the reduction in the investment in a cattle partnership — $123,000. These amounts are net of tax reductions of $1,553,000 and $137,000, respectively. The 1971 extraordinary item consists of foreign currency exchange rate losses, $936,000, and the write-downs to market value of Whittington Oil Co., Inc. securities, $155,000, and other investments, $49,000; these amounts are net of tax reductions of $999,000, $166,000 and $51,000, respectively.

(C) Earnings per common and common equivalent share were computed based on the weighted average number of common shares outstanding during the year, and the shares issued for an acquisition accounted for as a pooling of interests, and common stock equivalents consisting of Series B Convertible Preferred stock and common stock purchase warrants and options, if dilutive, reduced by the number of shares that could be purchased with the proceeds from the exercise of the warrants and options. The average number of common and common equivalent shares was as follows: 1967, 5,294,000 shares; 1968, 6,055,000 shares; 1969, 7,018,000 shares; 1970, 7,453,000 shares; and 1971, 7,883,000 shares.

Earnings per common share assuming full dilution were computed based on the weighted average of common and common equivalent shares, and on the assumption that the 5½% convertible subordinated debentures due 1991, and the 5¼% guaranteed subordinated debentures due 1989, were converted (eliminating the related interest expense, net of applicable income taxes, resulting in fully diluted earnings available for common stock of $2,910,000, $9,558,000, $12,619,000, $13,499,000, and $18,849,000 for the years 1967, 1968, 1969, 1970, and 1971, respectively), and that contingently issuable shares were issued, resulting in an average number of common shares as follows: 1967, 6,267,000 shares; 1968, 7,025,000 shares; 1969, 7,193,000 shares; 1970, 7,895,000 shares; and 1971, 8,475,000 shares.

(D) The following table shows the ratio of earnings to fixed charges for the years ended December 31, 1967 through 1971. The ratio of earnings to fixed charges represent the number of times that interest, debt expense, one-third of rentals and preferred dividends were covered by the sum of earnings before income taxes, interest, debt expense and one-third of rentals.

	Year Ended December 31,				
	1967	1968	1969	1970	1971
Net earnings before extraordinary items	5.42	7.98	4.71	3.53	3.59
Net earnings available for common stock	5.46	10.64	4.88	3.25	3.36

The following summary indicates the results of the Company's consolidated operations for the six months ended June 30, 1971 and 1972. The figures shown in the summary are unaudited and all adjustments, consisting only of normal recurring accruals, necessary for a fair presentation of the results shown have been made.

	Six Months Ended June 30,	
	1971(a)	1972
Total revenues	$61,000,000	$62,316,000
Net earnings	$ 8,854,000	$10,441,000
Net earnings — common stock	$ 8,833,000	$10,441,000
Earnings per common and common equivalent share	$1.12	$1.30
Earnings per common share assuming full dilution	$1.09	$1.17

(a) Restated to reflect the consolidation of the Company's insurance operations, the acquisition of Bankers National Life Insurance Company and Liberty on a pooling of interests basis and the rescission of the Diversified Land Company acquisition. The results shown in the summary do not include Northern Life Insurance Company.

14

EQUITY FUNDING LIFE INSURANCE COMPANY

Statement of Operations

The following statement of operations has been prepared on the basis of generally accepted accounting principles (adjusted basis) with respect to the four years ended December 31, 1971, and on the basis of accounting practices prescribed or authorized by the Insurance Department of the State of Illinois (statutory basis) with respect to the year ended December 31, 1967. The statement for the four years ended December 31, 1971, has been examined by Haskins & Sells, independent certified public accountants; the opinion of said firm, which as referred to therein is based, as to policy reserves, net deferred and uncollected life premiums, and accrued costs of recapture of reinsured policies on the opinion of independent consulting actuaries, and as to amounts applicable to certain accident and health business on the report of other independent accountants, appears elsewhere herein. The statement for the year ended December 31, 1967, has been examined by Arthur Young & Company, independent certified public accountants, as set forth in their report included elsewhere herein. This statement should be read in conjunction with its notes and the other Equity Life financial statements and the notes thereto, together with the above-mentioned opinions and reports, included elsewhere herein.

	Statutory Basis(a) Year Ended December 31,		Adjusted Basis(c) Year Ended December 31,		
	1967(b)	1968	1969	1970	1971
Premiums and Other Considerations (net of reinsurance ceded):					
Life	$ 811,719	$ 780,079	$ 3,130,791	$11,010,514	$16,839,624
Accident and health(e)	42,352	1,566,036	2,100,502	173,919	356,898
Considerations for supplementary contracts without life contingencies	—	—	144,052	10,166	—
Total	854,071	2,346,115	5,375,345	11,194,599	17,196,522
Coinsurance Considerations(d)	—	535,782	2,342,777	4,374,200	5,748,766
Investment Income:					
Interest on bonds	99,885	74,475	75,405	55,282	421,185
Interest on policy loans	11,260	734	1,965	2,253	2,922
Interest on certificates of deposit	—	8,410	248,221	89,514	178,677
Interest on mortgage loans	—	—	18,548	33,927	167
Interest on loans to parent company and its affiliates	—	55,342	28,750	497,989	57,052
Other	4,314	—	—	1,060	3,071
Total investment income	115,459	138,961	372,889	680,025	663,074
Investment expense	1,727	647	2,541	2,094	1,540
Net investment income	113,732	138,314	370,348	677,931	661,534
Other income:					
Service fees from parent company	—	205,651	89,820	100,000	—
Coinsurance renewal allowances(d)	—	—	—	—	686,323
Total income	967,803	3,225,862	8,178,290	16,346,730	24,293,145

Policy Benefits and Reserves:					
Death and other benefits under life policies	264,494	179,030	90,606	156,660	641,970
Benefits under accident and health policies(e)	14,793	101,929	383,704	19,277	87,606
Increase (decrease) in policy reserves:					
Life	(702,490)	58,794	(366,181)	3,257,850	4,524,633
Accident and health(e)	—	613,992	(574,580)	25,754	46,934
Supplementary contracts without life contingencies	—	—	118,101	(567)	(2,656)
Total	(423,203)	953,745	(348,350)	3,458,974	5,298,487
Remainder	1,391,006	2,272,117	8,526,640	12,887,756	18,994,658
Operating Expenses:					
Life commissions(g) (Note 3)	453,188	78,997	1,299,836	3,921,254	5,496,090
Accident and health commissions(e)	114	769,618	2,041,077	112,426	59,865
Other policy acquisition costs (including recapture costs) (Note 3)	—	25,765	859,988	1,115,667	2,306,911
Salaries and other general expenses	761,979	804,912	189,537	362,182	924,487
Taxes, licenses and fees	61,726	85,259	148,717	197,663	596,952
Increase (decrease) in loading on deferred and un- collected premiums	(25,007)	(28,664)	226,320	362,414	205,788
Total	1,252,000	1,735,887	4,765,475	6,071,606	9,590,093
	139,006	536,230	3,761,165	6,816,150	9,404,565
Dividends to life policyholders	219	—	—	—	—
Income before loss on sale of investments, etc.	138,787	536,230	3,761,165	6,816,150	9,404,565
Loss on sale of investments	—	6,905	631,750	41,504	—
Income before Federal income taxes and extraordinary credit	138,787	529,325	3,129,415	6,774,646	9,404,565
Provisions for Federal income taxes(f)	50,000	145,000	1,013,000	1,680,000	2,325,000
Income before extraordinary credit	88,787	384,325	2,116,415	5,094,646	7,079,565
Credit resulting from tax loss carryover(f)	50,000	145,000	410,000	—	—
Net income	$ 138,787	$ 529,325	$ 2,526,415	$ 5,094,646	$ 7,079,565

(See accompanying notes next page)

15

EQUITY FUNDING LIFE INSURANCE COMPANY

Notes to Statement of Operations

(a) The statement of operations for the year ended December 31, 1967 has been prepared on the basis of accounting practices prescribed or authorized by the Insurance Department of the State of Illinois (statutory basis), which practices differ in certain respects from generally accepted accounting principles. The more important differences applicable to the aforementioned statement pertain to the accounting for commissions and other acquisition costs applicable to the issuance of new policies which were charged to operations when incurred rather than amortized over the expected policy lives and to policy reserves which were based on statutory requirements. In the opinion of management of Equity Life, the effects of variances from generally accepted accounting principles on the statement of operations for the year ended December 31, 1967 are not practicably or reasonably determinable.

(b) In December 1967, Equity Life entered into an agreement with respect to the reinsurance of a block of business for a consideration of $600,000. As a result of this agreement, the provision in 1967 for aggregate life reserves was reduced approximately $1,142,000, premium income was decreased approximately $542,000 and income before Federal income taxes and extraordinary credit was increased approximately $600,000. Another reinsurance agreement was modified during 1967 to retroactively reinsure an additional block of business. The principal effect of this agreement was to reduce premium income for the year approximately $570,000 ($173,000 applicable to prior years) and to reduce expenses and provision for aggregate life reserves approximately $630,000 ($158,000 applicable to prior years). The net effect was to increase 1967 income before Federal income taxes and extraordinary credit approximately $60,000 of which a portion (not material) was attributable to the prior two years. The approximate effect on 1967 results of operations of the two foregoing agreements was to decrease premium income by $1,112,000 and to increase net income by $660,000.

(c) As of December 31, 1970, Equity Life adopted the practice of preparing its financial statements, other than those issued pursuant to requirements of insurance regulatory authorities, in conformity with generally accepted accounting principles, and restated its financial statements for 1968 and 1969 to conform to such practice. See Note 1 to Equity Life's financial statements elsewhere in this Prospectus for additional information. A reconciliation of net gain from operations, determined pursuant to statutory accounting and reporting requirements, and net income as reported herein is as follows:

		Year Ended December 31,		
	1968	1969	1970	1971
Statutory net gain from operations	$ 474,367	$2,928,876	$2,438,989	$3,424,929
Add (Deduct):				
Net change in deferred and accrued policy acquisition and recapture costs	179,629	354,143	5,710,678	6,991,390
Recalculation of policy reserve increase	39,391	99,718	(1,076,371)	(918,970)
Deferred Federal income taxes	—	(253,000)	(2,030,000)	(2,210,000)
Net realized loss on sale of investments	(6,905)	(631,750)	(41,504)	—
Other	(157,157)	28,428	92,854	(207,784)
Total	54,958	(402,461)	2,655,657	3,654,636
Net income reported herein	$ 529,325	$2,526,415	$5,094,646	$7,079,565

(d) During 1968, an aggregate cash consideration of $535,782 was received pursuant to the terms of two coinsurance agreements and policy reserves of about $96,000 were assumed by a coinsurer under one of the agreements. Also a $250,000 expense allowance was received pursuant to the terms of a 1967 coinsurance agreement.

BANKERS NATIONAL LIFE INSURANCE COMPANY

Statement of Operations
(Statutory Statement)

The following statement reflects the results of operations of Bankers and the results of its operations allocable to its stockholders for the periods indicated, stated on the basis of the requirements of the Department of Insurance of the State of New Jersey. The statements for the five years ended December 31, 1971 have been examined by Joseph Froggatt & Co., independent certified public accountants (relying on the certification of the reserves for life policies and contracts by the Commissioner of Insurance of the State of New Jersey), and is included in reliance upon their report appearing elsewhere herein. This statement should be read in conjunction with the other financial statements of Bankers and the notes thereto appearing elsewhere herein.

				Year Ended December 31,	
	1967	1968	1969	1970	1971
Premiums and other considerations:					
Life	$26,646,322	$28,823,114	$28,890,703	$30,364,783	$29,139,911
Accident and health	1,358,382	1,410,070	1,375,839	1,460,730	1,673,920
Consideration for supplementary contracts and coupon accumulations	977,538	913,129	1,005,051	872,955	857,633
Total premiums and other considerations	28,982,242	31,146,313	31,271,593	32,698,468	31,671,464
Investment income:					
Interest on bonds — Note 3	2,420,718	2,706,997	3,278,578	4,172,715	5,040,090
Dividends — unaffiliated companies	279,486	301,102	357,043	296,391	274,247
Interest on mortgage loans — Note 4	2,640,730	2,813,246	2,815,069	3,007,460	2,917,798
Real estate income — Note 5	319,721	357,414	320,718	490,143	543,122
Interest on policy loans	556,635	603,215	725,060	885,240	963,843
Other investment income	12,093	34,428	31,007	53,723	261,827
Gross investment income	6,229,383	6,816,402	7,527,475	8,905,672	10,000,927
Investment expenses	551,979	699,893	716,037	1,036,620	1,161,626
Net investment income	5,677,404	6,116,509	6,811,438	7,869,052	8,839,301
Other income	50,440	70,036	407,811	31,176	116,325
Total	34,710,086	37,332,858	38,490,842	40,598,696	40,627,090
Death and other benefits	14,295,187	15,191,134	16,574,408	16,385,952	16,055,782
Increase in aggregate reserves for all policies	6,987,821	8,099,294	8,165,292	7,275,344	2,983,970
Increase in other reserves	817,221	668,523	45,568	1,786,203	4,871,629
Total	22,100,229	23,958,951	24,785,268	25,447,499	23,911,381
Balance	12,609,857	13,373,907	13,705,574	15,151,197	16,715,709
Expenses:					
Commissions	4,319,762	3,900,793	3,639,929	3,016,881	2,876,103
General insurance expenses	3,651,017	4,035,076	4,137,545	4,884,938	4,851,882
Insurance taxes, licenses and fees	739,323	882,754	941,838	1,024,012	973,045
Interest on funds held by the Company under reinsurance treaties	287,263	347,553	626,388	631,061	452,583
Increase (decrease) in loading on deferred and uncollected premiums	57,715	(144,032)	(132,183)	(101,217)	(171,200)
Total expenses	9,055,080	9,022,144	9,213,517	9,455,675	8,982,413
Net income from insurance and investments	3,554,777	4,351,763	4,492,057	5,695,522	7,733,296
Dividends to policyholders — Note 17	1,945,475	1,750,123	1,746,252	1,781,753	1,634,663
Net income before provision for income taxes	1,609,302	2,601,640	2,745,805	3,913,769	6,098,633
Provision for income taxes — Note 10	519,140	584,816	739,982	1,095,673	1,559,800
Net income — Note 14	$ 1,090,162	$ 2,016,824	$ 2,005,823	$ 2,818,096	$ 4,538,833

Numerical note references are to the Notes to Financial Statements of Bankers appearing elsewhere herein.

EQUITY FUNDING LIFE INSURANCE COMPANY

Notes to Statement of Operations — (Continued)

During the years 1969, 1970, and 1971, the Company entered into significant coinsurance agreements with respect to its new business. The Company's policy has been to reinsure substantial portions of its life business and it intends to continue that policy in the ordinary course of conducting its operations. Under these agreements, the Company retains the first-year premiums on ceded life business and receives considerations from the reinsurers, which, in general, are defined in the agreements as various first year allowances. The Company will not receive renewal premium income on the coinsured portion of its policies; however, it retains all policy fees and the reinsurers will pay the Company allowances of approximately 10% of the renewal premiums. The applicable policy acquisition and recapture costs have been charged against income. The foregoing new business coinsurance transactions are summarized as follows:

	Year Ended December 31,		
	1969	1970	1971
Premiums retained	$3,023,000	$5,479,000	$7,188,000
Coinsurance considerations	2,343,000	4,374,000	5,749,000
Policy acquisition and recapture costs	(2,132,000)	(4,298,000)	(6,536,000)
Excess of premiums and considerations over acquisition and recapture costs	$3,234,000	$5,555,000	$6,401,000

For additional information, see Notes 3 and 5 to the Equity Life financial statements and "Reinsurance" under the caption "Business — Insurance Sales and Operations" appearing elsewhere in this Prospectus.

(e) Substantially all of the accident and health business for 1968 and 1969 was produced by a nonrelated company under an agreement which, in general, provided that Equity Life's earnings thereunder would be a specified percentage of net premiums written. As of July 1, 1969, the business covered by the agreement was 100% coinsured and the reinsurer assumed the assets and liabilities related to the business.

Amounts included in the financial statements for 1968 and 1969 regarding this business are based on schedules of accounts which were submitted by the producing company.

(f) The provisions for Federal income taxes consist of the following:

	1967	1968	Year Ended December 31,		
			1969	1970	1971
Current (credit)			$ 350,000	$ (350,000)	$ 115,000
Charge equivalent to tax reduction resulting from utilization of tax operating loss carryforward	$50,000	$145,000	410,000		
Deferred			253,000	2,030,000	2,210,000
Total	$50,000	$145,000	$1,013,000	$1,680,000	$2,325,000

Deferred Federal income taxes relate primarily to the excess of deductions for life policy reserves and policy acquisition costs claimed for tax purposes over amounts charged against income for financial accounting purposes. See Note 6 to Equity Life's financial statements elsewhere in this Prospectus for additional information relating to Federal income taxes.

(g) Commissions paid to subsidiaries of Equity Life's parent were approximately $896,000, $3,046,000, $10,125,000, and $12,500,000 during the years ended December 31, 1968, 1969, 1970 and 1971.

(h) Numerical note references are to notes to the Equity Life financial statements.

BANKERS NATIONAL LIFE INSURANCE COMPANY

(Concluded)

Statement of Operations

(Statutory Statement)

Bankers has in force both participating and non-participating insurance. The net income allocated to participating insurance is determined by methods accepted by state regulatory authorities. Income and disbursements not identifiable with either participating or non-participating policies are allocated in accordance with generally accepted formulas and factors. Surplus gains and losses allocable to participating insurance are determined in a similar manner. The earnings on non-participating insurance are allocated to the stockholders. Provisions of the New Jersey statutes limit the amount Bankers may transfer to inure to the benefit of stockholders from participating insurance in any year to a maximum of $0.50 per thousand dollars of participating life insurance in force at the end of the year. Bankers' Charter also has restrictions on the amount of profits which may be allocated to stockholders out of the yearly profits arising from participating policies issued prior to January 1, 1948, but since 1959 the statutory limitation has been more restrictive.

The stockholders' portion of net income (non-participating insurance) adjusted for the transfer of amounts from participating insurance to stockholders is shown below:

	Year Ended December 31,				
	1967	1968	1969	1970	1971
Net income — statutory	$ 1,090,162	$ 2,016,824	$ 2,005,823	$ 2,818,096	$ 4,538,833
Deduct — Net income allocable to policyholders (participating insurance)	872,932	934,018	856,337	1,314,508	915,127
Net income allocable to stockholders (non-participating insurance)	217,230	1,082,806	1,149,486	1,503,588	3,623,706
Amounts transferred to stockholders from participating insurance	296.348	308,490	302,551	312,322	371,480
Net income allocable to stockholders	$ 513,578	$ 1,391,296	$ 1,452,037	$ 1,815,910	$ 3,995,186

BANKERS NATIONAL LIFE INSURANCE COMPANY

Adjusted Statement of Operations

(GAAP Basis)

The following statement shows the net income allocable, to stockholders retroactively adjusted to be in accordance with generally accepted accounting principles, as included in the preliminary draft prepared by the American Institute of Certified Public Accountants released in December 1970.

The Institute is considering comments on the exposure draft and is restudying the subject. The exposure draft has not been adopted by the American Institute of Certified Public Accountants and there is no assurance that it will be adopted, or that it will not be substantially revised before adoption. The following are major differences from reporting practices prescribed by regulatory authorities:

(1) Policy acquisition and issue expenses have been deferred using the natural expense reserve method and are being amortized by charges to income over the term of the policy (but not in excess of twenty years) instead of being charged to expense when incurred; (2) Policy reserves have been adjusted according to the natural benefit reserve method which takes into consideration, among other factors, interest assumptions, persistency assumptions and assumed mortality rates taken from a select and ultimate table which considers Company experience, the method being designed to provide liabilities adequate to discharge benefit obligations over the actuarially computed life of the policies; (3) Deferred Federal income taxes on income are provided for changes in deferred acquisition costs, reserve changes and other cases where there is a difference between the time a deduction is recorded in the statement of income and when it is reported for income tax purposes; (4) Gain on sale of investments, less applicable income tax, is included in net income; (5) Investments in subsidiaries have been included by the equity method as against including them at their statutory net worth. Reference is made to Notes (a), (b) and (c).

The statements for the five years ended December 31, 1971 have been examined by Joseph Froggatt & Co., independent certified public accountants, and should be read in conjunction with the financial statements appearing elsewhere herein, including the related notes and the report of the independent certified public accountants.

	Year Ended December 31,				
	1967	**1968**	**1969**	**1970**	**1971**
Net income (statutory)	$1,090,162	$2,016,824	$2,005,823	$2,818,096	$4,538,833
Retroactive adjustments resulting from adoption of generally accepted accounting principles:					
Deferred acquisition costs(a)	2,454,556	1,171,687	502,454	49,675	(888,389)
Policy reserves(b)	(1,148,476)	(737,554)	(339,015)	(178,221)	(264,840)
Income tax:					
Deferred(c)	(1,569,841)	(614,605)	(273,862)	(109,679)	476,667
Adjusted for prior years	(375,000)	(39,533)	(29,689)	(14,742)	445,369
Net gain (loss) on sale of investments(1)	8,062	(75,711)	537,867	423,041	1,366,265
Equity in gain (loss) of non-consolidated affiliates	(1,183)	(125,394)	(186,371)	(31,510)	(41,437)
Expenses of proposed merger (Fidelity Corporation)(2)	—	—	—	(219,127)	—
Other	99,284	(124,816)	(65,152)	(56,998)	(131,485)
Total additions (deductions)	(532,598)	(545,926)	146,232	(137,561)	962,150
Adjusted net income(c)	557,564	1,470,898	2,152,055	2,680,535	5,500,983
Deduct portion of net income and adjustments to net income allocable to participating policyholders	271,082	455,375	807,122	1,404,347	2,214,103
Adjusted net income allocable to stockholders (non-participating)	286,482	1,015,523	1,344,933	1,276,188	3,286,880
Amounts transferred to stockholders from participating insurance....	296,348	308,490	302,551	312,322	371,480
Adjusted net income allocable to stockholders	582,830	1,324,013	1,647,484	1,588,510	3,658,360
Adjusted net income(c)	$ 582,830	$1,324,013	$1,647,484	$1,588,510	$3,658,360

Adjusted Statement of Operations (Continued)

(GAAP Basis)

(1) Net gain (loss) on sale of investments includes a portion allocable to stockholders as follows: 1967, $2,413; 1968, ($26,113); 1969, $106,906; 1970, $39,922, and 1971, $465,943.

(2) Expenses of the proposed merger (Fidelity Corporation) in the amount of $219,127 previously reported in 1970 as an extraordinary item are included herein as general expenses.

(a) Deferred Acquisition Costs:

Deferred acquisition costs represent life insurance policy acquisition costs which are capitalized and amortized in proportion to the incidence of the present value of premium payments over the term of the policies involved, but not in excess of twenty years. Costs so capitalized are charged immediately to income upon surrender or default in premium payment with respect to a given policy. For Federal income tax purposes deferred acquisition costs are charged to income during the period incurred, reducing the amount of tax which would otherwise be payable. A deferred Federal income tax has been provided as a result of this timing difference.

(b) Adjustment to Policy Reserves:

The policy reserves shown in the supplemental statements with respect to life policies and contracts were computed on the net level premium method using assumptions with respect to rates of interest, mortality and termination. In some instances the reserves so computed are the same as reserves used in previous reports and reports to regulatory authorities. This is the case with respect to all participating policies, non-participating group policies, non-participating policies on a paid-up basis, annuity contracts, and disability and accidental death benefit coverages. The mortality tables and assumed rates of interest most generally used for this group of policies are the Commissioners 1958 Standard Ordinary Mortality Table 2¼%, 3%, 3½%; the Commissioners 1941 Standard Ordinary Mortality Table 2½%, 3%; American Men Ultimate 3%; American Experience 3½% and other miscellaneous tables.

The reserves on non-participating policies, on a premium paying basis, were recomputed utilizing the assumptions inherent in the calculation of gross premiums at the time such policies were issued. For non-participating policies issued in the years 1964 and later, the most generally representative set of assumptions is as follows:

Mortality — Intercompany select experience for male, medically examined lives between the years 1955 and 1959 with a conservative graduation into the ultimate experience table.

Interest — 4½% per year graded down to 4%.

Termination — Linton BA withdrawal table for permanent coverages.
Linton C withdrawal table for term coverages.

For non-participating policies issued in the years prior to 1964 the assumptions used were as follows:

Mortality — 90% of intercompany select experience between the years 1946 and 1949, grading into ultimate experience.

Interest — 4% per annum.

Termination — Linton BA withdrawal table for permanent coverages.
Linton C withdrawal table for term coverages.

21

Adjusted Statement of Operations (Continued)

(GAAP Basis)

Policy reserves used for Federal income tax purposes differ from reserves calculated in accordance with generally accepted accounting principles. A deferred Federal income tax has been provided on this difference. Reference is made to Deferred Federal Income Taxes in Note (c) below.

(c) Provision for Deferred Federal Income Tax:

Provision has been made for deferred Federal income taxes with respect to timing differences between income as reported for tax return purposes and income as reported in accordance with generally accepted accounting principles. The most significant differences relate to deferred acquisition costs which are expensed for annual statement and tax reporting purposes but capitalized in the supplemental statements; and, deductions with respect to policy reserves which are recalculated on a Natural Benefit Reserve basis. The reserve for deferred taxes on the timing differences has been computed on the basis of the full corporate rate for the years 1970 and prior in effect in the year the items of adjustment occurred with further provision for subsequent amortization. Other provisions have been made for deferred tax credits with respect to deductions unused for tax purposes, and other miscellaneous timing differences. This represents maximum provision for applicable taxes which may be payable in future years. Reference is made to Note 10.

The calculation of the necessary provision for deferred Federal income tax for the current year affects the benefits of the Phase III reduction in effective tax rates. (See explanation in Note 10 of Notes to Financial Statements.) The provision for 1970 (and prior years) did not consider the Phase III reduction. As a consequence, the reversal of certain prior years timing differences will result in a reduction of the deferred tax reserve at the full corporate rate rather than the reduced rate used in calculation of the current year's addition to the Deferred tax reserve. Net income for the year 1971 has been benefited because of this reduction in the amount of $324,239.00.

Should be read in conjunction with the Notes to Financial Statements which are made a part hereof.

EQUITY FUNDING CORPORATION OF AMERICA AND SUBSIDIARIES

Pro-Forma Consolidated Financial Statements

The accompanying pro-forma consolidated statement of earnings for the year ended December 31, 1971 gives effect to the acquisition of Northern Life Insurance Company ("Northern") as if it had been consummated as of January 1, 1971. The accompanying pro-forma consolidated balance sheet as of December 31, 1971 gives effect to the acquisition of Northern as if it had been consummated as of that date. These statements are not necessarily indicative of the results of operations as they might have been had the acquisition been consummated at the beginning of 1971, or the financial position at December 31, 1971 had the acquisition been consummated at that date. These statements should be read in conjunction with the financial statements and related notes of Equity Funding Corporation of America and Subsidiaries, and Northern Life Insurance Company included elsewhere herein.

Pro-Forma Consolidated Statement of Earnings
(Unaudited)

		For the Year Ended December 31, 1971		
	EFCA	Northern	Adjustments	Pro-Forma Consolidated
REVENUES				
Insurance-premiums and commissions	$ 62,482,000	$15,774,000		$ 78,256,000
Securities	14,824,000			14,824,000
Real estate	18,996,000			18,996,000
Natural resources	10,532,000			10,532,000
Investment management	1,712,000			1,712,000
Interest and investment income	20,314,000	6,866,000		27,180,000
Other	1,281,000	9,000		1,290,000
Earnings from Liberty Savings & Association	810,000			810,000
Total Revenues	130,951,000	22,649,000		153,600,000
COSTS AND EXPENSES				
Insurance:				
Insurance benefits	16,959,000	12,786,000		29,745,000
Increase in reserves	14,657,000	1,076,000		15,733,000
Commissions	10,260,000	1,650,000		11,910,000
	41,876,000	15,512,000		57,388,000
Securities commissions	5,021,000			5,021,000
Real estate, cost of sales	17,472,000			17,472,000
Natural resources, cost of sales	7,236,000			7,236,000
Interest and amortization of debt expense	9,325,000		$ 2,426,000(2)	11,751,000
Selling, general and administrative expenses	19,907,000	3,319,000	263,000(3)	23,489,000
Dividends and income allocable to policyholders	3,478,000	1,049,000		4,527,000
Minority interest			244,000(4)	244,000
Total Costs and Expenses	104,315,000	19,880,000	2,933,000	127,128,000
Earnings Before Income Taxes (Loss)	26,636,000	2,769,000	(2,933,000)	26,472,000
Income taxes	7,304,000	1,171,000	(1,356,000) (5)	7,119,000
Earnings Before Extraordinary Items	19,332,000	1,598,000	(1,577,000)	19,353,000
Extraordinary items, less applicable income taxes	(1,140,000)	—		(1,140,000)
Net Earnings	18,192,000	1,598,000	(1,577,000)	18,213,000
Dividends on Preferred Stock	(21,000)	—	—	(21,000)
Net Earnings Available for Common Stock	$ 18,171,000	$ 1,598,000	$(1,577,000)	$ 18,192,000
Earnings per common and common equivalent share:				
Earnings before extraordinary items				$2.45
Extraordinary items				(.14)
Net Earnings				$2.31
Earnings per common share assuming full dilution:				
Earnings before extraordinary items				$2.36
Extraordinary items				(.13)
Net Earnings				$2.23

See accompanying notes to Pro-Forma Consolidated Financial Statements.

BUSINESS

EFCA commenced operations in 1960 and until 1966 was engaged almost exclusively in the marketing of life insurance and mutual fund shares issued by others, either separately or in its *Equity Funding* Programs. During 1966 the Company formed Equity Growth Fund of America, Inc. ("Equity Growth Fund") and in 1968 it acquired the investment adviser and manager of Equity Progress Fund, Inc. ("Equity Progress Fund", formerly "Republic Technology Fund, Incorporated"). In 1969 the Company acquired the domestic assets of the investment adviser and manager of Fund of America, Inc. ("Fund of America"). Equity Growth Fund, Equity Progress Fund and Fund of America are registered investment companies under the Investment Company Act of 1940 (the "1940 Act") and their investment adviser and principal distributor are subsidiaries of the Company.

In 1967 the Company acquired Equity Funding Life Insurance Company ("Equity Funding Life", formerly "The Presidential Life Insurance Company of America"), and in 1971 it acquired Bankers National Life Insurance Company ("Bankers") and Equity Funding Life Insurance Company of New York ("Equity Funding Life New York", formerly "Palisades Life Insurance Company"). On June 29, 1972, the Company acquired a 91.2% interest in Northern Life Insurance Company. See "Certain Recent Acquisitions".

During 1967, EFCA also acquired Crown Savings and Loan Association ("Crown"), a savings and loan association, and in 1971, it completed the acquisition of Liberty Savings and Loan Association ("Liberty"), into which Crown has been merged. Since 1969, the Company, also has become involved in real estate and cattle operations, oil and gas exploration, and certain stock exchange brokerage activities.

In the first year of the Company's operations it had approximately 150 sales representatives and 7 sales offices located in California. As a result of internal growth, and certain of the above and other acquisitions, EFCA now has approximately 4,000 sales representatives with approximately 130 sales offices located in 39 states, and over 240 insurance general agents. The Company has keyed its development to the marketing capabilities of its sales force which it continually seeks to improve through training methods, performance standards and product line expansion.

MARKETING — FINANCIAL SERVICES PRODUCTS

Sales Organization

The Company markets its financial services products through its own nationwide sales organization of approximately 4,000 sales representatives and through over 240 insurance general agents who have contracts with its insurance subsidiaries. Most of the sales representatives are dually licensed to sell both life insurance and mutual fund shares. During 1971, 31% of the Company's life insurance sales (exclusive of Northern Life Insurance Company's sales) were made in California, 9% in Pennsylvania and 7% in New Jersey, and approximately 29% of its mutual fund share sales, including mutual funds sold under contractual plans, were effected in New York and approximately 22% of mutual fund sales were made in California. The Company sells primarily to middle-income customers.

Sales representatives are compensated on a commission basis under agreements appointing them independent contractors. In addition, they may earn commission bonuses based on their individual production. Stock options granted and to be granted by the Company as an incentive to certain sales representatives and supervisors are described under "The Offering — III. Stock Option Plans".

EFCA produces and continually up-dates its own sales development programs that include training in insurance and mutual funds, *Equity Funding* Programs, limited partnership investments as well as sales presentations and methods. It maintains marketing schools in Los Angeles and near New York City which conduct training courses on a full-time basis. In addition, regional training programs are conducted periodically. The Company has recently installed an analytical and predictive data system to assist it in its evaluation of the sales performance and potential career productivity of each of its sales representatives. The Company maintains an active recruiting program for new sales representatives and has historically experienced a turnover of about 20% annually in its sales force.

Insurance Sales and Operations*

General. The Company, through subsidiaries, acts as a general agent for various insurance companies, but its objective is to place all of its life and accident and health insurance with its own insurance subsidiaries. During 1971, EFCA's insurance subsidiaries accounted for 68% of total premiums due, net of lapses, and 81% of new business in that year.

The insurance policies sold by the Company primarily are individual whole life and endowment policies, which accounted for 48% of premiums due in 1971. Individual term life, accident and health and other individual policies accounted for 34%, and group life and accident and health policies accounted for 18% of premiums due in 1971. The Company sells fire and casualty insurance issued by unaffiliated insurers, but this phase of business has not been significant to date. Under its general agency agreements, the Company is entitled to first year and renewal commissions.

The following table reflects pertinent information with respect to the Company's total life insurance sales, including policies written by its insurance subsidiaries and by unaffiliated insurers, for the five years ended December 31, 1971:

Year	Premiums In Force Beginning of Year	Premiums Due During Year	Premiums Terminated During Year	Premiums Paid and In Force at End of Year
1967	$ 44,608,454	$ 59,353,233	$ 6,272,673	$ 53,085,560
1968	53,085,560	72,548,315	7,474,482	65,073,833
1969	65,073,833	88,517,382	9,771,682	78,745,700
1970	78,745,700	105,995,281	11,323,442	94,671,839
1971	94,671,839	125,600,900	9,832,224	115,768,676

Insurance Subsidiaries. Bankers was incorporated in New Jersey in 1927, Equity Funding Life in Illinois in June 1959, and Equity Funding Life New York in New York in 1964. All are legal reserve life, accident and health insurance companies and, collectively, are authorized to do business in all states, the District of Columbia and Puerto Rico. Of the life insurance written by these subsidiaries which is presently in force, approximately 16% was written in California, 10% in New Jersey, 9% in Pennsylvania, 8% in Illinois and 6% in New York.

The subsidiaries in the insurance group offer a broad line of individual and group whole life and endowment, term, credit life, and accident and health insurance policies. Premium rates are believed by the Company to be generally competitive with similar types of insurance written by other companies. The policies written by Equity Funding Life and Equity Funding

---

* Does not include information as to sales or operations of Northern Life Insurance Company which is described under "Certain Recent Acquisitions".

life New York are non-participating. Bankers writes on both a participating and non-participating basis, and writes some annuity contracts on a non-participating basis. Under a participating policy the insured pays a higher premium than under a comparable non-participating policy with the expectation of achieving a lower ultimate cost through the receipt of policy holder dividends.

Operations. The following table sets forth certain information with respect to the combined operations of the Company's insurance subsidiaries for the periods indicated.

	1967	1968	1969	1970	1971
Premiums and other considerations (net of reinsurance ceded) Life — Individual —					
Non-participating	$ 13,585,419	$ 14,519,196	$ 17,276,457	$ 25,185,118	$ 39,478,152
Participating	6,529,204	6,174,400	5,854,729	5,581,963	5,651,481
Group — Non-participating	4,950,158	6,473,657	6,659,458	8,638,158	5,510,766
Participating	2,153,883	1,957,474	1,908,218	1,784,164	2,050,660
Accident and health	1,387,483	2,976,106	3,492,384	1,640,537	2,161,394
Annuities	713,298	1,034,250	871,634	938,925	1,552
Supplementary contracts and dividend and coupon accumulations	977,538	913,129	1,149,103	883,120	857,633
Total	$ 30,296,983	$ 34,048,212	$ 37,211,983	$ 44,651,985	$ 55,711,638
Life Insurance: In Force Beginning of Year —					
Whole Life and Endowment	$ 633,064,422	$ 742,228,052	$ 806,916,718	$ 934,229,815	$1,358,504,341
Term and Other Policies	187,229,404	168,567,017	211,781,231	384,364,704	697,779,987
Group — Credit	690,289,264	729,497,930	860,058,160	937,619,091	1,001,591,855
Group — Other	280,742,139	327,238,535	375,460,877	405,159,203	439,636,303
Total in Force Beginning of Year	1,791,325,229	1,967,531,534	2,254,216,986	2,661,372,813	3,497,512,486
Paid for New Business — Direct:					
Whole Life and Endowment	214,453,594	180,853,404	264,993,448	563,316,698	547,845,835
Term and Other Policies	23,530,056	66,867,028	218,951,880	389,798,012	681,091,357
Group — Credit	113,373,734	221,100,351	169,432,695	189,826,805	182,971,632
Group — Other	40,318,282	48,434,376	41,662,367	51,156,938	138,386,999
Total Direct New Business	391,675,666	517,255,159	695,040,390	1,194,098,453	1,550,295,823
Reinsurance Assumed:					
Whole Life and Endowment	—	—	6,197,000	6,125,182	106,041,006
Term and Other Policies	37,630,604	19,375,935	3,795,992	4,367,376	—
Group — Other	—	—	—	—	123,933,875
Total Reinsurance Assumed	37,630,604	19,375,935	9,992,992	10,492,558	229,974,881
Total Paid for New Business	429,306,270	536,631,094	705,033,382	1,204,591,011	1,780,270,704
Terminations —					
Whole Life and Endowment	103,731,088	110,048,979	143,877,351	145,167,354	200,873,213
Term and Other Policies	51,779,233	35,919,288	49,175,651	80,750,105	119,106,196
Group — Credit	74,165,068	90,540,121	91,871,764	125,854,041	220,636,921
Group — Other	23,424,576	12,937,254	12,952,789	16,679,838	101,177,707
Total Terminations	253,099,965	249,445,642	297,877,555	368,451,338	641,794,037
In Force End of Year —					
Whole Life and Endowment	742,228,052	806,916,718	934,229,815	1,358,504,341	1,811,517,969
Term and Other Policies	168,567,017	211,781,231	384,364,704	697,779,987	1,259,765,148
Group — Credit	729,497,930	860,058,160	937,619,091	1,001,591,858	963,926,566
Group — Other	327,238,535	375,460,877	405,159,203	439,636,303	600,779,470
Total in Force End of Year	1,967,531,534	2,254,216,986	2,661,372,813	3,497,512,489	4,635,989,153
Reinsurance Ceded —					
Individual	122,864,767	182,108,365	474,901,898	784,722,117	1,301,657,082
Group — Credit	588,606,117	702,813,002	773,419,017	827,555,069	806,760,109
Group — Other	400,500	2,277,750	20,456,618	22,304,871	147,624,691
Total Reinsurance Ceded	711,871,384	887,199,117	1,268,777,533	1,634,582,057	2,256,041,882
Net in Force End of Year — After Reinsurance Ceded	$1,255,660,150	$1,367,017,869	$1,392,595,280	$1,862,930,429	$2,379,947,271

31

The following table shows for the periods indicated, the amount of new insurance written during each period by EFCA's insurance subsidiaries, and the amount of insurance in force at the end of each period segregated as between participating and non-participating policies:

	1967	1968	1969	1970	1971
Paid for New Business:					
Whole Life and Endowment —					
Non-participating	$ 199,682,367	$ 170,932,183	$ 259,573,180	$ 558,192,561	$ 629,191,096
Participating	3,326,124	2,366,869	3,253,855	4,449,704	17,475,446
Term and Other Policies —					
Non-participating	27,375,109	69,104,129	213,105,253	384,362,175	677,576,579
Participating	380,830	370,405	803,194	2,884,772	3,514,778
Group — Credit —					
Non-participating	105,802,496	208,501,278	161,344,491	182,208,152	172,786,242
Participating	7,571,238	12,599,073	8,031,860	7,618,653	10,185,390
Group — Other —					
Non-participating	2,551,516	6,395,668	40,214,649	20,111,747	153,752,366
Participating	54,150,500	21,411,600		29,723,055	1,295,500
Reinstatements and Increase....	28,466,090	44,449,889	18,706,900	15,040,192	114,493,307
Total Paid for New Business....	$ 429,306,270	$ 536,131,094	$ 705,033,382	$1,204,591,011	$1,780,270,704
In Force End of Year (including reinsurance ceded)					
Whole Life and Endowment —					
Non-participating	$ 533,774,679	$ 606,972,107	$ 742,257,958	$1,171,524,118	$1,599,537,707
Participating	208,453,373	199,944,611	191,971,907	186,980,223	211,980,262
Term and Other Policies —					
Non-participating	148,317,101	192,874,397	366,480,553	678,437,490	1,240,851,910
Participating	20,249,916	18,906,834	17,884,101	19,342,497	18,913,238
Group — Credit —					
Non-participating	647,836,186	791,268,507	868,960,297	932,035,903	898,134,858
Participating	81,661,744	68,789,653	68,658,794	69,555,952	65,791,708
Group — Other —					
Non-participating	44,907,842	46,122,068	78,572,902	90,783,438	135,516,817
Participating	282,330,693	329,338,809	326,586,301	348,852,825	465,262,653
Total in Force End of Year	$1,967,531,534	$2,254,216,986	$2,661,372,813	$3,497,512,446	$4,635,989,153

The following table shows certain mortality and general expense information pertaining to the combined operations of the insurance subsidiaries.

	1967	1968	1969	1970	1971
Ratio of voluntary terminations to mean number of individual policies in force	11.0%	8.5%	7.0%	6.1%	3.8%
Ratio — Actual to expected mortality for individual life insurance policies	74.4%	57.8%	54.4%	60.9%	48.2%
Ratio of statutory general insurance expenses to premiums and other considerations	14.8%	14.6%	13.8%	14.8%	11.2%

The average face amount of ordinary life policies (non-group policies) sold in the years 1969, 1970 and 1971 was $20,888, $24,301 and $30,141.

Underwriting Policy.   The insurance subsidiaries generally require medical examinations of applicants before issuing individual life insurance. Policies may be issued up to specified amounts without a medical examination, in reliance upon a questionnaire covering physical condition and medical history. These amounts vary according to the age of the applicant and the type of insurance applied for. Also, policies solicited through associations and corporations, as well as in connection with pension plans may be issued up to prescribed limits without medical examinations or other evidence of insurability. Medical examinations are not usually required for group life and group health insurance. In accordance with general industry practice the insurance group subsidiaries accept some substandard risks for which a higher premium is charged. At December 31, 1971, less than 2% of the individual life insurance in force was represented by substandard risks.

Group credit life insurance is written by Bankers in connection with small loans made by one consumer finance company. The average coverage on any one life is usually less than $2,500. Evidence of insurability is normally not required on this type of insurance.

Reinsurance.   As is customary in the insurance industry, the insurance subsidiaries cede portions of their insurance to various reinsurance companies which assume the risk under the insurance they accept. The ceding insurer, however, remains contingently liable as to the ceded insurance should the reinsurer be unable to meet its obligation. The maximum amount of insurance retained on any one life by any of the insurance group subsidiaries is $100,000.

In the past Equity Funding Life has ceded substantial amounts of life insurance and it presently intends to continue this policy in the future although the proportionate amount of new business retained in recent periods has increased as follows: 1969—10%, 1970—40%, and 1971—50%. it is expected that 60% of its new business will be retained in the current year.

The Company's insurance group subsidiaries are parties to various reinsurance agreements with unaffiliated reinsurers. The table below shows, for the periods indicated, the approximate face-amount of life insurance ceded and the coinsurance considerations received by the insurance group subsidiaries.

Period	Approximate Face Amount Ceded	Reinsurance Considerations
1969	$239,000,000	$ 2,343,000
1970	435,000,000	4,374,000
1971	625,000,000	5,749,000

The effect of ceding insurance is to realize, as current income, coinsurance considerations and to forego the profits or losses in subsequent periods prior to any recapture of the business coinsured. As a general rule, a small portion of each of the policies reinsured is retained by the ceding insurer which also retains, as an expense allowance, a portion of all renewal premiums attributed to policies reinsured. The Company's insurance group subsidiaries have the right to recapture certain reinsured business during various periods ranging from 8 to 15 years from the date of cession. (See Note 5 and Note 13 to the Financial Statements of Equity Funding Life and Bankers in this connection.)

Bankers and Equity Funding Life also assume reinsurance. The total face amount assumed at December 31, 1971 was $23,000,000.

Most of Banker's group credit life insurance and a portion of its group credit disability insurance is reinsured with affiliates of a consumer finance company. Bankers is holding assets in respect of funds left on deposit by one of such affiliates which may be recovered in whole or in part at any time. The deposit amounted to approximately $1,225,000 at June 30, 1972. Bankers pays interest on the deposit. On August 2, 1971, effective as of January 1, 1971, Bankers reinsured with such affiliates most of its group credit disability insurance not previously reinsured, and in connection therewith Bankers transferred approximately $4.9 million of assets to the reinsurers who assumed the reserve liability on such insurance.

Accounting Principles. Equity Funding Life has restated its financial statements since 1968, other than those issued pursuant to the requirements of insurance regulatory authorities, in conformity with generally accepted accounting principles ("GAAP") and Bankers, in order to show the effect of applying GAAP to its financial statements, has prepared its Supplemental Statements and its Statement of Sources and Uses of Funds shown herein in conformity with GAAP as indicated in the report of Joseph Froggatt & Co., independent certified public accountants, set forth elsewhere herein. The accounts of Equity Funding Life since 1968 and the Supplemental Statements and Statement of Sources and Uses of Funds of Bankers shown herein have been adjusted in accordance with a preliminary draft dated December 1970 of proposed accounting principles for life insurance companies prepared by the Committee on Insurance Accounting and Auditing of the American Institute of Certified Public Accountants. It is not known whether, when or in what form the proposed accounting principles may be adopted by the American Institute of Certified Public Accountants.

Financial statements of Equity Funding Life for years prior to 1968 and financial statements of Bankers, other than such Supplemental Statements and its Statement of Changes in Financial Position, have been prepared in accordance with statutory practices and principles prescribed for life insurance companies. Under statutory accounting treatment, in the year in which a life insurance policy is written, costs and expenses, together with reserves required by law, generally, exceed the amount of the first year's premium and are required to be charged as expenses in that year, although premium income is taken into earnings over the periods in which the policies are in effect. Certain assets designated as "non-admitted assets", together with a "mandatory securities valuation reserve", must be deducted from surplus. Assets designated as "admitted assets" must be stated at values permitted to be reported to the domiciliary state regulatory authority. See Note 1 of Notes to Financial Statements of Bankers and Note 1 of Notes to Financal Statements of Equity Funding Life elsewhere herein.

The effect of GAAP on a life insurance company is to match the life insurance company's expenses with its income. Since life insurance companies experience high first year acquisition costs in relation to their expenses in renewal years, a conversion to GAAP tends to increase profits on new business and reduce profits on renewal business. For a company, such as Equity Funding Life, which has in recent periods experienced a significant increase in new business, conversion to GAAP basis would increase reported earnings. In addition, under a GAAP basis, certain assets are included in the insurance company's balance sheet which are not admitted in a company's statutory financial reports. Significant changes resulting from its conversion to GAAP are described in Notes 1, 3, 4 and 6 to Equity Funding Life's financial statements and the effect of a conversion to GAAP is described in the introductory paragraph to the Adjusted Statement of Operations of Bankers, and in the Notes to such statement, as well as in Note 1 and Note 20 of the Notes to Financial Statements of Bankers.

The presentation of the financial statements shown herein on a GAAP basis does not affect the manner in which Bankers and Equity Funding Life are required to report to their respective domiciliary state regulatory authorities, and in general such reports determine the rights of each insurance company under state insurance laws with respect to such matters as payment of dividends to stockholders, maintenance of policy reserves and investment of funds.

Reserves. Equity Funding Life and Bankers are required under the laws of their respective domiciliary states to provide reserves, differing in the case of Equity Funding Life from those shown in the accompanying financial statements, to meet obligations to their policyholders. These statutory reserves are carried as liabilities and, together with future valuation net premiums and interest, are calculated to be sufficient to meet policy obligations as they mature. The various actuarial factors used to compute statutory reserves are based upon interest rates, mortality tables and rates of morbidity prescribed by statute and are valued in accordance with standard industry methods. See Note (f) of the Notes to the Statement of Operations of Equity Funding Life and Note (c) of the Notes to the Adjusted Statement of Operations of Bankers elsewhere herein.

Equity Funding Programs

The *Equity Funding* Programs enable participants to finance their insurance premiums through loans from the Company which are secured by mutual fund shares purchased by the participant for cash. The Company requires a minimum annual premium of $300 and the investment in shares must equal at least 2.5 times each premium loan. Thus the minimum initial investment in mutual fund shares is $750. It is intended that loans and the refinancing of previous borrowings recur annually for a period of ten years, unless the Program is sooner terminated. A Program may be terminated at any time by a Participant, by the Company on the anniversary date or in the event of a participant's inability to meet minimum collateral requirements of 135% of the amount borrowed. Most policies financed in the Programs are ordinary life policies.

Since May 1, 1972, all of the life insurance policies sold in the Programs have been written by the Company's insurance subsidiaries. During the past three years about 46% of the mutual fund shares sold in the Programs have been issued by funds managed by EFCA.

The following table indicates the percentage of gross insurance and mutual fund commission income represented (i) by the sale of *Equity Funding* Programs and (ii) by the sale of insurance and mutual fund shares independent of the Programs for the five years ended December 31, 1971:

	1967	1968	1969	1970	1971
Program sales	45%	52%	35%	44%	53%
Non-Program sales	55%	48%	65%	56%	47%

Programs initiated after August 31, 1969, are subject to regulations of the Federal Reserve Board which limit insurance premiums loans to an amount not in excess of 40% of the value of the mutual fund shares pledged for each borrowing. Under such regulations, the amount which may be loaned in a Program may be reduced, or loans may be precluded, by action of the Board. Program participants, as well as the Company, could be adversely affected by any such action.

The following table sets forth statistical information, for the periods indicated, concerning the sale and termination of Programs:

Equity Funding Programs Sold.	1967	1968	1969	1970	1971
Number of Programs Sold(1)	3,912	5,783	9,354	11,139	13,813
Amount of Premiums Financed in First Year Programs Sold(1)	$ 2,071,778	$ 3,164,048	$ 5,694,476	$ 7,583,097	$ 9,775,513
Amount of Mutual Funds Purchased in Financing of First Year Premiums	$ 13,687,157	$ 19,253,232	$ 35,259,256	$ 36,224,454	$ 42,967,289
Face Amount of Life Insurance Policies Sold	$116,262,182	$172,774,122	$296,587,278	$528,520,003	$798,652,769
Premium Loans Outstanding at End of Period(2)	$ 25,094,811	$ 36,311,037	$ 51,188,119	$ 63,324,413	$ 88,615,732
Total Number of Programs in Effect at Year End	12,020	16,682	23,939	31,892	41,121
Equity Funding Programs Terminated.					
Termination of Programs Sold During Period Indicated, as of December 31, 1971(3)	1,569	1,897	2,285	1,086	89
Amount of Annual Premiums Involved in Terminations(4)	$ 841,579	$ 1,042,490	$ 1,375,938	$ 703,563	$ 60,905
Face Amount of Life Insurance Involved in Terminations(4)	$ 47,353,952	$ 56,755,228	$ 70,544,018	$ 46,453,738	$ 4,505,415
Total Number of Programs Terminated During Year	369	1,121	2,097	3,186	4,584

(1) Includes Programs involving accident and health insurance and fire and casualty but the sale of Programs with such insurance is not significant.

(2) Including interest and renewal premiums financed.

(3) Since the introduction of the Programs in 1960, a total of 254 forced liquidations occurred through 1971 due to inadequate collateral of which 140 occurred in 1970, and 102 occurred in 1971.

(4) "Terminations" refer only to the financing arrangements and not necessarily to a termination of the related life insurance policy.

The average face amount of the life insurance policies sold in all Programs is approximately $40,000. The average amount of the first year loan made to participants is approximately $700.

The Company finances loans made to participants in its Equity Funding Programs through the sale of debt securities, including Custodial Collateral Notes (the "Custodial Notes"), to unaffiliated lenders, including banks, and from cash generated in its operations. The Custodial Notes are issued pursuant to a Custodial Collateral Note Agreement (the "Custodial Agreement") with a custodian bank which also acts as agent for Program participants. Among the banks involved in such financing arrangements are some of the banks participating in the Revolving Credit Agreement of June 29, 1972. All of the Custodial Notes are secured by notes receivable from Program participants and the accumulated mutual fund shares pledged thereunder. The Custodial Agreement contains collateral requirements for the pledged shares which are coextensive with those provided for in the participants' notes. Notes receivable from Program participants at June 30,

1972 amounted to approximately $103,525,000. Of such amount, $31,306,000 secured an equal amount of Custodial Notes, bearing an average interest rate of 5½% per annum. See "Capitalization".

Funds to finance loans made by the Company to maintain Programs sold prior to October 1963 (the "old Programs") are obtained, in part, through demand or short-term bank borrowings secured by the mutual fund shares of participating investors thereunder. Of the total shares pledged by such participants to the Company at June 30, 1972, approximately $4,575,000 secured demand or short-term borrowings in the amount of $2,713,000, bearing an average interest of 6½%. No representation can be made as to applicable interest rates on any of the Company's future borrowings.

Currently, the average per annum rate of interest charged investors under the old Programs is 7¾%. Interest under Programs started after October 1963 but before May 1966 has been, and will be, charged at the constant rate of 6% per annum. Interest on loans to participants in Programs commenced after April 1966 is based on a formula related to the prime interest rate in effect in New York City and at this time does not exceed 7¾% per annum. Interest charged by the Company is subject to limitations of state law.

Although the Company does not now anticipate any material difficulty in obtaining funds for financing loans made in the Programs, there is, of course, no assurance that this will be the case in the future.

Securities Sales and Distribution

Mutual Funds. Mutual fund shares are marketed principally through the Company's subsidiary, Equity Funding Securities Corporation ("Equity Securities"), which has selling agreements with the distributors of a large number of mutual funds. At present, about 50% of its total mutual fund sales is in shares of Equity Growth Fund, Equity Progress Fund and Fund of America. All of the mutual fund shares sold by the Company are redeemable at any time at net asset value.

EFC Distributors Corporation ("EFC Distributors"), a subsidiary of the Company, acts as the principal distributor for shares of Equity Growth Fund, Equity Progress Fund and Fund of America under agreements which may be terminated by either of the respective parties thereto, without penalty, upon not more than 60 days' notice. Such agreements must be approved at least annually by the directors of the respective mutual funds, including a majority of the directors who are not "interested persons" within the meaning of the 1940 Act.

Shares of Equity Growth Fund, Equity Progress Fund and Fund of America are sold to EFC Distributors at their net asset value, and are offered to the public at net asset value plus a sales charge of 8.75% of the offering price on single purchases of less than $25,000. A 7% discount on such purchases is reallowed dealers, including subsidiaries of the Company, and the balance of the sales charge is retained by EFC Distributors. The amount of the sales charge, including the dealers discount, is reduced in larger transactions. Under each of its distribution agreements, EFC Distributors bears a portion of the expenses of such funds.

EFC Sponsors Corporation ("EFC Sponsors"), a subsidiary of the Company, sells and sponsors contractual plans for the accumulation of shares of Fund of America and National Investors Corporation. As the sponsor of such plans, EFC Sponsors receives sales commissions applicable to the plan which range from 8.7% to 1% of the total payments made, depending upon the plan purchased. EFC Sponsors also receives fees for certain administrative and investor services which have been delegated to it.

The following table sets forth pertinent information concerning the sale of mutual fund shares by the Company for the five years ended December 31, 1971.

Year	Mutual Fund Shares and Contractual Plans Sold(1)	Gross Commissions(2)	Commission Expenses	Net Commissions
1967	$ 36,235,687	$ 2,043,964	$ 1,006,705	$ 1,037,259
1968	64,450,778	5,001,777	2,061,166	2,940,611
1969	202,165,256	19,954,887	7,880,604	12,074,283
1970	125,607,166	12,746,247	4,816,280	7,929,967
1971	108,158,702	10,373,431	3,924,517	6,448,917

(1) Based on offering price of mutual fund shares and payments under contractual plans, including applicable sales charges. The marked increase in mutual fund and contractual plans sold in 1969 was in large part due to the acquisition as of January 1, 1969, of substantially all of the domestic assets of the former principal distributor for Fund of America which had also sponsored and sold contractual plans. Such plans were not offered by the Company prior thereto. See "Certain Recent Acquisitions".

(2) Includes gross commissions attributable to the sale of contractual plans (including commissions on plans sold in prior years) in 1969 of $6,948,528, in 1970 of $5,490,736 and in 1971 of $3,882,363.

On December 14, 1970, Federal legislation was enacted into law which may result in a lowering in the amount of sales commissions on mutual fund shares. Further, as a result of such law, the Company restructured its front-end sales commission arrangement on contractual plans, effective June 14, 1971, so that not more than 20% of any one year's payments by an investor is deducted for sales commissions and the sales commission deducted from the payments during the first four years of the contractual plan does not exceed an average of 16%. Because the Company realized approximately 50% of the total charges applicable to a plan in the first year under plans sold before June 14, 1971, the new law will significantly affect the amount of the first year commissions received on contractual plan sales. In 1969, 1970 and for the six months ended June 30, 1971, the Company's first year commissions on contractual plan sales which would have been affected by following the new sales commission arrangement now in effect amounted to $2,918,000, $1,995,000 and $852,000, respectively. During the six months ended December 31, 1971, first year commissions on contractual plan sales amounted to $721,000.

Limited Partnership Investments. Since 1970, the Company has formed two real estate and two cattle limited partnerships in which it has publicly sold a total of $26,237,000 of limited partnership interests. A third real estate limited partnership was formed in 1972 and a public offering of $6,500,000 of limited partnership interests therein is currently being made on a best efforts basis. In addition, a fourth real estate limited partnership was recently formed and a public offering of $6,000,000 of limited partnership interests is planned, also on a best efforts basis, subject to compliance with various governmental regulations. The general partner of all such limited partnerships is a subsidiary of EFCA. In the past, the Company has also sold interests in oil and gas limited partnership which it has formed. There can be no assurance whether, or the extent to which, limited partnership interests will be sold by the Company in the future.

The National Association of Securities Dealers, Inc. and certain States have recently proposed rules which would regulate the distribution of the type of limited partnership interests which have been offered by EFCA. In addition, proposed revisions to the Federal tax laws as they apply to real estate, cattle and similar limited partnerships are now before Congress. No representations can be made at this time whether, or in what form, such rules or revisions may become effective. However, in their present form, they could have an adverse effect on the distribution of such limited partnership interests to an extent not now ascertainable.

Other Securities Activities.   North American Equity Corporation ("NAEC"), a subsidiary of the Company, is a member of the Midwest, Pacific Coast and Philadelphia-Baltimore-Washington Stock Exchanges. Substantially all of NAEC's business is restricted to the handling of transactions for institutions and others engaged in the securities business. NAEC commenced its present operations in December 1969.

NAEC's total commission income in 1970 and 1971, amounted to $1,620,504 and $2,375,379, and is included in securities revenues in the Company's Consolidated Statement of Earnings. This was derived from transactions executed for mutual funds managed by the Company's subsidiary, EFC Management Corporation ("EFC Management"), and for unaffiliated persons.

Under the advisory and management agreements between Equity Growth Fund, Fund of America and Equity Progress Fund, and EFC Management, the fee otherwise payable by such funds to EFC Management is reduced by 50% of that portion of the "net income after taxes", as defined, of NAEC which is attributable to any "reciprocal business" of NAEC resulting from stock exchange transactions effected for the fund. NAEC may effect transactions for the above funds on the New York or American Stock Exchanges through members of such exchanges who may direct brokerage business originated with their customers to NAEC if such business (reciprocal business) can be executed on a regional stock exchange of which NAEC is a member.

On August 3, 1972, the Securities and Exchange Commission proposed a rule which would require securities exchanges registered with the Commission to adopt rules limiting membership to persons conducting at least 80% of their securities business with unaffiliated customers or in certain specified transactions. It is not known at this time whether, when or in what form any such rules may finally be adopted. Adoption of the rule as proposed by the Commission would result in the exclusion of NAEC from exchange membership thereby causing the Company to terminate NAEC's present operations. Also, the Commission has determined to reduce the point at which commission rates on all orders of institutional size will be subject to competitive rates. To the extent that such rates are reduced by competition, the amount of NAEC's income may be decreased notwithstanding the continuance of its membership on an exchange.

Bishops Bank and Trust Company ("Bishops Bank"), a Bahamian subsidiary of the Company, was acquired by the Company in 1969. Bishops Bank is principally engaged in the overseas marketing and distribution of foreign commercial securities to institutional investors. Its income is included in the Company's securities revenues and is derived from underwriting fees, income on securities held for resale and the resale of such securities. Bishops Bank has offices in Nassau, Mexico, Venezuela and Argentina. It has also served as a derivative source of foreign capital for the Company.

ASSET MANAGEMENT

As a result of the Company's marketing of financial services products offered by its subsidiaries or companies it manages, EFCA manages assets consisting principally of the securities investments of its insurance group subsidiaries, the portfolio of investments of the mutual funds it manages and the assets of the real estate and cattle limited partnerships managed by EFCA.

Insurance Subsidiaries Assets*

At December 31, 1971, Equity Funding Life, Bankers and Equity Funding Life New York had investments in bonds, mortgage loans, loans to policyholders and corporate stocks and other securities having an aggregate book value of $168,479,000 and a market value of $168,208,000.

The following table shows, on a combined basis, the cash and invested assets of the Company's insurance group subsidiaries for the periods indicated.

| | 1970 | | 1971 | |
	Amount	Percent of Total	Amount	Percent of Total
Bonds	$ 79,954,759	48.1%	$ 92,899,396	52.7%
Stocks	4,492,618	2.7	5,003,570	2.8
Mortgage Loans	49,420,449	29.7	46,076,502	26.1
Real Estate Company Occupied	5,381,843	3.2	5,397,450	3.1
Other	1,556,962	.9	1,102,670	.6
Policy Loans	18,993,684	11.4	19,495,609	11.1
Cash and Certificates on Deposits	5,340,326	3.2	6,294,588	3.6
Collateral Loan	1,350,000	.8	—	—
Totals	$166,490,641	100.0%	$176,269,785	100.0%

The following table shows for the periods indicated, on a combined basis, the cash and invested assets at the end of each period, net investment income and net investment yield on average cash and invested assets of the Company's insurance group subsidiaries.

	Cash and Invested Assets	Net Investment Income	Net Investment Yield
1967	$132,072,590	$5,893,977	4.70%
1968	148,762,223	6,363,473	4.60
1969	158,888,863	7,282,733	4.81
1970	166,490,641	8,647,031	5.35
1971	176,269,785	9,629,887	5.61

The following table sets forth for the periods indicated, the insurance group subsidiaries' admitted assets and stockholders' equity and the ratio of stockholders' equity to total liabilities and participating policyholders' surplus, all determined on a statutory basis with GAAP adjustments shown in the note to the table.

	1967	1968	1969	1970	1971
Admitted Assets(1)	$142,041,441	$160,171,510	$172,094,813	$184,495,126	$199,198,731
Stockholder's Equity(1)	12,316,284	16,905,745	18,659,843	19,797,783	22,192,856
Ratio of stockholder's equity to total liabilities and participating policyholders' surplus(1)	8.7%	10.5%	10.8%	10.7%	11.1%

(1) The figures shown above are on a statutory basis. The following are corresponding figures shown on a generally accepted accounting principles basis:

Assets	$156,724,658	$179,025,985	$192,052,212	$213,433,627	$237,639,325
Stockholder's Equity	12,813,206	18,285,394	22,199,434	27,223,904	35,747,485
Ratio of stockholder's equity to total liabilities and participating policyholders' surplus	8.9%	11.4%	13.1%	14.6%	17.7%

* Does not include information as to operations of Northern Life Insurance Company which is described under "Certain Recent Acquisitions".

Mutual Fund Management

The Company began its mutual fund management operations in 1967. The approximate asset value of the funds under the Company's management, at year end, since that time are as follows: 1967 — $15,418,000, 1968 — $75,475,000, 1969 — $194,862,000, 1970 — $174,116,000, and 1971 — $210,554,000.

EFC Management manages the assets of Equity Growth Fund, Equity Fund and Fund of America. The fees charged by EFC Management are determined by formulae related to the value of the assets managed. On June 30, 1972 the total mutual fund net assets managed by the Company amounted to $221,253,068. During 1970 and 1971, the revenues of the Company derived from mutual fund management were $772,965 and $856,859, respectively.

EFC Management's agreements with Equity Growth Fund, Fund of America and Equity Progress Fund may be terminated by either of the respective parties thereto, including the stockholders of such funds, without penalty, upon not more than 60 days' nor less than 30 days' notice. The agreements must be approved annually by Boards of Directors of the funds, including a majority of directors who are not "interested persons" within the meaning of the Investment Company Act of 1940, as amended.

Limited Partnership Management

Real Estate Partnerships.   EFC Property Management, Inc. ("EFC Property"), a subsidiary of the Company, is the general partner and manager of Equity Properties Limited 1970 ("EPL-70"), Equity Properties Limited 1971 ("EPL-71") and Equity Properties Limited 1972 ("EPL-72"), in which limited partnership interests were (and with respect to EPL-72, are currenty being) publicly sold by EFCA. A fourth limited partnership, Equity Properties Limited — 1972-B ("EPL-72B"), of which EFC Properties is also the general partner, was recently formed and a public offering of limited partnership interests therein is planned. EFC Property manages a total of 20 apartment projects, containing 2,087 apartment units, located in Arizona and California, most of which are managed for EPL-70 and EPL-71 and will manage any apartment projects constructed by EPL-72 and EPL-72B. For its services, EFC Property receives a fee related to the annual gross income of such apartment projects and has a limited interest in the proceeds of any sale of the apartment projects owned by EPL-70 and EPL-71 and has a similar interest in the sale of any apartment projects owned by EPL-72 or EPL-72B. During 1970 and 1971, EFC Property received or accrued a total of $150,142 and $698,780 in management fees from EPL-70 and EPL-71, of which $84,648 and $387,306 was paid as commissions for the sale of EPL-70 and EPL-71 limited partnership interests.

If during the five-year period ending December 31, 1975, operating cash income to EPL-70 is inadequate, the Company has undertaken to pay to EPL-70 sufficient cash so that the partnership will have cash available for distribution to the limited partners, after applying receipts from operations and payment of its expenses (including management fees, all other operating expenses and mortgage obligations), in and amount equal is 6.43% of each limited partner's investment. Payments by the Company for 1971 were $208,000. In addition, the Company has agreed, for a two-year period commencing January 1, 1972, if operating cash income is inadequate, to pay all operating expenses and mortgage obligations of EPL-71, and to assure limited partners a minimum cash distribution of 6% per annum of their investments. Commitments similar to those applicable to EPL-71 have been made by the Company to EPL-72 and EPL-72B.

As previously noted, EPL-72 is currently making a public offering of $6,500,000 of limited partnership interests. EPL-72B whose business is similar to that of EPL-70, EPL-71 and EPL-72 has filed a registration statement with the Securities and Exchange Commission covering a pro-

41

posed public offering of a maximum of $6,000,000 of limited partnership interests to be offered subject to the satisfaction of various regulatory requirements. Assuming the completion of such offering and the offering by EPL-72, and the realization of adequate mortgage financing, as to which no representation can be made, EPL-72 and EPL-72B propose to acquire a total of 14 apartment projects containing approximately 1,891 apartments located in Phoenix and Tucson, Arizona, Southern California and the San Francisco Bay area, which are to be managed by EFC Property. It is expected that EFC Property will be compensated for its services, and will have a limited interest in any sale of such apartment projects, under arrangements similar to those it has with EPL-71.

Cattle Partnerships. Subsidiaries of the Company (the "cattle subsidiaries") act as general partner and manager of Ankony Breeding Systems — 1970 ("Ankony Breeding Systems") and Ankony Cattle Systems — 1971 ("Ankony Cattle Systems"). Ankony Breeding Systems owns a breeding herd of 15,054 cattle. In connection with Ankony Breeding Systems, the Company:

(i) has advanced $2,800,000 to Ankony Breeding Systems for operating expenses, at 6.50% interest, payable at December 31, 1977;

(ii) has guaranteed repayment of any principal balance, up to a maximum amount of $4,000,000 of notes issued by Ankony Breeding Systems to purchase its herd;

(iii) has undertaken, until December 31, 1980, (a) to insure the performance of Ankony Angus Corporation ("Ankony"), the Company's principal cattle subsidiary, under its operating agreement with Ankony Breeding Systems and (b) to advance, or arrange for others to advance, such funds as may be required to conduct Ankony Breeding System's cattle business, excluding funds to purchase cattle.

As of June 30, 1972, Ankony Cattle Systems owns a herd of 4,777 registered Black Angus and 85,192 feeder cattle which, together with the progeny thereof, secure indebtedness of Ankony Cattle Systems incurred in connection with the acquisition of the herd. The Company has guaranteed any deficiency under certain lines of credit incurred by Ankony Cattle Systems to unaffiliated lenders. As of June 30, 1972, $21,401,054 was owed by Ankony Cattle Systems to several lenders at interest rates ranging from 6.25% to 8.50%. The indebtedness is expected to be paid from the sale of feeder cattle during 1972, but there is no assurance that the proceeds of sale will be sufficient for that purpose. In addition, the Company has agreed to guarantee the performance of Ankony to Ankony Cattle Systems.

The cattle subsidiaries are compensated for their services to Ankony Breeding Systems and Ankony Cattle Systems under arrangements with those partnerships pursuant to which fees were received by the cattle subsidiaries in 1970 and 1971 in the aggregate amounts of $247,704 and $308,296. The cattle subsidiaries act as general partners and managers for two private cattle partnerships, and in certain cases share in the profits of the partnerships they manage.

CONSTRUCTION AND DEVELOPMENT, CATTLE, OIL AND GAS, AND SAVINGS AND LOAN BUSINESSES

The Company also is engaged in residential construction and development, proprietary cattle and oil and gas businesses, and owns a savings and loan association.

Construction and Development

The Company commenced its construction and development operations in July 1969, with the acquisition of a company engaged in the construction and sale of apartment projects in Southern

California. As of June 30, 1972, Equity Funding Development Corporation ("Development"), the Company's principal real estate subsidiary, has developed, constructed and sold 21 apartment projects in California and Arizona with 2,125 apartment units. Seven of these projects were sold, for a total price of $12,475,000, to EPL-70. Development has also sold nine projects, containing 957 apartments, to EPL-71 for an aggregate purchase price of $16,970,000 to be paid from the proceeds of EPL-71's completed public offering of $6,000,000 of limited partnership units and from anticipated mortgage financing. All the projects for EPL-71 are expected to be completed by September 1, 1972.

Development has entered into an agreement with EPL-72 and is expected to enter into an agreement with EPL-72B for the construction of their apartment projects. The agreements are subject to the completion of the proposed public offerings and the availability of suitable mortgage finance as to which no representation can be made.

Cattle Business

The Company conducts its proprietary cattle operations through Ankony. Ankony and its predecessors have been engaged in the business of breeding, buying and selling high quality registered Black Angus cattle, for more than 30 years. Virtually all of the Company's natural resources revenues is accounted for by Ankony.

At June 30, 1972, Ankony owned 2,670 cattle and approximately 27,020 acres, and leased approximately 10,670 acres, at farms and ranches located in eight states. Ankony also has grazing and other cattle maintenance agreements at various locations.

Substantially all of Ankony's revenues have been derived from the sale of cattle to the limited partnerships managed by the Company's subsidiaries. Additional revenues have been derived from fees for managing the partnership and maintaining the cattle. No representations can be made as to the extent of future revenues from these partnerships or whether additional partnerships will be formed by the Company.

In 1970, Ankony Breeding Systems purchased a breeding herd of approximately 13,000 cattle from Ankony and one of the private partnerships managed by Ankony for $8,000,000 represented by non-recourse notes secured by such cattle and currently bearing interest at the rate of 5¾% per annum, of which $1,000,000 was paid in 1970, and $2,000,000 was paid in 1971, with the balance maturing from 1975 through 1977. The purchase price included a mark-up of approximately $4,100,000 after giving effect to certain acquisition and related costs. In connection with Ankony Breeding Systems, the Company has guaranteed repayment of any principal balance, up to a maximum amount of $4,000,000 of the above note and has furnished certain guarantees and undertakings as previously described.

In 1971, Ankony Cattle Systems purchased 3,538 Black Angus cattle from Ankony for $4,000,000. The purchase price is represented by a non-recourse note payable in ten annual $400,000 installments commencing on December 31, 1971, which currently bears interest at the rate of 6¼% per annum. The note is secured by the cattle purchased by Ankony Cattle Systems and the progeny thereof. The purchase price included a mark-up of $1,915,231.

Oil and Gas Exploration

The Company formed Equitex Petroleum Corporation ("Equitex Petroleum") in September 1968, to enter into oil and gas exploration overseas, primarily in Africa and the Middle East. Equitex Petroleum owns a 10% undivided interest in nine off-shore oil and gas licenses granted by the Government of Israel covering an aggregate of approximately 800,000 acres off the Mediterranean coast of that country, and a 25% undivided interest in an off-shore oil and gas concession covering approximately 2,475,000 acres in the southern area of the Red Sea off the coast of Ethiopia. In August 1969, the Company also acquired all the outstanding capital stock of Traserco, Inc. ("Traserco"). Traserco is the owner of an undivided 23.75% interest in various oil and gas concessions previously granted by the government of Ecuador and now owned by a consortium of which Traserco is a member. The concessions cover approximately 2,147,000 acres in the Gulf of Guayaquil off the coast of Ecuador.

Eight wells have been completed on the Ecuadorian concessions, of which three, Amistad No. 1, Amistad No. 3 and Amistad No. 4 have reported substantial flows of natural gas. Amistad No. 2, drilled two miles northeast of Amistad No. 1 as a confirmation well, was a dry hole. Four other exploration wells, Playas No. 1, Esperanza No. 1, Domito No. 1 and Tiburon No. 1, each of which was drilled on different structures were abandoned as dry holes after failing to establish production in commercial quantities. The consortium is planning additional confirmation and exploratory drilling. The full amount and nature of the gas located in the Amistad structure are not presently determinable. The consortium is discussing with other companies the development, liquification, transportation and marketing of any natural gas which may be produced from the Ecuadorian concessions, but there can be no assurance as to whether or when any such arrangements will be consummated, or if consummated, that they will be profitable. Accordingly, Amistad No. 1, Amistad No. 3 and Amistad No. 4 have been temporarily suspended.

Six test wells have been drilled on the Israel properties at widely separated locations and all were abandoned after failing to encounter oil and gas in commercial quantities. The current phase of the test program in Israel has been completed and the licensees are reviewing and evaluating all geological and geophysical data obtained to date. Exploration activities in the Company's Ethiopian concession area presently consist primarily of geological and geophysical studies to determine structural and stratigraphic conditions. An unaffiliated company has an option, currently exercisable until October 1, 1972, to earn a 30% interest in the Company's interest in return for undertaking to drill an exploratory well on the Company's concessions at its own risk and expense.

The Ecuadorian government recently promulgated certain decrees and other provisions that require the renegotiation by June 6, 1973 of previously granted concessions, including those held by Traserco's consortium. The changes that will result from such renegotiation are uncertain at this time, but could have an adverse effect on the Company which is not now ascertainable. Also, all of the Company's overseas oil and gas operations are affected by laws, regulations and policies of the United States government which are applicable to oil and gas imports and are subject to periodic review and change.

At this time, the concession interests of Traserco and Equitex Petroleum should be regarded as speculative. The Company had invested approximately $8,377,000 as of June 30, 1972 in these overseas exploration ventures. The existing and any future exploration and drilling commitments of Traserco and Equitex have been guaranteed by the Company.

Since 1968, the Company has formed four oil and gas limited partnerships, two of which are still in existence, to engage in oil and gas drilling programs but none of the partnerships' activities have resulted in any significant income to the Company. The partnerships' oil and gas operations are located in Colorado, Louisiana, Oklahoma and Saskatchewan, Canada. No representations can be made as to the extent to which the Company may participate in these activities in the future. Effective at year end 1970, the Company acquired interests of the 1968 oil and gas limited partnership previously formed by it, in exchange for 64,120 shares of its common stock and cancellation of $234,240 of debt owed to the Company. See "Certain Transactions" in this connection.

44

Savings and Loan Association

Organization and Offices.   Liberty was incorporated in California in 1924 and was merged with Crown in April 1971. It is a stock-type savings and loan association with offices located in the western section of Los Angeles, adjacent to Beverly Hills, in El Monte and North Hollywood, California. Like other savings and loan associations, Liberty furnishes a savings medium for deposits and provides home financing by lending money on the security of first mortgages or trust deeds for purchasing, constructing, improving or refinancing residential real property.

Assets.   The following table sets forth the total assets, unpaid principal balance of loans, amount of outstanding deposits and aggregate of general reserves, undivided profits, capital and surplus of Liberty for the five years ended December 31, 1971.

Year Ended December 31,	Total Assets	Unpaid Principal Balance of Loan Portfolio	Total Deposits (Investment Certificates)	General Reserves, Undivided Profits, Capital and Surplus
1967	$101,997,435	$85,192,088	$84,474,158	$6,743,381
1968	107,954,787	89,799,088	89,607,778	7,287,885
1969	108,460,458	90,243,631	78,135,409	8,126,810
1970	108,634,017	88,198,890	80,424,445	8,093,881
1971	118,516,492	95,208,438	88,194,777	8,159,271

Interest Rates on Savings Accounts.   Interest on savings accounts has been paid by Liberty since its organization. Since July 1, 1967, Liberty has paid interest at the rate of 5% per annum and a bonus on its minimum term accounts. Such rate and bonus are the maximum permitted under governmental regulations. Liberty also issues definite-rate definite-term certificates at interest rates of 5¼% to 7½% per annum payable quarterly. All other savings and loan associations in the Los Angeles area presently maintain the same interest rates as are currently paid by Liberty.

Home Financing.   The principal source of income for the association is loans made upon the security of residential real property. This income consists of interest paid by borrowers, origination fees and other loan fees. Substantially all of the loans on real estate made by Liberty are long-term conventional uninsured loans on single-family residences or other residential or commercial property. It also makes some "pass book" loans. As of December 31, 1971, Liberty's real estate loans had an aggregate unpaid principal balance of $95,001,921 and an approximate average yield of 7.1%. All but $10,879,316 of such balance was represented by conventional uninsured loans on property having original terms averaging 25 years.

Scheduled Items.   A savings and loan association's "scheduled items" are those assets which by regulatory definition are of a sub-standard nature. In substantially all cases scheduled items are the result of protracted loan delinquency, real estate acquired through loan delinquency and below normal standard loans made "to facilitate" the sale of real estate acquired through loan delinquency. Scheduled items can cause an association to suffer various regulatory penalties. The following table sets forth the scheduled items experience of Liberty during the past three years ended December 31, 1971.

Year Ended December 31,	Delinquent Loans	Real Estate Acquired	Loans to Facilitate	Specified Assets	Ratio to Specified Assets
1969	$217,305	$1,385,867	$5,507,174	$93,545,547	7.60%
1970	229,125	967,100	6,013,158	91,503,307	7.88%
1971	475,065	2,218,412	2,081,932	96,049,829	4.97%

The higher ratio of scheduled items to specified assets of Liberty in 1969 and 1970 resulted primarily from delinquent loans converted to real estate through foreclosures and subsequently sold on loans to facilitate sale of real estate. Economic conditions in the greater Los Angeles area and Liberty's underwriting policies during 1964 to 1969 were the primary causes of these loan delinquencies.

In October 1971, the FHLB regulations were changed to allow savings and loan associations to exclude from scheduled items 80% of loans made to facilitate the sale of residential real estate in certain circumstances. At December 31, 1971, the ratio of scheduled items to specified assets were reduced by 1.64% due to the change.

Federal Savings and Loan Insurance Corporation.   The deposits of Liberty are insured by the the Federal Savings and Loan Insurance Corporation up to a maximum of $20,000 for any one depositor. Because its accounts are insured, Liberty is required to maintain a Federal insurance reserve which must be used solely for the purpose of absorbing losses, and amounts allocated to this reserve may not be used as a source for payment of dividends on their guarantee stock or for payment of interest on deposits.

Federal Home Loan Bank System.   Liberty is a member of the Federal Home Loan Bank System, which functions in a reserve credit capacity for home-financing institutions. As a member, it is required under the Federal Home Loan Bank Act to acquire and hold shares of capital stock in the Federal Home Loan Bank of San Francisco in an amount equal to at least 1% of the aggregate of the unpaid principal of its home mortgage loans, home-purchase contracts and similar obligations. Advances from the Federal Home Loan Bank of San Francisco may be obtained upon the security of that Bank's stock held by Liberty, certain of its home mortgages or certain other obligations in an amount not in excess of its line of credit with the Bank, unless this line of credit is otherwise extended or restricted by the Federal Home Loan Bank Board. At the present time, Liberty may borrow under this line of credit up to 50% of the aggregate amount of deposits to meet withdrawals from outstanding accounts. In addition to borrowings to meet withdrawals, certain borrowings are available for expansion purposes. Because of its scheduled items ratio, at present Liberty may borrow only up to an additional 9½% of deposits for expansion purposes. The current rate of interest on substantially all of the borrowings under this line of credit is 6⅞%. As of July 15, 1972, Liberty had borrowings from the Federal Home Loan Bank of $5,809,900, of which $5,114,900 was for savings withdrawals and $695,000 was for expansion purposes.

Liberty is required to maintain 7% of its savings accounts and borrowings due within one year in liquid assets. Liquid assets consist of cash (including certificates of deposit and bankers acceptances), U.S. government obligations and Federal agency obligations, subject to certain limitations. If an association fails to maintain the liquidity required, monetary penalties are assessed by the Federal Home Loan Bank based on the amount of the deficiency calculated. As of June 30, 1972, Liberty's ratio of liquid assets to savings accounts and borrowings due within one year was 8.93%.

Loan and Investment Limitations. The California Savings and Loan Association Law provides, in part, that an association may make only certain authorized investments and loans. Authorized investments, subject to certain limitations, include real property, United States obligations, certain federal agency and municipal obligations and certain other bonds and securities. Loans on real property are limited to those made on the security of first mortgages or first trust deeds, although additional security may be taken. Loans secured by deposits and other prescribed instruments also are permitted.

California law requires each association to appropriate part of its profits to a loan reserve until such reserve equals at least 5% of its unpaid loans secured by real property. This reserve is independent of other reserves required by California or federal law or regulations, but amounts appropriated thereto may be included in calculating the amounts in such other reserves. At June 30, 1972, Liberty's reserves for this purpose were 5.4%.

REGULATION

EFCA is engaged primarily in regulated businesses. Each of its insurance subsidiaries is subject to regulation and supervision, principally for the benefit of policyholders, by the insurance departments of the states in which they are incorporated and the jurisdictions in which they are licensed to do business. Although different in each state, such regulations generally establish supervisory agencies with administrative powers over the activities of insurance companies relating, among other things, to the granting and revoking of licenses to transact business, the licensing of agents and general agents, the regulation of trade practices, the approval of policy and contract forms, the approval of reinsurance treaties, the maintenance of specified reserves, the character of investments and the form and content of required financial statements.

The insurance subsidiaries are also required to file detailed annual reports with the supervisory agencies in each jurisdiction in which they do business and their accounts are subject to examination at any time by such agencies. They are subject to examination by the insurance departments of their states of incorporation and are examined by those departments periodically. The last examination for Bankers and Equity Funding Life covered the period ending December 31, 1968, for Northern Life Insurance Company covered the period ending December 31, 1970 and for Equity Funding Life New York covered the period ending December 31, 1971.

In addition, the insurance laws of the respective states of incorporation of each of the Company's insurance subsidiaries require the registration of insurers doing business in such states, which are members of an "insurance holding company system"; subject material transactions by registered insurers with their affiliates to requirements that the terms thereof be fair and reasonable and that the books, accounts and records of each party be so maintained as to clearly and accurately disclose the nature and details of the transactions; and confer broad examination and enforcement powers on the Commissioner. Bankers' Charter provides for the payment of dividends to stockholders and participating policyholders from surplus. A portion of the yearly profits of Bankers after provision for reserves, contingency funds and current liabilities must be allocated by the directors of Bankers to the participating policyholders. The insurance laws of New Jersey also provide, in this connection, that no profits on participating policies or contracts in excess of 50¢ per year per thousand dollars of participating life insurance in force at the end of the year shall inure to the benefit of the stockholders. Under amendments to the New Jersey insurance laws, effective January 1, 1972, it is provided that no profits on participating policies or contracts in excess of the larger of (a) 10% of such profits before payment of policyholders dividends or (b) 50¢ per year per thousand dollars of participating life insurance in force at the end of the year, shall inure to the benefit of the stockholders. Also, the insurance laws of New Jersey, Illinois and Washington require notice of extraordinary dividends, in New York the insurance laws require notice of all dividends and each such state authorizes the Commissioner or Superintendent of Insurance in his discretion to disapprove such dividends. (See Notes 14 and 19 of Notes to Financial Statements of Bankers.)

The New Jersey Insurance Commissioner approved the merger between E-B Insurance Company ("E-B"), an EFCA subsidiary, and Bankers on August 9, 1971. In addition, on September 7, 1971 the New York Superintendent of Insurance approved the acquisition by the Company of control of Equity Funding Life New York. The approvals of the New Jersey Commissioner and the New York Superintendent are subject to several conditions and restrictions relating, among other things, to the operations of Bankers and Equity Funding Life New York following the merger and cover such matters as capitalization, places of business, books and records, financial statements, replacement of existing insurance policies, reporting, marketing, employees, policy holders and relationships with the Company. Violations of such conditions and restrictions could result in various sanctions including, subject to any rights to a hearing and judicial review, divestiture of Equity Funding Life New York and the suspension of *Equity Funding Program* sales in New York. The Company intends to comply, and to cause Bankers and Equity Funding Life New York to comply, fully with the conditions and restrictions imposed by the New Jersey Commissioner and the New York Superintendent.

Certain of the Company's broker-dealer subsidiaries are subject to regulation by the Securities and Exchange Commission (the "Commission") under the Securities Exchange Act of 1934 and by state and quasi-governmental agencies. The Commission requires such subsidiaries to report regularly with respect to their capital and other aspects of their business, and to conform to the rules and regulations promulgated under the various securities laws, which change from time to time. As members of the National Association of Securities Dealers, Inc., a registered securities association, such subsidiaries are also subject to the supervision of that organization. NAEC is subject to the rules and regulations of the stock exchanges of which it is a member.

Liberty is subject to California statutes and to supervision and regulation of the California Savings and Loan Commissioner, Federal Home Loan Bank Board ("FHLB") and Federal Savings and Loan Insurance Corporation, which conducts periodic examinations of savings and loan associations and their parents. Because of its ownership of Liberty, the Company is a registered diversified savings and loan holding company under Section 408 of the National Housing Act, as amended, and is subject to provisions of such Act and regulations thereunder which prohibit and restrict various activities involving savings and loan associations and their affiliates, including the payment of dividends by the association in certain circumstances.

CERTAIN RECENT ACQUISITIONS

Independent Securities

On August 21, 1970, the Company completed the acquisition, from unaffiliated parties, of Independent Securities Corporation, a California corporation ("Independent Securities") in consideration of the payment by the Company of 150,000 shares of its Common Stock, valued at $20.50 per share. The Company also agreed to issue additional shares of its Common Stock upon the exercise of 1969 Incentive Stock Options (maximum of 1,300 shares) and Warrants (maximum of 30,900 shares exercisable at $68 per share) granted to holders of stock options and warrants previously issued by Independent Securities. Independent Securities is engaged in the separate sale of mutual fund shares and life insurance and at the time of the acquisition was represented by approximately 2,000 salesmen. Independent Securities had twelve sales offices located in various western states, substantially all of which have been merged into the Company's existing sales offices.

Liberty

The Company acquired Crown in January 1968. Pursuant to the terms of a Merger Agreement of July 9, 1970, between the Company, Crown and Liberty, the Company on April 9, 1971, issued 64,974 shares of its Series B Convertible Voting Preferred Stock, $100 stated value, for distribution to the stockholders of Liberty, none of whom were affiliated with the Company. The Preferred Stock is convertible into shares of the Company's Common Stock, at a price of $35 per share of Common Stock. The number of shares issuable upon any conversion is subject to adjustment in certain events to prevent dilution. The Agreement provides that the Company may redeem all or any part of the shares of Preferred Stock at any time by paying in cash the stated value for each share, and must redeem (by paying in cash the stated value for each share) at least 10% of the outstanding shares of Preferred Stock by the end of the first year, an additional 15% by the end of the second year, 20% by the end of the third year, 25% by the end of the fourth year and the balance by the end of the fifth year. Conversions of Preferred Stock may be credited by the Company against the required redemptions. As of June 30, 1972 an aggregate of 40,412 shares of Preferred Stock have been converted into Common Stock of the Company and it has credited such amount against the required redemptions. The holders of Preferred Stock will not be entitled to any dividends, but in the event of liquidation, dissolution or winding up of the Company, they are preferred over the holders of the Company's Common Stock as to assets in an amount equal to stated value.

Bankers

Pursuant to an Agreement and Plan of Reorganization ("Agreement"), dated May 26, 1971, as amended on August 23, 1971, among the Company, its subsidiary E-B and Bankers, E-B was merged into Bankers on October 15, 1971, and Bankers has become a wholly-owned subsidiary of the Company. Under the terms of the Agreement, a total of 1,600,000 shares of the Company's Common Stock, valued at $39.20 per share, has been issued for distribution to the stockholders of Bankers in exchange for their shares of Bankers Capital Stock.

Other Acquisitions

Substantially all of the domestic assets of the former principal distributor and manager of Fund of America, which also distributed mutual fund accumulation plans now sold by EFC Sponsors, were acquired by the Company from unaffiliated persons as of January 1, 1969. The purchase price consisted of 27,367 shares of Common Stock of the Company, valued at $71.03 per share, $2,025,000 principal amount of the Company's non-interest notes due April 1, 1970 (subsequently reduced to $1,200,000 and paid), $6,264,866 in cash and the assumption of certain liabilities. The assets acquired by the Company amounted to approximately $7,700,000, of which approximately $4,500,000 was represented by receivables, and the liabilities assumed amounted to approximately $4,400,000, as of December 31, 1968. Among other assets acquired by the Company were 29 sales offices, most of which have been combined with those of the Company.

The Company also acquired from unaffiliated persons as of January 1, 1969, all of the assets, properties and goodwill of several cattle breeding and raising businesses which now form part of Ankony. The purchase price consisted of (i) 92,909 shares of Common Stock of the Company, valued at $69.93 per share, (ii) the Company's 7%, $1,000,000 promissory note (which has been paid), and (iii) a total cash payment of $5,300,000.

Acquisition of Northern Life Insurance Company

Acquisition Transaction. Pursuant to a Purchase and Sale Agreement, dated June 9, 1972, between the Company and Nationwide Corporation, an Ohio corporation unaffiliated with the Company ("Nationwide"), the Company, on June 29, 1972, acquired 91.2% of the outstanding shares of capital stock of Northern Life Insurance Company, a Washington insurance corporation ("Northern") for $39,200,000. The purchase price consisted of approximately $31,200,000 in cash and $8,000,000 of the Company's unsecured promissory notes bearing interest at 7¼% per annum and due June 29, 1973 — $2,000,000, 1974 — $3,000,000 and 1975 — $3,000,000. The Company acquired 875,625 shares in this transaction at a per share cost of $44.79, and has agreed that it will, no later than October 27, 1972, arrange for the holders of the 8.8% minority interest in Northern (represented by 84,375 shares) to have the opportunity to receive the same price per share for their shares as the price paid to Nationwide. On or about September 15, 1972 Northern intends to offer to redeem the outstanding 84,375 shares held by this minority interest at a price of $44.79 per share, payable in cash.

General. Northern was incorporated in the State of Washington in 1906, as a legal reserve stock life and accident and health insurer. It writes individual ordinary life insurance on both a participating and non-participating basis. Accident and health insurance and annuity contracts are written on a non-participating basis. Northern also writes group life and accident and health insurance. It is licensed to do business in 21 states, located on the West Coast and in the Mid-West. Of Northern's life insurance presently in force, excluding reinsurance accepted, approximately 27% was written in California, 26% in Washington and 8% in Oregon.

Northern writes a variety of insurance to meet personal and corporate needs. During 1971, Northern's premium income was derived approximately 68% from the sale of individual ordinary life insurance and annuity contracts, 12% from individual accident and health insurance, 11% from group accident and health policies and 9% from other group life insurance policies. During 1971, about 40% of Northern's individual life insurance sales was on a non-participating basis. Approximately 11% of premium income from new sales of ordinary life insurance policies for the six-months ended June 30, 1972 was in the military market.

	1967	1968	1969	1970	1971
Admitted Assets (1)	$124,264,390	$127,507,266	$124,190,084	$125,887,789	$131,283,287
Stockholders' Equity (1)	21,499,013	22,123,006	22,034,593	22,456,221	23,202,873
Ratio of Stockholders' Equity to Total Liabilities and Participating Policyholders' Surplus (1)	17.3%	17.4%	17.7%	17.8%	17.7%

(1) The figures shown above are on a statutory basis. The following are corresponding figures shown on a generally accepted accounting principles basis:

	1967	1968	1969	1970	1971
Admitted Assets	$132,862,270	$135,930,100	$137,892,843	$140,034,263	$145,982,577
Stockholders' Equity	26,896,561	27,687,102	29,592,843	30,436,172	31,460,511
Ratio of Stockholders' Equity to Total Liabilities and Participating Policyholders' Surplus	20.2%	20.4%	21.5%	21.7%	21.6%

Reinsurance. Northern's maximum retention limit on any one life is $100,000. Northern is a member of the Northwest Reinsurance Conference, which consists of four companies. Northern both reinsures and assumes reinsurance through the Conference, and reinsures with other reinsurance companies. Northern also assumes other reinsurance, principally through participation in the Federal Employees Group Life Insurance policy and the Servicemen's Group Life Insurance policy. The total volume assumed under these policies at June 30, 1972 was $117,460,213.

Accounting Principles and Reserves. Northern has restated its financial statements since 1967, other than those issued pursuant to the requirements of insurance regulatory authorities, in conformity with generally accepted accounting principles in accordance with the preliminary draft dated December 1970 of proposed accounting principles for life insurance companies prepared by the American Institute of Certified Public Accountants. Reference is made to "Accounting Principles" at page 34 and "Reserves" at page 35, concerning the general provisions of statutory accounting principles, the effect of GAAP, and reserves of life insurance companies. Northern is required under the laws of Washington to provide reserves, differing from those shown in its financial statements herein, to meet obligations to its policy holders. See Notes (1) and (4) of the Notes to the Consolidated Financial Statements of Northern.

GENERAL INFORMATION REGARDING THE COMPANY
Employees
Apart from its sales representatives, who are independent contractors, the Company has approximately 1,400 employees, none of whom is covered by collective bargaining arrangements. The Company believes its relationship with employees to be excellent.

Competition
The Company operates in highly competitive industries in virtually all of its activities, and in many cases competes with companies which have been established longer than the Company and its subsidiaries and have greater financial resources. There are over 2,000 life insurance companies in the United States, many of which have been in business for a longer time, offer more diversified lines of insurance and have greater assets than the Company's insurance subsidiaries. The mutual fund industry also is highly competitive.

Properties
Except as noted below, the Company and its subsidiaries presently rent all of their sales offices, executive offices and certain equipment from non-affiliated lessors under leases of varying terms at monthly rentals totaling approximately $290,000.

Bankers owns its home office building which is located in Parsippany, New Jersey, contains approximately 110,000 square feet of floor space and is situated on a tract of land containing 30 acres. The building was recently completed, is of modern design and is well maintained.

Northern owns its fourteen-story home office building which is located in Seattle, Washington. It contains approximately 183,000 square feet of floor space situated on ¼ acre of land. The building was recently completed, is of modern design and is well-maintained. Northern also owns a one-story concrete building located in Seattle, Washington, containing 39,497 square feet of floor space on 1½ acres of land, which is currently leased for commercial purposes, as well as unimproved real estate consisting of approximately four acres in Bellevue, Washington.

The Company owns long-term ground and building net leases, with respect to property located in Los Angeles, California, in which Liberty's home office is located. The Company has an option to purchase the building in 1978, 1983 or 1988 for $2,050,000. The building is of modern design and contains 46,000 square feet, of which Liberty occupies approximately 13,000 square feet; the balance is subleased. The building was completed in 1965 and has been well maintained.

The Company also owns a modern three-story office building located in El Monte, California, which houses a branch office of Liberty. The building was completed in 1962 and contains about 21,200 square feet of floor space of which approximately one-third is utilized by Liberty as a branch office and the remainder by several tenants under leases of varying terms. A second branch office of Liberty is located in leased premises.

The land and facilities owned or leased by Ankony and the apartment projects being built by the Company, have been described elsewhere in the prospectus.

The Current Economic Stabilization Program

Phase II of the President's economic stabilization program began on November 14, 1971. The program, which is administered by the Cost of Living Council ("COLC"), a Pay Board and a Price Commission, continues restraints on prices, rents, wages and salaries for an indefinite period. Interest rates and dividends are not currently subject to mandatory controls under the program. Under the current regulations of the COLC, it would appear that insurance premiums (except as noted hereinafter), mutual fund and contractual plan sales charges, mutual fund advisory fees, real estate commissions, fees charged for the management of cattle and oil and gas programs, other types of management fees including the management of realty, rental rates for certain apartment complexes and securities brokerage commissions, as well as all forms of employees' compensation are covered by the program. The COLC has exempted from the program at this time the following categories of products and services, among others: insurance premiums charged for life insurance policies (except credit-life insurance purchased or renewed after November 13, 1971, including ordinary, term and group policies, and individual endowments or annuities); securities; live cattle; unimproved real estate as well as real estate with improvements completed prior to August 15, 1971; and rentals on industrial and nonresidential commercial property, as well as on residential rental property on which construction is completed, and which is offered for rent for the first time, after August 15, 1971.

On November 15, 1971, the President's Committee on Interest and Dividends issued Guidelines that companies are expected to observe in paying dividends in 1972. Under the Guidelines, "Cash dividends on any class of common stock to be paid in 1972 should be declared at such rates that the aggregate annual payment per share (adjusted for stock splits and issuance of stock dividends) will not exceed by more than 4 per cent the highest aggregate annual payment per share in any of the company's fiscal years ending in 1969, 1970, or 1971 (adjusted through

December 31, 1971 for stock splits and issuance of stock dividends)." Stock dividends and stock splits are not restricted by the Guidelines.

While EFCA believes that its business will not be adversely affected by the current stabilization program or by other related legislative measures recommended by the President, the ultimate impact of the foregoing program or measures or any others which may be adopted cannot now be predicted.

MANAGEMENT

The Executive Officers and Directors of the Company are as follows:

Name	Position
Stanley Goldblum*	President and Chairman of the Board of Directors
Dov Amir	Executive Vice President — Natural Resources Operations
Yura Arkus-Duntov*	Executive Vice President — Investment Management Operations and Director
Herbert Glaser*	Executive Vice President — Real Estate and International Operations and Director
Fred Levin*	Executive Vice President — Insurance Operations and Marketing and Director
Samuel B. Lowell*	Executive Vice President — Corporate Operations and Finance and Director
Marvin A. Lichtig	Executive Vice President — Administrative Services and Treasurer
R. W. Loeb	Executive Vice President — General Counsel and Secretary
Robert R. Bowie	Director
Gale Livingston	Director
Nelson Loud	Director
Judson Sayre	Director

* Member of Executive Committee.

Stanley Goldblum has been President and a director of the Company since 1960. He was elected Chairman of the Board of Directors in 1969.

Dov Amir joined the Company in June 1968 as President of Equity Resources. He has served in his present capacity since April 1969. From September 1967 through May 1968, Mr. Amir was privately engaged in natural resources activities, including oil and gas, mining and chemicals.

Yura Arkus-Duntov was elected a Vice President of the Company in August 1967 and has served in his present capacity since April 1969. He has been a director of the Company since 1969.

Herbert Glaser joined the Company in November 1968 as Executive Vice President — General Counsel and has served in his present and related capacities since April 1969. Prior to joining the Company, Mr. Glaser was engaged in the private practice of law. He has been a director of the Company since 1962.

Fred Levin joined Equity Funding Life in 1964 as Secretary and Counsel. In 1968, he was named President of Equity Life and in April 1969 was elected Executive Vice President — Insurance. He has served in his present capacity since November 1969. He was elected a director of the Company in 1971.

Samuel B. Lowell joined the Company in May 1969 as Controller and has served in his present capacity since April 1970. Prior to his association with the Company, he had served as Treasurer of a subsidiary of Dart Industries, Inc., a diversified company, since April 1968. For more than five years prior to April 1968, Mr. Lowell was a certified public accountant associated with Haskins & Sells. He was elected a director of the Company in 1971.

Marvin A. Lichtig has served in his present capacities since joining the Company in May 1969. Prior thereto he was associated with Wolfson, Weiner, Ratoff & Lapin (subsequently combined with Seidman & Seidman), the Company's auditors, since 1961, and had been a partner in that firm since January 1967.

R. W. Loeb joined the Company in July 1969 as Vice President and General Counsel and has served in his present capacities since May 1970. Prior to his association with the Company, he had served as Vice President — Legal of Commonwealth United Corporation for approximately one year, and was engaged in the private practice of law for more than five years prior thereto.

Robert R. Bowie, a director of the Company since 1970, has been Clarence Dillon Professor of International Affairs and Director of the Center for International Affairs, Harvard University since 1957. From August 1966 until March 1968, Professor Bowie was on leave from Harvard University, serving as Counselor, United States Department of State.

Gale Livingston, a director of the Company since 1971, has been associated with subsidiaries of Litton Industries, Inc. ("Litton"), in executive capacities for a number of years. He presently is President of Litton International Corporation, Aero Service Corporation, Westrex Company and Vice President of Professional Service and Equipment Group, all wholly-owned subsidiaries of Litton.

Nelson Loud, a director of the Company since 1964, is Chairman of the Board of The Loud Consulting Corporation, Financial Consultants; Chairman of the Board, ASG Industries, Inc., manufacturers and fabricators of flat glass and flat glass products. Prior to August 1, 1970 Mr. Loud was a Senior Partner of New York Securities Co., the predecessor partnership of New York Securities Co. Incorporated. Mr. Loud is a director of several other corporations.

Judson Sayre, a director of the Company since 1971, has been an independent business financial consultant since 1965 and before that served in various executive positions with Borg-Warner Corporation.

Certain of the Company's executive officers also serve in executive capacities with EFCA's subsidiaries.

Remuneration

The table below sets forth, with respect to the year ended December 31, 1971, information as to the amount of direct remuneration accrued or paid, and the number of shares of Common Stock delivered under the Company's Employee Stock Bonus Plan for (i) each director and each of the four highest paid officers of the Company whose direct aggregate remuneration, accrued or received, exceeded $30,000 and (ii) all directors and officers of the Company as a group.

Name	Capacity in Which Remuneration Was Received	Direct Remuneration	Shares Received Under Employee Stock Bonus Plan(1)
Stanley Goldblum	President	$100,000	5,000
Herbert Glaser	Executive Vice President	70,000	4,000
Fred Levin	Executive Vice President	70,000	4,000
S. B. Lowell	Executive Vice President	70,000	4,000
Yura Arkus-Duntov	Executive Vice President	52,500	1,250
All Directors and Officers as a group (14 persons)		593,958	21,500

(1) The closing price of the Company's Common Stock on the New York Stock Exchange on January 4, 1971, the effective date of receipt of the shares, was $23⅞.

Employee Stock Bonus Plan

The Company maintains an Employee Stock Bonus Plan for the benefit of Company employees, all of whom will be eligible to participate in the Plan. The Plan was adopted by the Board of Directors of the Company in December 1970 and approved by the stockholders of the Company at an annual meeting held in May 1971. It is administered by an Administrative Committee appointed by the Board of Directors of the Company and presently consisting of Messrs. Goldblum, Loud, Livingston and Arkus-Duntov. The Committee determines as of the last day of any year whether bonuses are to be granted under the Plan (the "Plan Year"), those employees who shall participate in the Plan for such Plan Year, as well as the number of Units to be credited to the account of each participant. No participant may be granted Units for any one Plan Year which shall exceed 5,000 Units, and the maximum number of Units to be allocated to all participants for any one Plan Year shall not exceed more than one-half of 1% of the number of shares of Common Stock outstanding on the last day of such Plan Year. Each Unit consists of four shares of Common Stock, and the shares are scheduled for issuance in four equal instalments beginning January 1 of the year following the Plan Year (except for the 1970 Plan Year) and on January 1 of each of the three succeeding years. Except in the event of death or retirement, no participating employee will be entitled to any instalment unless he is employed by the Company on the date upon which such instalment is scheduled to be paid. Thus, termination by a participant for any reason other than retirement or death shall result in a forfeiture of benefits. Also if a participant engages in a business competitive with the Company after retirement, any remaining benefits will be forfeited. The payment of instalments over a four year period is designed to insure continued employment of the employee for the benefit of the Company during that period. A total of 500,000 shares of the Company's Common Stock is reserved for issuance under the Plan. The number of shares reserved under the Plan and the number to be issued to any participant at any instalment date, will be subject to adjustment upon the occurrence of certain events to prevent dilution. The value of Units issued under the Plan will be taxable to the participating employee and deductible by the Company.

All of the shares awarded for the 1970 and 1971 Plan Years have been issued, but only 60,555 shares have been delivered (including the shares shown in the table above) to the participating employees. The remaining 95,665 shares are being held in escrow and will be delivered pursuant to the terms of the Plan. The tabulation below shows the grants of Units made to officers named under "Remuneration" and to all officers and directors as a group under the 1970 and 1971 Plan Years.

Name	Title	Units Granted 1970 Plan Year	Units Granted 1971 Plan Year
Stanley Goldblum	President; Chairman of the Board	5,000	2,500
Herbert Glaser	Executive Vice President — Real Estate and International Operations	4,000	2,000
Fred Levin	Executive Vice President — Insurance Operations and Marketing	4,000	2,000
S. B. Lowell	Executive Vice President — Corporate Operations and Finance	4,000	2,000
Yura Arkus-Duntov	Executive Vice President — Investment Management Operations	1,250	625
All Directors and Officers as a group (22 persons)		21,500	14,200

PRINCIPAL STOCKHOLDERS

As of April 7, 1972, the amount of stock owned beneficially by all officers and directors as a group was 387,788 shares, or approximately 4.9% of the Common Stock then outstanding. On such date Stanley Goldblum beneficially owned approximately 3.2% of the outstanding Common Stock of the Company. Mr. Goldblum may be deemed to be a "parent" of the Company as defined in the Rules and Regulations under the Act, by virtue of his stock ownership and management position.

Fidelity Corporation ("Fidelity") and The Central National Insurance Company of Omaha, a wholly-owned subsidiary of Fidelity, two of the Selling Stockholders hereunder, own 469,093 shares and 110,000 shares, respectively, of the Company's Common Stock or a total of 7.4% of the presently outstanding shares which were acquired by Fidelity on October 15, 1971 in exchange for stock of Bankers.

CERTAIN TRANSACTIONS

Included among the shares of the Company's Common Stock offered by Selling Stockholders under this registration statement are 4,943 shares offered by Nelson Loud and 1,471 shares offered by Gale Livingston, directors of the Company. The Company has agreed to indemnify such directors against certain liabilities, including liabilities under the Act in connection with such registration.

During 1968, Equity Resources Limited Partnership 1968 (a limited partnership formed by the Company, the general partner of which is a subsidiary of the Company) publicly offered limited partnership interests in units of not less than $10,000 each. Funds for the purchase of some of the units were provided by the Company to qualified investors (including persons affiliated with the Company) through collateralized loans maturing five years from the respective dates thereof and bearing interest at the rate of 7½% per annum. The total amount of such loans was $2,115,000, of which $855,000 was represented by loans made to persons who were at that time officers or directors of the Company. These persons included: Stanley Goldblum — $300,000 loan; Gale Livingston — $50,000 loan; Nelson Loud — $50,000 loan; Herbert Glaser — $40,000 loan; Yura Arkus-Duntov — $30,000 loan; John S. Pennish — $60,000 loan; Charles J. Helfrich — $30,000 loan; and Jerome Evans — $30,000 loan. In December 1970 and January 1971, the Company made an offer to purchase the limited partnership interests from all the limited partners in exchange (1) for shares of the Company's Common Stock having a market value of approximately $7,320 for each $10,000 unit of limited partnership interest, or (ii) for cancellation of $7,320 indebtedness for each $10,000 unit. None of the present officers or directors of the Company, except Gale Livingston, a director, has an outstanding indebtedness to the Company arising from the purchase in 1968 of these limited partnership interests, all such loans having been satisfied either through acceptance of the purchase offer through the cancellation of debt and/or separate payments. The loan to Mr. Livingston is collateralized by 1,471 shares of the Company's Common Stock which he received in the purchase offer, plus limited partnership interests in a publicly held cattle partnership of which a subsidiary of the Company acts as general partner. Messrs. Pennish, Helfrich and Evans are no longer associated with the Company and all except for Messrs. Helfrich and Pennish have repaid their loans.

In 1969, Mr. Stanley Goldblum purchased a $250,000 limited partnership interest and Mr. and Mrs. Herbert Glaser purchased a $100,000 limited partnership interest in a limited partnership (the "1969 Cattle Partnership"), which included other investors, and which had a total capitalization of $1,600,000. A subsidiary of the Company is the general partner of this partnership. As of July 1, 1969, the 1969 Cattle Partnership acquired an aggregate of 480 head of cattle from Ankony, and from an earlier cattle limited partnership of which Ankony is the general partner. The purchase price for the cattle was $1,200,000 payable in installments over a five year period with 5¼% interest thereon. The sellers' adjusted cost basis for the cattle was approximately $277,000. Ankony manages the 1969 Cattle Partnership's herd for $500 per cow unit per year and is required to purchase at $500 per calf each bull offspring produced from the herd. As of June 30, 1972, the 1969 Cattle Partnership was indebted to the Company in the amount of $480,000.

In January 1970, Fred Levin, an officer of the Company exercised an option granted to him under the 1967 Qualified Stock Option Plan for 2,101 shares of the Company's Common Stock at a price of $35,170. Certain officers of the Company, as described below, have, from time to time, effected home mortgage loans with Liberty. All of these loans were made (i) in the ordinary course of the subsidiary's savings and loan business; (ii) on substantially the same terms, including interest rates and collateral, as those prevailing at that time for comparable transactions with non-affiliated persons; (iii) do not involve more than the normal risk of collectibility; and (iv) are collateralized in each case by security exceeding the amount of the loan.

Name and Title	Date of Loan	Term of Mortgage Loan and Interest Rate	Original Loan Balance	Approximate Loan Balance June 1972
Dov Amir Executive Vice President	Feb. 1972	30-Yr.–7%	$125,000	$124,600
Bradford Erickson Vice President	Nov. 1971	30-Yr.–7%	100,000	99,500
Fred Levin Executive Vice President	Sept. 1969	30-Yr.–8.5%	77,000	(A)
S. B. Lowell Executive Vice President	April 1971	30-Yr.–7%	85,000	84,000
Jerrold Monkarsh Vice President	July 1971	30-Yr.–7%	56,000	55,400
Michael Sultan Vice President	May 1971	30-Yr.–7%	51,200	50,600
Lawrence Williams Vice President	April 1971	30-Yr.–7.5%	54,500	53,500

(A) Mortgage loan paid in full in December, 1971.

DESCRIPTION OF COMMON STOCK

Each share of Common Stock, $.30 par value, of the Company entitles its holder to share ratably in any dividend paid. See "Dividends" in this connection as to certain limitations on the payment of cash dividends. Stockholders are entitled to cumulative voting in the election of directors, and one vote per share on all other matters. Subject to any rights of the holders of any outstanding preferred stock of the Company, in the event of any dissolution, liquidation or winding-up of the Company, each holder of Common Stock is entitled to his pro rata share of the assets of the Company legally available therefor. The Common Stock has no pre-emptive rights. The shares of Common Stock outstanding are, and those to be issued upon exercise of options or warrants or upon any conversion of the 5¼% Guaranteed (Subordinated) Debentures due 1989, will be fully paid and nonassessable shares.

The Company furnishes annual reports containing certified financial statements to its stockholders and makes public quarterly reports setting forth pertinent information concerning its interim operations.

The Transfer Agent and Registrar for the Company's Common Stock is United California Bank, 108 West Sixth Street, Los Angeles, California 90014 and the Co-Transfer Agent and Co-Registrar is First National City Bank, 111 Wall Street, New York, New York 10015.

LITIGATION

In May and June 1969, the Company was served with two substantially identical complaints in actions brought by Lavinia V. Funnell and Richard Weiner, plaintiffs (U.S. Dist. Ct. S.D.N.Y.), against IOS, Ltd. ("IOS"), its subsidiary IPC and various affiliated individuals and the Company, its subsidiaries, EFC Management, EFC Distributors, IPC Sponsors and RMF Corporation (the former manager of Equity Progress Fund) and Yura Arkus-Duntov, Stanley Goldblum and Herbert Glaser, officers and directors of the Company, and certain other affiliated individuals and corporations, including as derivative defendants only, Fund of America, Equity Growth Fund and Equity Progress Fund. Plaintiffs allege that the defendants have violated various provisions of the Securities Act of 1933, Securities Exchange Act of 1934 and Investment Company Act of 1940 in the management of each of the mutual funds named in the complaints and in the sale of shares issued by such funds. Judgments are sought against the defendants on behalf, and for the benefit, of Fund of America, Equity Growth Fund and Equity Progress Fund, and the other mutual funds named in the complaints, (a) returning to such funds certain fees, commissions, profits and other emoluments, (b) rescinding the management and distribution contracts between Fund of America, Equity Growth Fund and Equity Progress Fund, and subsidiaries of the Company, (c) restraining and enjoining defendants and their agents from continuing the alleged acts complained of, (d) declaring certain brokerage methods contrary to statutory requirements and (e) certain other relief.

On July 21, 1971 and on August 3, 1971, two substantially identical derivative actions, *Halbfinger* v. *Bleakney* (U.S. Dist. Ct., S.D.N.Y.) and *Levinkind* v. *Winters* (U.S. Dist. Ct., E.D.N.Y.), were commenced on behalf of Fund of America against IPC, which prior to April 1969 was the manager and the distributor for Fund of America, its parent, IOS, and various individuals affiliated with these companies and the Company, EFC Management, EFC Distributors, IPC Sponsors Corp. (now EFC Sponsors) and various affiliated individuals including Messrs. Goldblum, Arkus-Duntov and Glaser. Both suits concern the sale in April 1969 of certain assets of IPC to the Company, the proxy statement used in connection with the meeting in March 1969 of the stockholders of Fund of America and the approval by such stockholders at that meeting of a new investment advisory contract with EFC Management and underwriting and sponsorship agreements with EFC Distributors and IPC Sponsors Corp. Plaintiffs seek to require IOS and IPC and its affiliated defendants to pay to Fund of America approximately $7,000,000, which amount is allegedly the profit received by IPC from the sale of assets to the Company, on the theory that such sum constitutes the proceeds from the sale of a fiduciary office. The Company and its affiliated defendants are charged with participating in the sale and it is claimed that they are jointly and severally liable for restitution of IPC's alleged profits. All defendants also are charged with being jointly and severally liable to Fund of America for the profits derived from the investment advisory, underwriting and sponsorship agreements with the Company's subsidiaries which plaintiffs contend are void; and for alleged receipt by IPC of illegal "kickbacks" while its subsidiary acted as investment adviser. The complaints further allege that the proxy statement for the March 1969 meeting was materially false and misleading in that it failed to disclose that Fund of America was allegedly entitled to IPC's profit from the sale of assets, that IPC was allegedly receiving "kickbacks" and that the Company had allegedly participated in similar "kickback" arrangements which are not specified in the complaint.

61

On September 9, 1971, all parties served in the *Funnel-Weiner* and *Halbfinger* actions consented to a consolidation order, entered on December 29, 1971 under which an amended and supplemental complaint was ordered to be filed in the *Funnel* and *Weiner* actions and lead counsel was appointed for *Funnel-Weiner* and for *Halbfinger*. The new complaint in *Funnel-Weiner* added an alleged cause of action based upon Fund of America's purchase of certain unregistered securities; such new complaint did not include Equity Growth Fund and Equity Progress Fund as derivative parties.

It is the opinion of the Company's special counsel, Paul, Weiss, Rifkind, Wharton & Garrison, that the claims in the amended and supplemental complaint in the *Funnel-Weiner* consolidated action and the claims in the *Halbfinger* and *Levenkind* complaints are without merit as they pertain to the Company, its subsidiaries and its affiliated individuals.

The Company is involved as a defendant in various other lawsuits none of which individually or in the aggregate, in the opinion of the Company's General Counsel, R. W. Loeb, Esq., will have a material adverse effect on the operations or property of the Company taken as a whole.

LEGAL OPINIONS

Legal matters in connection with the sale of the securities offered hereby will be passed on for the Company by R. W. Loeb, Esq., Executive Vice President-General Counsel of the Company. Freedman, Levy, Kroll & Simonds, Washington, D. C., special counsel to the Company, will pass upon matters relating to the Securities Act of 1933. Mr. Loeb holds an option for the purchase of 6,080 shares of the Company Common Stock under the Company's 1968 Qualified Stock Option Plan and has been awarded 9,000 shares of Common Stock under the Company's Employee Stock Bonus Plan, of which 3,500 shares have been delivered to him.

EXPERTS

The consolidated balance sheet of the Company as of December 31, 1971 and related consolidated statement of earnings and the consolidated statement of additional paid-in capital and retained earnings of the Company for the five years then ended, and the consolidated statement of changes in financial position for the three years then ended included in this Prospectus and the related schedules included in the Registration Statements have been examined by Seidman & Seidman and by Wolfson, Weiner, Ratoff & Lapin, independent certified public accountants, as stated in their respective opinions appearing elsewhere herein. The financial statements of Equity Funding Life at December 31, 1971 and for the four years then ended, included herein, and related schedules, have been examined by Haskins & Sells, independent certified public accountants, and for the year ended December 31, 1967, included herein, have been examined by Arthur Young & Company, independent certified public accountants, to the extent set forth in their opinion and report, respectively, appearing elsewhere herein. With respect to certain actuarial items, Haskins & Sells and Arthur Young & Company have relied upon the opinion of Milliman & Robertson, Inc., consulting actuaries, whose opinion is also set forth herein. Haskins & Sells also has relied upon the report, as set forth elsewhere herein, of Lybrand, Ross Bros. & Montgomery, independent certified public accountants, with respect to certain schedules of accounts relative to amounts included in Equity Funding Life's financial statements applicable to accident and health business transacted under certain agreements. The Balance Sheet, Statement of Operations, Statement of Capital Surplus, Statement of Surplus Allocable to Participating Policyholders, Statement of Unassigned Surplus allocable to stockholders, adjusted Statement of Operations, Adjusted Statement of Surplus Allocable to Policyholders and Adjusted Statement of Unassigned Surplus allocable to stockholders and Statement of Sources and Uses of Funds of Bankers have been examined by Joseph Froggatt & Co., independent certified public accountants, to the extent stated in their opinion herein. The Consolidated Balance Sheet as of December 31, 1971, and related Consolidated Statement of Operations, Consolidated Statement of Additional Paid-in-Capital and Retained Earnings and Consolidated Statement of Changes in Financial Position of Nothern and Subsidiary for the three years then ended have been examined by Peat, Marwick, Mitchell & Co., independent certified public accountants, as set forth in their report appearing elsewhere herein. The financial statements referred to above have been included in reliance upon such opinions and reports given upon the authority of such firms as experts.

THE OFFERINGS

The offerings covered by this Prospectus are as follows:

I. SELLING STOCKHOLDERS

The 801,871 shares of Common Stock offered hereby may be sold by the Selling Stockholders named below, from time to time in ordinary brokerage transactions or otherwise at the then current market prices over-the-counter or on a national securities exchange. The Selling Stockholders may be deemed to be "underwriters" within the meaning of the Securities Act of 1933 (the "Act").

The following table sets forth information as to the principal Selling Stockholders offering 1,000 shares or more of the Company's Common Stock, as of April 15, 1972, and after giving effect to the sale of their respective shares:

Selling Stockholder	Shares Owned	Shares to be Offered	Shares to be Owned After Sale
The "Independent Securities" Group			
Lombard Holdings, Inc.	3,749	3,749	—
Louis Marx, Jr.	1,545	1,545	—
Reece Investment Co.	2,060	2,060	—
Herbert N. Somekh	1,030	1,030	—
The "New York Securities" Group			
Nelson Loud	4,943	4,943	—
Jarvis J. Slade	13,353	13,353	—
Bradford Mills	2,548	2,548	—
F. Kenneth Melis	9,118	9,118	—
F. Kenneth Melis Foundation	1,444	1,444	—
F. Kenneth Melis, as Custodian for his children	768	768	—
Craig Severance	16,187	16,187	—
The "Crown" Group			
J. Howard Edgerton	7,000	7,000	—
Arthur E. Neelley	2,138	2,138	—
Frederick T. Burrill	2,030	2,030	—
Ray Hommes	8,073	8,073	—
Oliver M. Chatburn	1,021	1,021	—
Theodore Cummings	9,284	9,284	—

Selling Stockholder	Shares Owned	Shares to be Offered	Shares to be Owned After Sale
The "Traserco" Group			
Gale Livingston	1,471	1,471	—
William Garnett	2,200	2,200	—
The Bankers Group			
Ann L. Brundage	5,695	5,695	—
John D. Brundage	13,275	13,275	—
Fidelity Corporation (a)	469,093	469,093	—
Central National Insurance Company of Omaha (a)	110,000	110,000	—
May B. Lounsbury Estate	3,789	3,789	—
Ralph R. Lounsbury	5,598	5,598	—
Roberta L. Warren	2,682	2,682	—
The Ankony Group			
Myron M. Fuerst	2,970	2,966	4
James H. Leachman	13,076	12,815	261
Mildred H. Leachman	7,585	7,585	—
Lester J. Leachman	19,532	19,532	—
William A. Leachman	1,071	1,004	67
Kent M. Klineman	16,258	14,970	1,288
Others			
Wendell B. Christenson	5,033	4,980	53
Charles A. Dumbeck	2,611	1,385	1,226
Joseph Golan	3,500	3,500	—
Eugene Monkarsh	7,085	7,085	—
Jerrold Monkarsh	9,085	9,085	—
Forty-eight other persons offering less than 1,000 shares each (b)	16,958	16,870	88
Total	804,858	801,871	2,987

(a) The shares to be offered by Fidelity Corporation and Central National Insurance Company of Omaha, unless included in an underwritten public offering, or unless the Company has otherwise consented, may be sold publicly only in ordinary brokerage transactions on a national securities exchange or over-the-counter in an amount not in excess of 10,000 shares in any one trading day (except that a maximum of 25,000 shares may be sold on any one trading day if all of such shares are sold at a price not less than the last sale price regular way of the Company's Common Stock on the New York Stock Exchange on the next preceding trading day), and sales may not exceed one percent of the Company's outstanding shares in a six-month period. Similar restrictions apply to the sale of shares by the other members of the Bankers group.

(b) The names of the Shareholders offering less than 1,000 shares each are listed in Part II of the Registration Statement filed with the Securities and Exchange Commission.

II. WARRANTS (1974) AND COMMON STOCK ISSUABLE UPON EXERCISE OF WARRANTS (1974)

The 41,856 shares of Common Stock offered hereby are issuable upon the exercise of Common Stock Purchase Warrants (the "Bearer Warrants") originally attached to 7½% Guaranteed (Subordinated) Notes due 1974 (the "Notes") of Equity Funding Capital Corporation N. V. ("Equity Capital"). The Notes and Bearer Warrants were sold in November 1969, in bearer form, to investors who were represented to be neither nationals nor residents of the United States, nor residents of Canada.

Equity Capital is a Netherlands Antilles corporation. All of its outstanding stock is owned by EQF Capital, Inc., a wholly-owned subsidiary of the Company.

INDEX TO FINANCIAL STATEMENTS

REPORT OF INDEPENDENT CERTIFIED PUBLIC ACCOUNTANTS

Board of Directors and Shareholders
Equity Funding Corporation of America

We have examined the consolidated balance sheet of Equity Funding Corporation of America and subsidiaries as of December 31, 1971 and the related consolidated statements of earnings, additional paid-in capital and retained earnings, and changes in financial position for the year then ended. Our examination was made in accordance with generally accepted auditing standards, and accordingly included such tests of the accounting records and such other auditing procedures as we considered necessary in the circumstances. We have been furnished the opinion of independent actuaries that policy reserves and other actuarially determined amounts of life insurance subsidiaries are fairly stated.

In our opinion, which as to actuarially determined amounts in the statements of life insurance subsidiaries is based on the aforementioned reports of independent actuaries, the statements mentioned present fairly the consolidated financial position of Equity Funding Corporation of America and subsidiaries at December 31, 1971 and the consolidated results of their operations and changes in financial position for the year then ended, in conformity with generally accepted accounting principles applied on a basis consistent with that of the preceding year.

SEIDMAN & SEIDMAN
(As successors to the practice of
WOLFSON, WEINER, RATOFF & LAPIN)

Los Angeles, California
March 21, 1972, except for Note 11,
which is as of April 13, 1972

REPORT OF INDEPENDENT CERTIFIED PUBLIC ACCOUNTANTS

Board of Directors and Shareholders
Equity Funding Corporation of America

We have examined the consolidated statements of earnings, additional paid-in capital and retained earnings of Equity Funding Corporation of America and subsidiaries for the four years ended December 31, 1970, and the consolidated statement of changes in financial position for the two years then ended. Our examination was made in accordance with generally accepted auditing standards, and accordingly included such tests of the accounting records and such other auditing procedures as we considered necessary in the circumstances.

In our opinion, such consolidated financial statements present fairly the consolidated results of operations of Equity Funding Corporation of America and subsidiaries for the four years ended December 31, 1970, and the consolidated changes in financial position for the two years then ended, in conformity with generally accepted accounting principles applied on a consistent basis.

WOLFSON, WEINER, RATOFF & LAPIN
(Subsequently combined with
SEIDMAN & SEIDMAN)

March 25, 1971
Los Angeles, California

EQUITY FUNDING CORPORATION OF AMERICA AND SUBSIDIARIES

Consolidated Balance Sheet (Note 1)

December 31, 1971

Assets

Cash and Short-Term Investments		$ 39,593,000
Investments — principally of insurance subsidiaries (Note 2):		
Bonds (market value $89,198,000)	$ 92,899,000	
Mortgage loans	46,077,000	
Loans to life insurance policyholders	19,496,000	
Other loans	12,269,000	
Corporate stock and other securities (market value $19,813,000)	17,261,000	
TOTAL INVESTMENTS		188,002,000
Funded Loans and Accounts Receivable (Note 3)		88,616,000
Contracts, Notes and Loans Receivable, of which $10,767,000 matures within one year		34,162,000
Insurance Premiums in Course of Collection		9,925,000
Accounts and Commissions Receivable		17,897,000
Inventories and Properties held for resale (Notes 4 and 6)		5,632,000
Deferred Policy Acquisition and Recapture Costs (Note 12)		40,636,000
Property and Equipment, at cost, less accumulated depreciation and amortization of $1,820,000 (Notes 5 and 6)		27,351,000
Other Assets		12,782,000
Excess Cost Over Net Assets of Consolidated Subsidiaries (Note 1)		23,032,000
Equity in Liberty Savings and Loan Association, including excess cost over net assets of $908,000		9,067,000
TOTAL ASSETS		$496,695,000

See accompanying notes to consolidated financial statements.

EQUITY FUNDING CORPORATION OF AMERICA AND SUBSIDIARIES

Consolidated Balance Sheet (Continued) (Note 1)

December 31, 1971

Liabilities

Insurance Reserves and Claims	$148,250,000
Notes and Loans Payable:	
Short term	7,038,000
Funded loans and accounts receivable (Note 3)	26,934,000
Long-Term Debt, of which $17,510,000 matures within one year (Note 6)	49,728,000
Amounts Due and Allocable to Policyholders	19,704,000
Accounts and Commissions Payable	16,283,000
Accrued Expenses and Other Liabilities	11,506,000
Income Taxes, of which $33,322,000 is deferred (Notes 7 and 12)	34,903,000
Subordinated Debt (Note 6)	64,687,000
Commitments and Contingent Liabilities (Note 8)	—

Shareholders' Equity (Note 9)

Preferred Stock	$ 3,649,000	
Common Stock	2,314,000	
Additional Paid-In Capital	61,156,000	
Retained Earnings	50,555,000	
	117,674,000	
Less Common Stock held in Treasury, at cost	12,000	
		117,662,000
TOTAL LIABILITIES AND SHAREHOLDERS' EQUITY		$496,695,000

See accompanying notes to consolidated financial statements.

EQUITY FUNDING CORPORATION OF AMERICA AND SUBSIDIARIES

Consolidated Statement of Additional Paid-In Capital and Retained Earnings

	1967	1968	1969	1970	1971
	Restated	Restated	Restated	Restated	Year Ended December 31
ADDITIONAL PAID-IN CAPITAL:					
Balance at beginning of year	$(3,307,000)	$ 2,855,000	$13,577,000	$41,770,000	$54,553,000
Excess of proceeds or market value over par value of stock issued for the employee stock bonus plan, and exercises of options and warrants, and sale of stock	4,706,000	8,730,000	757,000	1,131,000	2,397,000
Excess of market value over par value of stock issued as a dividend	1,456,000	1,992,000	5,880,000	5,688,000	—
Excess of market value over par value of stock issued in acquisitions	—	—	6,609,000	1,974,000	1,382,000
Excess of market value of Series 'B' Preferred Stock over par value of stock issued on conversions	—	—	—	—	2,824,000
Proceeds of issuance of common stock purchase warrants	—	—	—	3,990,000	—
Excess of exercise price over par value of stock issued on conversions of debentures	—	—	14,947,000	—	—
Balance at end of year	$ 2,855,000	$13,577,000	$41,770,000	$54,553,000	$61,156,000
RETAINED EARNINGS:					
Balance at beginning of year	$12,511,000	$13,676,000	$20,791,000	$27,149,000	$33,060,000
Net earnings for the year	2,786,000	9,285,000	12,527,000	12,870,000	18,192,000
Dividends on preferred stock	—	—	—	(42,000)	(21,000)
Dividends on common stock	(1,619,000)	(2,170,000)	(6,169,000)	(6,917,000)	(676,000)
Adjustment for minority interest	(2,000)	—	—	—	—
Balance at end of year	$13,676,000	$20,791,000	$27,149,000	$33,060,000	$50,555,000

See accompanying notes to consolidated financial statements.

EQUITY FUNDING CORPORATION OF AMERICA AND SUBSIDIARIES

Consolidated Statement of Changes in Financial Position

	Year Ended December 31		
	1969	**1970**	**1971**
	Restated	Restated	
SOURCE OF FUNDS:			
Earnings Before Extraordinary Items	$ 11,891,000	$ 13,891,000	$ 19,332,000
Items Not Requiring the Use of Funds:			
Depreciation and amortization	2,012,000	3,420,000	2,596,000
Deferred income taxes	6,103,000	5,430,000	5,313,000
Equity in undistributed earnings of Liberty Savings and Loan Association	(839,000)	35,000	(60,000)
FUNDS PROVIDED BY OPERATIONS	19,167,000	22,776,000	27,181,000
Earnings from extraordinary items	230,000	—	—
Item Not Requiring the Use of Funds:			
Deferred income taxes	294,000	—	—
Funds Provided by Extraordinary item	524,000	—	—
Funds Provided by Net Earnings	19,691,000	22,776,000	27,181,000
Proceeds from long-term debt, notes and loans payable	48,815,000	52,142,000	49,744,000
Sales, repayments and maturities of investments	18,001,000	25,976,000	28,927,000
Increases in insurance reserves and amounts allocable to policyholders	9,204,000	13,565,000	9,354,000
Increase (decrease) in other liabilities	8,936,000	(3,649,000)	4,529,000
Sale of property and equipment	2,494,000	6,141,000	4,301,000
Funds provided from the issuance of stock ..	22,540,000	1,149,000	2,220,000
TOTALS	$129,681,000	$118,100,000	$126,256,000
APPLICATION OF FUNDS:			
Increase in investments	$ 42,592,000	$ 36,978,000	$ 36,688,000
Increase in receivables	25,146,000	35,083,000	28,509,000
Retirement of long-term debt	16,554,000	12,811,000	19,947,000
Increase in cash	8,721,000	4,909,000	18,738,000
Increase in deferred acquisition costs	1,264,000	6,662,000	11,284,000
Additions to property and equipment	15,746,000	14,083,000	10,238,000
Cash dividends	260,000	1,157,000	697,000
Increase in inventories and other assets	2,350,000	6,417,000	155,000
Excess of cost over net assets of acquisitions	17,048,000	—	—
TOTALS	$129,681,000	$118,100,000	$126,256,000

See accompanying notes to consolidated financial statements.

EQUITY FUNDING CORPORATION OF AMERICA AND SUBSIDIARIES

Notes to Consolidated Financial Statements

1. Principles of Consolidation, Acquisition and Disposition of Subsidiaries:

The consolidated financial statements include the accounts of the Company and all of its subsidiaries after elimination of intercompany accounts, except for Liberty Savings and Loan
Association (an unconsolidated subsidiary) which is stated at cost, plus equity in undistributed
earnings since acquisition.

The accounts of life insurance companies have been stated on the basis of generally accepted
accounting principles, which differ materially in some respects from those followed in reports to
regulatory authorities, in accordance with guidelines contained in the Exposure Draft dated
December 1970 prepared by the Committee on Insurance Accounting and Auditing of the American
Institute of Certified Public Accountants entitled "Audits of Life Insurance Companies".

During 1971, the Company acquired the outstanding guaranteed stock of Liberty Savings and
Loan Association for approximately $6,500,000 in preferred stock. On April 12, 1971, the operations
of Crown Savings and Loan Association were merged into Liberty Savings and Loan Association.
Condensed financial statements of Liberty Savings and Loan Association are as follows:

Condensed Balance Sheet

December 31, 1971

Assets

Cash and bank certificates of deposit	$ 6,820,000
U.S. Government and other obligations, at amortized cost (market, $6,893,000)	6,986,000
Loans receivable	95,208,000
Property held for sale, at cost, less valuation allowance, $404,000	3,549,000
Other assets	5,953,000
Total assets	$118,516,000

Liabilities

Savings accounts	$ 88,195,000
Advances from Federal Home Loan Bank	16,947,000
Other liabilities and deferred income	5,215,000
Total liabilities	110,357,000

Shareholders' Equity

Guarantee capital stock	517,000
Additional paid-in capital	5,000
Retained earnings:	
Appropriated to general reserves	6,530,000
Unappropriated	1,107,000
Total shareholders' equity	8,159,000
Total liabilities and shareholders' equity	$118,516,000

EQUITY FUNDING CORPORATION OF AMERICA AND SUBSIDIARIES

Notes to Consolidated Financial Statements (Continued)

Condensed Statement of Earnings

	Year ended December 31,		
	1969	1970	1971
Income:			
Interest	$6,773,000	$7,071,000	$7,102,000
Other	507,000	514,000	975,000
Total income	7,280,000	7,585,000	8,077,000
Expenses:			
Interest	5,095,000	5,508,000	5,772,000
Other	1,058,000	1,304,000	1,227,000
Total expenses	6,153,000	6,812,000	6,999,000
Earnings before income taxes	1,127,000	773,000	1,078,000
Income taxes	288,000	251,000	263,000
Net earnings	$ 839,000	$ 522,000	$ 815,000

The Company also acquired Bankers National Life Insurance Company of Parsippany, New Jersey for 1,600,000 shares of the Company's common stock. The acquisitions of "Liberty" and "Bankers" have been accounted for as a pooling of interests, and accordingly, the consolidated financial statements have been restated for the periods prior to 1971.

In September 1971, the Company rescinded its acquisition agreement to acquire Diversified Land Company and a 51% interest in New Era Development Corporation. An amount of $2,316,000 due from "Diversified" (advances from the Company) is included in the consolidated balance sheet as a receivable. The rescission was mutually agreed to on March 1, 1972 but was effective as of December 31, 1971. Therefore, the accounts of "Diversified" are not included in the accompanying financial statements.

The amount by which the Company's investments in consolidated subsidiaries exceeded the net book values on dates of acquisition is not being amortized since the Company anticipates no diminution in value.

2. Investments:

Investments are stated in the consolidated balance sheet as follows:

Bonds — at amortized cost

Loans — at unpaid principal balances, which balances as to policy loans do not exceed the cash value of the underlying policies

Corporate stocks and other securities — at cost.

3. Funded Loans and Accounts Receivable:

Under the Company's method of operations, funded loans and accounts receivable represent, in the aggregate, the amount that clients owe as a result of the various "Equity Funding" Insurance Premium Funding Programs offered by the Company, and net contracts receivable, together with

EQUITY FUNDING CORPORATION OF AMERICA AND SUBSIDIARIES

Notes to Consolidated Financial Statements (Continued)

loans and receivables where "Equity Funding" Programs have terminated and where the respective shares have not been liquidated.

The Funded Loans and Accounts Receivable are offset, in part, by the contra Notes Payable on Funded Loans and Accounts Receivable. The difference, in the amount of $61,682,000, is held by the Company.

Of the total issued collateral assigned by clients as security to the Company, $52,204,000 is being used to secure notes payable in the amount of $26,934,000 held by various lending institutions.

4. Inventories and Properties Held for Resale:

Inventories are stated at the lower of cost or market (generally on a specific item basis) and consist of the following:

	January 1, 1971	December 31, 1971
	Restated	
Land and construction in process	$3,699,000	$3,163,000
Property held for resale	2,616,000	1,103,000
Cattle and feed	64,000	880,000
Other	786,000	486,000
	$7,165,000	$5,632,000

5. Property and Equipment:

Property and equipment, at cost, consist of the following:

Real estate and leasehold improvements	$12,542,000
Furniture, fixtures and equipment	4,059,000
Breeding herd	1,613,000
Exploration and development of natural resources	10,957,000
	29,171,000
Less accumulated depreciation and amortization	1,820,000
	$27,351,000

It is the policy of the Company to provide for depreciation primarily on a "straight-line" basis predicated on the estimated useful lives of the individual items in the various classes of assets. The principal estimated useful lives used in computing depreciation are as follows:

Breeding herd	3 to 8 years
Buildings and improvements	20 to 50 years
Exploration and development of natural resources	Unit of production
Leasehold improvements	3 to 10 years
Office furniture and equipment	5 to 10 years

EQUITY FUNDING CORPORATION OF AMERICA AND SUBSIDIARIES

Notes to Consolidated Financial Statements (Continued)

Expenditures for additions, major renewals and betterments are capitalized and expenditures for maintenance and repairs are charged to income as incurred. Upon sale or retirement of items of property and equipment, the costs and related accumulated depreciation are eliminated from the accounts, and the resulting gain or loss, if any, is reflected in income. Equipment becoming obsolete or unusable is written down to salvage value.

6. Long-Term and Subordinated Debt:

Notes payable secured by contracts receivable, inventory of land, land and buildings, security interests in cattle and buildings in process of construction (bearing interest between 5 and 10% per annum) maturing between February 1972 and January 1, 2000 .... $ 4,961,000

Notes payable secured by custodial collateral notes in the amount of $5,000,000 bearing interest between 7 and 8½% per annum maturing September 8, 1972 5,168,000

Note payable secured by 200,000 shares of Equity Funding Life Insurance Company (a wholly-owned subsidiary) bearing interest of 8⅝% per annum maturing January 1975 5,480,000

Unsecured notes payable bearing interest between 6¼ and 8% per annum maturing between January 1, 1972 and January 1, 1975 15,909,000

9½% debentures (authorized $40,000,000, issued $22,000,000 less unamortized discount of $3,790,000, the balance may be issued at any time up to October 14, 1976) due 1990, redeemable through sinking fund operation commencing with 1976 as follows:

    4% of principal outstanding October 15, 1976

    "Base Amount" for the period 1976-1980

    6% of the "Base Amount" 1981-1985

    10% of the "Base Amount" 1986-1989

    The balance is due at maturity.

As a part of the indenture agreement, the Company may not, in the aggregate, have senior debt exceeding 200% of the sum of the tangible net assets and subordinated debt (as defined in the indenture) so long as any of these debentures shall be outstanding 18,210,000

TOTAL LONG-TERM DEBT $49,728,000

5½% convertible subordinated debentures due 1991 redeemable through sinking fund operation commencing with 1982 as follows:

    Prior to December 1, in each year commencing with the year 1982 and including the year 1990, an amount in cash sufficient to redeem on such date not less than 10 nor more than 20% of the principal amount thereof outstanding at the close of business on December 1, 1981.

These debentures are convertible into the Company's common stock at $36.75 per share, subject to adjustment in certain events $38,500,000

5¼% guaranteed (subordinated) debentures due 1989. The debentures are subject to optional redemption at fixed percentages from February 1972 to maturity. The debentures also are subject to redemption in part on February 1, 1980 and on each February 1st thereafter to and including February 1, 1988 through the operation of a sinking fund at the rate of 10% of the aggregate principal amount of the debentures outstanding on November 30, 1979. The debentures are convertible into common stock of the Company at $49.52 per share 22,917,000

EQUITY FUNDING CORPORATION OF AMERICA AND SUBSIDIARIES

Notes to Consolidated Financial Statements (Continued)

7½% guaranteed (subordinated) notes due 1974. The notes may be applied at face value in payment of the exercise price of originally attached warrants	3,270,000
TOTAL SUBORDINATED DEBT	$64,687,000

Long-term and subordinated debt maturing each of the next five years ended December 31, is as follows:

1972	$17,510,000
1973	$ 2,625,000
1974	$ 6,196,000
1975	$ 2,401,000
1976	$ 450,000

7. Income Taxes:

The provision and the liability for Federal and State income taxes have been computed on the accrual basis. The Company reports on the cash basis for income tax purposes. Also, for income tax purposes, certain items, consisting primarily of intangible drilling costs, are deducted in the year paid, whereas for financial reporting purposes the costs are capitalized. The Company is of the opinion that this difference is of a permanent nature, and therefore results in a reduction of the normal tax provision. The deferred portion of the income tax liability has been separately stated. In 1971, the Internal Revenue Service completed its examination of the Company's consolidated tax returns for the years 1965 through 1968. No material changes were required as a result of the examination.

8. Commitments and Contingent Liabilities:

Leases:

The Company leases offices and equipment at monthly rentals totalling approximately $258,000 plus property taxes and insurance in some instances. The leases expire in the years 1972 through 1980.

Litigation:

The Company has been advised by counsel that its potential liability with respect to the various lawsuits in which it is involved will not have a material adverse effect upon the operations or property of the Company taken as a whole.

Guarantees:

The Company and certain subsidiaries have guaranteed loans, notes and commitments under their limited partnership operations. At December 31, 1971 the Company is unaware of any defaults in connection with these guarantees (See "Capitalization—Revolving Credit Agreement", Construction and Development, Cattle, Oil and Gas, and Savings and Loan Business—Real Estate Partnerships", "Cattle Business" and "Oil and Gas Exploration").

88

EQUITY FUNDING CORPORATION OF AMERICA AND SUBSIDIARIES

Notes to Consolidated Financial Statements (Continued)

9. Shareholders' Equity:

Preferred stock, authorized 2,000,000 shares of no par value:

Series A:

All shares issued were cancelled as of December 31, 1971.

Series B ($100 stated value):

64,974 shares issued	$6,497,000
(28,484) shares converted into common stock	(2,848,000)
36,490 shares outstanding	$3,649,000

Liquidation preference — $100 per share

Redemption rights —

10% within 1st year following issuance

15% within 2nd year following issuance

20% within 3rd year following issuance

25% within 4th year following issuance

Balance within 5th year following issuance

Annual Dividend rate — none

Voting Rights — one per share

Convertible into common at a conversion price of $35.00 per share.

Common stock, authorized 30,000,000 shares of $.30 par value:

Balance at beginning of year	$2,241,000
Issue of stock upon conversion of Series B Preferred Stock	24,000
Issue of stock for employee bonus plan and exercise of stock options	31,000
Issue of stock — other	18,000
Balance at end of year	$2,314,000
Shares issued at end of year	7,712,063
Less shares reacquired and held in treasury	5,278
Shares outstanding at end of year	7,706,785

Stock options:

The Company has issued common stock purchase options to certain employees, district and branch managers and agents of the Company. Information as of December 31, with respect to outstanding options granted under the plans is as follows (adjusted for all stock splits and stock dividends through December 31, 1971):

89

EQUITY FUNDING CORPORATION OF AMERICA AND SUBSIDIARIES

Notes to Consolidated Financial Statements (Continued)

	Number of Shares	Option Price(1) Per Share	Option Price(1) Total
Production Options	201,202	$20.13-$70.96	$ 7,997,104
Incentive Options	62,823	$14.75-$62.01	2,537,188
Qualified Options	200,333	$13.29-$74.51	8,402,974
Recruiting Options	710	$20.13-$61.03	25,571
Other Options	16,221	$24.44-$29.21	469,723
	481,289		$19,432,560

(1) Market values at date of grant were the same as the option

   Additional information with respect to common stock purchase options as of December 31, 1971:

	Number of Shares	Option Price Per Share	Option Price Total	Market Value Per Share	Market Value Total
1967 Qualified Stock Option Plan:					
Shares under option at December 31, 1971	9,586	$16.41-$55.87	$ 253,944	$16.41-$55.87	$ 253,944 (a)
Options which became exercisable during 1971	None	—	—	—	—
Options exercised during 1971	4,794	$16.41-$25.11	$ 79,809	$30.38-$45.13	$ 159,436 (c)
1968 Qualified Stock Option Plan:					
Shares under option at December 31, 1971	158,095	$15.00-$74.51	$7,247,891	$15.00-$74.51	$7,247,891 (a)
Options which became exercisable during 1971	40,874	$15.00-$74.51	$1,723,561	$23.88-$45.13	$1,414,623 (b)
Options exercised during 1971	4,677	$15.00-$26.00	$ 76,575	$30.38-$41.38	$ 157,643 (c)
Bankers Qualified Stock Option Plans:					
Shares under option at December 31, 1971	32,652	$13.29-$32.48	$ 901,139	$13.29-$32.48	$ 901,139 (a)
Options which became exercisable during 1971	8,699	$24.44-$32.48	$ 285,068	$39.25	$ 341,436 (d)
Options exercised during 1971	None	—	—	—	—
1968 Incentive Stock Option Plan:					
Shares under option at December 31, 1971	25,460	$25.11-$60.79	$ 811,400	$25.11-$60.79	$ 811,400 (a)
Options which became exercisable during 1971	6,630	$25.11-$60.79	$ 207,538	$23.88-$44.75	$ 177,161 (b)
Options exercised during 1971	3,185	$25.11-$36.16	$ 84,968	$30.38-$45.88	$ 126,113 (c)

90

EQUITY FUNDING CORPORATION OF AMERICA AND SUBSIDIARIES

Notes to Consolidated Financial Statements (Continued)

	Number of Shares	Option Price		Market-Value	
		Per Share	Total	Per Share	Total
1969 Incentive Stock Option Plan:					
Shares under option at December 31, 1971....	37,363	$14.75-$62.01	$1,725,788	$14.75-$62.01	$1,725,788 (a)
Options which became exercisable during 1971	5,438	$52.99-$62.01	$ 312,800	$23.88-$42.88	$ 175,998 (b)
Options exercised during 1971	None	—	—	—	—
1968 Production Stock Option Plan:					
Shares under option at December 31, 1971....	50,264	$25.11-$41.45	$1,365,284	$25.11-$41.45	$1,365,284 (a)
Options which became exercisable during 1971	13,683	$25.11-$41.45	$ 369,038	$23.88	$ 326,750 (b)
Options exercised during 1971	5,151	$25.11-$41.45	$ 131,694	$28.62-$45.13	$ 200,433 (c)
1969 Production Stock Option Plan:					
Shares under option at December 31, 1971....	83,802	$51.50-$70.96	$5,129,858	$51.50-$70.96	$5,129,858 (a)
Options which became exercisable during 1971	16,176	$51.50-$70.96	$ 993,690	$23.88-$41.75	$ 442,887 (b)
Options exercised during 1971	None	—	—	—	—
1970 Production Stock Option Plan:					
Shares under option at December 31, 1971....	67,136	$20.13-$23.88	$1,501,962	$20.13-$23.88	$1,501,962 (a)
Options which became exercisable during 1971	5,219	$20.13	$ 105,058	$39.88	$ 208,134 (b)
Options exercised during 1971	93	$20.13	$ 1,872	$32.25-$41.38	$ 3,310 (c)
1969 Recruiting Stock Option Plan:					
Shares under option at December 31, 1971....	710	$20.13-$61.03	$ 25,571	$20.13-$61.03	$ 25,571 (a)
Options which became exercisable during 1971	450	$20.13-$53.43	$ 16,936	$23.88-$43.25	$ 17,560 (b)
Options exercised during 1971	None	—	—	—	—

91

EQUITY FUNDING CORPORATION OF AMERICA AND SUBSIDIARIES

Notes to Consolidated Financial Statements (Continued)

	Number of Shares	Option Price		Market-Value	
		Per Share	Total	Per Share	Total
Bankers Stock Option Plan for Key General Agents:					
Shares under option at December 31, 1971....	16,221	$24.44-$29.21	$ 469,723	$24.44-$29.21	$ 469,723 (a)
Options which became exercisable during 1971	5,407	$24.44-$29.21	$ 156,374	$39.25	$ 212,225 (d)
Options exercised during 1971	None	—	—	—	—

(a) At the dates options were granted.

(b) At the dates options became exercisable.

(c) At the dates options were exercised.

(d) At the date of acquisition of Bankers.

Warrants:

As of December 31, 1971, warrants to purchase common stock were outstanding as follows: 550,000 shares at $25.25, 41,856 shares at $58.46 and 30,900 shares at $68.00.

Other:

On May 24, 1971, an Employee Stock Bonus Plan was approved by the shareholders. Pursuant to terms and conditions contained in the Plan (i) 21,500 shares have been issued directly to various employees as compensation, and (ii) 64,500 shares have been issued and placed in escrow for future payment to the various employees when conditions required under the Plan have been met. (See "Management — Employee Stock Bonus Plan".)

10. Dividend Restriction on Retained Earnings:

As of December 31, 1971, $46,889,000 was available for payment of dividends out of consolidated retained earnings of $50,555,000. The difference, in the amount of $3,666,000, is restricted as a result of a surplus deficit of one of the Company's life insurance subsidiaries at the date of its acquisition by the Company. However, only $17,668,000 of the retained earnings available for dividends may be paid in cash because of provisions contained in an indenture agreement.

11. Subsequent Events:

Subsequent to December 31, 1971, the Company reached an agreement in principle to acquire a 91% interest in Northern Life Insurance Co., of Seattle, Washington, from Nationwide Corp., Columbus, Ohio, for $39,200,000, of which $31,200,000 would be paid in cash, with the remainder in term notes. Completion of the acquisition is subject to approval of a definitive agreement by the boards of directors of the companies, and the approval of regulatory agencies, including the Insurance Commissioner of the State of Washington. (See "Certain Recent Acquisitions — Acquisition of Northern Life Insurance Company".)

OPINION OF INDEPENDENT CERTIFIED PUBLIC ACCOUNTANTS

Equity Funding Life Insurance Company:

We have examined the balance sheet of Equity Funding Life Insurance Company as of December 31, 1971, the related statement of operations for the four years then ended, and the related statements of additional paid-in capital, retained earnings, and changes in financial position for the three years then ended. Our examination was made in accordance with generally accepted auditing standards, and accordingly included such tests of the accounting records and such other auditing procedures as we considered necessary in the circumstances. The policy reserves (exclusive of accident and health reserves as of December 31, 1968), net deferred and uncollected life premiums, and accrued costs of recapture of reinsured policies were confirmed by an opinion of Milliman & Robertson, Inc., independent consulting actuaries. As to amounts included in the statement of operations for the two years ended December 31, 1969 applicable to accident and health business transacted under the agreement referred to in Note e to such statement (which amounts constitute substantial portions of the accident and health totals), we were furnished with the report of other independent accountants on their examination of the "schedules of accounts" relating to such business.

In our opinion, based on our examination and the aforementioned opinion of independent consulting actuaries and report of other independent accountants, the above-mentioned financial statements present fairly the financial position of the Company at December 31, 1971 and the results of its operations and the changes in its financial position for the stated periods then ended, in conformity with generally accepted accounting principles applied on a consistent basis, after giving retroactive effect to the change, in which we concur, in financial reporting practices described in Note 1.

HASKINS & SELLS

Los Angeles, California
March 10, 1972

REPORT OF INDEPENDENT CERTIFIED PUBLIC ACCOUNTANTS

Presidential Life Insurance Agency, Inc.
Beverly Hills, California

We have examined the schedules of accounts for the period March 7, 1968 to December 31, 1968 and the year ended December 31, 1969, relating to accident and health insurance solicited by Presidential Life Insurance Agency, Inc., for Equity Funding Life Insurance Company (formerly The Presidential Life Insurance Company of America) under an agency agreement dated March 1, 1968, as amended. Our examination was made in accordance with generally accepted auditing standards, and accordingly included such tests of the accounting records and such other auditing procedures as we considered necessary in the circumstances.

In our opinion the aforementioned schedules of accounts (not separately presented in this prospectus) of the Presidential Life Insurance Agency, Inc., present fairly the information set forth for the period March 7, 1968 to December 31, 1968, and the year ended December 31, 1969, in conformity with accounting practices prescribed or permitted by the Insurance Department of Illinois, applied on a consistent basis.

LYBRAND, ROSS BROS. & MONTGOMERY

Philadelphia, Pennsylvania
March 12, 1970

REPORT OF CERTIFIED PUBLIC ACCOUNTANTS

The Board of Directors
Equity Funding Life Insurance Company

We have examined the statement of operations of The Presidential Life Insurance Company of America (now Equity Funding Life Insurance Company) for the year ended December 31, 1967. Our examination was made in accordance with generally accepted auditing standards, and accordingly included such tests of the accounting records and such other auditing procedures as we considered necessary in the circumstances. The amounts of aggregate reserves for life insurance policies at December 31, 1966 were certified by the Department of Insurance of the State of Illinois and the amounts of actuarial items reflected in the financial statements at December 31, 1967 were certified by consulting actuaries and were not independently verified by us.

The Company maintains its accounts in accordance with accounting practices authorized by the Department of Insurance of the State of Illinois. Material differences between such practices and those required by generally accepted accounting principles are set forth in Note (a) to the Statement of Operations.

In our opinion, based upon our examination and the certifications referred to in the first paragraph, the statement mentioned above presents fairly the results of operations of Equity Funding Life Insurance Company for the year ended December 31, 1967, in conformity with accounting practices authorized by the Department of Insurance of the State of Illinois applied on a basis consistent with that of the preceding year.

ARTHUR YOUNG & COMPANY

Chicago, Illinois
March 12, 1968

OPINION OF INDEPENDENT CONSULTING ACTUARIES

The Board of Directors
Equity Funding Life Insurance Company

We have examined the calculations of policy reserves (exclusive of accident and health reserves as of December 31, 1968), net deferred and uncollected life premiums and accrued costs of recapture of reinsured policies of Equity Funding Life Insurance Company for the five years ended December 31, 1971. Our examination included such tests of the actuarial bases and methods and such other procedures as we considered necessary in the circumstances.

In our opinion, the above mentioned items have been calculated in conformity with generally accepted actuarial methods applied on a consistent basis, after giving retroactive effect to the change, in which we concur, in the recalculation of policy reserves referred to in Note 1.

MILLIMAN & ROBERTSON, INC.
by Gilbert E. Kerns
Fellow, Society of Actuaries

Pasadena, California
March 10, 1972

OPINION OF INDEPENDENT CONSULTING ACTUARIES

The Board of Directors
Equity Funding Life Insurance Company

In our opinion, the amounts of deferred and uncollected premiums and aggregate reserve for insurance policies included in the financial statements of Equity Funding Life Insurance Company for the year ended December 31, 1967 was computed in accordance with applicable state insurance regulations and represent adequate provisions for such items.

MILLIMAN & ROBERTSON, INC.
By Gilbert E. Kerns
Fellow, Society of Actuaries

Pasadena, California
March 19, 1971

EQUITY FUNDING LIFE INSURANCE COMPANY

Balance Sheet

December 31, 1971

Assets

Investments (Note 2):

Bonds	$ 7,663,931
Bank certificates of deposit	5,003,617
Policy loans	90,361
Total	12,757,909
Cash	574,344
Net Deferred and Uncollected Premiums	798,007
Deferred Policy Acquisition and Recapture Costs (Note 3)	16,559,942
Accrued Interest	82,511
Amounts Due from Reinsurers	3,683,571
Other Assets	1,013,689
TOTAL	$35,469,973

Liabilities and Stockholder's Equity

Policy Reserves (Note 4):

Life	$ 7,898,075
Accident and health	117,633
Supplementary contracts without life contingencies	114,878
Total	8,130,586
Accrued Costs of Recapture of Reinsured Policies (Note 5)	3,242,434
Policy and Contract Claims	115,630
Amounts Payable to Reinsurers	1,685,471

Other Liabilities:

Federal income taxes	115,000
Premium taxes and general expenses	357,762
Miscellaneous	12,670
Total	485,432
Deferred Federal Income Taxes (Note 6)	4,213,000

Commitments and Contingent Liabilities (Note 4)

Stockholder's Equity:

Common stock—authorized, 5,000,000 shares of $2 par value each; issued and outstanding, 500,000 shares	1,000,000
Additional paid-in capital	7,062,000
Retained earnings (Note 1)	9,535,420
Total	17,597,420
TOTAL	$35,469,973

See notes to the Equity Life financial statements.

EQUITY FUNDING LIFE INSURANCE COMPANY

Notes to Financial Statements (Continued)

6. Federal Income Taxes:

The Company is subject to Federal income tax under the Life Insurance Company Income Tax Act of 1959, as amended. In 1970 and 1971, the Company incurred losses for Federal income tax purposes and, as of December 31, 1971, the Company had an operating loss carryforward of approximately $2,300,000 available to offset future taxable income, if any. Of that amount, $1,600,000 expires in 1975 and $700,000 in 1976. A portion of the 1970 loss gave rise to a claim for refund of $350,000.

Deferred Federal income taxes relate primarily to the excess of deductions for life policy reserves and policy acquisition costs claimed for tax purposes over amounts charged against income for financial accounting purposes.

Under the provisions of the above-mentioned Income Tax Act, the portion of life insurance company gain from operations not currently subject to tax together with certain special deductions are accumulated in a memorandum "Policyholders Surplus Account" for tax purposes. The tax basis "Policyholders Surplus Account" was eliminated at December 31, 1971 as a result of the payment of a $2,435,000 cash dividend to the Company's parent. Federal income tax of approximately $115,000 was incurred on this distribution. The Company's "Policyholders Surplus Account", recomputed in accordance with generally accepted accounting principles applied in the accompanying financial statements, aggregated approximately $9,000,000 at December 31, 1971, including additions thereto of about $900,000 in 1969, $3,300,000 in 1970 and $4,600,000 in 1971. No Federal income tax was incurred on the aforementioned dividend on this basis of reporting inasmuch as such distribution was absorbed by another tax surplus account. A provision for Federal income taxes of approximately $4,300,000 at December 31, 1971 would be required with respect to the recomputed balance of the "Policyholders Surplus Account" when and if such "account" exceeds a prescribed maximum or distributions are made therefrom.

The Company has a long-term capital loss carryforward of approximately $600,000 at December 31, 1971 which expires principally in 1974.

SUMMARIZED FINANCIAL INFORMATION

Equity Funding Corporaton of America and Subsidiaries

Consolidated Statement of Earnings	Three Months Ended March 31	
	1972	1971
Revenues		
Insurance-premiums and commissions		
(includes coinsurance for 1972 of $1,600,000)	$15,763,000	$13,842,000
Securities	3,495,000	4,414,000
Real estate	4,391,000	4,696,000
Natural resources	1,387,000	1,582,000
Investment management	650,000	382,000
Interest and investment income	5,392,000	4,527,000
Other	279,000	65,000
Earnings from Liberty Savings and Loan Association	186,000	101,000
Total Revenues	31,543,000	29,609,000
Costs and Expenses		
Insurance:		
Insurance benefits	5,301,000	4,818,000
Increase in reserves	2,021,000	1,834,000
Commissions	3,063,000	2,975,000
	10,385,000	9,627,000
Securities commissions	1,103,000	1,501,000
Real estate, cost of sales	3,894,000	4,243,000
Natural resources, cost of sales	1,221,000	937,000
Interest and amortization of debt expense	2,799,000	2,274,000
Selling, general and administrative expenses	4,260,000	4,313,000
Dividends and income allocable to policyholders	474,000	546,000
Total Costs and Expenses	24,136,000	23,441,000
Earnings Before Income Taxes	7,407,000	6,168,000
Income taxes, including $1,529,000 deferred for 1972	2,265,000	1,801,000
Net Earnings	$ 5,142,000	$ 4,367,000
Earnings Per Common Share (Exhibit 1 Attached)		
Earnings Per Common and Common Equivalent Share	$.64	$.55
Earnings Per Common Share-Assuming Full Dilution	$.58	$.53
Cash Dividend Per Share	—0—	$.10

4 & 5

QUARTERLY
REPORT

Equity Funding Corporation of America and Subsidiaries

Consolidated Statement of Earnings	Six Months Ended June 30	
	1972	1971
		(Restated)
Revenues		
Insurance-premiums and commissions (includes coinsurance for 1972 of $3,600,000)	$32,290,000	$28,085,000
Securities	7,347,000	8,141,000
Real estate	6,478,000	10,898,000
Natural resources	2,872,000	3,408,000
Investment management	1,297,000	817,000
Interest and investment income	11,032,000	9,004,000
Other	599,000	262,000
Earnings from Liberty Savings and Loan Association	401,000	385,000
Total Revenues	62,316,000	61,000,000
Costs and Expenses		
Insurance:		
Insurance benefits	9,467,000	9,740,000
Increase in reserves	3,098,000	4,063,000
Commissions	6,386,000	5,181,000
Policy acquisition costs	1,930,000	350,000
	20,881,000	19,334,000
Securities commissions	2,381,000	2,849,000
Real estate, cost of sales	5,761,000	9,869,000
Natural resources, cost of sales	2,538,000	2,416,000
Interest and amortization of debt expense	5,569,000	4,373,000
Selling, general and administrative expenses	8,966,000	8,684,000
Dividends and income allocable to policyholders	1,238,000	1,148,000
Total Costs and Expenses	47,334,000	48,673,000
Earnings Before Income Taxes	14,982,000	12,327,000
Income taxes, including $3,290,000 deferred for 1972	4,541,000	3,473,000
Net Earnings	$10,441,000	$ 8,854,000
Earnings Per Common Share		
Earnings Per Common and Common Equivalent Share	$1.30	$1.12
Earnings Per Common Share-Assuming Full Dilution	$1.17	$1.09

Equity Funding Corporation of America and Subsidiaries

Consolidated Balance Sheet	*June 30*
	1972

Assets

Cash and short-term investments	$ 33,280,000
Investments — principally of insurance subsidiaries	
Bonds	143,707,000
Mortgage loans	86,233,000
Loans to life insurance policyholders	32,941,000
Other loans	18,582,000
Corporate stocks and other securities	26,082,000
Real Estate	1,827,000
Total Investments	309,372,000
Funded loans and accounts receivable	103,525,000
Contracts, notes and loans receivable, of which $11,127,000 matures within one year	37,867,000
Insurance premiums in course of collection	15,292,000
Accounts and commissions receivable	27,087,000
Inventories and properties held for resale	6,284,000
Deferred policy acquisition and recapture costs	52,866,000
Property and equipment, at cost, less accumulated depreciation and amortization of $2,432,000	33,566,000
Other assets	12,797,000
Excess of cost over net assets of consolidated subsidiaries	23,860,000
Equity in Liberty Savings and Loan Association including excess cost over net assets of $908,000	9,468,000
Total Assets	$665,264,000

6 & 7

	June 30 1972
Liabilities	
Insurance reserves and claims	$234,205,000
Notes and loans payable:	
Short-term	10,317,000
Funded loans and accounts receivable	34,019,000
Long -Term Debt, of which $8,617,000 matures within one year	99,055,000
Amounts due and allocable to policyholders	24,228,000
Accounts and commissions payable	13,433,000
Accrued expenses and other liabilities	12,263,000
Income taxes, of which $36,724,000 is deferred	38,381,000
Subordinated debt	64,687,000
Minority interest	3,764,000
Shareholders' Equity	
Preferred stock-authorized 2,000,000 shares, $100 stated value, issued 24,562 shares	2,456,000
Common stock-authorized 30,000,000 shares, $.30 par value, issued 7,923,976 shares	2,377,000
Additional paid-in capital	65,857,000
Retained earnings	60,230,000
	130,920,000
Less common stock held in treasury, at cost	(8,000)
	130,912,000
Total Liabilities and Shareholders' Equity	$665,264,000

4 & 5

Equity Funding Corporation of America and Subsidiaries

Consolidated Statement of Earnings	Nine Months Ended September 30	
	1972	1971
		(Restated)
Revenues		
Insurance-premiums and commissions (includes coinsurance of $5,544,000 for 1972 and $4,146,000 for 1971)	$ 54,809,000	$ 42,673,000
Securities	11,569,000	11,437,000
Real estate	12,317,000	11,083,000
Natural resources	3,735,000	4,886,000
Investment management	2,192,000	1,163,000
Interest and investment income	18,644,000	14,078,000
Other	1,035,000	438,000
Earnings from Liberty Savings and Loan Association	604,000	577,000
Total Revenues	104,905,000	86,335,000
Costs and Expenses		
Insurance:		
Insurance benefits	15,743,000	13,242,000
Increase in reserves	11,852,000	7,444,000
Commissions	9,693,000	7,602,000
Policy acquisition costs	2,219,000	434,000
	39,507,000	28,722,000
Securities commissions	3,832,000	3,839,000
Real estate, cost of sales	11,365,000	10,071,000
Natural resources, cost of sales	3,248,000	3,451,000
Interest and amortization of debt expense	9,057,000	6,760,000
Selling, general and administrative expenses	14,034,000	13,016,000
Dividends and income allocable to policyholders	1,962,000	1,852,000
Total Costs and Expenses	83,005,000	67,711,000
Earnings Before Income Taxes	21,900,000	18,624,000
Income taxes, including $4,621,000 deferred for 1972	6,415,000	5,441,000
Net Earnings	$ 15,485,000	$ 13,183,000
Earnings Per Common Share		
Earnings Per Common and Common Equivalent Share	$1.93	$1.66
Earnings Per Common Share-Assuming Full Dilution	$1.73	$1.62

Equity Funding Corporation of America and Subsidiaries

Consolidated Balance Sheet	September 30 1972
Assets	
Cash and short-term investments	$ 26,808,000
Investments—principally of insurance subsidiaries:	
Bonds	151,027,000
Mortgage loans	82,976,000
Loans to life insurance policyholders	33,257,000
Other loans	23,046,000
Corporate stocks and other securities	25,555,000
Real estate	1,865,000
Total Investments	317,726,000
Funded loans and accounts receivable	111,694,000
Contracts, notes and loans receivable, of which $11,774,000 matures within one year	38,325,000
Insurance premiums in course of collection	15,921,000
Accounts and commissions receivable	28,936,000
Inventories and properties held for resale	5,710,000
Deferred policy acquisition and recapture costs	58,329,000
Property and equipment, at cost, less accumulated depreciation and amortization of $2,676,000	33,187,000
Other assets	12,098,000
Excess cost over net assets acquired of consolidated subsidiaries	23,855,000
Equity in Liberty Savings and Loan Association including excess cost over net assets acquired of $908,000	9,671,000
Total Assets	$682,260,000

6 & 7

	September 30 1972
Liabilities	
Insurance reserves and claims	$246,346,000
Notes and loans payable:	
Short-term	10,900,000
Funded loans and accounts receivable	39,372,000
Long-Term Debt, of which $3,749,000 matures within one year	97,705,000
Amounts due and allocable to policyholders	21,491,000
Accounts and commissions payable	11,676,000
Accrued expenses and other liabilities	12,011,000
Income taxes, of which $38,169,000 is deferred	39,760,000
Subordinated debt	64,687,000
Minority interest	2,332,000
Shareholders' Equity	
Preferred stock-authorized 2,000,000 shares, $100 stated value, issued 24,500 shares	2,450,000
Common stock-authorized 30,000,000 shares, $.30 par value, issued 7,925,257 shares	2,378,000
Additional paid-in capital	65,886,000
Retained earnings	65,274,000
	135,988,000
Less common stock held in treasury, at cost	(8,000)
	135,980,000
Total Liabilities and Shareholders' Equity	$682,260,000

Sources of Financial Materials on Equity Funding

Equity Funding made enough public issues of its securities and acquisitions during its history to provide an unusually continuous series of highly detailed prospectuses. These provide substantially more financial and operating information than its annual reports. Space limitations in this volume prevent reproducing more than a small portion of these materials. Since those interested in further investigation of Equity Funding will find these documents of considerable value, this listing is provided.

Prospectuses contain five years' comparative income statements restated for acquisitions (but only a single year's balance sheet). Each prospectus also has about the same complete information (usually for the five previous years) on insurance and funding plan operations as in the prospectus dated September 11, 1972, included here. Thus they are particularly useful in developing the type of calculations made by the trustee in his report.

Listing applications are comparatively brief, but they contain the details of particular acquisitions, including recent financial statements of the *acquired* company.

Prospectuses are, in theory, available from the original underwriter. They will often be found in other stock brokerage and accounting firm libraries. Listing applications are available from each stock exchange (by number) and are also found in financial libraries.

Note that many of the institutions involved in litigation over Equity Funding are often less than eager to make their files available.

Significant Prospectuses of Equity Funding

Date of Prospectus	Contains Audited Financial Statements for Year Ended	Contains Unaudited Income Statement for Period Ended	Comment
12-14-64	12-31-63	9-30-64	
5-12-65	12-31-64	—	
12-21-65	12-31-64	9-30-65	
11-4-66	12-31-65	6-30-66	
5-25-67	12-31-66	—	
6-18-68	12-31-67	—	Filed with Amex listing application No. 6647, dated 6-28-68
1-22-69	12-31-67	9-30-68	
11-6-69	12-31-68	6-30-69	Filed with Amex Listing application No. 7976, dated 10-10-69
11-14-69	12-31-68	6-30-69	Filed with Amex listing application No. 8081, dated 11-14-69
12-9-70	12-31-69	6-30-70	Filed with NYSEX listing application No. A30376, dated 12-10-70
9-24-71	12-31-70	—	
12-7-71	12-31-70	6-30-70	
9-11-72	12-31-71	—	

Significant Listing Applications of Equity Funding

Acquisition of	Number	Date
Presidential Life Insurance	AMEX 6044	8-6-67
Crown Savings and Loan Association	AMEX 6194	1-9-68
Investors Planning Corp.	AMEX 7334	3-20-69
Ankony Angus	AMEX 7685	6-19-69
Diversified Land	AMEX 8599	6-22-70
Independent Securities Corp.	AMEX 8689	8-11-70
Liberty Savings & Loan	NYSEX A30690	3-15-71
Bankers National Life	NYSEX B702	10-12-71

Proxy Statements

Equity Funding: 9-10-71 — Special proxy statement in connection with acquisition of Bankers National Life Insurance, included in NYSEX Listing Application B702, dated 10-12-71

Bankers Life: 4-27-70 — Special proxy statement in connection with merger with Equity Funding

Stock Prices and Trading Volume, 1965 through March 27, 1973

The following information is provided to give a range of information on the market activity in Equity Funding shares, from the time the company went public until the stock was suspended from trading by the New York Stock Exchange.

All prices given represent actual prices at the time. That is, no adjustments have been made retroactively for splits, stock dividends, etc. Major stock splits are indicated in the footnotes. Volume figures are given only for the later periods in the company's history. Note that the volume in the last two days of trading was equal to 15 percent of the total shares outstanding.

Equity Funding Corporation of America Share Price and Trading Volume for Selected Dates and Periods 1965 to March 27, 1973[1]

Period Ended or Date	High/Low	Volume (100's of shares)
First Quarter 1965	9⅝/7¼	—
Second Quarter 1965	9¾/6⅝	—
Third Quarter 1965	9⅜/6⅞	—
Fourth Quarter 1965	10½/7⅜	—
First Quarter 1966	20¼/10½	—
Second Quarter 1966	21/14	—
Third Quarter 1966	15½/8½[2]	—
November 30, 1966[3]	14⅛/13¾	—
Month of December 1966	15/10½	—

Period Ended or Date	High/Low	Volume (100's of shares)
Month of January 1967	17⅛/11⅛	—
Month of February 1967	24⅜/16½	—
Month of March 1967	33¾/24⅜	—
Second Quarter 1967	40½/27⅜	—
Third Quarter 1967	46⅝/36	—
Fourth Quarter 1967	54⅞/38	—
December 29, 1967	52¾/52⅛	—
January 2, 1968[4]	39/35⅝	—
First Quarter 1968	49⅝/31⅝	—
Second Quarter 1968	65⅛/36⅞	—
Third Quarter 1968	85/57¾	—
September 26, 1968[5]	84⅛/81	—
Third Quarter 1968	85/57¾	—
Month of October 1968	92½/82	—
November 1, 1968	90⅜/86⅛	—
November 4, 1968	87¼/84¼	—
November 5, 1968	Holiday	—
November 6, 1968[6]	46½/43¼	—
November 7 to 29, 1968	64¼/44⅝	—
Month of December 1968	66/52⅛	—
First Quarter 1969	75/47⅛	—
Second Quarter 1969	81⅝/65	—
Third Quarter 1969	74⅛/49⅝	—
Fourth Quarter 1969	76⅛/53	—
October 1969	76⅛/61	—
November 1969	72/63	—
December 1969	69/53	—
December 31, 1969	55¼/54	—
First Quarter 1970	59/38½	15,801
April 1970	52½/26½	5,828
May 1970	28⅝/12¾	19,144
June 1970	25⅛/16¾	29,758
Third Quarter 1970	31/17	48,894
October 1 to 16, 1970	30/24½	5,719
October 19, 1970[7]	24⅞/24¼	439
October 20 to December 31, 1970	26⅞/21⅝	—
Fourth Quarter 1970	30/21⅝	21,362
Month of January 1971	29¾/23⅞	8,479
Month of February 1971	35⅜/29¾	11,914
Month of March 1971	43⅜/33¾	8,844
First Quarter 1971	43⅜/23⅞	29,237
Second Quarter 1971	47/36½	17,937
Third Quarter 1971	45⅜/33⅜	21,353
Month of October 1971	43⅜/32⅝	10,625
Month of November 1971	36¾/27¾	7,368
Month of December 1971	38⅜/31½	10,718
Fourth Quarter 1971	43⅝/27¾	28,711

Period Ended or Date	High/Low	Volume (100's of shares)
First Quarter 1972	43/31¾	25,780
Second Quarter 1972	46½/35¼	18,103
July 1972	39⅝/33⅜	5,331
August 1972	42⅜/37⅛	3,931
September 1972	37⅞/34½	2,585
Third Quarter 1972	42⅜/33⅜	11,847
October 1972	37¼/32¼	3,666
November 1972	40/35¼	4,045
December 1972	41⅛/35½	5,263
Fourth Quarter 1972	41⅛/32¼	12,974
Week of January 1, 1973	37¼/35½	692
Week of January 8, 1973	35¾/31¼	1,211
January 15, 1973	34¾/32¼	992
January 22, 1973	33⅜/29¾	705
January 29, 1973	30/26½	1,970
Month of January 1973	37¼/26½	4,659
Week of February 5, 1973	28½/27⅛	1,311
February 12, 1973	30¼/28	1,077
February 19, 1973	29⅜/25	1,017
February 26, 1973	26¼/23½	1,049
Month of February 1973	30¼/23½	5,044
Week of March 5, 1973	28⅜/25⅝	493
March 12, 1973	28⅝/27½	447
March 13, 1973	27⅜/27¼	143
March 14, 1973	27⅜/27	150
March 15, 1973	26⅞/25½	453
March 16, 1973	25⅝/25	107
Week of March 12, 1973	28⅝/25	1,300
March 19, 1973	25/23	1,238
March 20, 1973	23½/23⅛	144
March 21, 1973	23⅜/19¼	5,240
March 22, 1973	20¼/19¾	596
March 23, 1973	20¼/18⅞	1,137
Week of March 19, 1973	25/18⅞	8,355
March 26, 1973	19¾/16⅜	7,684
March 27, 1973	17½/14⅜	3,072
March 28, 1973	TRADING SUSPENDED	

Notes

[1] Equity Funding's first public offering of shares was in December 1964.

[2] The quotes for 1965 and 1966 through the third quarter are from the National Quotation Bureau and represent prices between dealers. They do not reflect retail mark-ups, mark-downs, or commissions.

[3] First day of listing of Equity Funding on the American Stock Exchange. Prices subsequently reflect AMEX quotes.

[4] Prices reflect a 3-for-2 stock split on January 2, 1968.

[5] Warrants of Equity Funding were issued and traded to November 4, 1968. They opened at 41¾ on September 26, 1968, and closed November 4, 1968, at 43⅜.

[6] Prices reflect a 2-for-1 split on November 6, 1968.

[7] First day of listing of Equity Funding on the New York Stock Exchange. Prices subsequently reflect NY Stock Exchange quotes. Warrants were traded on the American Stock Exchange.

EPILOGUE

In early 1977, tentative settlements were announced in cases related to many of the major defendants in the Equity Funding case. If approved by U. S. District Court Judge Malcolm Lucas, these settlements could result in the payment of approximately sixty million dollars to former shareholders of Equity Funding.

The bulk of the funds, some $39 million, would come from accounting firms that handled the auditing of Equity Funding and its life insurance company. Those included in the proposed settlement are: Wolfson, Weiner & Co., Wolfson, Weiner, Ratoff & Lapin, Seidman & Seidman, and Haskins & Sells.

Other potential settlements include:

$5 million from Pennsylvania Life Co. which, among other things, allegedly discovered the existence of the fraudulent practices and demanded money for its silence.

$3,467,500 from Bache Halsey Stuart, Inc. and New York Securities Co., Inc. These two firms acted as the underwriters of Equity Funding's public offerings and as such, the suit charged, were responsible for the inaccurate information in the prospectuses.

$3,450,000 would be received from Joseph Froggatt & Co., the auditors of Bankers National Life Insurance Co., an Equity Funding subsidiary.

$3 million is expected from Milliman and Robertson, Inc., the actuarial firm whose opinions were included in various Equity Funding publications and who allegedly received finder's fees for helping Equity Funding sell its insurance policies to other insurance companies.

$2 million from the Estate of Michael R. Riordan, one of the founders of Equity Funding and Chairman of the Board until his death in 1969.

$50,000 from the brokerage firm of Dishy, Easton and Co. This small, New York company had several business deals with Equity Funding.

Various former officers and directors filed settlements totalling $77,381. Herbert Glaser (former Director, Assistant Secretary, & Executive Vice-President) would pay $25,000. Defendants Arkus-Duntov (former Director, Vice-President, and Executive Vice-President), Gale Livingston (former Director), and Nelson Loud (former Director) each agreed to pay $10,000. In addition to the money, the defendants have assigned all of their claims and rights to shares of Orion Capital Corporation to the plaintiffs. Settlements have also been filed for seventeen other former employees, including Samual B. Lowell and Fred Levin, both of whom are serving prison terms. Payments of $22,381 from some of these former officials were part of the agreement.

While the total settlement is close to 56 million dollars, this translates into a recovery of only 15 to 20 cents on the dollar for most investors. An additional four million dollars could be available to those stockholders who purchased their shares in the period between March 15, 1973 and March 27 of that year when the scandal was made public. The settlement is the result of allegations that certain people were aware of the conditions within Equity Funding during this interval and yet continued to trade the stock. Mcre than 250 defendants would pay a total of $3,250,000, with an additional $750,000 coming from the accounting firm settlement.

In a related action, U. S. District Court Judge Harry Pregerson, authorized payment of $10.2 million to attorneys and others involved in the bankruptcy. The largest fee, $5.76 million, was awarded to the firm of O'Melveny and Myers of Los Angeles, who acted as general counsel to the trustee. Robert Loeffler, the Equity Funding trustee, was authorized fees of $1 million.

The resolution of these suits in no way ends the Equity Funding case. At press time, Peat, Marwick, Mitchell & Co. and Stanley Goldblum were among the major defendants who had not yet agreed to settlements.